STUDY GUIDE FOR

Lippincott Williams & Wilkins'

COMPREHENSIVE
Medical Assisting

THIRD EDITION

Judy Kronenberger, RN, CMA, MEd
Associate Professor, Medical Assistant Technology
Sinclair Community College
Dayton, Ohio

Laura Southard Durham, BS, CMA
Medical Assisting Technologies Program Coordinator
Forsyth Technical Community College
Winston-Salem, North Carolina

Denise Woodson, MA, MT(ASCP)SC
Academic Coordinator
Health Professions and Nursing
Smarthinking, Inc.
Richmond, Virginia

D1224038

Wolters Kluwer | Lippincott Williams & Wilkins
Health

Philadelphia • Baltimore • New York • London
Buenos Aires • Hong Kong • Sydney • Tokyo

Executive Editor: John Goucher
Managing Editor: Kevin C. Dietz
Senior Marketing Manager: Nancy Bradshaw
Production Editor: Beth Martz
Compositor: Maryland Composition

Copyright 2009 Lippincott Williams & Wilkins, a Wolters Kluwer business.

351 West Camden Street
Baltimore, Maryland 21201-2436 USA

530 Walnut Street
Philadelphia, Pennsylvania 19106-3640 USA

All rights reserved. This book is protected by copyright. No part of this book may be reproduced in any form or by any means, including photocopying, or utilized by any information storage and retrieval system without written permission from the copyright owner.

The publisher is not responsible (as a matter of product liability, negligence, or otherwise) for any injury resulting from any material contained herein. This publication contains information relating to general principles of medical care that should not be construed as specific instructions for individual patients. Manufacturers' product information and package inserts should be reviewed for current information, including contraindications, dosages, and precautions.

Printed in the United States of America

Library of Congress Cataloging-in-Publication Data

Kronenberger, Judy.
   Study guide for LWW's comprehensive medical assisting / Judy Kronenberger, Laura Southard Durham, Denise Woodson.
      p. cm.
   A companion study guide for Lippincott Williams & Wilkins' comprehensive medical assisting. 3rd ed. c2008.
   ISBN 978-0-7817-7005-7
   1. Medical assistants. I. Durham, Laura Southard. II. Woodson, Denise. III. Kronenberger, Judy. Lippinscott Williams & Wilkin's comprehensive medical assisting. IV. Title. V. Title: Study guide for Lippincott Williams and Wilkin's comprehensive medical assisting.
   R728.8.K76 2009
   610.73'7069--dc22   2007048364

The publishers have made every effort to trace the copyright holders for borrowed material. If they have inadvertently overlooked any, they will be pleased to make the necessary arrangements at the first opportunity.

To purchase additional copies of this book, call our customer service department at (800) 638-3030 or fax orders to **(301) 223-2320**. International customers should call **(301) 223-2300.**

Visit Lippincott Williams & Wilkins on the Internet: http://www.LWW.com. Lippincott Williams & Wilkins customer service representatives are available from 8:30 am to 6:00 pm, EST.

7 8 9 10

DRC0411

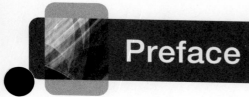

Preface

Welcome to the completely revised *Study Guide* to accompany *Lippincott Williams & Wilkins' Comprehensive Medical Assisting 3e*. This Study Guide is a learning resource that will help you to apply your knowledge of the information in the textbook, create Work Products that will establish a winning Portfolio, and master the skills needed to become a successful medical assistant. To help you get the most out of your studies, we've included a variety of exercises that will help reinforce the material you learned and build your critical thinking skills. This *Study Guide* is unique in a number of ways and offers features that most Medical Assisting study guides do not.

The *Study Guide* is divided into three sections that coincide with the Texbook: Administrative, Clinical, and Laboratory. Each section contains exercises that will reinforce your skills and knowledge of the Medical Assisting field. Each chapter includes the following:

- **Chapter Checklist**—This feature will guide you as you work through the chapter and begin to create your Portfolio.
- **Learning Objectives**—Listed at the beginning of each chapter and highlighted within the Chapter Notes.
- **Chapter Notes**—This feature includes the text headings in the left column and blank spaces for note-taking in the right column.
- **Content Review**—This feature is divided into two parts: Foundations Knowledge and Application. The Foundation section contains Key Terms, Matching Exercises, and Re-

view Questions. The Application section features Critical Thinking Practice questions; Patient Education questions; and Documentation Practice exercises.

- **Active Learning Exercises**—These exercises require you to become an active participant in your learning and will allow you to apply your recently acquired knowledge and skills to the medical assisting profession. Active Learning exercises will help you retain new information, build confidence, and show you how to gather information and learn from sources other than the textbook.
- **Professional Journal Page(s)**—Each chapter will include a Journal page that will encourage you to Reflect, Ponder, Solve, and Experience.
- **Skill Practice**—These exercises include Skill Practice Activities, Forms, Work Products, and Competency Evaluation Forms.
- **Chapter Self-Assessment Quiz**—These quizzes are comprised of multiple-choice questions consistent with the certification exam format.
- **Skill Sheets**—These are included for every procedure in the textbook. Each form has a place for students to complete a self-evaluation, partners to evaluate them, and, finally, for the instructor's evaluation.

This *Study Guide* has been developed in response to numerous requests from students and instructors for a concise, understandable, and interactive resource that covers the skills necessary to become successful in the Medical Assisting field.

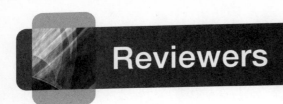

Reviewers

Lippincott Williams & Wilkins greatfully acknowledges the contributions of the following reviewers for their valuable comments and suggestions:

Gerry Brasin, CMA, AS, CPC
Education Coordinator
Premier Education Group
Springfield, MA

Sherry Brewer, CMA-AC, BS
Preceptor
Medical Assisting Department
Cuyahoga Community College
Cleveland, OH

Patricia Donahue, MS
Associate Professor
Office and Computer Programs Department
Monroe Community College
Rochester, NY

Sharon Harris-Pelliccia, BS, RPAC
Department Chair, Medical Studies
Mildred Elley
Latham, NY

Joyce Minton, MA
Program Director
Medical Assisting Department
Wilkes Community College
Wilkesboro, NC

Brigitte Niedzwiecki, RN, BSN, MSN
Medical Assistant Program Director
Chippewa Valley Technical College
Eau Claire, WI

Marianne Van Deursen, BS
Medical/Dental Assisting Director
Continuing Ed
Warren County Community College
Washington, NJ

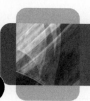

Contents

PART V

Career Strategies

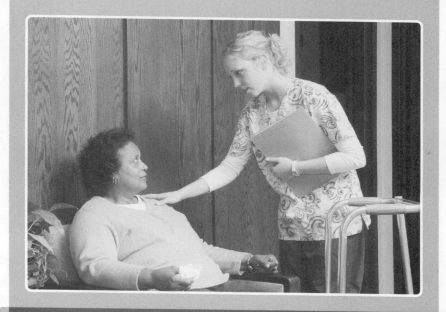

Introduction to Medical Assisting

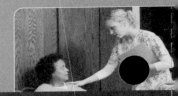

Medicine and Medical Assisting

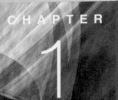

Chapter Checklist

☐ Read textbook chapter and take notes within the Chapter Notes outline. Answer the Learning Objectives as you reach them in the content, and then check them off.

☐ Work the Content Review questions—both Foundational Knowledge and Application.

☐ Perform the Active Learning exercise(s).

☐ Complete Professional Journal entries.

☐ Complete Skill Practice Activity(s) using Competency Evaluation Forms and Work Products, when appropriate.

☐ Take the Chapter Self-Assessment Quiz.

☐ Insert all appropriate pages into your Portfolio.

Learning Objectives

1. Spell and define the key terms.
2. Summarize a brief history of medicine.
3. Identify the key founders of medical science.
4. Explain the system of health care in the United States.
5. Discuss the typical medical office.
6. List medical specialties a medical assistant may encounter.
7. List settings in which medical assistants may be employed.
8. List the duties of a medical assistant.
9. Describe the desired characteristics of a medical assistant.
10. Identify members of the health care team.
11. Explain the pathways of education for medical assistants.
12. Discuss the importance of program accreditation.
13. Name and describe the two nationally recognized accrediting agencies for medical assisting education programs.
14. Explain the benefits and avenues of certification for the medical assistant.
15. List the benefits of membership in a professional organization.

Chapter Notes

Note: Bold-faced headings are the major headings in the text chapter; headings in regular font are lower-level headings (i.e., the content is subordinate to, or falls "under," the major headings). Make sure you understand the key terms used in the chapter, as well as the concepts presented as Key Points.

TEXT SUBHEADINGS	NOTES
Introduction _____	

Key Term: multiskilled health professional
Key Point:
• You have selected a fascinating and challenging career, one of the fastest growing specialties in the medical field.

☐ **LEARNING OBJECTIVE 1:** Spell and define the key terms.

History of Medicine _____

Ancient Medical History _____

Key Term: caduceus
Key Point:
• Some of these early medications played a key role in the development of our modern pharmacology.

☐ **LEARNING OBJECTIVE 2:** Summarize a brief history of medicine.

Modern Medical History _____

Key Point:
• Great minds collaborated to advance medical and scientific theories and perform experiments that led to discoveries of enormous benefit in the fight against disease.

☐ **LEARNING OBJECTIVE 3:** Identify the key founders of medical science.

Strides in the Prevention of Disease Transmission _____

Possibilities in Surgery _____

Women in Medicine _____

Important Discoveries _____

_____

_____

Recent Medical History _____

_____

Key Term: medical assistant
Key Points:
- Throughout the next three decades, public health protection improved and advancements continued. Government legislation mandated clean water, and citizens reaped the benefits of preventive medicine and education about health issues.
- New discoveries will continue to expand the parameters of medicine as further research in recombinant DNA, transplantation, immunizations, diagnostic procedures, and so forth push back the boundaries of health care and make today's therapies seem as primitive as those we have just covered.

The American Health Care System _____

_____

Key Term: outpatient
Key Point:
- The allied health care arena has grown quickly. New professions have been added to the health care team, and each one is an important part of a patient's total care.

☐ **LEARNING OBJECTIVE 4:** Explain the system of health care in the United States.

The Medical Office _____

_____

Key Point:
- The patient's health care encounter can be pleasant or unpleasant, depending on the skills and the attitude of the team.

☐ **LEARNING OBJECTIVE 5:** Discuss the typical medical office.

Medical Specialties _____

_____

Key Term: specialty

☐ **LEARNING OBJECTIVE 6:** List medical specialties a medical assistant may encounter.

The Medical Assisting Profession _____

_____

_____

What Is a Medical Assistant? _____

_____

Key Terms: clinical; administrative

☐ **LEARNING OBJECTIVE 7:** List settings in which medical assistants may be employed.

Duties of a Medical Assistant _____

_____

Key Term: laboratory

Administrative Duties _____

_____

_____

Clinical Duties _____

_____

_____

Laboratory Duties _____

_____

☐ **LEARNING OBJECTIVE 8:** List the duties of a medical assistant.

Characteristics of a Professional Medical Assistant _____

_____

Key Point:
• Medical assistants play a key role in creating and maintaining a professional image for their employers.

☐ **LEARNING OBJECTIVE 9:** Describe the desired characteristics of a medical assistant.

Members of the Health Care Team _____

_____

Key Term: multidisciplinary
Key Point:
• A multidisciplinary team is a group of specialized professionals who are brought together to meet the needs of the patient.

☐ **LEARNING OBJECTIVE 10:** Identify members of the health care team.

Health Care Providers _____

_____

_____

Physicians _____

_____

_____

Physicians Assistants _____

_____

Key Point:
• Their scope of practice corresponds to the supervising physician's practice.

Nurse Practitioners _____

_____

_____

The Nursing Profession _____

_____

Key Term: inpatient
Key Point:
• Nurses work with physicians and implement various patient care needs in the **inpatient** or hospital setting.

Allied Health Professionals _____

_____

_____

The History of Medical Assisting _____

_____

Key Point:
• The need for a highly trained professional with a background in administrative and clinical skills led to the formation of an alternative field of allied health care.

Medical Assisting Education _____

_____

Key Term: externship
Key Point:
• After you finish school, your education should not stop.

☐ **LEARNING OBJECTIVE 11:** Explain the pathways of education for medical assistants.

Medical Assisting Program Accreditation _____

_____

Key Term: accreditation

☐ **LEARNING OBJECTIVE 12:** Discuss the importance of program accreditation.

The Commission of Accreditation of Allied Health Education Programs _____

_____

The Accrediting Bureau of Health Education Schools _____

_____

Key Term: certification

☐ **LEARNING OBJECTIVE 13:** Name and describe the two nationally recognized accrediting agencies for medical assisting education programs.

Medical Assisting Certification _____

_____

☐ **LEARNING OBJECTIVE 14:** Explain the benefits and avenues of certification for the medical assistant.

Certified Medical Assistant _____

_____

Key Terms: recertification; continuing education unit

_____

Registered Medical Assistant _____

_____

Medical Assisting and Related Allied Health Associations _____

_____

Association Membership _____

_____

☐ **LEARNING OBJECTIVE 15:** List the benefits of membership in a professional organization.

_____

American Association of Medical Assistants _____

_____

Key Point:
• The purpose of the AAMA is to promote the professional identity and stature of its members and the medical assisting profession through education and credentialing.

_____

American Medical Technologists _____

_____

Key Point:
• The AMT and its governing body are set up similarly to the AMAA, with local, state, and national affiliations, opportunities for continuing education, professional benefits, and a professional journal.

_____

Professional Coder Associations _____

_____

The American Health Information Management Association _____

_____

Employment Opportunities _____

_____

Key Point:
• Because of the flexible, multiskilled nature of their education, medical assistants can work in a variety of health care settings.

_____

Content Review

FOUNDATIONAL KNOWLEDGE

1. A Brief History

Place the following list of events in the correct order in the table, with 1 being the oldest event, and 6 being the most recent.

a. Moses is appointed the first public health officer.

b. Hippocrates turns medicine into a science.

c. Egyptians perform the first skull surgeries.

d. The bubonic plague sweeps Europe and Asia and kills millions.

e. The Greek physician Galen is the first to document a patient's pulse.

f. The Renaissance fosters great strides in medicine.

1.	2.	3.
4.	5.	6.

2. Great Thinkers

Modern history is filled with notable individuals who made great breakthroughs in the field of medicine. Without their efforts, many of us wouldn't be alive today! In the chart below, draw a line to match the scientist with his or her contribution to medicine.

Scientist	Contribution to Medicine
1. Andreas Vesalius	**a.** Founder of modern nursing
2. Edward Jenner	**b.** Discovered x-rays
3. Louis Pasteur	**c.** Discovered the smallpox vaccine
4. Florence Nightingale	**d.** "Father of Modern Anatomy"; wrote the first relatively correct anatomy book
5. Wilhelm Konrad Roentgen	**e.** Invented pasteurization, which eliminated bacterial transmission

3. My Country, My Health Care

What is the purpose of the Centers for Medicare and Medicaid Services?

_____

_____

4. The following are three specialists who may employ medical assistants. Describe what each does.

a. allergist: _____

b. internist: _____

c. gynecologist: _____

5. Name That Task

As a medical assistant, you must be "multiskilled," or skilled at completing many different tasks. Almost all the tasks you will complete fall into one of two categories: administrative and clinical. But what's the difference between administrative and clinical tasks? Read each selection below and determine whether the task requires your clinical or administrative skills, then place a check in the appropriate column.

Task	Administrative	Clinical
a. preparing patients for examinations		
b. maintaining medical records		
c. ensuring good public relations		
d. obtaining medical histories		
e. preparing and sterilizing instruments		
f. screening sales representatives		

6. You've Got Character
Read the following scenario and answer the question below.

Mrs. Esposito approaches Jan, a medical assistant, at the front desk. Jan has recently treated Mrs. Esposito's son, Manuel, for a foot injury. Mrs. Esposito asks Jan if she may have her son's medical records to show Manuel's soccer coach that he will be unable to play for the rest of the season. Jan explains to Mrs. Esposito that because her son is 18 and legally an adult, she must have his permission to release his medical records. Mrs. Esposito is furious, but Jan calmly explains that the physician would be happy to write a note for Manuel to give to his soccer coach explaining his injuries. Mrs. Esposito thanks her for this information and apologizes for becoming angry.

From the list below, circle the **two** characteristics of a professional medical assistant that Jan exhibited in the above scenario.

Accuracy	Good interpersonal skills
Ability to respect patient confidentiality	Ability to work as a team player
Honesty	Initiative and responsibility

7. Name That Person
I am generally regarded as the team leader. I am responsible for diagnosing and treating the patient. Who am I?

_____

_____

8. Review the list of job titles below. Circle those that are considered allied health professionals.

Dentist	Electrocardiograph Technician	Nurse
Health Information Technologist	Medical Assistant	Physician Assistant
Nuclear Medical Technician	Nutritionist	Physical Therapist
Nurse Practitioner	Pharmacist	Risk Manager

9. What Came Next. . . ?
Medical assisting has been practiced as a profession for less than 100 years, so the profession has grown rapidly to meet the needs of patients. Read the following events in the left column and place them in the correct order in the right column, with 1 being the oldest event and 5 being the most recent.

a. The American Association of Medical Assistants (AAMA) was founded.	**1.**
b. The Board of Trustees of the AAMA approved the current definition of medical assisting.	**2.**
c. A certification examination for CMA was conducted and set the standards for medical assistant education.	**3.**
d. Dr. M. Mandl opened the first school for medical assistants.	**4.**
e. Illinois recognized the AAMA as a not-for-profit educational organization.	**5.**

10. Julia is a student in her last year of a medical assisting program. What must she complete before graduating?

   a. Certification

   b. An associate's degree

   c. An externship

   d. Curriculum

11. Who is eligible to take the RMA examination? Circle all that apply.

   a. Medical assistants who have been employed as medical instructors for a minimum of five years

   b. Medical assistants who have been employed in the profession for a minimum of five years

   c. Graduates from ABHES-accredited medical assisting programs

   d. Graduates from CAAHEP-accredited medical assisting programs

12. Sign Me Up!

   As a medical assistant wishing to learn more about the medical field, you may decide to join a national organization, such as the American Association of Medical Assistants. Can you name three of the six benefits of association membership?

   1. _____

   2. _____

   3. _____

13. Employment

   Complete the following sentence with the correct word from the word bank.

   Medical assistants work under the direct supervision of a licensed _____.

nurse	medical assisting instructor
health care provider	medical office manager

14. Jamie would like to become a medical assistant and asks for your advice. Describe his educational options and suggest what program might be best for him.

   _____

   _____

15. You feel strongly about attending a program that has accreditation. Your friend also wants to attend school to become a medical assistant and doesn't understand why accreditation is important. What would you tell him?

   _____

   _____

16. Name the two nationally recognized accrediting agencies.

   1. _____

   2. _____

17. The AAMA and AMT have developed certification examinations that test the knowledge of a graduate and indicate entry-level competency. Review the information about the interested applicants in the chart below and indicate if they are eligible for the CMA or RMA exam or both.

Interested Applicants	Eligible for the CMA Exam	Eligible for the RMA Exam
1. Jorge graduated from an ABHES-accredited medical assisting program.		
2. Carla graduated from a CAAHEP-accredited medical assisting program.		
3. Jason has been working as a medical assistant for almost six years.		

18. List three settings in which a medical assistant may be employed.

a. _____

b. _____

c. _____

19. Match the following key terms to their definitions.

Key Terms

a. caduceus _____

b. medical assistant _____

c. outpatient _____

d. specialty _____

e. clinical _____

f. administrative _____

g. laboratory _____

h. multidisciplinary _____

i. inpatient _____

j. externship _____

k. accreditation _____

l. certification _____

m. recertification _____

Definitions

1. completed by a CMA every 5 years by either taking the examination again or by acquiring 60 CEU's

2. describing a medical facility where patients receive care but are not admitted overnight

3. a subcategory of medicine that a physician chooses to practice upon graduation from medical school

4. referring to a team of specialized professionals who are brought together to meet the needs of the patient

5. regarding a medical facility that treats patients and keeps them overnight, often accompanied by surgery or other procedure

6. a medical symbol showing a wand or staff with two serpents coiled around it

7. voluntary process that involves a testing procedure to prove an individual's baseline competency in a particular area

8. regarding tasks that involve direct patient care

9. an educational course during which the student works in the field gaining hands-on experience

10. a multiskilled health care professional who performs a variety of tasks in a medical setting

11. a nongovernmental professional peer review process that provides technical assistance and evaluates educational programs for quality based on pre-established academic and administrative standards

12. regarding tasks that involve scientific testing

13. regarding tasks that focus on office procedures

20. True or False? Determine whether the following statements are true or false. If false, explain why.

a. The Hippocratic Oath is still a part of medical school graduation ceremonies.

b. The makeup of the medical team is the same for every office.

c. Recertification can only be obtained by taking the examination again.

d. The purpose of the AAMA is to promote the professional identity and stature of its members and the medical assisting profession through education and credentialing.

APPLICATION

Critical Thinking Practice

1. Why is the ability to respect patient confidentiality essential to the role of the medical assistant?

_____

_____

2. The medical office in which you work treats a variety of patients, from all ages and backgrounds. Why should you work with a multidisciplinary health care team? What are the benefits to the patients?

_____

_____

Patient Education

1. You are preparing a patient for her examination, but the physician is running behind schedule. The patient is becoming anxious and asks you to perform the examination, instead of the physician. You tell her that you will go check how much longer the physician will be. But she responds, "Can't you just perform the exam? Aren't you like a nurse?" How should you respond?

_____

_____

Documentation

1. The patient who asked you to perform the examination now refuses to wait for the physician. Even though she has a serious heart condition requiring monthly check-ups, she leaves without being treated by the physician. You need to write a note that will be included in her chart and in an incident report. What would you say?

_____

_____

Active Learning

1. Many of the Roman and Greek gods and goddesses were symbols of health and medicine. Research on the Internet for information about caduceus. Write a paragraph explaining when and why modern Western culture adopted this symbol. Then, draw your own symbol for medical assisting and explain what each part represents.

2. Talk with a grandparent or another older adult, and ask him or her to tell you about a medical discovery that he or she remembers well. Create a "before and after" chart, explaining what life was like before the discovery, and the changes and benefits that came about after the discovery.

3. Review the list of specialists who employ medical assistants in textbook Table 1-2. Choose one specialist that interests you the most. Perform research on what kinds of procedures the specialist performs. Then consider what kinds of tasks a medical assistant employed by this specialist might perform. Write a letter to this specialist explaining why you would want to work in this kind of office. Be sure to include specific references to the tasks and procedures that interest you based on your research.

Professional Journal

REFLECT

(Prompts and Ideas: Are you concerned about meeting the patient needs and the standards of day-to-day operations in a medical office? Are you concerned about your ability to complete clinical and administrative tasks? Think about the medical office that you visit as a patient. In what ways does the medical assistant keep the office running smoothly? What changes would you like to see?)

_____

_____

_____

_____

PONDER AND SOLVE

1. Scope of practice for medical assistants can vary from state to state. In some states, certified medical assistants are not allowed to perform invasive procedures, such as injections or laboratory testing. Why is it important to understand your scope of practice before beginning work in a new medical office?

_____

_____

2. What are the ways in which an externship prepares you for your career as a medical assistant?

_____

_____

_____

_____

_____

_____

_____

Chapter Self-Assessment Quiz

1. The earliest recorded evidence of medical history dates to the early:
   a. Greeks.
   b. Romans.
   c. Egyptians.
   d. Christians.
   e. Chinese.

2. Which of the following is true of the Middle Ages?
   a. Medicine focused on comforting patients rather than finding cures for disease.
   b. The establishment of universities helped spread the practice of medicine.
   c. Vesalius wrote the first relatively correct anatomy textbook.
   d. Advances in sanitation promoted good personal hygiene practices.
   e. Anton von Leeuwenhoek invented the microscope.

3. Marie and Pierre Curie revolutionized the principles of:

   a. nursing.

   b. disease.

   c. infection.

   d. physics.

   e. radioactivity.

4. The medical assistant's role will expand over time because of:

   a. a growing population.

   b. the risk of disease and infection.

   c. advances in medicine and technology.

   d. a financial boom.

   e. more effective training programs.

5. What drives the management practices of the outpatient medical facility?

   a. The desire to compete with other medical facilities

   b. The need to adhere to government rules and regulations

   c. The attempt to fit into mainstream medical opinion

   d. The effort to retain medical employees

   e. The focus on hiring specialized health care workers

6. Which of the following tasks is the administrative team responsible for in the medical office?

   a. Physical examinations

   b. Financial aspects of the practice

   c. Laboratory test processing

   d. Minor office surgery

   e. Drawing blood

7. Which of the following is a clinical duty?

   a. Scheduling appointments

   b. Obtaining medical histories

   c. Handling telephone calls

   d. Filing insurance forms

   e. Implementing ICD-9 and CPT coding for insurance claims

8. Empathy is the ability to:

   a. care deeply for the health and welfare of patients.

   b. keep your temper in check.

   c. show all patients good manners.

   d. remain calm in an emergency.

   e. feel pity for sick patients.

9. If a patient refers to you as a "nurse," you should:

   a. call the physician.

   b. ignore the mistake.

   c. politely correct him.

   d. send him home.

   e. ask the nurse to come into the room.

10. A group of specialized people who are brought together to meet the needs of the patient is called:

   a. multiskilled.

   b. multifaceted.

   c. multitasked.

   d. multidisciplinary.

   e. multitrained.

11. A medical assistant falls into the category of:

   a. nurse.

   b. physician assistant.

   c. medical office manager.

   d. allied health professional.

   e. office manager.

12. The discovery of which vaccine opened the door to an emphasis on preventing disease rather than simply trying to cure preventable illnesses?

   a. Smallpox

   b. Cowpox

   c. Puerperal fever

   d. Typhoid

   e. Influenza

13. In 1991, which group approved the current definition of medical assisting?

   a. The U.S. Department of Health and Education

   b. The Health Management Organization

   c. The American Medical Technologists

   d. The American Association of Medical Assistants

   e. The State Department of Health

14. All accredited programs must include a(n):

   a. medical terminology course.

   b. computer course.

   c. externship.

   d. certification examination.

   e. multidisciplinary program.

15. What is the requirement for admission to the CMA examination?

  a. Successful completion of 60 CEUs

  b. Successful completion of an externship

  c. Graduation from high school

  d. Graduation from an accredited medical assisting program

  e. Successful completion of a GED program

16. An oncologist diagnoses and treats:

  a. disorders of the musculoskeletal system.

  b. disorders of the ear, nose, and throat.

  c. pregnant women.

  d. the aging population.

  e. benign and malignant tumors.

17. A CMA is required to recertify every:

  a. 1 year.

  b. 2 years.

  c. 5 years.

  d. 10 years.

  e. 15 years.

18. Which organization offers the RMA examination?

  a. American Medical Technologists

  b. American Association of Medical Assistants

  c. American Academy of Professional Coders

  d. American Health Information Management Association

  e. American Board of Medical Specialties

19. Which of the following is a benefit of association membership?

  a. Time off from work

  b. Networking opportunities

  c. Hotel expenses

  d. Free health insurance

  e. Externship placement

20. Which specialist diagnoses and treats disorders of the stomach and intestine?

  a. Endocrinologist

  b. Gastroenterologist

  c. Gerontologist

  d. Podiatrist

  e. Internist

2

Law and Ethics

☐ Read textbook chapter and take notes within the Chapter Notes outline. Answer the Learning Objectives as you reach them in the content, and then check them off.

☐ Work the Content Review questions—both Foundational Knowledge and Application.

☐ Perform the Active Learning exercise(s).

☐ Complete Professional Journal entries.

☐ Complete Skill Practice Activity(s) using Competency Evaluation Forms and Work Products, when appropriate.

☐ Take the Chapter Self-Assessment Quiz.

☐ Insert all appropriate pages into your Portfolio.

1. Spell and define the key terms.
2. Identify the two branches of the American legal system.
3. List the elements and types of contractual agreements and describe the difference in implied and express contracts.
4. List four items that must be included in a contract termination or withdrawal letter.
5. List six items that must be included in an informed consent form and explain who may sign consent forms.
6. List five legally required disclosures that must be reported to specified authorities.
7. Describe the four elements that must be proven in a medical legal suit.
8. Describe four possible defenses against litigation for the medical professional.
9. Explain the theory of respondeat superior, or law of agency, and how it applies to the medical assistant.

10. List ways that a medical assistant can assist in the prevention of a medical malpractice suit.
11. Outline the laws regarding employment and safety issues in the medical office.
12. List the requirements of the Americans with Disabilities Act relating to the medical office.
13. Differentiate between legal issues and ethical issues.
14. List the seven American Medical Association principles of ethics.
15. List the five ethical principles of ethical and moral conduct outlined by the American Association of Medical Assistants.
16. Describe the purpose of the Self-Determination Act.
17. List 10 opinions of the American Medical Association's Council pertaining to administrative office procedures.

Note: Bold-faced headings are the major headings in the text chapter; headings in regular font are lower-level headings (i.e., the content is subordinate to, or falls "under," the major headings). Make sure you understand the key terms used in the chapter, as well as the concepts presented as Key Points.

TEXT SUBHEADINGS   **NOTES**

Introduction _____

_____

Key Term: fraud

_____

☐ **LEARNING OBJECTIVE 1:** Spell and define the key terms.

_____

The American Legal System _____

_____

Key Term: litigation
Key Point:
• Our legal system is in place to ensure the rights of all citizens.

_____

Sources of Law _____

_____

Key Terms: common law; stare decisis; precedents
Key Point:
• The foundation of our legal system is our rights outlined in the Constitution and the laws established by our Founding Fathers.

_____

Branches of the Law _____

_____

Key Term: civil law

_____

☐ **LEARNING OBJECTIVE 2:** Identify the two main branches of the American legal system.

_____

Public Law _____

_____

_____

Private or Civil Law _____

_____

Key Terms: tort; breach

_____

The Rise in Medical Legal Cases _____

_____

Key Term: malpractice

Physician-Patient Relationship _____

_____

Rights and Responsibilities of the Patient and Physician _____

_____

Key Point:
• In any contractual relationship, both parties have certain rights and responsibilities.

Contracts _____

_____

Key Term: contract
Key Point:
• A contract is not valid unless all three elements are present.

Implied Contracts _____

_____

Key Term: implied contracts

Expressed Contracts _____

_____

Key Term: expressed contracts

☐ **LEARNING OBJECTIVE 3:** List the elements and types of contractual agreements and describe the difference in implied and expressed contracts.

Termination or Withdrawal of the Contract _____

_____

Key Terms: protocol; locum tenens
Key Point:
• Clear documentation is essential.

☐ **LEARNING OBJECTIVE 4:** List four items that must be included in a contract termination or withdrawal letter.

Consent _____

Key Terms: consent; durable power of attorney
Key Point:
• The law requires that patients must **consent** or agree to being touched, examined, or treated by the physician or agents of the physician involved in the contractual agreement.

Implied Consent _____

Key Term: implied consent

Informed or Expressed Consent _____

Key Terms: informed consent; expressed consent; emancipated minor
Key Point:
• Never coerce (force or compel against his or her wishes) a patient into signing a consent form.

☐ **LEARNING OBJECTIVE 5:** List six items that must be included in an informed consent form and explain who may sign consent forms.

Refusal of Consent _____

Key Point:
• Patients may refuse treatment for any reason.

Releasing Medical Information _____

Key Point:
• Although the medical record itself belongs to the physician, the information belongs to the patient.

Legally Required Disclosures _____

_____

Key Term: legally required disclosures

Vital Statistics _____

_____

Medical Examiner's Reports _____

_____

Infectious or Communicable Diseases _____

_____

National Childhood Vaccine Injury Act of 1986 _____

_____

Abuse, Neglect, or Maltreatment _____

_____

Key Point:
• Health care workers, teachers, and social workers who report suspected abuse are not identified to the parents and are protected against liability.

Violent Injuries _____

_____

Key Point:
• Health care providers have the legal duty to report suspected criminal acts. Injuries resulting from weapons, assault, attempted suicide, and rape must be reported to local authorities.

Other Reports _____

_____

☐ **LEARNING OBJECTIVE 6:** List five legally required disclosures that must be reported to specified authorities.

Specific Laws and Statutes that Apply to Health Professionals _____

_____

Medical Practice Acts _____

_____

Key Terms: licensure; fee splitting
Key Point:
• As a medical assistant, it is your responsibility to report illegal or unethical behavior or signs of incompetence in the medical office.

Licensure, Certification, and Registration _____

_____

Key Terms: registered; certification
Key Point:
• The physician-employer has the sole responsibility of setting any limits on the duties of a medical assistant.

Controlled Substances Act _____

_____

Good Samaritan Act _____

_____

Basis of Medical Law _____

_____

Tort Law _____

_____

Key Terms: plaintiff; defendant

Negligence and Malpractice (Unintentional Torts) _____

_____

Key Terms: negligence; expert witness; res ipsa loquitur
Key Point:
• In a legal situation, the standard of care determines what a reasonable professional would have done.

Duty _____

_____

Dereliction of Duty _____

_____

_____

Direct Cause _____

_____

_____

Damage _____

_____

Key Term: damages

Jury Awards _____

_____

☐ **LEARNING OBJECTIVE 7:** Describe the four elements that must be proven in a medical legal suit.

Intentional Torts _____

_____

Key Term: intentional tort

Assault and Battery _____

_____

Key Terms: assault; battery
Key Point:
• By law, a conscious adult has the right to refuse medical care.

Duress _____

_____

Key Term: duress

Invasion of Privacy _____

_____

Defamation of Character _____

_____

Key Terms: defamation of character; libel; slander

Fraud _____
_____
_____

Tort of Outrage _____
_____
_____

Undue Influence _____
_____
_____

The Litigation Process _____
_____

Key Terms: depositions; bench trial; appeal

Defenses to Professional Liability Suits _____
_____

Key Point:
• The objective of all court proceedings is to uncover the truth.

Medical Records _____
_____

Key Point:
• The best and most solid defense the caregiver has is the medical record.

Statute of Limitations _____
_____

Key Term: statute of limitations

Assumption of Risk _____
_____

Key Point:
• A signed consent form indicating that the patient was informed of all of the risks of a procedure proves this point.

Res Judicata _____

_____

Key Term: res judicata

Contributory Negligence _____

_____

Key Terms: contributory negligence; comparative negligence

Comparative Negligence _____

_____

☐ **LEARNING OBJECTIVE 8:** Describe four possible defenses against litigation for the medical professional.

Defense for the Medical Assistant _____

_____

_____

Respondeat Superior or Law of Agency _____

_____

Key Term: respondeat superior
Key Points:
- The physician is responsible for your actions as a medical assistant as long as your actions are within your scope of practice.
- Never hesitate to seek clarification from a physician. If you are not sure about something, such as a medication order, ask!

☐ **LEARNING OBJECTIVE 9:** Explain the theory of respondeat superior, or law of agency, and how it applies to the medical assistant.

☐ **LEARNING OBJECTIVE 10:** List ways that a medical assistant can assist in the prevention of a medical malpractice suit.

Employment and Safety Laws _____

_____

_____

Civil Rights Act of 1964, Title VII _____

_____

_____

Sexual Harassment _____

_____

Key Point:
• In the medical office setting, the office manager must be alert for signs of harassment and should have in place a policy for handling complaints.

Americans with Disabilities Act _____

_____

Key Point:
• The law is designed to protect employees, not to require unreasonable accommodations.

Occupational Safety and Health Act _____

_____

Key Term: blood-borne pathogens
Key Point:
• Universal or standard precautions are designed to protect health care workers from blood and body fluids contaminated with HIV, hepatitis, or any contagious "bugs" by requiring that those in direct contact with patients use protective equipment (e.g., gloves, gowns, face mask).

Other Legal Considerations _____

_____

☐ **LEARNING OBJECTIVE 11:** Outline the laws regarding employment and safety issues in the medical office.

☐ **LEARNING OBJECTIVE 12:** List the requirements of the Americans with Disabilities Act to the medical office.

Medical Ethics _____

_____

Key Terms: ethics; bioethics

☐ **LEARNING OBJECTIVE 13:** Differentiate between legal issues and ethical issues.

American Medical Association (AMA) Code of Ethics _____

_____

☐ **LEARNING OBJECTIVE 14:** List the seven American Medical Association principles of ethics.

Medical Assistant's Role in Ethics _____

_____

> **Key Point:**
> • The care you give patients must be objective, and personal opinions about options must not be shared.

Patient Advocacy _____

_____

> **Key Point:**
> • Your primary responsibility as a medical assistant is to be a patient advocate at all times.

Patient Confidentiality _____

_____

> **Key Term:** confidentiality
> **Key Point:**
> • Whatever you say to, hear from, or do to a patient is confidential.

Honesty _____

_____

> **Key Point:**
> • Treating the patient with dignity, respect, and honesty in all interactions will build trust in you and your professional abilities.

American Association of Medical Assistants (AAMA) Code of Ethics _____

_____

_____

Principles _____

_____

_____

☐ **LEARNING OBJECTIVE 15:** List the five ethical principles of ethical and moral conduct outlined by the American Association of Medical Assistants.

Bioethics _____

_____

_____

> **Key Term:** bioethics

American Medical Association (AMA) Council on Ethical and Judicial Affairs _____

_____

_____

Social Policy Issues _____

_____

_____

Allocation of Resources _____

_____

_____

Clinical Investigations and Research _____

_____

_____

Obstetric Dilemmas _____

_____

_____

Stem Cell Research _____

_____

_____

Organ Transplantation _____

_____

_____

Withholding or Withdrawing Treatment _____

_____

Key Term: advance directive
Key Point:
• Today, everyone is encouraged to participate in his or her own end-of-life decisions.

☐ **LEARNING OBJECTIVE 16:** Describe the purpose of the Self-Determination Act.

Professional and Ethical Conduct and Behavior _____

_____

Key Point:
• No health care professional should engage in any act that he or she feels is ethically or morally wrong.

Ethical Issues in Office Management _____

_____

_____

☐ **LEARNING OBJECTIVE 17:** List 10 opinions of the American Medical Association's Council pertaining to administrative office procedures.

Content Review

FOUNDATIONAL KNOWLEDGE

1. The Branches of Law

Supply the appropriate branch of law below.

a. Branch of Law: _____

Focuses on issues between the government and its citizens

b. Branch of Law: _____

Focuses on issues between private citizens

2. All About Public Law

Public law is divided into four subgroups. In the chart below, decide which type of law is represented and place a check mark in the appropriate box.

Types of Laws	Criminal Law	Constitutional Law	Administrative Law	International Law
a. civil rights laws				
b. Internal Revenue Service				
c. trade agreements				
d. rape				
e. murder				
f. abortion				
g. extradition				
h. Food and Drug Administration				
i. burglary				
j. Board of Medical Examiners				

Physician-Patient Contract

3. Dr. Read places the following ad in a local newspaper on July 14:

Notice: From September 1, Dr. Michael Read will no longer be treating patients on Fridays at Lucas Surgery, 114 Chestnut Street, Northeast, MD. Queries should be directed to (443) 380-9900.

One of Dr. Read's patients, Mrs. Jones, calls the office the following day and tells them that because Dr. Read will not be in his office on Fridays, he will have to come and treat her at home instead. Who is legally correct? Explain your answer.

4. Mr. De Souza calls the physician's office to request an appointment with Dr. Phillips. The receptionist tells him that there is an available slot next Tuesday at 4 PM and asks him if he would like to take it. At this point in the conversation, which part of the physician-patient contract has Mr. De Souza already completed?

    a. Offer and acceptance

    b. Offer

    c. Offer, acceptance, and consideration

5. Dr. Duke has decided to terminate patient Mrs. Akon. The office manager drafted the following letter to Mrs. Akon. However, when you review the letter, you find that there are errors. Read the letter below and then explain the three problems with this letter in the space below.

Dear Mrs. Akon,

Because you have consistently refused to follow the dietary restrictions and to take the medication necessary to control your high blood pressure, I feel I am no longer able to provide your medical care. This termination is effectively immediately.

Because you do not seem to take your medical condition seriously, I'm not sure that any other physician would want to treat you either. I will hold on to your medical records for 30 days and then they will be destroyed.

                                          Sincerely,
                                          Anthony Duke, MD

    a. _____

    b. _____

    c. _____

I Consent

6. Which of the following must be included in a patient consent form? Circle all that apply.

    a. Name of the physician performing the procedure

    b. Alternatives to the procedure and their risks

    c. Date the procedure will take place

    d. Probable effect on the patient's condition if the procedure is not performed

    e. Potential risks from the procedure

    f. Patient's next of kin

    g. Any exclusions that the patient requests

    h. Success rate of the procedure

7. Some situations require a report to be filed with the Department of Health with or without the patient's consent. Read the scenarios in the chart below and decide which ones are legally required disclosures.

Scenario	Legally Required Disclosure	No Action Needed
a. A 35-year-old woman gives birth to a healthy baby girl.		
b. A physician diagnoses a patient with meningococcal meningitis.		
c. A 43-year-old man falls off a ladder and breaks his leg. He spends three weeks in the hospital.		
d. A teenager is involved in a hit-and-run accident. He is rushed to the hospital, but dies the next day.		
e. A 2-year-old girl is diagnosed with measles.		
f. A man is diagnosed with a sexually transmitted disease and asks the physician to keep the information confidential.		
g. A woman visits the physician's office and tells him she has mumps, but when he examines her, he discovers it is influenza.		

8. Lawsuits

Mrs. Stevens visits Dr. Johnson's office with neck pain. Dr. Johnson examines her and recommends that she see a specialist. Several months later, Mrs. Stevens sues Dr. Johnson for malpractice, claiming that when he examined her, he made her neck pain worse. In court, she provides pictures of her neck that show severe bruising. A specialist confirms that muscle damage has restricted Mrs. Stevens from going about her daily life. Which of the four elements needed in a medical lawsuit has Mrs. Stevens failed to prove? Circle all that apply.

a. Duty

b. Dereliction of duty

c. Direct cause

d. Damage

9. Mr. Saunders visits Dr. Finnegan with chronic insomnia and tells him that the over-the-counter medication he is using is not working. Dr. Finnegan prescribes Mr. Saunders a stronger sedative and warns him of the possible side effects. The interaction is documented in Mr. Saunders' medical record. Nine months later, Mr. Saunders files a malpractice suit against Dr. Finnegan, claiming that he has become dependent on the sleep medication. List two possible defenses Dr. Finnegan could use in court and explain what they mean.

_____

_____

10. You are a medical assistant in a busy office, and the physician has been called away on an emergency. Some of the patients have been waiting for over 2 hours, and one of them urgently needs a physical check-up for a job application. Although you are not officially qualified, you feel confident that you are able to carry out the examination by yourself. Six months later, the patient files a malpractice suit because you failed to notice a lump in her throat that turned out to be cancerous. Describe the law of agency and explain whether it would help you in the lawsuit.

_____

_____

11. List five ways that medical assistants can help to avoid a medical malpractice suit.

a. _____

b. _____

c. _____

d. _____

e. _____

Laws to Protect

12. Which of these laws protects you from exposure to blood-borne pathogens and other body fluids in the workplace?

a. Civil Rights Act of 1964

b. Self-Determination Act of 1991

c. Occupational Safety and Health Act

d. Americans with Disabilities Act

13. The Americans with Disabilities Act (ADA) prohibits discrimination against people with disabilities in employment practice. Take a look at the scenarios in this chart and assess whether or not the ADA is being followed correctly. Place a check mark in the appropriate box.

Scenario	ADA correctly followed	ADA incorrectly followed
a. A physician's office extends an offer of employment to a man in a wheelchair, but says that due to a shortage of parking, the office cannot offer him a parking space in the garage.		
b. A 46-year-old woman is refused a position on the basis that she is HIV positive.		
c. A mentally ill man with a history of violence is refused a job in a busy office.		
d. A small office with ten employees chooses a healthy woman over a disabled woman because the office cannot afford to adapt the facilities in the workplace.		
e. An office manager at physician's office sends letters to hearing-impaired patients because she is unable to contact them by telephone.		
f. A job applicant with a severe speech impediment is rejected for a position as an emergency room receptionist.		

A Matter of Ethics

14. What is the difference between medical ethics and medical laws?

_____

_____

15. Fill in the missing terms from the AMA Code of Ethics with the words from the list below.

The physician shall:

a. Practice _____ medical care with compassion while respecting human dignity.

b. Remain honest in dealings with patients and colleagues; expose colleagues with _____ _____ or who are incompetent or who engage in _____ and _____.

c. Adhere to all _____ and when needed, be a voice to _____ in the best interest of patient care.

d. Respect the rights of patients and other health care professionals; safeguard patient _____ except within the provisions of the law.

e. Continue appropriate education to remain current; request _____ and obtain the knowledge and skills of other health professionals when needed.

f. Be free to select whom to treat, where to establish a _____, and whom to associate with except in _____ _____.

g. Participate in activities to enhance the _____.

Missing Words

character deficiencies	community	fraud	confidentiality	practice
emergency situations	deception	competent	laws	consultation lawmakers

16. List three principles of the American Association of Medical Assistants Code of Ethics.

a. _____

b. _____

c. _____

17. When a patient is hospitalized, the patient has the right to decide when to terminate treatment. What is the name of the act that allows hospitalized patients to make this decision?

_____

_____

18. As a medical assistant, you will be involved in some administrative issues. Read the following scenarios and assess whether the American Medical Association standards for office management are being met. Place a check mark in the appropriate box.

Scenario	Standards Met	Standards Not Met
a. Dr. Benson tells his medical assistant to cancel Mrs. Burke's tests because she recently lost her job and will be unable to pay for them.		
b. Mr. Grant canceled his appointment with less than 24 hours' notice. He was charged a fee as noted in a sign by the receptionist's desk.		
c. Mrs. O'Malley asks Dr. Gokool to help her fill out an insurance form. The form is a four-page document that takes Dr. Gokool an hour to fill out. Dr. Gokool charges Mrs. O'Malley $15 for filling out the form.		
d. Dr. Harris dies suddenly, and his staff tell patients that the office will close and that copies of their medical records will be transferred to another physician.		
e. Mr. Davies owes the physician's office several thousand dollars. He is moving and asks the office to transfer his medical records to his new physician. The office refuses on the grounds that Mr. Davies has not paid his bill.		
f. Mrs. Jones comes into the office for a vaccination. The physician tells the medical assistant to charge her $10 less than other patients because she is elderly and cannot afford the standard charges.		

19. Match the following key terms to their definitions.

Key Terms

a. abandonment _____

b. slander _____

c. assault _____

d. battery _____

e. bioethics _____

f. tort _____

g. civil law _____

h. common law _____

i. defamation of character _____

j. defendant _____

k. deposition _____

l. durable power of attorney _____

m. emancipated minor _____

n. fee splitting _____

o. fraud _____

p. libel _____

q. litigation _____

r. locum tenens _____

s. malpractice _____

Definitions

1. a deceitful act with the intention to conceal the truth

2. process of filing or contesting a lawsuit

3. traditional laws outlined in the Constitution

4. a theory meaning that the previous decision stands

5. a person under the age of majority but married or self-supporting

6. previous court decisions

7. a branch of law that focuses on issues between private citizens

8. the righting of wrongs suffered as a result of another person's wrongdoing

9. a substitute physician

10. an arrangement that gives the patient's representative the ability to make health care decisions for the patient

11. sharing fees for the referral of patients to certain colleagues

12. the accuser in a lawsuit

13. failure to take reasonable precautions to prevent harm to a patient

14. the accused party in a lawsuit

15. a doctrine meaning "the thing speaks for itself"

16. the unauthorized attempt to threaten or touch another person without consent

17. the physical touching of a patient without consent

18. malicious or false statements about a person's character or reputation

19. written statements that damage a person's character or reputation

t. negligence _____

u. plaintiff _____

v. precedents _____

w. res ipsa loquitur _____

x. res judicata _____

y. respondeat superior _____

z. stare decisis _____

20. a process in which one party questions another party under oath

21. an action by a professional health care worker that harms a patient

22. a doctrine meaning "the thing has been decided"

23. a doctrine meaning "let the master answer," also known as the law of agency

24. moral issues that affect a patient's life

25. withdrawal by a physician from a contractual relationship with a patient without proper notification

26. oral statements that damage a person's character or reputation

20. True or False? Determine whether the following statements are true or false. If false, explain why.

a. If a patient is in a life-threatening situation, it is important to obtain the patient's consent before beginning treatment.

_____

_____

b. A minor cannot sign a consent form unless he or she is in the armed services.

_____

_____

c. A bench trial does not involve a jury.

_____

_____

d. In court, the burden of proof is on the defendant.

_____

_____

APPLICATION

Critical Thinking Practice

1. A family member calls to inquire about a patient's condition. You know that the patient has not given written consent for information to be passed on, but you recognize the person's voice and remember that she came in with the patient the previous day. Explain what you would say and why.

_____

_____

2. You are running late and have several tasks that need to be done immediately. You are dealing with a patient who needs to sign a consent form for a surgical procedure. The patient does not speak English very well, and you are not entirely sure that the patient understands what he is signing. List three things you should do, and explain why they are important.

_____

_____

Patient Education

1. You have a patient who has just been diagnosed with a sexually transmitted disease. After the physician leaves the office, the patient turns to you and begs you to keep the information confidential. It is obvious that the patient is worried and embarrassed. Explain how you would inform the patient about legally required disclosures and what you would say.

_____

_____

Documentation

1. Dr. Mason tells you that he needs to terminate a relationship with Mr. Stevens because he has not been keeping his appointments. He asks you to draft the letter. Write a letter to Mr. Stevens, including the correct legal information required to terminate successfully a physician-patient relationship without fear of litigation.

Active Learning

1. Research two recent medical malpractice cases on the Internet. Write a brief outline of each case and make a record of whether the tort was intentional or unintentional, and what the outcome of the case was. Compare the cases to see if there is a common theme, and draw a chart to show your findings.

2. Visit a physician's office and make a list of steps that have been taken to comply with the law. For example, if the physician charges for canceling appointments without notice, there is probably a sign by the reception desk to warn patients of the fee. How many other legal requirements can you find? Are there any that are missing?

3. As technology develops, new laws have to be written to protect the rights of patients who use it. Stem cell research is a particularly gray area, and has raised many interesting ethical dilemmas. Research some recent legal cases regarding stem cell research, and write a report on some of the ethical issues the cases have raised.

Professional Journal

REFLECT

(Prompts and Ideas: Have you or a loved one ever been mistreated by a medical professional? Have you ever been unsure of what you were signing, or not had a procedure properly explained to you? Do you have any personal beliefs that you would find difficult to keep to yourself as a medical professional?)

_____

_____

_____

PONDER AND SOLVE

1. One of your friends is also training to be a medical assistant and has applied for a job at the physician's office where you work. You know that your friend attends anti-abortion rallies and is vehemently opposed to abortion. The physician's office you work in carries out the procedure on a regular basis. What do you do?

_____

_____

_____

2. A 50-year-old patient has just been told that his cancer has returned for the third time. He tells you that he can't face any more treatment and just wants to die peacefully. His 23-year-old daughter is devastated by her father's decision and begs you to make him change his mind. What do you do?

_____

_____

_____

_____

_____

_____

EXPERIENCE

Skills related to this chapter include:

1. Monitoring Federal and State Regulations, Changes, and Updates (Procedure 2-1).

Record any common mistakes, lessons learned, and/or tips you discovered during your experience of practicing and demonstrating these skills:

_____

_____

_____

_____

_____

_____

_____

Skill Practice

PERFORMANCE OBJECTIVE:

1. Monitor federal and state health care legislation (Procedure 2-1).

Name_____ Date _____ Time _____

| Procedure 2-1: | MONITORING FEDERAL AND STATE REGULATIONS, CHANGES, AND UPDATES |

EQUIPMENT: Computer, Internet connection, search engine or website list

KEY: 4 = Satisfactory   0 = Unsatisfactory   NA = This step is not counted

PROCEDURE STEPS	SELF	PARTNER	INSTRUCTOR
1. Using a search engine, go to the homepage for your state government (Example: www.nc.gov) and/or other related sites such as: Centers for Disease Control and Prevention (CDC), Occupational Safety and Health Act (OSHA), your state medical society, and the American Medical Association (AMA).	☐	☐	☐
2. Input keywords such as: Health care finances, allied health professionals, outpatient medical care, Medicare, etc.	☐	☐	☐
3. Create and enforce a policy for timely dissemination of information received by fax or e-mail from outside agencies.	☐	☐	☐
4. Circulate information gathered to all appropriate employees with an avenue for sharing information. Any information obtained should be shared.	☐	☐	☐
5. Post changes in policies and procedures in a designated area of the office.	☐	☐	☐

CALCULATION

Total Possible Points: _____
Total Points Earned: _____ Multiplied by 100 = _____ Divided by Total Possible Points = _____ %

Pass   **Fail**
☐   ☐   Comments:

Student's signature _____ Date _____
Partner's signature _____ Date _____
Instructor's signature _____ Date _____

Work Product

Document Appropriately.

Britney Smith is a 16-year-old patient who comes for her routine gynecological exam with her mother. Her mother waits in the reception area while Britney has her appointment. You are directed to collect a urine sample from Britney Smith. She refuses to give a sample. If you are currently working in a medical office, use a blank paper patient chart from the office. If this is not available to you, use the space below to write a note recording her refusal of the urine test.

_____

_____

Chapter Self-Assessment Quiz

1. The branch of law concerned with issues of citizen welfare and safety is:

   a. private law.

   b. criminal law.

   c. constitutional law.

   d. administrative law.

   e. civil law.

2. Which branch of law covers injuries suffered because of another person's wrongdoings resulting from a breach of legal duty?

   a. Tort law

   b. Contract law

   c. Property law

   d. Commercial law

   e. Administrative law

3. Scientific advances are among the causes of the rise in malpractice claims because:

   a. complications and risks for new procedures have escalated.

   b. patients complain more often for receiving outdated treatments.

   c. the high costs for new technology are unaffordable for most patients.

   d. the medical community is too specialized and does not share information.

   e. physicians are able to cure more patients than in the past.

4. The Health Insurance Portability and Accountability Act of 1996 deals with the patient's right to:

   a. privacy.

   b. choose a physician.

   c. get information prior to a treatment.

   d. interrupt a treatment considered disadvantageous.

   e. refuse treatment.

5. Which of the following can lead a patient to file a suit for abandonment against a physician?

   a. The physician verbally asks to end the relationship with the patient.

   b. A suitable substitute is not available for care after termination of the contract.

   c. The patient disagrees with the reasons given by the physician for the termination.

   d. Termination happens 35 days after the physician's withdrawal letter is received.

   e. The physician transfers the patient's medical records to another physician of the patient's choice.

Scenario: A man is found lying unconscious outside the physician's office. You alert several colleagues, who go outside to assess the man's condition. It is clear that he will be unable to sign a consent form for treatment.

6. How should the physician handle the unconscious man?

a. Implied consent should be used until the man can give informed consent.

b. A health care surrogate should be solicited to provide informed consent.

c. The hospital administration should evaluate the situation and give consent.

d. The physician should proceed with no-risk procedures until informed consent is given.

e. The physician should wait for a friend or family member to give consent on the patient's behalf.

7. Once the man wakes up and gives his expressed consent to a treatment, this implies that he:

a. no longer needs assistance.

b. verbally agrees in front of witnesses on an emergency treatment.

c. authorizes the physician to exchange patients' information with other physicians.

d. trusts the physician with emergency procedures that can be deemed necessary at a later time.

e. is now familiar with the possible risks of the procedure.

End Scenario

8. A diagnosis of cancer must be reported to the DHHS to:

a. alert the closest family members.

b. protect the patient's right to treatment.

c. investigate possible carcinogens in the environment.

d. check coverage options with the insurance company.

e. provide research for a national study.

9. What is the difference between licensure and certification?

a. Licensure is accessible to medical assistants.

b. Certification standards are recognized nationally.

c. Licensure indicates education requirements are met.

d. Certification limits the scope of activity of a physician.

e. Licensure allows a professional to practice in any state.

10. The Good Samaritan Act covers:

a. emergency care provided by a medical assistant.

b. compensated emergency care outside the formal practice.

c. sensible emergency practice administered outside the office.

d. emergency practice administered in the hospital to uninsured patients.

e. emergency care administered in the physician's office before the patient is registered.

11. The term *malfeasance* refers to:

a. failure to administer treatment in time.

b. administration of inappropriate treatment.

c. administration of treatment performed incorrectly.

d. failure to administer treatment in the best possible conditions.

e. the physical touching of a patient without consent.

12. Which tort pertains to care administered without the patient's consent?

a. Duress

b. Assault

c. Tort of outrage

d. Undue influence

e. Invasion of privacy

13. The statute of limitation indicates:

a. the privacy rights of a minor receiving care.

b. the risks that are presented to a patient before treatment.

c. the responsibilities of a physician toward his or her patients.

d. the right of a physician to have another physician care for his patients while out of the office.

e. the time span during which a patient can file a suit against a caregiver.

14. The court may assess contributory negligence when a(n):

a. team of physicians incorrectly diagnoses the patient.

b. physician's malpractice is aggravated by the patient.

c. patient does not follow the physician's prescribed treatment properly.

d. patient gives inaccurate information that leads to wrong treatment.

e. physician is entirely responsible for the patient's injury.

15. Which of these best describes the principle of patient advocacy?

a. A medical assistant must adhere to his or her own code of conduct.

b. A medical assistant must act first and foremost in the interest of the patient.

c. A medical assistant must make sure the patient's information remains confidential.

d. A medical assistant must make sure to act as a mediator between the physician and the patient.

e. A medical assistant should only perform procedures that agree with his personal ethics.

16. Which of these is the basic principle of bioethics?

   a. All patients are entitled to the best possible treatment.

   b. Moral issues must be evaluated according to the patient's specific circumstances.

   c. Members of the medical community should never compromise their religious beliefs.

   d. The medical community must agree on a code of moral standards to apply to controversial cases.

   e. Moral issues are guidelines that the medical community is legally bound to follow.

17. What is AMA's regulation on artificial insemination?

   a. Both husband and wife must agree to the procedure.

   b. The donor has the right to contact the couple after the child is born.

   c. The procedure can only be performed legally in certain states.

   c. A donor can be selected only after the husband has tried the procedure unsuccessfully.

   d. The couple requesting the procedure has the right to gain information about possible donors.

18. What does the Self-Determination Act of 1991 establish?

   a. The physician has the last word on interruption of treatment.

   b. A person has the right to make end-of-life decisions in advance.

   c. The physician must follow advance directives from a patient verbatim.

   d. Family members cannot make decisions about terminating a patient's treatment.

   e. If a patient cannot make his own decision, a close family member can do so on his behalf.

19. Which of these patients would be unable to sign a consent form?

   a. A 17-year-old requesting information about a sexually transmitted disease

   b. A pregnant 15-year-old

   c. A 16-year-old boy who works full-time

   d. A 17-year-old girl who requires knee surgery

   e. A married 21-year-old

20. In a comparative negligence case, how are damages awarded?

   a. The plaintiff receives damages based on a percentage of their contribution to the negligence.

   b. The defendant does not have to pay the plaintiff anything.

   c. The plaintiff and defendant share 50% of the court costs and receive no damages.

   d. The plaintiff has to pay damages to the defendant for defamation of character.

   e. The plaintiff receives 100% of the damages awarded.

3

Communication Skills

Chapter Checklist

☐ Read textbook chapter and take notes within the Chapter Notes outline. Answer the Learning Objectives as you reach them in the content, and then check them off.

☐ Work the Content Review questions—both Foundational Knowledge and Application.

☐ Perform the Active Learning exercise(s).

☐ Complete Professional Journal entries.

☐ Complete Skill Practice Activity(s) using Competency Evaluation Forms and Work Products, when appropriate.

☐ Take the Chapter Self-Assessment Quiz.

☐ Insert all appropriate pages into your Portfolio.

Learning Objectives

1. Spell and define the key terms.
2. List two major forms of communication.
3. Explain how various components of communication can affect the meaning of verbal messages.
4. Define active listening.
5. List and describe the six interviewing techniques.
6. Give an example of how cultural differences may affect communication.
7. Discuss how to handle communication problems caused by language barriers.
8. List two methods that you can use to promote communication among hearing-, sight-, and speech-impaired patients.
9. Discuss how to handle an angry or distressed patient.
10. List five actions that you can take to improve communication with a child.
11. Discuss your role in communicating with a grieving patient or family member.
12. List the five stages of grief as outlined by Elisabeth Kubler-Ross.
13. Discuss the key elements of interdisciplinary communication.

Chapter Notes

Note: Bold-faced headings are the major headings in the text chapter; headings in regular font are lower-level headings (i.e., the content is subordinate to, or falls "under," the major headings). Make sure you understand the key terms used in the chapter, as well as the concepts presented as Key Points.

TEXT SUBHEADINGS	NOTES
Introduction _____	_____

Key Term: messages
Key Point:
- In your role, you must accurately and appropriately share information with physicians, other professional staff members, and patients.

☐ **LEARNING OBJECTIVE 1.** Spell and define the key terms.

Basic Communication Flow _____

Key Terms: feedback; clarification

Forms of Communication _____

Verbal Communication _____

Key Terms: paralanguage; nonlanguage
Key Points:
- You need good verbal communication skills when performing such tasks as making appointments, providing patient education, making referrals, and sharing information with the physician.
- The ability to write clearly, concisely, and accurately is important in the health care profession.

Nonverbal Communication _____

Key Terms: cultures; therapeutic; demeanor
Key Point:
- A patient's face can sometimes reveal inner feelings, such as sadness, happiness, fear, or anger, that may not be mentioned explicitly during a conversation.

☐ **LEARNING OBJECTIVE 2:** List two major forms of communication.

☐ **LEARNING OBJECTIVE 3:** Explain how various components of communication can affect the meaning of verbal messages.

Active Listening _____

Key Point:
• To listen actively, you must give your full attention to the patient with whom you are speaking. Interruptions should be kept to a minimum.

☐ **LEARNING OBJECTIVE 4:** Define active listening.

Interview Techniques _____

Key Point:
• To conduct either type of interview, you must use effective techniques: listen actively, ask the appropriate questions, and record the answers.

Reflecting _____

Key Term: reflecting

Paraphrasing or Restatement _____

Key Term: paraphrasing

Asking for Examples or Clarification _____

Asking Open-Ended Questions _____

Key Point:
• The best way to obtain specific information is to ask open-ended questions that require the patient to formulate an answer and elaborate on the response.

Summarizing _____

_____

Key Term: summarizing
Key Point:
• Briefly reviewing the information you have obtained, or summarizing, gives the patient another chance to clarify statements or correct misinformation.

Allowing Silences _____

_____

☐ **LEARNING OBJECTIVE 5:** List and describe the six interviewing techniques.

Factors Affecting Communication _____

_____

_____

Cultural Differences _____

_____

Key Points:
• The way a person perceives situations and other people is greatly influenced by cultural, social, and religious beliefs or firmly held convictions.
• To help avoid miscommunication and offending patients, you must be sensitive to these differences in all of your patient interactions.

☐ **LEARNING OBJECTIVE 6:** Give an example of how cultural differences may affect communication.

Stereotyping and Biased Opinions _____

_____

Key Terms: bias; discrimination; stereotyping
Key Point:
• As a health care professional, you are expected to treat all patients impartially, to guard against discriminatory practices, remain nonjudgmental, avoid stereotypes, and have a professional demeanor.

Language Barriers _____

_____

☐ **LEARNING OBJECTIVE 7:** Discuss how to handle communication problems caused by language barriers.

Special Communication Challenges _____

Key Point:
• Patients must feel that they are part of the process even if their condition requires involvement by family members or other caregivers.

Hearing-Impaired Patients _____

Key Terms: anacusis; presbyacusis

Sight-Impaired Patients _____

Key Point:
• Patients who can't see lose valuable information from non-verbal communication.

Speech Impairments _____

Key Terms: dysphasia; dysphonia

☐ **LEARNING OBJECTIVE 8:** List two methods that you can use to promote communication among hearing-, sight-, and speech-impaired patients.

Mental Health Illnesses _____

Key Point:
• Your communication should be professional, nonjudgmental, and encouraging when appropriate.

Angry or Distressed Patients _____

Key Point:
• The key to communicating with upset patients is to prevent an escalation of the problem.

☐ **LEARNING OBJECTIVE 9:** Discuss how to handle an angry or distressed patient.

Children _____

_____

_____

☐ **LEARNING OBJECTIVE 10:** List five actions that you can take to improve communication with a child.

Communicating with a Grieving Patient or Family Member _____

_____

Key Terms: grief; mourning
Key Point:
- Empathy can help you recognize a patient's fear and discomfort so you can do everything possible to provide support and reassurance.

☐ **LEARNING OBJECTIVE 11:** Discuss your role in communicating with a grieving patient or family member.

☐ **LEARNING OBJECTIVE 12:** List the five stages of grief as outlined by Elisabeth Kubler-Ross.

Establishing Positive Patient Relationships _____

_____

_____

Proper Form of Address _____

_____

Key Point:
- These terms denigrate the individual's dignity and put the interaction on a personal, not professional, level.

Professional Distance _____

_____

Key Point:
- You should not become too personally involved with patients because doing so may jeopardize your ability to be objective.

Teaching Patients _____

_____

_____

Professional Communication _____

_____

_____

Communicating with Peers _____

_____

Key Point:
• Involvement in local community organizations and support groups is also beneficial to promoting you and your profession.

_____

Communicating with Physicians _____

_____

_____

Communicating with Other Facilities _____

_____

☐ **LEARNING OBJECTIVE 13:** Discuss the key elements of interdisciplinary communication.

Content Review

FOUNDATIONAL KNOWLEDGE

Communication Skills

1. The two main forms of communication are verbal communication and nonverbal communication. Read each form of communication below and place a check mark to indicate whether it represents verbal or nonverbal communication.

Communication	Verbal	Nonverbal
a. A patient sighs while explaining her symptoms.		
b. A patient shrugs his shoulders after being told he needs to lose weight.		
c. A patient's eyes dart around the room during an explanation of a procedure.		
d. A physician writes "take two aspirin every eight hours."		
e. A mother is given a sheet of paper describing what to expect of her baby during months 6–9.		
f. A physician puts her hand on a patient's shoulder before delivering test results.		

2. The physician has recommended that your patient Valerie schedule a mammogram because he is concerned about a lump in her breast. You explain the procedure to the patient and provide her with the information she needs to make her appointment. When you ask if she has any questions, she says no. However, you notice that there are tears in Valerie's eyes. What is the problem with this interaction, and how should you respond?

_____

_____

3. Explain what it means to listen actively.

_____

_____

Interviewing Patients

4. Physicians use the information obtained during a patient interview to help them assess the patient's health. Patients will be more willing to provide information during a professionally conducted interview. Read each of the following statements describing patient interviews. Answer *yes* if the statement describes a correct interview practice; answer *no* if it describes an incorrect interview practice. Provide an explanation on how to correct the problem for all *no* answers.

	Yes	No
a. Patient interviews can be conducted in an exam room or in the waiting room.		
b. Answering a phone call in the middle of a new patient interview is acceptable if it is a call you have been waiting for.		
c. It is important to maintain eye contact with the patient, so you do not write any patient responses down until the interview is over.		
d. You confirm which blood pressure medication and what dosage the patient is taking.		
e. There is nothing wrong with skipping questions in a patient interview that may make the patient feel uncomfortable.		
f. Introducing yourself to the patient is a nice way to start an interview.		

5. Conducting patient interviews is a major part of a medical assistant's job. It is important that you're familiar with the interview techniques. Match the name of each interview technique below with its correct description.

Interview Techniques

a. reflecting
b. paraphrasing
c. clarification
d. asking open-ended questions
e. summarizing
f. allowing silences

Descriptions

1. asking the patient to give an example of the situation being described
2. taking a moment to gather your thoughts and let the patient gather her thoughts
3. repeating what you have heard the patient say, using open-ended statements
4. asking the patient a question that begins with *what, when,* or *how.*
5. repeating what you have heard, using your own words
6. briefly reviewing the information obtained so the patient can correct any misinformation

6. **Next Question, Please**

When conducting patient interviews, you'll need to ask a lot of questions to learn a patient's medical history, family history, and social history, as well as information about medications and body functions. Fill in the chart below with one question in each category that you could ask a patient during an interview.

Area of Questioning	Sample Question
Past medical history	
Family history	
Body system review	
Social history	
Medications	

7. **Culture Clash**

Why is it important to be aware of cultural differences among people?

_____

_____

8. Explain how bias and stereotyping on the part of a medical assistant could hinder patient care.

_____

_____

9. Sharing Bad News

A young patient named Sumaja has just received news that she has breast cancer. She is becoming distressed. The medical assistant does the following things for the patient (see table below). Determine whether these were the appropriate ways to handle the situation. If it was an inappropriate action, explain why.

Action	Right	Wrong
a. Giving Sumaja information about breast cancer to read at home		
b. Providing Sumaja with phone numbers for places to call for more information		
c. When Sumaja asked if she might die, telling Sumaja that her case is not that bad and that she should be fine		
d. Giving Sumaja information on treatment options		
e. Telling Sumaja which treatment options will work best for her		

10. The Language Barrier

You are helping a new medical assistant learn how to conduct patient interviews. One of his patients is a Spanish-speaking woman who came to the office with her son and daughter. The following are some of the steps he took to get information. Write correct or incorrect after reading each statement. If you answer _incorrect,_ explain what the medical assistant should have done.

a. He spoke in a normal tone and volume. _____

b. He spoke directly to the translator. _____

c. When asking a question about eyesight, he pointed to his eyes. _____

d. He used abbreviations and slang terms for medical tests. _____

e. He asked the woman's son to be the interpreter and her daughter to wait outside. _____

f. He used complex medical language to explain procedures. _____

g. He used a Spanish-English phrase book. _____

11. Keep Your Cool

A patient comes into an already crowded waiting room and asks how long her wait will be to see the doctor. When you tell her it will be approximately one hour, she starts yelling at you. She claims that you don't know how to schedule appointments correctly and that perhaps you should be replaced. You start to get angry. How should you respond?

_____

_____

12. Are You Up for the Challenge?

Your office treats some hearing-impaired patients. Place a check mark next to the suggestions that will help you to communicate with a hearing-impaired patient.

Suggestion	Yes	No
a. Gently touch the patient to get her attention.		
b. Exaggerate your facial movements.		
c. Eliminate all distractions.		
d. Enunciate clearly.		

e. Use short sentences with short words.		
f. Speak loudly.		
g. Write things down on note pads.		
h. Turn toward the light so your face is illuminated.		
i. Talk directly face-to-face with the patient, not at an angle.		

13. Mr. Webb comes into the office with his 10-year-old daughter for a checkup. He mentions that she got sunburned over the weekend, and it is blistering on her back and shoulders. Which response would be appropriate? Explain.

   a. "I will tell the doctor you are concerned about the sunburn."

   b. "Everyone with coloring like you gets sunburned. You should be more careful in the sun and use more sunscreen."

   _____

   _____

14. Children can be challenging to communicate with because their levels of comprehension vary with their ages. Read the following suggestions to help facilitate communication with children. Circle the suggestions that are most helpful.

   a. Tell children when you need to touch them and what you are going to do.

   b. Talk loudly and sternly so the child will stay focused on you and not other distractions in the office.

   c. If you think a child may be frightened, it is best to work quickly and let him or her be surprised by what you do.

   d. Rephrase questions until the child understands.

   e. Be playful to help gain a child's cooperation.

   f. When dealing with adolescents, it is always best to have a parent present.

   g. Keeping an interview professional and nonjudgmental will help keep adolescents communicating.

   h. Try to speak to children at their eye level.

15. Explain how the TDD phone system works, and list two ways in which it can be beneficial to a medical office.

   Explanation: _____

   Benefit 1: _____

   Benefit 2: _____

16. **Good Grief!**

   The five stages of grief as outlined by Elisabeth Kubler-Ross are denial, anger, bargaining, depression, and acceptance. Fill in one of the five stages of grief for each statement below.

   a. The doctor must have gotten my test results mixed up. _____

   b. I have terminal brain cancer. _____

   c. If I survive this, I will change the way I live my life for the better. _____

   d. I hate this doctor; I am going to find a new one. _____

   e. I don't care if the treatment might help me live a little longer. _____

17. A patient who you have known for five years has just been diagnosed with advanced terminal cancer. List three things you can do as a medical assistant to be supportive.

   a. _____

   b. _____

   c. _____

18. A patient calls the office with symptoms and a condition that you are not familiar with. She has used some terms that you do not understand. When you relay the message to the physician, how should you communicate the patient's problem?

_____

_____

19. Match the following key terms to their definitions.

Key Terms

a. anacusis _____

b. bias _____

c. clarification _____

d. cultures _____

e. demeanor _____

f. discrimination _____

g. dysphasia _____

h. dysphonia _____

i. feedback _____

j. grief _____

k. messages _____

l. mourning _____

m. nonlanguage _____

n. paralanguage _____

o. paraphrasing _____

p. presbyacusis _____

q. reflecting _____

r. stereotyping _____

s. summarizing _____

t. therapeutic _____

Definitions

1. information

2. something that is beneficial to a patient

3. a group of people who share a way of life and beliefs

4. holding an opinion of all members of a particular culture, race, religion, or age group based on oversimplified or negative characterizations

5. loss of hearing associated with aging

6. difficulty speaking

7. sounds that include laughing, sobbing, sighing, or grunting to convey information

8. the response to a message

9. restating what a person said using your own words or phrases

10. removal of confusion or uncertainty

11. formation of an opinion without foundation or reason

12. a demonstration of the signs of grief

13. complete hearing loss

14. briefly reviewing information discussed to determine the patient's comprehension

15. great sadness caused by a loss

16. voice tone, quality, volume, pitch, and range

17. the way a person looks, behaves, and conducts himself

18. a voice impairment that is caused by a physical condition, such as oral surgery

19. the act of not treating a patient fairly or respectfully because of his cultural, social, or personal values

20. repeating what one heard using open-ended questions

20. True or False? Determine whether the following statements are true or false. If false, explain why.

a. When the office is busy, it is okay to refer to patients by their medical condition, for example, stomach pain in room 1.

_____

_____

b. If an elderly patient does not have a ride home, a staff member in the office should offer her one.

_____

_____

c. When talking with patients, do not reveal too many personal details about your life.

_____

_____

d. It is inappropriate to carry on personal conversations with other staff members in front of a patient.

_____

_____

APPLICATION

Critical Thinking Practice

1. There is a medical assistant in your office who is easily distracted when interviewing patients. You have observed her doodling on paper and taking incomplete notes. The office manager has told her she needs to practice her active listening skills. At break time she complains to you, saying, "I don't know why this active listening is so important!" Think of a creative way to show your co-worker why active listening is a skill needed by medical assistants.

_____

_____

2. A patient's husband recently died in a car accident. She comes into the office because she needs to have a test for strep throat since she has had a fever and sore throat for two days. While there, she tells you that she is having trouble sleeping and is losing weight because she hasn't had an appetite since her husband died. You feel terrible for her, but don't know how to act or what to say. Explain why it is better to show empathy for a grieving patient rather than sympathy.

_____

_____

_____

Patient Education

1. Mr. Rivera's wife died a year ago. Since that time, Mr. Rivera has stopped seeing friends and participating in social activities. He visits the cemetery several times a week. Mr. Rivera asks if his feelings of sadness and depression will ever go away. He wonders if he will ever feel any differently. What would you say to Mr. Rivera? How would you explain the grief process?

_____

_____

Documentation

1. You need to document the conversation that you had with Mr. Rivera in his chart. Write a narrative chart note describing your interaction with Mr. Rivera.

_____

_____

Active Learning

1. Patients who have been told they have a terminal illness will likely go through a grieving process. Their families will be grieving, too. There are resources available to patients and their families, and grief counselors can help them work through the grieving process. You have been asked to prepare a handout for patients on the benefits of grief counselors.
   - Use the Internet to research what grief counselors do and how they can help terminally ill patients.
   - Imagine yourself as a family member of the patient and create a list of questions you would ask a grief counselor.
   - Contact a grief counselor (through a local hospice program or hospital) and interview him or her.
   - Prepare a one-page handout to be given to patients and their families about the benefits of grief counselors.

2. Practice active listening with a partner. Have your partner tell you a detailed story that you have never heard before or explain a topic that you are unfamiliar with. After he or she has finished, wait silently for 2 minutes. Then try to repeat the story or steps back to your partner. Next, reverse roles and let your partner listen while you tell a story or explain a concept.

3. If you work in a pediatric office, you will certainly spend a good deal of time communicating with children. To help strengthen your communication skills with children, find a local preschool or elementary school teacher who has experience working with children. Interview this teacher about his or her communication techniques and write a list of ten tips for communicating with children.

Professional Journal

REFLECT

(Prompts and Ideas: Have you ever had trouble communicating with medical professionals for yourself or a loved one? What could you have done differently? What could they have done differently?)

_____

_____

_____

_____

_____

_____

PONDER AND SOLVE

1. You are helping a 7-year-old patient with a nebulizer for his asthma. While you are doing this, a coworker comes in the room and starts talking about her weekend. She asks why you and your girlfriend left the party early and tells you everything that went on after you left. You know this is not appropriate for a patient to hear. How would you stop your coworker, and what would you say to her later in private?

_____

_____

_____

_____

_____

2. Mrs. Saltz is a very independent 70-year-old woman. She has trouble hearing, but does not acknowledge her hearing problem. The doctor has given her verbal instructions on how to take her medications, but you are not sure she completely understood him. What would you say to Mrs. Saltz? What else can you do?

_____

_____

_____

_____

_____

_____

Chapter Self-Assessment Quiz

1. Laughing, sobbing, and sighing are examples of:

   a. kinesics.

   b. proxemics.

   c. nonlanguage.

   d. paralanguage.

   e. clarification.

2. Hearing impairment that involves problems with either nerves or the cochlea is called:

   a. anacusis.

   b. conductive.

   c. presbyacusis.

   d. sensorineural.

   e. dysphasia.

3. Sally needs to obtain information from her patient about the medications he is taking. Which of the following open-ended questions is phrased in a way that will elicit the information that Sally needs?

   a. Are you taking your medications?

   b. What medications are you taking?

   c. Have you taken any medications?

   d. Did you take your medications today?

   e. Have you taken medications in the past?

4. Which of the following shows the five stages of grief in the correct sequence?

   a. Denial-anger-bargaining-depression-acceptance

   b. Acceptance-depression-bargaining-anger-denial

   c. Anger-denial-depression-acceptance-bargaining

   d. Denial-bargaining-anger-depression-acceptance

   e. Bargaining-anger-acceptance-depression-denial

5. "Those people always get head lice." This statement is an example of:

   a. culture.

   b. demeanor.

   c. discrimination.

   d. stereotyping.

   e. prejudice.

6. What can you do as a medical assistant to communicate effectively with a patient when there is a language barrier?

   a. Find an interpreter who can translate for the patient.

   b. Raise your voice so the patient can focus more on what you are saying.

   c. Give the patient the name and address of a physician who speaks the same language.

   d. Assess the patient and give the physician your best opinion about what is bothering the patient.

   e. Suggest that the patient find another physician who is better equipped to communicate with the patient.

7. When dealing with patients who present communication challenges, such as hearing-impaired or sight-impaired patients, it is best to:

   a. talk about the patient directly with a family member to find out what the problem is.

   b. conduct the interview alone with the patient because he needs to be able to take care of himself.

   c. address the patient's questions in the waiting room, where other people can try to help the patient communicate.

   d. refer the patient to a practice that specializes in working with hearing- and sight-impaired patients.

   e. make sure the patient feels like he is part of the process, even if his condition requires a family member's help.

8. A hearing-impaired patient's test results are in. It is important that the patient gets the results quickly. How should you get the results to the patient?

   a. Mail the test results Priority Mail.

   b. Call the patient on a TDD/TTY phone and type in the results.

   c. Drive to the patient's house at lunchtime to deliver the results.

   d. Call an emergency contact of the patient and ask him or her to have the patient make an appointment.

   e. Send the patient a fax containing the test results.

9. Which of the following statements about grieving is true?

    a. The grieving period is approximately 30 days.

    b. Different cultures and individuals demonstrate grief in different ways.

    c. The best way to grieve is through wailing because it lets the emotion out.

    d. The five stages of grief must be followed in that specific order for healing to begin.

    e. Everyone grieves in his own way, but all of us go through the stages at the same time.

10. Proxemics refers to the:

    a. pitch of a person's voice.

    b. facial expressions a person makes.

    c. physical proximity that people tolerate.

    d. the combination of verbal and nonverbal communication.

    e. the ability of a patient to comprehend difficult messages.

11. Which of the following situations would result in a breach of patient confidentiality?

    a. Shredding unwanted notes that contain patient information

    b. Discussing a patient's lab results with a co-worker in the hospital cafeteria

    c. Keeping the glass window between the waiting room and reception desk closed

    d. Shutting down your computer when you leave every night

    e. Paging the physician on an intercom to let him know a patient is waiting on the phone for results

12. "Those results can't be true. The doctor must have mixed me up with another patient." This statement reflects which of the following stages of grieving?

    a. Anger

    b. Denial

    c. Depression

    d. Bargaining

    e. Acceptance

13. Which of the following statements about communication is correct?

    a. Communication can be either verbal or nonverbal.

    b. Written messages can be interpreted through paralanguage.

    c. Verbal communication involves both oral communication and body language.

    d. Body language is the most important form of communication.

    e. Touch should be avoided in all forms of communication because it makes the recipient of the message uncomfortable.

14. During a patient interview, repeating what you have heard the patient say, using an open-ended statement is called:

    a. clarifying.

    b. reflecting.

    c. summarizing.

    d. paraphrasing.

    e. allowing silences.

15. What should you do during a patient interview if there is silence?

    a. Silence should not be allowed during a patient interview.

    b. Immediately start talking so the patient does not feel awkward.

    c. Fill in charts that need to be completed until the patient is ready.

    d. Wait for the physician to arrive to speak with the patient.

    e. Gather your thoughts and think of any additional questions you have.

16. The physician is behind schedule, and a patient is angry that her appointment is late. The best way to deal the patient is to:

    a. tell her anything that will calm her down.

    b. ignore her until the problem is solved.

    c. threaten that the physician will no longer treat her if she continues to complain.

    d. keep her informed of when the physician will be able to see her.

    e. ask her why it is such a big deal.

17. Why is it helpful to ask open-ended questions during a patient interview?

   a. They let the patient give yes or no answers.

   b. They let the patient develop an answer and explain it.

   c. They let the patient respond quickly using few words.

   d. They provide simple answers that are easy to note in the chart.

   e. They let the patient give his own feelings and opinions on the subject.

18. Difficulty with speech is called:

   a. dysphasia.

   b. dysphonia.

   c. nyctalopia.

   d. strabismus.

   e. myopia.

19. Adrian Makey is a 65-year-old man who recently had a mild heart attack. The medical assistant is the first person he encounters on his first visit to Dr. Liu's cardiology office. Which greeting by the medical assistant would be most professional?

   a. Hi, Adrian, how are you feeling?

   b. Hi, Gramps, how are you feeling?

   c. Hi, sweetie, how are you feeling?

   d. Hi, Mr. Makey, how are you feeling?

   e. Hi, Adrian Makey, how are you feeling?

20. The limit of personal space is generally considered to be a:

   a. 1-foot radius.

   b. 3-foot radius.

   c. 5-foot radius.

   d. 10-foot radius.

   e. 15-foot radius.

Patient Education

☐ Read textbook chapter and take notes within the Chapter Notes outline. Answer the Learning Objectives as you reach them in the content, and then check them off.

☐ Work the Content Review questions—both Foundational Knowledge and Application.

☐ Perform the Active Learning exercise(s).

☐ Complete Professional Journal entries.

☐ Complete Skill Practice Activity(s) using Competency Evaluation Forms and Work Products, when appropriate.

☐ Take the Chapter Self-Assessment Quiz.

☐ Insert all appropriate pages into your Portfolio.

1. Spell and define the key terms.
2. Explain the medical assistant's role in patient education.
3. Define the five steps in the patient education process.
4. Identify five conditions that are needed for patient education to occur.
5. Explain Maslow's hierarchy of human needs.
6. List five factors that may hinder patient education and at least two methods to compensate for each of these factors.
7. Discuss five preventive medicine guidelines that you should teach your patients.

8. Explain the kinds of information that should be included in patient teaching about medication therapy.
9. Explain your role in teaching patients about alternative medicine therapies.
10. List and explain relaxation techniques that you and patients can learn to help with stress management.
11. Describe how to prepare a teaching plan.
12. List potential sources of patient education materials.
13. Locate community resources and list ways of organizing and disseminating information.

Note: Bold-faced headings are the major headings in the text chapter; headings in regular font are lower-level headings (i.e., the content is subordinate to, or falls "under," the major headings). Make sure you understand the key terms used in the chapter, as well as the concepts presented as Key Points.

TEXT SUBHEADINGS   **NOTES**

Introduction _____

_____

> **Key Point:**
> • Patient education is performed under the direction of the physician.

☐ **LEARNING OBJECTIVE 1:** Spell and define the key terms.

The Patient Education Process _____

_____

☐ **LEARNING OBJECTIVE 2:** Explain the medical assistant's role in patient education.

Assessment _____

_____

> **Key Term:** assessment
> **Key Point:**
> • **Assessment** requires gathering information about the patient's present health care needs and abilities.

Planning _____

_____

> **Key Term:** learning objectives
> **Key Point:**
> • Learning goals and objectives that are established with input from the patient are most meaningful.

Implementation _____

_____

> **Key Term:** implementation
> **Key Point:**
> • **Implementation** is the process used to perform the actual teaching.

Evaluation _____

_____

Key Term: evaluation
Key Point:
• **Evaluation** is the process that indicates how well patients are adapting or applying new information to their lives.

Documentation _____

_____

Key Term: documentation
Key Point:
• Documentation is essential because from a legal viewpoint, procedures are only considered to have been done if they are recorded.

☐ **LEARNING OBJECTIVE 3:** Define the five steps in the patient education process.

Conditions Needed for Patient Education _____

_____

☐ **LEARNING OBJECTIVE 4:** Identify five conditions that are needed for patient education to occur.

Maslow's Hierarchy of Needs _____

_____

Key Points:
• Maslow arranged human needs in the form of a pyramid, with basic needs at the bottom and the higher needs at the top.
• If possible, you should involve family members or significant others in the teaching process.

☐ **LEARNING OBJECTIVE 5:** Explain Maslow's hierarchy of human needs.

Environment _____

_____

Key Point:
• For patients to acquire knowledge, they must feel relaxed and comfortable.

Equipment _____

_____

Key Term: psychomotor
Key Point:
• Always provide written step-by-step instructions.

Knowledge _____

_____

Key Point:
• Never guess or imply that you know something that you do not know.

Resources _____

_____

Key Point:
• The more techniques that are used, the more the patient will learn and retain.

Factors That Can Hinder Education _____

_____

_____

Existing Illnesses _____

_____

_____

Communication Barriers _____

_____

Key Point:
• Any barriers to communication must be resolved before you can start teaching the patient.

Age _____

_____

Key Point:
• The age of the patient plays a very important part in the amount and type of education that you can do.

Educational Background _____

_____

_____

Physical Impairments _____

_____

_____

Other Factors _____

_____

Key Point:
• It is important that you assess the patient's readiness to learn and either try to remove or work around any obstacles that may be present.

☐ **LEARNING OBJECTIVE 6:** List five factors that may hinder patient education and at least two methods to compensate for each of these factors.

Teaching Specific Health Care Topics _____

_____

_____

Preventive Medicine _____

_____

Key Points:
• Preventing health problems is the key to living a long, healthy life.
• Fall prevention tips should be taught to all older patients or any patient who has a problem with maintaining balance or uses an ambulation device (cane, walker).

☐ **LEARNING OBJECTIVE 7:** Discuss five preventive medicine guidelines that you should teach your patients.

Lifestyle Changes _____

_____

_____

Medications _____

_____

Key Point:
• A patient's medication regimen should be reviewed at each visit to be sure the patient is taking the right medication in the right way.

☐ **LEARNING OBJECTIVE 8:** Explain the kinds of information that should be included in patient teaching about medication therapy.

Alternative Medicine _____

_____

Key Term: alternative

Acupuncture _____

_____

_____

Acupressure _____

_____

_____

Hypnosis _____

_____

_____

Yoga _____

_____

_____

Herbal Supplements _____

_____

Key Term: placebo
Key Point:
• Patients should be advised to verify the training and credentials of the practitioner they are using and to ascertain that the practitioner is appropriately licensed.

☐ **LEARNING OBJECTIVE 9:** Explain your role in teaching patients about alternative medicine therapies.

Stress Management _____

_____

Key Term: stress

Positive and Negative Stress _____

_____

_____

Psychological Defense Mechanisms _____

_____

Key Point:
• Humans employ the use of defense mechanisms to cope with the painful and difficult problems life can bring.

Relaxation Techniques _____

_____

_____

☐ **LEARNING OBJECTIVE 10:** List and explain relaxation techniques that you and patients can learn to help with stress management.

Patient Teaching Plans _____

_____

_____

Developing a Plan _____

_____

Key Point:
• To ensure that teaching is done logically, always use the education process to help you formulate a plan in your mind.

☐ **LEARNING OBJECTIVE 11:** Describe how to prepare a teaching plan.

Selecting and Adapting Teaching Material _____

_____

☐ **LEARNING OBJECTIVE 12:** List potential sources of patient education materials.

Developing Your Own Material _____

_____

_____

Locating Community Resources and Disseminating Information _____

_____

Key Term: disseminates

☐ **LEARNING OBJECTIVE 13:** Locate community resources and list ways of organizing and disseminating information.

Content Review

FOUNDATIONAL KNOWLEDGE

Personal Ownership

1. Patients should be encouraged to take an active approach to their health and health care education. To educate patients effectively, which of the following must you do? Circle all that apply.

   a. Help patients accept their illness.

   b. Expect patients to follow your instructions without further explanation.

   c. Involve patients in the process of gaining knowledge.

   d. Provide patients with positive reinforcement.

   e. Give patients the most in-depth professional textbooks you can find.

2. Write a sentence explaining why, as a medical assistant, you must set aside your own personal feelings and life experiences when educating patients.

   _____

   _____

Educating Patients

3. Dr. Lin has created a lifestyle modification plan for her patient, Mr. Ramirez. Draw a line to match the name of each step of the patient education process on the left to the corresponding step taken by Dr. Lin and Mr. Ramirez on the right.

Name of Step	Step in Action
1. Assessment	**a.** Dr. Lin explains to Mr. Ramirez how to exercise properly and eat a healthy diet.
2. Planning	**b.** Mr. Ramirez visits with Dr. Lin to determine how his weight loss is progressing.
3. Implementation	**c.** Mr. Ramirez meets with Dr. Lin to discuss his weight problem and how it is affecting his health.
4. Evaluation	**d.** Dr. Lin records the dates and times of his appointments with Mr. Ramirez.
5. Documentation	**e.** Mr. Ramirez understands why he needs to lose weight, and together they create a weight loss schedule.

4. Suppose you want to teach a patient about the need to adopt a low-sugar diet because of diabetes, but the patient doesn't believe that diabetes is a serious health problem. If education is to be effective, then which of the following must the patient accept? Circle all that apply.

   a. Diabetes has to be managed.

   b. There is a correlation between high sugar intake and diabetes.

   c. Diabetes isn't as serious as other diseases.

   d. Diabetes management requires dietary changes.

   e. It is possible to consume large quantities of high-sugar foods, but only occasionally.

5. Ms. Jasinski is an elderly patient who has recently lost several relatives and friends. She lives alone and feels disconnected from others and, as a result, her health has begun to deteriorate. Brian, a medical assistant, gives Ms. Jasinski a friendly hug when he sees her during patient visits. He talks to her and listens to her stories. He has also encouraged her to join a senior citizens' group. Which of Maslow's hierarchy of needs has Brian helped fulfill for Ms. Jasinski?

   a. physiological

   b. safety and security

   c. affection and belonging

   d. self-actualization

6. List the five factors that can hinder patient education.

a. _____

b. _____

c. _____

d. _____

e. _____

7. Age Isn't Just a Number

Luis is an 8-year-old boy living with HIV. As a medical assistant, it is important to explain his symptoms and how the illness will be treated. You want to be honest with Luis, but you're not sure how much to explain to him. Which of the following might you do when preparing to talk with Luis? Place a check mark in the table below to answer "Yes" or "No." If your answer is "No," briefly explain why.

	Yes	No, because . . .
a. Discuss HIV with his parents; they are solely responsible for explaining his medical condition to him.		
b. Communicate with his parents; they understand Luis' developmental stage.		
c. Consider Luis' age when determining what is and isn't appropriate to say.		
d. Take Luis to a psychiatrist; he can deal with Luis' emotional reactions, and you cannot.		

8. Taking Action Against Illness

Maria is the mother of a 3-month-old baby. Though Maria's baby is healthy, you understand that infants are often susceptible to illness because their immune systems are not fully developed. Which preventive health care tip would you recommend for Maria's baby?

_____

_____

9. Speaking of Medication . . .

Read the following paragraph and fill in each blank with the appropriate word or words from the word bank below. Note: Not all of the words will be used.

I was diagnosed with heart disease, and my physician prescribed 2 mg of the (1.) _____ name drug, Coumadin™ (warfarin sodium). The medical assistant explained that this medication was (2.) _____ to me because it inhibits reactions that lead to blood clotting. She explained the (3.) _____ as one tablet every day. Possible (4.) _____ include headache and fever. She also told me to watch for bleeding or abnormal bruising, as these may be signs of an adverse (5.) _____.

Word Bank

a. side effects	d. reaction	g. brand
b. dosage	e. prescribed	h. medicated
c. route	f. activities	

10. A Common Myth

Many patients believe that over-the-counter medications are 100% safe at all times. In a sentence or two, explain why this is a misconception.

_____

_____

11. Survey Says . . .

When educating patients about medications, it's important to include information regarding alternative medicines. Surveys have shown that about _____% of all Americans have used some form of unconventional medicine.

a. 12

b. 51

c. 75

d. 90

e. 25

12. Assessing Alternatives

As a medical assistant, it is your job to assess whether a patient is using any alternative therapies. In one or two sentences, explain what information should be included in your assessment.

_____

_____

Don't Stress Out!

13. Fill in the chart below with three more possible side effects of illness and injury.

Potential Side Effects:
- Physical pain
- Stress of treatments, procedures, and possible hospitalization
- Changes in relationships with family and friends
-
-
-

14. There are two types of stress; one is good for us and the other is bad. Fill in the chart below with the differences and similarities between positive and negative stress.

Positive Stress	Both	Negative Stress

15. Which of the following is a relaxation technique that you can suggest to patients?

a. visualization

b. sublimation

c. hypnosis

d. self-actualization

e. acupressure

A Master Plan

16. List the five elements included in every teaching plan.

a. _____

b. _____

c. _____

d. _____

e. _____

17. List three potential sources of patient education materials.

a. _____

b. _____

c. _____

18. List three places that patients can find information about financial assistance and transportation.

a. _____

b. _____

c. _____

19. Match the following key terms to their definitions.

Key Terms

a. alternative _____

b. assessment _____

c. coping mechanisms _____

d. dissemination _____

e. documentation _____

f. evaluation _____

g. implementation _____

h. learning objectives _____

i. noncompliance _____

j. placebo _____

k. planning _____

l. psychomotor _____

m. stress _____

Definitions

1. involves using the information you have gathered to determine how you will approach the patient's learning needs

2. skill that requires the patient to physically perform a task

3. the process that indicates how well patients are adapting or applying new information to their lives

4. produced by illness or injury and may result in physiological and psychological effects

5. includes procedures or tasks that will be discussed or performed at various points in the program to help achieve the goal

6. the process of distributing information on community resources

7. includes recording of all teachings that occurred

8. the patient's inability or refusal to follow a prescribed order

9. involves gathering information about the patient's present health care needs and abilities

10. psychological defenses employed to help deal with the painful and difficult problems life can bring

11. the power of believing that something will make you better when there is no chemical reaction that warrants such improvement

12. the process used to perform the actual teaching

13. an option or substitute to the standard medical treatment, such as acupuncture

20. True or False? Determine whether the following statements are true or false. If false, explain why.

a. Patients benefit from the use of teaching aids that they can take home and use as reference material.

_____

_____

b. If a patient asks you a question and you're not sure of the answer, then you should give your best guess.

_____

_____

c. A patient must have his basic needs met before self-actualization may occur.

_____

_____

d. Visualization is a relaxation technique that involves deep-breathing and physical exercise.

_____

_____

APPLICATION

Critical Thinking Practice

1. A patient wants to use alternative medicine in addition to medicine prescribed by the physician. What should you do?

_____

_____

2. A patient in your care is suffering physiologic effects from negative stress brought on by chronic back pain. What types of coping strategies would you recommend to the patient and why?

_____

_____

Patient Education

1. Julia is an 8-year-old patient who has been diagnosed with type 1 diabetes. The medical office has a preprinted teaching plan entitled "Living with Type 2 Diabetes." Should you use this plan or develop your own? Explain.

_____

_____

Documentation

1. You have completed the patient education with your 8-year-old patient Julia from the previous question. Give an example of a chart note that you might write following your discussion with her about diabetes.

_____

_____

Active Learning

1. Juggling school with other commitments may occasionally cause negative stress in your life. Make a list of how you experience stress in your daily life. Then, choose one of the three relaxation techniques discussed in this chapter. Practice that technique and then write a paragraph describing the "pros" and "cons" of the chosen technique.

2. Develop a teaching plan for a family member or friend. For example, if your mother has asthma, then do research on the Internet to find information and resources about asthma. Remember to include all of the elements of a teaching plan. Practice your teaching techniques by educating a family member or friend about a particular illness or disease.

3. Choose a health concern that may require external support. For example, a patient fighting cancer may wish to join a support group or other organization for help. Search the Internet for local, state, and national agencies that provide information, support, and services to patients with your chosen need. Then, compile this information in an informative and creative brochure, pamphlet, or other learning tool.

Professional Journal

REFLECT

(Prompts and Ideas: Are you concerned about your ability to educate patients effectively? What challenges do you foresee, and how do you plan to deal with those challenges? Think about the most effective teachers you have had. What made them so good?)

_____

_____

_____

_____

_____

_____

_____

PONDER AND SOLVE

1. The evaluation phase of the patient education process will indicate how well the patient is adapting new information to her life. If a patient has been compliant, but the teaching still hasn't worked, what might you do next to improve the results?

_____

_____

_____

_____

_____

_____

2. How can understanding Maslow's hierarchy of needs help you provide better care to patients?

_____

_____

_____

_____

_____

_____

EXPERIENCE

Skills related to this chapter include:

1. Instructing a Hearing-Impaired Patient (Procedure 4-1).

2. Locating Community Resources and Disseminating Information (Procedure 4-2).

Record any common mistakes, lessons learned, and/or tips you discovered during your experience of practicing and demonstrating these skills:

_____

_____

_____

_____

_____

_____

_____

Skill Practice

PERFORMANCE OBJECTIVES:

1. Instruct individuals according to their needs (Procedure 4-1).
2. Locate community resources (Procedure 4-2).

Name _____ Date _____ Time _____

Procedure 4-1:	INSTRUCTING A HEARING-IMPAIRED PATIENT

EQUIPMENT/SUPPLIES: Patient's chart, Internet, printer, paper

STANDARDS: Given the needed equipment and a place to work, the student will perform this skill with _____% accuracy in a total of _____ minutes. (*Your instructor will tell you what the percentage and time limits will be before you begin.*)

KEY: 　4 = Satisfactory 　　0 = Unsatisfactory 　　NA = This step is not counted

PROCEDURE STEPS	SELF	PARTNER	INSTRUCTOR
1. Use the patient's chart to identify the patient's communication barrier and assess the tools needed.	☐	☐	☐
2. Used an online map service and print a map of the specific route.	☐	☐	☐
3. Use the suggestions listed in Chapter 3 for communicating with the hearing-impaired to explain the appointment and directions to the patient.	☐	☐	☐
4. Speak clearly in a low tone facing the patient.	☐	☐	☐
5. Make sure the patient understood.	☐	☐	☐

CALCULATION

Total Possible Points: _____
Total Points Earned: _____ Multiplied by 100 = _____ Divided by Total Possible Points = _____%

Pass　　**Fail**
☐　　　☐　　| Comments: |

Student's signature _____ Date _____
Partner's signature _____ Date _____
Instructor's signature _____ Date _____

Name _____ Date _____ Time _____

Procedure 4-2:	**LOCATING COMMUNITY RESOURCES AND DISSEMINATING INFORMATION**

EQUIPMENT/SUPPLIES: Phone book, Internet, newspaper

STANDARDS: Given the needed equipment and a place to work, the student will perform this skill with _____% accuracy in a total of _____ minutes. (*Your instructor will tell you what the percentage and time limits will be before you begin.*)

KEY: 4 = Satisfactory   0 = Unsatisfactory   NA = This step is not counted

PROCEDURE STEPS	SELF	PARTNER	INSTRUCTOR

1. Assess the patient's needs for the following:
  a. Education
  b. Someone to talk to
  c. Financial information
  d. Support groups
  e. Home health needs
	☐	☐	☐

2. Check the local telephone book for local and state resources.	☐	☐	☐
3. Check for websites for the city and/or county in which the patient lives.	☐	☐	☐
4. Be prepared with materials already on hand.	☐	☐	☐
5. Give the patient the contact information in writing.	☐	☐	☐
6. Document actions and the information given to the patient.	☐	☐	☐
7. Instruct the patient to contact the office if he has any difficulty.	☐	☐	☐

CALCULATION

Total Possible Points: _____
Total Points Earned: _____ Multiplied by 100 = _____ Divided by Total Possible Points = _____%

Pass   **Fail**
☐   ☐   Comments:

Student's signature _____ Date _____
Partner's signature _____ Date _____
Instructor's signature _____ Date _____

Chapter Self-Assessment Quiz

1. During assessment, the most comprehensive source from which to obtain patient information is the:

   a. physician's notes.

   b. immunization record.

   c. medical record.

   d. family member.

   e. nurse.

2. If a patient is not following physician's orders, you should determine:

   a. how long the order hasn't been followed.

   b. why the order is not being followed.

   c. how to make the patient follow the order.

   d. why the patient agreed to follow the order.

   e. if the physician has another suggestion for new orders.

3. Which of the following is an example of a psychomotor skill that a patient may perform?

   a. Telling the physician about his symptoms

   b. Explaining how a part of the body is feeling

   c. Walking around with a crutch

   d. Watching television in the waiting room

   e. Listening to a physician's instructions

4. Which part of Maslow's pyramid is the point at which a patient has satisfied all basic needs and feels he has control over his life?

   a. Safety and security

   b. Esteem

   c. Self-actualization

   d. Affection

   e. Physiologic

5. Noncompliance occurs when the patient:

   a. experiences a decrease in symptoms healed.

   b. forgets to pay his bill.

   c. refuses to follow the physician's orders.

   d. requests a new medical assistant to assist the physician.

   e. agrees with the physician.

6. The power of believing that something will make you better when there is no chemical reaction that warrants such improvement is:

   a. self-relaxation.

   b. positive stress.

   c. acupuncture.

   d. placebo.

   e. visualization.

7. Patient education should consist of multiple techniques or approaches so:

   a. the patient can apply her new knowledge to real-life events.

   b. the patient will learn and retain more.

   c. the patient will understand that there are many ways to look at an issue.

   d. the patient will know where you stand on her health care options.

   e. the patient will have a wider choice of treatments.

8. One mental health illness that can hinder patient education is:

   a. diabetes.

   b. Lyme disease.

   c. obstructive pulmonary disease.

   d. Alzheimer disease.

   e. anemia.

9. Health assessment forms that assess a patient's education level may also help you determine a patient's ability to:

   a. read.

   b. listen.

   c. communicate.

   d. respond.

   e. evaluate.

10. Before developing a medication schedule, you should evaluate the patient's:

   a. prescribed medication.

   b. side effects.

   c. changes in bodily functions.

   d. daily routine.

   e. bowel movements.

11. Which is an example of a recommended preventive procedure?

   a. Regular teeth whitening

   b. Childhood immunizations

   c. Daily exercise

   d. Yearly lung cancer evaluations

   e. Occasional antibiotics

12. Which of the following is true of herbal supplements?

   a. A medical assistant can recommend that a patient start taking herbal supplements without the physician's approval.

   b. A health store clerk is a good source of information on supplements.

   c. Products that claim to detoxify the whole body are generally effective.

   d. Supplements will not interfere with blood sugar levels because they are not medication.

   e. Patients should be advised that because a product is natural does not mean it is safe.

13. One example of a physiologic response to negative stress is:

   a. elevated mood.

   b. hunger pangs.

   c. headache.

   d. profuse bleeding.

   e. energy boost.

14. In Maslow's hierarchy of needs, air, water, food, and rest are considered:

   a. affection needs.

   b. safety and security needs.

   c. esteem needs.

   d. self-actualization needs.

   e. physiologic needs.

15. Breathing exercises can be done:

   a. at the gym.

   b. in the medical office.

   c. at home.

   d. anywhere.

   e. at work.

16. Humans use defense mechanisms to:

   a. cope with painful problems.

   b. increase their sense of accomplishment.

   c. decrease effects of chronic physical pain.

   d. learn to get along well with others.

   e. explain complicated emotions to medical staff.

17. Support groups give patients the opportunity to:

   a. exchange and compare medical records.

   b. meet and share ideas with others who are experiencing the same issues.

   c. spread the good word about the medical office.

   d. obtain their basic physiologic needs.

   e. learn more about malpractice suits.

18. When selecting teaching material, you should first:

   a. choose preprinted material.

   b. create your own material.

   c. assess your patient's general level of understanding.

   d. let the patient find a book from the clinic library.

   e. ask the patient to create a list of specific questions.

19. Acupressure is different from acupuncture because:

   a. it does not use needles.

   b. it is not an alternative medicine.

   c. it cannot be used with cancer patients.

   d. it does not require any licensure.

   e. it is less effective.

20. If your community doesn't have a central agency for information and resources, then you should create a(n):

   a. hierarchy of needs.

   b. teaching plan.

   c. telephone directory.

   d. information sheet.

   e. flowchart.

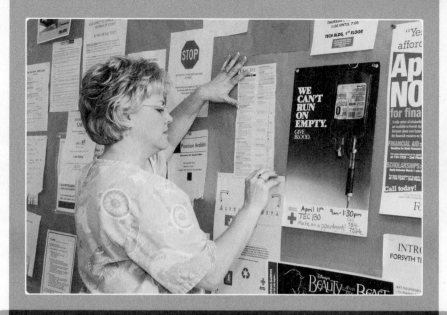

II

The Administrative Medical Assistant

Fundamentals of Administrative Medical Assisting

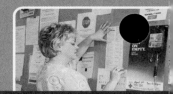

The First Contact: Telephone and Reception

Chapter Checklist

☐ Read textbook chapter and take notes within the Chapter Notes outline. Answer the Learning Objectives as you reach them in the content, and then check them off.

☐ Work the Content Review questions—both Foundational Knowledge and Application.

☐ Perform the Active Learning exercise(s).

☐ Complete Professional Journal entries.

☐ Complete Skill Practice Activity(s) using Competency Evaluation Forms and Work Products, when appropriate.

☐ Take the Chapter Self-Assessment Quiz.

☐ Insert all appropriate pages into your Portfolio.

Learning Objectives

1. Spell and define the key terms.
2. Explain the importance of displaying a professional image to all patients.
3. List six duties of the medical office receptionist.
4. List four sources from which messages can be retrieved.
5. Discuss various steps that can be taken to promote good ergonomics.
6. Describe the basic guidelines for waiting room environments.
7. Describe the proper method for maintaining infection control standards in the waiting room.

8. Discuss the five basic guidelines for telephone use.
9. Describe the types of incoming telephone calls received by the medical office.
10. Discuss how to identify and handle callers with medical emergencies.
11. Describe how to triage incoming calls.
12. List the information that should be given to an emergency medical service dispatcher.
13. Describe the types of telephone services and special features.

Chapter Notes

Note: Bold-faced headings are the major headings in the text chapter; headings in regular font are lower-level headings (i.e., the content is subordinate to, or falls "under," the major headings). Make sure you understand the key terms used in the chapter, as well as the concepts presented as Key Points.

TEXT SUBHEADINGS	NOTES

Introduction _____

_____

_____

☐ **LEARNING OBJECTIVE 1:** Spell and define the key terms.

_____

Professional Image _____

_____

_____

Importance of a Good Attitude _____

_____

> **Key Term:** attitude
> **Key Point:**
> • Ask yourself how you would feel in a similar situation, how you would want to be treated.

The Medical Assistant as a Role Model _____

_____

_____

Courtesy and Diplomacy in the Medical Office _____

_____

> **Key Term:** diplomacy
> **Key Point:**
> • Courtesy and diplomacy are fundamental to successful human relations.

First Impressions _____

_____

> **Key Point:**
> • The patient's perception of the medical office is based in part on the impression you make.

☐ **LEARNING OBJECTIVE 2:** Explain the importance of displaying a professional image to all patients.

Reception _____

_____

_____

The Role of a Receptionist _____

_____

Key Term: receptionist

_____

Duties and Responsibilities of the Receptionist _____

_____

_____

Prepare the Office _____

_____

Key Point:
• The office should be left in a professional manner.

_____

Retrieve Messages _____

_____

Key Point:
• No matter how a message has been sent, however, all information must be treated confidentially and handled according to HIPAA regulations.

_____

Prepare the Charts _____

_____

_____

Welcome Patients and Visitors _____

_____

_____

Register and Orient Patients _____

_____

_____

Manage Waiting Time _____

_____

_____

☐ **LEARNING OBJECTIVE 3:** List six duties of the medical office receptionist.

☐ **LEARNING OBJECTIVE 4:** List four sources from which messages can be retrieved.

Ergonomic Concerns for the Receptionist _____

_____

Key Term: ergonomic

☐ **LEARNING OBJECTIVE 5:** Discuss various steps that can be taken to promote good ergonomics.

The Waiting Room Environment _____

_____

General Guidelines for Waiting Rooms _____

_____

Key Term: closed captioning

Guidelines for Pediatric Waiting Rooms _____

_____

Americans with Disabilities Act Requirements _____

_____

Key Point:
• The ADA Title III act requires that all public accommodations be accessible to everyone.

☐ **LEARNING OBJECTIVE 6:** Describe the basic guidelines for waiting room environments.

Infection Control Issues _____

_____

Key Point:
• Handwashing is the most important practice for preventing the transmission of diseases.

☐ **LEARNING OBJECTIVE 7:** Describe the proper method for maintaining infection control standards in the waiting room.

The End of the Patient Visit _____

_____

Key Point:
• As patients leave the office, they should feel they have been well cared for by a competent and courteous staff.

Telephone _____

_____

_____

Importance of the Telephone in the Medical Office _____

_____

Key Point:
- You must be able to use the tone and quality of your voice and speech to project a competent and caring attitude over the telephone.

Basic Guidelines for Telephone Use _____

_____

_____

Diction _____

_____

Key Term: diction

Pronunciation _____

_____

_____

Expression _____

_____

_____

Listening _____

_____

_____

Courtesy _____

_____

Key Point:
- Remember, all information about and conversations with patients are confidential.

☐ **LEARNING OBJECTIVE 8:** Discuss the five basic guidelines for telephone use.

Routine Incoming Calls _____

_____

_____

Appointments _____
_____
_____

Billing Inquiries _____
_____
_____

Diagnostic Test Results _____
_____
_____

Routine and Satisfactory Progress Reports _____
_____
_____

Test Results _____
_____
_____

Unsatisfactory Progress Reports and Test Results _____
_____

Key Point:
• Never discuss unsatisfactory test results with a patient unless the doctor directs you to do so.

Prescription Refills _____
_____

Key Point:
• If there is any doubt, tell the pharmacy or the patient that you will check with the doctor and call back.

Other Calls _____
_____
_____

☐ **LEARNING OBJECTIVE 9:** Describe the types of incoming telephone calls received by the medical office.
_____

Challenging Incoming Calls _____
_____
_____

Unidentified Callers _____
_____
_____

Irate Patients _____

_____

_____

Medical Emergencies _____

_____

Key Points:
- As a medical assistant, you must be able to differentiate between routine calls and emergencies.
- Determine the patient's name, location, and telephone number as quickly as possible in case you are disconnected or the patient is unable to continue the conversation.

☐ **LEARNING OBJECTIVE 10:** Discuss how to identify and handle callers with medical emergencies.

Triaging Incoming Calls _____

_____

Key Term: triage

☐ **LEARNING OBJECTIVE 11:** Describe how to triage incoming calls.

Taking Messages _____

_____

Key Point:
- The minimum information needed for a telephone message includes the name of the caller, date, and time of the call; telephone number where the caller can be reached; a short description of the caller's concern; and the person to whom the message is routed.

Outgoing Calls _____

_____

_____

General Guidelines for Outgoing Calls _____

_____

Key Point:
- You should prepare for your calls carefully, have all information gathered, and know what you want to say before you dial the number.

Calling Emergency Medical Services _____

_____

> **Key Term:** emergency medical service (EMS)
> **Key Point:**
> • Reassure other patients in the waiting room. If the patient has any family members present, offer them assistance and reassurance.

☐ **LEARNING OBJECTIVE 12:** List the information that should be given to an emergency medical service dispatcher.

Services and Special Features _____

_____

_____

Telecommunication Relay Systems _____

_____

> **Key Term:** teletypewriter (TTY)

☐ **LEARNING OBJECTIVE 13:** Describe the types of telephone services and special features.

Content Review

FOUNDATIONAL KNOWLEDGE

1. A Lasting Impression

It's important for medical assistants to portray a professional image to patients and coworkers. Review the unprofessional actions below and explain what the medical assistant can do to correct each one and make a lasting professional impression.

a. Jacinda wears flowery perfume every day.

_____

b. Jorge's uniform has a hole at the seam and is wrinkled.

_____

c. Kate has beautiful long nails that are polished with bright red nail polish.

_____

Job Duties

2. Circle the six duties of a medical receptionist in the list below.

Prepare the office	Clean the examination rooms	Retrieve messages
Welcome patients and visitors	Update patient information in charts	Write prescriptions

| Prepare the charts | Register and orient patients | Manage waiting time |
| Create marketing materials | File paperwork for payroll | Call patients with test results |

3. Each morning a receptionist needs to collect messages. There are four different sources the receptionist needs to check to retrieve messages. Read the description of each message and then decide where the receptionist is most likely to find each message.

Message Retrieval System

a. Answering service

b. Voice mail system

c. E-mail

d. Fax machine

Descriptions

1. Dr. Orr's office sent a referral for patient Billy Waters.
2. Mr. Patel has a question about a blood test.
3. TGI health insurance has a question about a patient's billing charges.
4. The blood lab sent the results for five patients.
5. Lighthouse Nursing Home wants to tell the physician about a patient who fell out of bed early in the morning.
6. Mrs. Wright needs an appointment for her son who is complaining of an earache.
7. A pharmaceutical representative would like to discuss the release date of a new drug.
8. Mrs. Paul needs a prescription refill for her prenatal vitamins.

A Safe and Comfortable Place to Work

4. List four things a receptionist at a physician's office might do to avoid getting injured on the job.

a. _____

b. _____

c. _____

d. _____

5. The waiting room should be a comfortable and safe place for patients to wait. Review the list of guidelines below and determine which contribute to a comfortable and safe waiting room environment. Place a check in the "Yes" column for those guidelines that contribute to a comfortable and safe waiting room and place a check in the "No" column for those that do not.

Task	Yes	No
a. Sofas are preferable because they fit more people.		
b. Provide only chairs without arms.		
c. Bright, primary colors are more suitable and cheery.		
d. The room should be well ventilated and kept at a comfortable temperature.		
e. Soothing background music is acceptable.		
f. Reading material, like current magazines, should be provided.		
g. Patients should be allowed to control the television.		
h. In an office for adults, anything can be watched on the television.		
i. Closed captioning should be offered to patients with hearing impairments who want to watch television.		

6. Infection control is important to prevent the spread of disease among patients. List three things a medical assistant can do to help with infection control.

a. _____

b. _____

c. _____

7. A patient comes into the office with a severe bloody nose. He leaves bloody tissues in the waiting room and got blood on a magazine and a chair. Your supervisor says to you, "Come on! Get some gloves. We've got to clean this right away." Why do you need gloves? Why is it important that the waiting room be cleaned immediately?

_____

_____

8. Tatiana works as a receptionist in a busy medical office. During her review, her supervisor discusses her telephone skills and points out what telephone skills she has mastered and areas that need some improvement. Fill in the Comments section on the review sheet below. State one thing she is doing right for each "Satisfactory" mark and one thing she could do to improve each "Needs Improvement" mark.

Skill	Satisfactory	Needs Improvement	Comments
a. Courtesy	X		
b. Diction	X		
c. Expression		X	
d. Listening	X		
e. Pronunciation		X	

9. List four things you can do to maintain patient confidentiality within the reception area and waiting room.

a. _____

b. _____

c. _____

d. _____

Best Phone Practices

10. As a receptionist, you'll be answering incoming calls. Review the statements below and place a check in the "True" column for those that are true and place a check in the "False" column for those that are false.

Incoming Calls	True	False
a. Always ask new patients for their phone number in case you need to call them back.		
b. Always give patients an exact quote for services if asked.		
c. Patient information cannot be given to anyone without the patient's consent.		
d. All laboratory results phoned into the office must be immediately brought to the physician's attention.		
e. When a nursing home calls with a satisfactory report about a patient you should take the information down, record it in the patient's chart, and place it on the physician's desk for review.		
f. Never discuss unsatisfactory test results with a patient unless the doctor directs you to do so.		
g. Medical assistants are not allowed to take care of prescription refill requests.		

11. A woman calls the office frantic because she thinks she is having a heart attack. What information should you try to get first from the caller?

_____

_____

12. You are training a new receptionist. She doesn't understand why triaging calls is important. How would you explain this to her?

_____

_____

13. Triage the following calls:

    a. Line 1: A school nurse calls with a question about a medical form.

    b. Line 2: A mother calls about her child who is having an asthma attack.

    c. Line 3: A father calls with a question about his daughter's medication.

    d. Line 4: A patient calls complaining about a sore throat.

_____

_____

14. A patient in your office is having trouble breathing. You have been asked to call EMS. What five pieces of information will you need before you make the call?

    a. _____

    b. _____

    c. _____

    d. _____

    e. _____

15. Below are the steps that a receptionist should take to prepare the office for patient and other employee arrivals. However, they are not listed in the correct order. Review the steps and then place them in the correct order in which they should be performed.

    a. Turn on computers, printers, copiers, and other electronic devices.

    b. Disengage the alarm system.

    c. Restock your desk with necessary forms and office supplies.

    d. If the office uses a drop box to leave specimens for evening pickups, check the box to ensure that the specimens were taken.

    e. Turn on appropriate lights.

    f. Unlock doors as appropriate.

16. Dr. Porter is in a meeting, but he has instructed you to communicate with him via cell phone when you get the test results back for a certain patient. However, he does not like to have his cell phone ring while he is in meetings. How will you communicate with him?

_____

_____

17. It is an exceptionally hot day in spring. Because the air conditioner is not on yet, you take a chair from the waiting room and prop the door open with it. You also move the boxes that were delivered earlier away from the window so the air comes in. How is this a violation of the Americans with Disabilities Act?

_____

_____

18. Explain how a teletypewriter can help a hearing-impaired person communicate with a physician's office.

_____

_____

19. Match the following key terms to their definitions.

Key Terms

a. attitude _____

b. closed captioning _____

c. diction _____

d. diplomacy _____

e. emergency medical service (EMS) _____

f. ergonomic _____

g. receptionist _____

h. teletypewriter (TTY) _____

i. triage _____

Definitions

1. a person who performs administrative tasks and greets patients as they arrive at an office

2. the art of handling people with tact and genuine concern

3. a group of health care workers who care for sick and injured patients on the way to a hospital

4. printed words displayed on a television screen to help people with hearing disabilities or impairments

5. describing a workstation designed to prevent work-related injuries

6. the style of speaking and enunciating words

7. the sorting of patients into categories based on their level of sickness or injury

8. a state of mind or feeling regarding some matter

9. a special machine that allows communication on a telephone with a hearing-impaired person

20. True or False? Determine whether the following statements are true or false. If false, explain why.

a. An ergonomic workstation is nice, but not essential, for a medical office receptionist.

_____

_____

b. Jewelry such as dangling earrings and large rings are not appropriate for employees in a medical office.

_____

_____

c. Information about patients should never be transmitted using a fax machine.

_____

_____

d. It is not appropriate to have a television in a medical office waiting area.

_____

_____

APPLICATION

Critical Thinking Practice

1. You work as the office receptionist in a pediatrician's office. The physician has requested the purchase of new videos that can be used as teaching tools for parents. What kind of videos should you consider purchasing?

_____

_____

2. You receive a call from a patient who complains of being short of breath. What questions will you ask to determine whether this is an emergency?

_____

_____

Patient Education

1. Mrs. Gonzalez calls to schedule her annual check-up. She is put on hold, and when the receptionist comes back to her call, she is upset that she was placed on hold. When she comes in for her appointment, she says that the receptionist should deal with every call individually and that no one should be placed on hold. How would you explain the phone call triage system to her?

_____

_____

Documentation

1. Ms. Wheeler calls the office in the morning complaining of dizziness and nausea. She comes in for a 10:30 AM appointment. While she's in the waiting room, she faints and falls on the floor. She wakes up and says that she is still dizzy. The physician asks you to call for an ambulance to take Ms. Wheeler to the local hospital. Write a narrative note describing the situation to be included in the patient's chart.

_____

_____

Active Learning

1. You have accepted a job as the receptionist for a physician opening a new office. She asks you to develop a plan for the waiting room and to make a list of all the necessary furniture and equipment she will need to purchase. Type up a plan including a brief description of the room, and then research the costs of the furniture and equipment on your list to provide the physician with a budget.

2. Working with two classmates, role-play a medical emergency in the physician's office waiting room. Have one person play the role of the patient, the second person play the role of the receptionist, and the third person play the role of the EMS call operator. The patient should describe his or her condition, and the receptionist is responsible for conveying these details to EMS. Switch roles so that everyone gets a chance to play each role.

3. Many individuals with disabilities rely on service animals to assist them with daily activities. A number of patients in your office have service animals and routinely bring them in to the office. The new receptionist says that it is against the law to have animals in a place of business. Visit the website for the U.S. Department of Justice/Americans with Disabilities Act at www.usdoj.gov/crt/ada. Research any rules that apply to service animals in businesses and organizations. Then create a pamphlet for your office educating staff about this topic.

Professional Journal

Reflect

(Prompts and Ideas: Think about your past experiences as a patient. What do you like about the waiting rooms at medical offices you have visited in the past? What do you dislike? Have you ever had a negative experience with medical office staff either over the phone or in the reception area? How did it make you feel? What do you wish you could change about the experience?)

_____

_____

_____

_____

_____

PONDER AND SOLVE

1. Mr. Johnson is a difficult patient and frequently makes angry phone calls to the office. Today, he called yelling that his prescription refill had not been called in by the office. He demanded to speak to the person responsible, who is Nurse Karen. Nurse Karen had to leave early. What should you do?

_____

_____

_____

_____

2. Your office shows videos about healthy living, exercise, and nutrition throughout the day. It seems that most of the adults watch and enjoy the programming. One crowded afternoon, a patient comes up to the desk to complain that the programming is distracting and he would prefer having the television turned off. However, there are people in the room watching the television. What would you say to the upset patient?

_____

_____

_____

_____

_____

EXPERIENCE

Skills related to this chapter include:

1. Handling Incoming Calls (Procedure 5-1).
2. Calling Emergency Medical Services (Procedure 5-2).
3. Explaining General Office Policies (Procedure 5-3).

Record any common mistakes, lessons learned, and/or tips you discovered during your experience of practicing and demonstrating these skills:

_____

_____

_____

_____

_____

_____

Skill Practice

PERFORMANCE OBJECTIVES:

1. Handle incoming calls (Procedure 5-1).
2. Call Emergency Medical Services (Procedure 5-2).
3. Explain general office policies (Procedure 5-3).

Name_____ Date _____ Time _____

Procedure 5-1:	**HANDLING INCOMING CALLS**

EQUIPMENT/SUPPLIES: Telephone, telephone message pad, writing utensil (pen or pencil), headset (if applicable)

STANDARDS: Given the needed equipment and a place to work, the student will perform this skill with _____% accuracy in a total of _____ minutes. (*Your instructor will tell you what the percentage and time limits will be before you begin.*)

KEY: 4 = Satisfactory   0 = Unsatisfactory   NA = This step is not counted

PROCEDURE STEPS	SELF	PARTNER	INSTRUCTOR
1. Gather the needed equipment.	☐	☐	☐
2. Answer the phone within two rings.	☐	☐	☐
3. Greet caller with proper identification (your name and the name of the office).	☐	☐	☐
4. Identify the nature or reason for the call in a timely manner.	☐	☐	☐
5. Triage the call appropriately.	☐	☐	☐
6. Communicate in a professional manner and with unhurried speech.	☐	☐	☐
7. Clarify information as needed.	☐	☐	☐
8. Record the message on a message pad. Include the name of caller, date, time, telephone number where the caller can be reached, description of the caller's concerns, and person to whom the message is routed.	☐	☐	☐
9. Give the caller an approximate time for a return call.	☐	☐	☐
10. Ask the caller whether he or she has any additional questions or needs any other help.	☐	☐	☐
11. Allow the caller to disconnect first.	☐	☐	☐
12. Put the message in an assigned place.	☐	☐	☐
13. Complete the task within 10 minutes.	☐	☐	☐

CALCULATION

Total Possible Points: _____
Total Points Earned: _____ Multiplied by 100 = _____ Divided by Total Possible Points = _____%

Pass   **Fail**
☐   ☐   Comments:

Student's signature _____ Date _____
Partner's signature _____ Date _____
Instructor's signature _____ Date _____

Name_____ Date _____ Time _____

Procedure 5-2:	**CALLING EMERGENCY MEDICAL SERVICES**

EQUIPMENT/SUPPLIES: Telephone, patient information, writing utensil (pen, pencil)

STANDARDS: Given the needed equipment and a place to work, the student will perform this skill with _____% accuracy in a total of _____ minutes. (*Your instructor will tell you what the percentage and time limits will be before you begin.*)

KEY: 4 = Satisfactory   0 = Unsatisfactory   NA = This step is not counted

PROCEDURE STEPS	SELF	PARTNER	INSTRUCTOR
1. Obtain the following the information before dialing: patient's name, age, sex, nature of medical condition, type of service the physician is requesting, any special instructions or requests the physician may have, your location, and any special information for access.	☐	☐	☐
2. Dial 911 or other EMS number.	☐	☐	☐
3. Calmly provide the dispatcher with the above information.	☐	☐	☐
4. Answer the dispatcher's questions calmly and professionally.	☐	☐	☐
5. Follow the dispatcher's instructions, if applicable.	☐	☐	☐
6. End the call as per dispatcher instructions.	☐	☐	☐
7. Complete the task within 10 minutes.	☐	☐	☐

CALCULATION

Total Possible Points: _____
Total Points Earned: _____ Multiplied by 100 = _____ Divided by Total Possible Points = _____%

Pass   **Fail**
☐   ☐   Comments:

Student's signature _____ Date _____
Partner's signature _____ Date _____
Instructor's signature _____ Date _____

Name _____   Date _____   Time _____

Procedure 5-3:   EXPLAIN GENERAL OFFICE POLICIES

EQUIPMENT/SUPPLIES: Patient's chart, office brochure

STANDARDS: Given the needed equipment and a place to work, the student will perform this skill with _____% accuracy in a total of _____ minutes. (*Your instructor will tell you what the percentage and time limits will be before you begin.*)

KEY: 4 = Satisfactory   0 = Unsatisfactory   NA = This step is not counted

PROCEDURE STEPS	SELF	PARTNER	INSTRUCTOR
1. Assess the patient's level of understanding.	☐	☐	☐
2. Review important areas and highlight these in the office brochure.	☐	☐	☐
3. Ask the patient if he or she understands or has any questions.	☐	☐	☐
4. Give the patient the brochure to take home.	☐	☐	☐
5. Put in place a procedure for updating information and letting patients know of changes.	☐	☐	☐

CALCULATION

Total Possible Points: _____
Total Points Earned: _____ Multiplied by 100 = _____ Divided by Total Possible Points = _____%

Pass   **Fail**
☐   ☐   Comments:

Student's signature _____ Date _____
Partner's signature _____ Date _____
Instructor's signature _____ Date _____

Chapter Self-Assessment Quiz

1. Which of the following creates a professional image?
   a. Arguing with a patient
   b. Clean, pressed clothing
   c. Brightly colored fingernails
   d. Referring to physicians by first name
   e. Expensive flowery perfume

2. How can you exercise diplomacy?
   a. Treat patients as they treat you.
   b. Treat patients as you would like to be treated.
   c. Ignore patients who complain about their illnesses.
   d. Answer patients' questions about other patients they see in the waiting room.
   e. Disclose confidential information if a patient or relative asks for it tactfully.

3. When preparing the charts for the day, the charts should be put in order by:
   a. age.
   b. last name.
   c. chart number.
   d. reason for visit.
   e. appointment time.

4. The receptionist should check phone messages:
   a. at night before leaving.
   b. in the morning when coming in.
   c. when on the phone and knows a call has gone to voice mail.
   d. only after breaks, because each call coming in should be answered.
   e. when the office opens, after breaks, and periodically throughout the day.

5. Triaging calls is important because:
   a. it reduces the amount of time that callers wait.
   b. it places the calls in order of most urgent to least urgent.
   c. it lets the receptionist take care of the calls as quickly as possible.
   d. it puts the calls in time order so the receptionist knows who called first.
   e. it makes it easier for the receptionist to see which calls will be the easiest to handle.

6. There is a sign in the pediatrician's office that says "Do not throw dirty diapers in the garbage." Which of the following choices best explains the reason for the sign?
   a. Dirty diapers cannot be recycled.
   b. Dirty diapers are biohazard waste.
   c. Dirty diapers could leave an offensive odor.
   d. Dirty diapers could make the garbage too heavy.
   e. Dirty diapers take up too much room in the garbage.

7. Chewing gum or eating while on the phone could interfere with a person's:
   a. diction.
   b. attitude.
   c. ergonomics.
   d. expression.
   e. pronunciation.

8. Which of the following activities should a receptionist do in the morning to prepare the office for patients?
   a. Vacuum the office.
   b. Stock office supplies.
   c. Disinfect examination rooms.
   d. Turn on printers and copiers.
   e. Clean the patient restrooms.

9. Which of the following statements about telephone courtesy is correct?
   a. If two lines are ringing at once, answer one call and let the other go to voice mail.
   b. If you are on the other line, it is acceptable to let the phone ring until you can answer it.
   c. If a caller is upset, leaving him or her on hold will help improve the caller's attitude.
   d. If you need to answer another line, ask if the caller would mind holding and wait for a response.
   e. If someone is on hold for more than 90 seconds, they must leave a message and someone will call them back.

10. An ergonomic workstation is beneficial because it:
    a. prevents injuries to employees.
    b. educates patients about disease.
    c. maintains patients' confidentiality.
    d. creates a soothing, relaxed atmosphere.
    e. prevents the spread of contagious diseases.

11. Which feature fosters a positive waiting room environment?

    a. Abstract artwork on the walls

    b. Only sofas for patients to sit in

    c. Soap operas on the waiting room television

    d. Prominent display of the office fax machine

    e. Patient education materials in the reception area

12. How does a physician's pager system work?

    a. The pager sends a typed message that can be read by the physician.

    b. The pager has a "listen only" mode so the physician can hear messages.

    c. The pager will beep every two minutes until the physician answers it.

    d. The pager calls the physician over an intercom, so he/she can pick up a phone and call.

    e. The pager informs the physician of calls, but it cannot communicate messages.

13. A five-year-old girl has just come into the office with her mother. She has the flu and is vomiting into a plastic bag. Which of the following should the receptionist do?

    a. Get the patient into an examination room.

    b. Call the hospital and request an ambulance.

    c. Tell her to sit near the bathroom so she can vomit in the toilet.

    d. Place a new plastic bag in your garbage can and ask the girl to use it.

    e. Ask the patient to wait outside and you will get her when it is her turn.

14. An angry patient calls the office demanding to speak to the physician. The physician is not in the office. What should the receptionist do?

    a. Page the physician immediately.

    b. Try to calm the patient and take a message.

    c. Give the caller the physician's cell phone number.

    d. Tell the patient to calm down and call back in an hour.

    e. Place the patient on hold until he or she has calmed down.

15. Which of the following statements about e-mail is true?

    a. Patient e-mails should be deleted from the computer.

    b. The receptionist does not generally have access to e-mail.

    c. Actions taken in regard to e-mail do not need to be documented.

    d. Patients should not e-mail the office under any circumstances.

    e. E-mails should not be printed because the wrong person could view them.

16. The best technique for preventing the spread of disease is:

    a. washing your hands after any contact with patients.

    b. placing very sick patients immediately in an exam room.

    c. removing all reading materials or toys from the waiting room.

    d. keeping the window to the reception area closed at all times.

    e. preventing patients from changing channels on the TV in the waiting room.

17. One way to ensure patient privacy in the reception area is to:

    a. take all the patient's information at the front desk.

    b. ask the patient's permission before placing her name on the sign-in sheet.

    c. use computers in examination rooms only.

    d. make telephone calls regarding referrals at the front desk.

    e. close the privacy window when you are not speaking with a patient.

18. When receiving a call from a lab regarding a patient's test results, you should post the information:

    a. as an e-mail to the physician.

    b. in the receptionist's notebook.

    c. in the front of the patient's chart.

    d. as an e-mail to the patient's insurance company.

    e. in the front of the physician's appointment book.

19. In case of an emergency in the physician's office, who is usually responsible for calling emergency medical service (EMS)?

    a. Physician

    b. Dispatcher

    c. Receptionist

    d. Clinical staff

    e. Patient's relatives

20. What is a benefit of the teletypewriter (TTY)?

    a. Physicians can have verbal orders recorded in print.

    b. EMS crews can send messages from remote locations.

    c. Patients with hearing or speech impairments can type messages.

    d. A receptionist can write messages to patients on a television screen.

    e. Clinical staff can communicate with hearing-impaired patients within the medical office.

6 Managing Appointments

103

Chapter Checklist

- [ ] Read textbook chapter and take notes within the Chapter Notes outline. Answer the Learning Objectives as you reach them in the content, and then check them off.
- [ ] Work the Content Review questions—both Foundational Knowledge and Application.
- [ ] Perform the Active Learning exercise(s).

- [ ] Complete Professional Journal entries.
- [ ] Complete Skill Practice Activity(s) using Competency Evaluation Forms and Work Products, when appropriate.
- [ ] Take the Chapter Self-Assessment Quiz.
- [ ] Insert all appropriate pages into your Portfolio.

Learning Objectives

1. Spell and define the key terms.
2. Describe the various systems for scheduling patient office visits, including manual and computerized scheduling.
3. Identify the factors that affect appointment scheduling.
4. Explain guidelines for scheduling appointments for new patients, return visits, inpatient admissions, and outpatient procedures.
5. List three ways to remind patients about appointments.
6. Describe how to triage patient emergencies, acutely ill patients, and walk-in patients.
7. Describe how to handle late patients.
8. Explain what to do if the physician is delayed.
9. Describe how to handle patients who miss their appointments.
10. Describe how to handle appointment cancellations made by the office or by the patient.

Chapter Notes

Note: Bold-faced headings are the major headings in the text chapter; headings in regular font are lower-level headings (i.e., the content is subordinate to, or falls "under," the major headings). Make sure you understand the key terms used in the chapter, as well as the concepts presented as Key Points.

TEXT SUBHEADINGS	NOTES
Introduction _____	
	Key Term: providers **Key Point:** • Your responsibility is to manage all of this while maintaining a calm, efficient, and polite attitude.
☐ **LEARNING OBJECTIVE 1:** Spell and define the key terms.	
Appointment Scheduling Systems _____	
Manual Appointment Scheduling _____	
The Appointment Book _____	
Establishing a Matrix _____	
	Key Term: matrix **Key Point:** • Along with the notations in a patient's chart, the pages of the appointment book provide documentation of a patient's visits and any changes, such as cancellations and rescheduled appointments.
Computerized Appointment Scheduling _____	
	Key Point: • Once the daily schedule is printed, this important document is referred to as the daily activity sheet or the day sheet and is the guide for everyone involved in the flow of patient care. Figure 6-2 shows a computer-generated daily activity sheet.
☐ **LEARNING OBJECTIVE 2:** Describe the various systems for scheduling patient office visits, including manual and computerized scheduling.	

Types of Scheduling _____

_____

_____

Structured Appointments _____

_____

                              Key Term: buffer

_____

Clustering _____

_____

                              Key Term: clustering

Wave and Modified Wave _____

_____

                              Key Term: wave scheduling system

Fixed Scheduling _____

_____

_____

Streaming _____

_____

                              Key Term: streaming

Double Booking _____

_____

                              Key Term: double booking

Flexible Hours _____

_____

_____

Open Hours _____

_____

_____

Factors That Affect Scheduling _____

_____

_____

Patients' Needs _____

_____

Key Terms: acute, chronic
Key Point:
• With a patient in an emotional state, even the slightest real or imagined miscommunication can lead to a negative response from the patient.

Providers' Preferences and Needs _____

_____

_____

Physical Facilities _____

_____

Key Point:
• You must thoroughly understand the requirements for procedures to be performed in the office to schedule appointments accurately.

☐ **LEARNING OBJECTIVE 3:** Identify the factors that affect appointment scheduling.

Scheduling Guidelines _____

_____

_____

New Patients _____

_____

Key Point:
• The information you exchange at this encounter is crucial, and entering the patient's data accurately is imperative.

Established Patients _____

_____

_____

☐ **LEARNING OBJECTIVE 4:** Explain guidelines for scheduling appointments for new patients, return visits, inpatient admissions, and outpatient procedures.

Preparing a Daily or Weekly Schedule _____

_____

_____

Patient Reminders _____

_____

_____

Appointment Cards _____
_____
_____
_____

Telephone Reminders _____
_____

Key Point:
- All new patients and patients with appointments scheduled in advance should receive a telephone reminder the day before their appointment.

Mailed Reminder Cards _____
_____

Key Term: tickler file

☐ **LEARNING OBJECTIVE 5:** List three ways to remind patients about appointments.

Adapting the Schedule _____
_____
_____

Emergencies _____
_____

Key Terms: STAT; constellation of symptoms
Key Point:
- When a patient calls with an emergency (Fig. 6-5), your first responsibility is to determine whether the problem can be treated in the office.

Patients Who Are Acutely Ill _____
_____

Key Point:
- Obtain as much information about the patient's medical problem as you can so your message to the physician will allow him or her to decide how soon the patient should be seen.

Walk-in Patients _____
_____
_____

☐ **LEARNING OBJECTIVE 6:** Describe how to triage patient emergencies, acutely ill patients, and walk-in patients.

Late Patients _____

_____

☐ **LEARNING OBJECTIVE 7:** Describe how to handle late patients.

Physician Delays _____

_____

Key Point:
- If patients are waiting in the office, inform them immediately if the physician will be delayed.

☐ **LEARNING OBJECTIVE 8:** Explain what to do if the physician is delayed.

Missed Appointments _____

_____

Key Point:
- Continued failure to keep appointments should be brought to the attention of the physician, who may want to call the patient personally (particularly if the patient is seriously ill) or send a letter expressing concern for the patient's welfare.

☐ **LEARNING OBJECTIVE 9:** Describe how to handle patients who miss their appointments.

Cancellations _____

_____

_____

Cancellations by the Office _____

_____

Key Point:
- These cancellations should be noted in the patient's medical record.

Cancellations by the Patient _____

_____

☐ **LEARNING OBJECTIVE 10:** Describe how to handle appointment cancellations made by the office or by the patient.

Making Appointments for Patients in Other Facilities _____

_____

Referrals and Consultations _____

_____

Key Terms: consultation; referral; precertification
Key Point:
• Be sure the physician you are calling is on the preferred provider list for the patient's insurance company.

Diagnostic Testing _____

_____

_____

Surgery _____

_____

_____

When the Appointment Schedule Does Not Work _____

_____

Key Point:
• Since the work flow of the office affects every staff member, involve all employees in your study.

Content Review

FOUNDATIONAL KNOWLEDGE

Know Your Schedule

1. Medical offices may either use a manual or computerized appointment scheduling system. There are characteristics specific to each type of system. In the table below, read each characteristic, and then decide which type of system it describes. Place a check in the appropriate column.

Characteristic	Manual	Computerized
a. An appointment book		
b. Feature that allows you to search the appointment database for the next available timeslot		
c. Easy access to billing information		
d. Matrix created by crossing out unavailable times		

2. Identify each type of scheduling system in the chart below.

Description	Type of Scheduling System
a. several patients are scheduled for the first 30 minutes of each hour	
b. appointments are given based on the needs of individual patients	
c. each hour is divided into increments of 15, 30, 45, or 60 minutes for appointments depending on the reason for the visit	
d. patients are grouped according to needs or problems	
e. two patients are scheduled for the same period with the same physician	

3. List four advantages to clustering patients.

a. _____

b. _____

c. _____

d. _____

Schedule S.O.S.

4. Mr. Gonzalez requests an appointment for 1 PM on Wednesday. You already have a patient scheduled on that day and time slot. What should you do?

_____

_____

5. Name the three factors that can affect scheduling.

a. _____

b. _____

c. _____

6. The allotted time for each service will vary among different medical offices. However, you can estimate how long each service should take when creating a schedule. Match each service below with the estimated amount of time needed for each one.

Service

a. blood pressure check

b. complete physical exam

c. dressing change

d. recheck

e. school physical

Estimated Time

1. 5 minutes

2. 10 minutes

3. 15 minutes

4. 30 minutes

5. 1 hour

7. Below are the steps for making a return appointment. Some of the steps are false or incomplete. Review each step and then decide if it is correct or incorrect. If incorrect, rewrite the statement to make it true and complete.

a. Carefully check your appointment book or screen before offering an appointment time. If a specific examination, test, or x-ray is to be performed on the return visit, avoid scheduling two patients for the same examination at the same time.

_____

_____

b. Ask the patient when he or she would like to return.

_____

_____

c. Write the patient's name and telephone number in the appointment book or enter the information in computer.

_____

_____

d. Transfer the information to an appointment card that you will mail out to the patient at a later date.

_____

_____

e. Double-check your book or screen to be sure there are no errors.

_____

_____

f. End your conversation with a pleasant word and a smile.

_____

_____

_____

8. Don't Forget. . .

List the three ways to remind patients about appointments.

a. _____

b. _____

c. _____

9. When a patient calls with an emergency, your first responsibility is to:

   a. determine if the patient has an appointment.
   b. decide whether the problem can be treated in the office.
   c. verify that the physician can see the patient.
   d. identify the patient's constellation of symptoms.

10. What should you do if the physician decides not to see a walk-in patient?

   a. Ask the patient to schedule an appointment to return later.
   b. Explain that the physician is too busy.
   c. Tell the patient to try a different medical office.
   d. Tell the patient to go to the hospital.

11. Tardy Party

Like the rabbit in "Alice in Wonderland," some patients always seem to be running just behind schedule. Patients who are routinely late might benefit by having their appointments _____ for a time at the _____ of the day.

   a. rescheduled; end
   b. suspended; beginning
   c. revoked; afternoon
   d. renewed; middle

12. Time on the Mind

Sometimes, the physician will be the person who is running late. Explain what you would do in each situation.
The physician calls in to the office to say he is delayed. What would you do if:

   a. Office hours have not yet begun.

_____

_____

b. Patients are waiting in the office.

_____

_____

13. No-Show

Sometimes, a patient may neglect to keep an appointment. When this happens, you should call the patient. What should you do if you are unable to reach the patient by phone?

_____

_____

14. When might you write a letter to a patient who has an appointment that you must cancel?

   a. when you can't reach the patient by phone
   b. when the physician leaves the office abruptly
   c. when you have advance notice from the physician
   d. when you want to use written communication

15. Maria has just called into the office to cancel her appointment for today. Explain what you should do.

_____

_____

16. When calling another physician's office for an appointment for your patient, you'll need to provide certain information. Review the list below and circle the information that you should provide to another physician's office.

Physician's name	Patient's name	Physician's telephone number	Insurance company's telephone number
Reason for the referral	Patient's allergies	Patient's Social Security number	Patient's address and telephone number
Patient's next of kin	Degree of urgency	Patient's insurance information	If patient needs a consultation or referral

17. If diagnostic testing requires preparation from the patient, what should you do?

_____

_____

18. Preadmission testing for surgery may include:

   a. _____

   b. _____

   c. _____

19. Match the following key terms to their definitions.

Key Terms

   a. acute _____
   b. buffer _____
   c. chronic _____
   d. clustering _____
   e. constellation of symptoms _____
   f. consultation _____
   g. double booking _____
   h. matrix _____
   i. precertification _____

Definitions

   1. a group of clinical signs indicating a particular disease process
   2. the practice of booking two patients for the same period with the same physician
   3. term used in the medical field to indicate that something should be done immediately
   4. a system for blocking off unavailable patient appointment times
   5. a flexible scheduling method that allows time for procedures of varying lengths and the addition of unscheduled patients, as needed
   6. referring to a longstanding medical problem
   7. grouping patients with similar problems or needs

j. providers _____

k. referral _____

l. STAT _____

m. streaming _____

n. tickler file _____

o. wave scheduling system _____

8. a method of allotting time for appointments based on the needs of the individual patient that helps minimize gaps in time and backups

9. extra time booked on the schedule to accommodate emergencies, walk-ins, and other demands on the provider's daily time schedule that are not considered direct patient care

10. health care workers who deliver medical care

11. referring to a medical problem with abrupt onset

12. request for assistance from one physician to another

13. approved documentation prior to referrals to specialists and other facilities

14. instructions to transfer a patient's care to a specialist

15. a file that provides a reminder to do a given task at a particular date and time

20. True or False? Determine whether the following statements are true or false. If false, explain why.

a. Fixed scheduling is the most commonly used method.

_____

_____

b. A medical office that operates with open hours for patient visits is open 24 hours a day, 7 days a week.

_____

_____

c. Most appointments for new patients are made in person.

_____

_____

d. Patients with medical emergencies need to be seen immediately.

_____

_____

APPLICATION

Critical Thinking Practice

1. An elderly patient walks into the medical office. His constellation of symptoms includes chest discomfort, shortness of breath, and nausea. He doesn't have an appointment. Explain what you would do.

_____

_____

2. The appointment book below is divided into half-hour increments. The spaces below each time slot are empty. Fill in the appointment book with the following information: Dr. Brown has hospital rounds from 8:00 AM to 9:00 AM He has the following appointments: Cindy Wallis at 9:30 AM; Bill Waters at 10:00 AM; Rodney Kingston at 10:30 AM

8:00	8:30	9:00	9:30	10:00	10:30

Janet Pele calls the office and requests an emergency morning appointment because of a high fever. Can you accommodate her? Explain.

_____

_____

Patient Education

1. Juan is consistently late for appointments. You've spoken with him several times. What should you do next? Explain what you will you say to him and the information you will provide him with.

_____

_____

Documentation

1. Write a narrative charting note describing your interactions with Juan from the question above.

_____

_____

Active Learning

1. Record all of the activities you take part in on a typical day. Then, practice scheduling by placing these activities in a matrix.

2. Pretend that you're a new patient. Make a list of questions you might have about the medical office. Now as a medical assistant, answer your questions. If you don't know the answer to a question, find out. Then tape this "Q and A" list somewhere around your desk, and use it when new patients come into the office.

3. If you work in a medical office, place a "suggestions box" in the waiting room. Patients can place their suggestions concerning waiting times, scheduling, etc., into the box anonymously and at their leisure. After two weeks, open the box and discuss the suggestions with your coworkers. Decide which suggestions are possible and discuss ways of implementing these changes. Create a report for the medical office discussing the suggestions and how they may be addressed.

Professional Journal

REFLECT

(Prompts and Ideas: Are you concerned about controlling the appointment schedule effectively? How will you keep track of appointments, missed patients, physician delays, etc? Think about the medical office that you visit as a patient. In what ways does the medical assistant keep the schedule running smoothly? What changes would you like to see?)

_____

_____

_____

_____

_____

_____

_____

PONDER AND SOLVE

1. Patients may come and go without your direct involvement in their care. Even so, why is it important for you to understand the reason for a patient's appointment?

_____

_____

_____

_____

_____

_____

2. Would you rather use a manual or computerized appointment scheduling system? Explain your reasons and give advantages and disadvantages for each.

_____

_____

_____

_____

_____

_____

_____

EXPERIENCE

Skills related to this chapter include:

1. Making an Appointment for a New Patient (Procedure 6-1).
2. Making an Appointment for an Established Patient (Procedure 6-2).
3. Making an Appointment for a Referral to an Outpatient Facility (Procedure 6-3).
4. Arranging for Admission to an Inpatient Facility (Procedure 6-4).

Record any common mistakes, lessons learned, and/or tips you discovered during your experience of practicing and demonstrating these skills:

_____

_____

_____

_____

_____

_____

_____

Skill Practice

PERFORMANCE OBJECTIVES:

1. Schedule an appointment for a new patient (Procedure 6-1).
2. Schedule an appointment for a return visit (Procedure 6-2).
3. Schedule an appointment for a referral to an outpatient facility (Procedure 6-3).
4. Arrange for admission to an inpatient facility (Procedure 6-4).

Name_____ Date _____ Time _____

Procedure 6-1:	**MAKING AN APPOINTMENT FOR A NEW PATIENT**

EQUIPMENT/ITEMS NEEDED: Patient's demographic information, patient's chief complaint, appointment book or computer with appointment software

STANDARDS: Given the needed equipment and a place to work, the student will perform this skill with _____ % accuracy in a total of _____ minutes. (*Your instructor will tell you what the percentage and time limits will be before you begin.*)

KEY: 4 = Satisfactory   0 = Unsatisfactory   NA = This step is not counted

PROCEDURE STEPS	SELF	PARTNER	INSTRUCTOR
1. Obtain as much information as possible from the patient, such as: • Full name and correct spelling • Mailing address (not all offices require this) • Day and evening telephone numbers • Reason for the visit • Name of the referring person	☐	☐	☐
2. Determine the patient's chief complaint or the reason for seeing the physician.	☐	☐	☐
3. Explain the payment policy of the practice. Instruct patients to bring all pertinent insurance information.	☐	☐	☐
4. Give concise directions if needed.	☐	☐	☐
5. Ask the patient if it is permissible to call at home or at work.	☐	☐	☐
6. Confirm the time and date of the appointment.	☐	☐	☐
7. Check your appointment book to be sure that you have placed the appointment on the correct day in the right time slot.	☐	☐	☐
8. If the patient was referred by another physician, call that physician's office before the appointment for copies of laboratory work, radiology, pathology reports, and so on. Give this information to the physician prior to the patient's appointment.	☐	☐	☐

CALCULATION

Total Possible Points: _____
Total Points Earned: _____ Multiplied by 100 = _____ Divided by Total Possible Points = _____%

Pass   **Fail**
☐   ☐   Comments:

Student's signature _____ Date _____
Partner's signature _____ Date _____
Instructor's signature _____ Date _____

Name _____ Date _____ Time _____

Procedure 6-2:	MAKING AN APPOINTMENT FOR AN ESTABLISHED PATIENT

EQUIPMENT: Appointment book or computer with appointment software, appointment card

STANDARDS: Given the needed equipment and a place to work, the student will perform this skill with _____ % accuracy in a total of _____ minutes. (*Your instructor will tell you what the percentage and time limits will be before you begin.*)

KEY: 4 = Satisfactory   0 = Unsatisfactory   NA = This step is not counted

PROCEDURE STEPS	SELF	PARTNER	INSTRUCTOR
1. Determine what will be done at the return visit. Check your appointment book or computer system before offering an appointment.	☐	☐	☐
2. Offer the patient a specific time and date. Avoid asking the patient when he or she would like to return, as this can cause indecision.	☐	☐	☐
3. Write the patient's name and telephone number in the appointment book or enter it in the computer.	☐	☐	☐
4. Transfer the pertinent information to an appointment card and give it to the patient. Repeat aloud the appointment day, date, and time to the patient as you hand over the card.	☐	☐	☐
5. Double-check your book or computer to be sure you have not made an error.	☐	☐	☐
6. End your conversation with a pleasant word and a smile.	☐	☐	☐

CALCULATION

Total Possible Points: _____
Total Points Earned: _____ Multiplied by 100 = _____ Divided by Total Possible Points = _____%

Pass   **Fail**
☐   ☐   Comments:

Student's signature _____ Date _____
Partner's signature _____ Date _____
Instructor's signature _____ Date _____

Name_____ Date_____ Time_____

Procedure 6-3:	MAKING AN APPOINTMENT FOR A REFERRAL TO AN OUTPATIENT FACILITY

EQUIPMENT: Patient's chart with demographic information; physician's order for services needed by the patient and reason for the services; patient's insurance card with referral information, referral form, and directions to office

STANDARDS: Given the needed equipment and a place to work, the student will perform this skill with _____ % accuracy in a total of _____ minutes. (*Your instructor will tell you what the percentage and time limits will be before you begin.*)

KEY: 　4 = Satisfactory 　　0 = Unsatisfactory 　　NA = This step is not counted

PROCEDURE STEPS	SELF	PARTNER	INSTRUCTOR
1. Make certain that the requirements of any third-party payers are met.	☐	☐	☐
2. Refer to the preferred provider list for the patient's insurance company. Allow the patient to choose a provider from the list.	☐	☐	☐
3. Have the following information available when you make the call: • Physician's name and telephone number • Patient's name, address, and telephone number • Reason for the call • Degree of urgency • Whether the patient is being sent for consultation or referral	☐	☐	☐
4. Record in the patient's chart the time and date of the call and the name of the person who received your call.	☐	☐	☐
5. Tell the person you are calling that you wish to be notified if your patient does not keep the appointment. If this occurs, be sure to tell your physician and enter this information in the patient's record.	☐	☐	☐
6. Write down the name, address, and telephone number of the doctor you are referring your patient to and include the date and time of the appointment. Give or mail this information to your patient. Be certain that the information is complete, accurate, and easy to read.	☐	☐	☐
7. If the patient is to call the referring physician to make the appointment, ask the patient to call you with the appointment date, then document this in the chart.	☐	☐	☐

CALCULATION

Total Possible Points: _____
Total Points Earned: _____ Multiplied by 100 = _____ Divided by Total Possible Points = _____%

Pass　**Fail**
☐　　☐　　Comments:

Student's signature _____ Date_____
Partner's signature _____ Date_____
Instructor's signature _____ Date_____

Name _____ Date _____ Time _____

Procedure 6-4:	ARRANGING FOR ADMISSION TO AN INPATIENT FACILITY

EQUIPMENT: Physician's order with diagnosis, patient's chart with demographic information, contact information for inpatient facility

STANDARDS: Given the needed equipment and a place to work, the student will perform this skill with _____ % accuracy in a total of _____ minutes. (*Your instructor will tell you what the percentage and time limits will be before you begin.*)

KEY: 4 = Satisfactory   0 = Unsatisfactory   NA = This step is not counted

PROCEDURE STEPS	SELF	PARTNER	INSTRUCTOR
1. Determine the place patient and/or physician wants the admission arranged.	☐	☐	☐
2. Gather information for the other facility, including demographic and insurance information.	☐	☐	☐
3. Determine any precertification requirements. If needed, locate contact information on the back of the insurance card and call the insurance carrier to obtain a precertification number.	☐	☐	☐
4. Obtain from the physician the diagnosis and exact needs of the patient for an admission.	☐	☐	☐
5. Call the admissions department of the inpatient facility and give information from step 2.	☐	☐	☐
6. Obtain instructions for the patient and call or give the patient instructions and information.	☐	☐	☐
7. Provide the patient with the physician's orders for their hospital stay, including diet, medications, bed rest, etc.	☐	☐	☐
8. Document time, place, etc. in patient's chart, including any precertification requirements completed.	☐	☐	☐

CALCULATION

Total Possible Points: _____
Total Points Earned: _____ Multiplied by 100 = _____ Divided by Total Possible Points = _____%

Pass   **Fail**
☐   ☐   Comments:

Student's signature _____ Date _____
Partner's signature _____ Date _____
Instructor's signature _____ Date _____

Chapter Self-Assessment Quiz

1. If your medical office uses a manual system of sched-uled appointments for patient office visits, you will need a(n):

   a. toolbar.

   b. appointment book.

   c. computer.

   d. buffer time.

   e. fixed schedule.

2. How much time should be blocked off each morning and afternoon to accommodate emergencies, late ar-rivals, and other delays?

   a. 5 to 10 minutes

   b. 10 to 20 minutes

   c. 15 to 30 minutes

   d. 45 minutes to one hour

   e. one to two hours

3. When scheduling an appointment, why should you ask the patient the reason she needs to see the doctor?

   a. To know the level of empathy to give the patient

   b. To anticipate the time needed for the appointment

   c. To confront the patient about his personal choices

   d. To manipulate the patient's needs

   e. To determine who should see the patient

4. Which of the following is an advantage to clustering?

   a. Efficient use of employee's time

   b. Increased patient time for the physician

   c. Reduced staff costs for the office

   d. Shorter patient appointments

   e. Greater need for specialists in the office

5. In fixed scheduling, the length of time reserved for each appointment is determined by the:

   a. physician's personal schedule.

   b. number of hours open on a given day.

   c. reason for the patient's visit.

   d. type of insurance provider.

   e. patient's age.

6. Double booking works well when patients are being sent for diagnostic testing because:

   a. it gives each patient enough time to prepare for testing.

   b. it leaves time to see both patients without keeping either one waiting unnecessarily.

   c. the physician enjoys seeing two patients at one time.

   d. it challenges the medical practice's resources.

   e. it gives the physician more "downtime."

7. Which of the following is a disadvantage to open hours?

   a. Patients with emergencies cannot be seen quickly.

   b. Scheduling patients is a challenge.

   c. Effective time management is almost impossible.

   d. Walk-ins are encouraged.

   e. Patient charts aren't properly updated.

8. You should leave some time slots open during the schedule each day to:

   a. allow patients to make their own appointments on-line.

   b. make the schedule more well rounded.

   c. leave some time for personal responsibilities.

   d. provide the staff some flex time.

   e. make room for emergencies and delays.

9. Most return appointments are made:

   a. before the patient leaves the office.

   b. before the patient's appointment.

   c. after the patient leaves the office.

   d. during the patient's next visit.

   e. when the patient receives a mailed reminder.

10. Reminder cards be mailed:

    a. the first day of every month.

    b. a week before the date of the appointment.

    c. the beginning of the year.

    d. with all billing statements.

    e. only when the patient requests one.

11. A condition that is abrupt in onset is described as:

    a. chronic.

    b. commonplace.

    c. lethal.

    d. acute.

    e. uncurable.

12. Who is authorized to make the decision whether to see a walk-in patient or not?

    a. Medical assistant

    b. Emergency medical technician

    c. Physician

    d. Reception

    e. Nurse

13. If you reschedule an appointment, you should note the reason for the cancellation or rescheduling in:

    a. the patient's chart.

    b. the patient's immunization record

    c. the patient's insurance card

    d. the patient's billing form.

    e. the office's appointment book.

14. If you have to cancel on the day of an appointment because of a physician's illness:

    a. send the patient an apology letter.

    b. give the patient a detailed excuse.

    c. e-mail the patient a reminder.

    d. call the patient and explain.

    e. offer the patient a discount at his next appointment.

15. If you find that your schedule is chaotic nearly every day, then you should:

    a. evaluate the schedule over time.

    b. keep that information private.

    c. tell your supervisor that you would like a new job.

    d. stop the old schedule and make a new one.

    e. let the patients know that the schedule isn't working.

16. An instruction to transfer a patient's care to a specialist is a(n):

    a. precertification.

    b. consultation.

    c. transfer.

    d. referral.

    e. payback.

17. Established patients are:

    a. patients who are new to the practice.

    b. patients who have been to the practice before.

    c. patients who are over the age of 65.

    d. patients who are chronically ill.

    e. patients with insurance.

18. A flexible scheduling method that schedules patients for the first 30 minutes of an hour and leaves the second half of each hour open is called:

    a. clustering.

    b. wave scheduling system.

    c. streaming.

    d. fixed schedule system.

    e. doublebooking.

19. A chronic problem is one that is:

    a. not very serious.

    b. occurring for a short period of time.

    c. longstanding.

    d. easily cured.

    e. difficult to diagnose.

20. Which of the following is true of a constellation of symptoms?

    a. It can only be assessed by a physician.

    b. It is only an emergency if a patient is having a heart attack.

    c. It means a patient is suffering from appendicitis.

    d. It is a group of clinical signs indicating a particular disease.

    e. It probably requires a call to emergency medical services.

Chapter Checklist

- ☐ Read textbook chapter and take notes within the Chapter Notes outline. Answer the Learning Objectives as you reach them in the content, and then check them off.
- ☐ Work the Content Review questions—both Foundational Knowledge and Application.
- ☐ Perform the Active Learning exercise(s).

- ☐ Complete Professional Journal entries.
- ☐ Complete Skill Practice Activity(s) using Competency Evaluation Forms and Work Products, when appropriate.
- ☐ Take the Chapter Self-Assessment Quiz.
- ☐ Insert all appropriate pages into your Portfolio.

Learning Objectives

1. Spell and define key terms.
2. Discuss the basic guidelines for grammar, punctuation, and spelling in medical writing.
3. Discuss the 11 key components of a business letter.
4. Describe the process of writing a memorandum.
5. List the items that must be included in an agenda.

6. Identify the items that must be included when typing minutes.
7. Cite the various services available for sending written information.
8. Discuss the various mailing options.
9. Identify the types of incoming written communication seen in a physician's office.
10. Explain the guidelines for opening and sorting mail.

Chapter Notes

Note: Bold-faced headings are the major headings in the text chapter; headings in regular font are lower-level headings (i.e., the content is subordinate to, or falls "under," the major headings). Make sure you understand the key terms used in the chapter, as well as the concepts presented as Key Points.

TEXT SUBHEADINGS	NOTES
Introduction _____	

☐ **LEARNING OBJECTIVE 1:** Spell and define key terms.

Guidelines for Producing Professional and Medical Documents _____

Basic Grammar and Punctuation Guidelines _____

Basic Spelling Guidelines _____

Key Point:
• Remember, spell check will not recognize words that are spelled correctly but misused.

Accuracy _____

Key Point:
• Inaccurate information in some letters can lead to injury of a patient and lawsuits and can harm the physician's practice.

Capitalization _____

Key Terms: BiCaps, intercaps
Key Point:
• Ask for clarification and mark the proof letter with a question mark for the physician to assist.

Abbreviations and Symbols _____

Key Point:
• When in doubt, spell it out.

Plural and Possessive _____

Numbers _____

_____

_____

☐ **LEARNING OBJECTIVE 2:** Discuss the basic guidelines for grammar, punctuation, and spelling in medical writing.

Professional Letter Development _____

_____

Key Point:
• The goal of professional writing is to get information communicated in a concise, accurate, and comprehensible manner.

Components of a Letter _____

_____

Key Terms: template; salutation; enclosure

☐ **LEARNING OBJECTIVE 3:** Discuss the eleven key components of a business letter.

Letter Formats _____

_____

Key Terms: full block; semiblock; block

Composing a Business Letter _____

_____

_____

Composition _____

_____

Key Point:
• The goal of composition is to ensure that your message is transmitted clearly, concisely, and accurately to your reader. As you did during preparation, focus on the message, not on the mechanics.

Editing _____

_____

_____

Proofreading _____

_____

Key term: proofread

Corrections _____

_____

Types of Business Letters _____

_____

Memorandum Development _____

_____

Key term: memorandum

Components of a Memorandum _____

_____

☐ **LEARNING OBJECTIVE 4:** Describe the process of writing a memorandum.

Composing Agendas and Minutes _____

_____

Agendas _____

_____

Key Term: agenda
Key Point:
• It allows the meeting participants to prepare any necessary reports before the meeting and to anticipate questions.

☐ **LEARNING OBJECTIVE 5:** List the items that must be included in an agenda.

Minutes _____

_____

Key Point:
• Record only motions, seconds, and the results of a vote.

☐ **LEARNING OBJECTIVE 6:** Identify the items that must be included when typing minutes.

Sending Written Communication _____

_____

Key Point:
• All attempts must be made to ensure patient confidentiality.

Facsimile Machines _____

_____

_____

Electronic Mail _____

_____

_____

United States Postal Service _____

_____

_____

☐ **LEARNING OBJECTIVE 7:** Cite the various services available for sending written information.

Addressing Envelopes _____

_____

Key Term: font

_____

Affixing Postage _____

_____

_____

USPS Mailing Options _____

_____

_____

USPS Special Services _____

_____

Key Point:
• It does not provide proof that the letter was received by the addressee.

_____

Other Delivery Options _____

_____

_____

☐ **LEARNING OBJECTIVE 8:** Discuss the various mailing options.

_____

Receiving and Handling Incoming Mail _____

_____

_____

Types of Incoming Mail _____

_____

☐ **LEARNING OBJECTIVE 9:** Identify the types of incoming written communication seen in a physician's office.

_____

Opening and Sorting Mail _____

_____

Key Point:
• Mail that pertains to patient care issues should be opened and handled appropriately.

_____

☐ **LEARNING OBJECTIVE 10:** Explain the guidelines for opening and sorting mail.

_____

Annotation _____

_____

Key Term: annotation

Content Review

FOUNDATIONAL KNOWLEDGE

1. Check Your Spelling

Read the following sentences. If the sentence is free of errors, write "correct" on the line. If the sentence contains errors, circle the problem and explain how you would fix the sentence.

a. The patient has a cold and is bothered by the postnasal drip.

_____

_____

b. The patient complained of constipation and has not had a bowl movement in three days.

_____

_____

c. The patient, Mrs. Philips, sought weight-loss advise from the physician.

_____

_____

d. The nurse applied antiseptic to the wounded elbow.

_____

_____

2. Capitalize

Review the list of terms below and place a check mark to indicate whether each term must always be capitalized.

Name	Always	Not always
a. Streptococcus		
b. Tylenol		
c. Benadryl		
d. Diagnosis		
e. Analgesic		
f. Merck		
g. Antihistamine		
h. Tampax		

3. Details, Details

Which charting note is written correctly?

a. Patient is a forty-four-year-old Hispanic man with two sprained fingers.

b. Patient is a 44-year-old hispanic man with 2 sprained fingers.

c. Patient is a 44-year-old Hispanic man with 2 sprained fingers.

d. Patient is a 44-year-old hispanic man with two sprained fingers.

4. Which of these statements is both clear and concise?

a. Mr. Jensen entered the office in the early evening complaining of stomach pain unlike any he had felt before.

b. Mr. Jensen complained of severe stomach pain.

c. Mr. Jensen came to the office complaining about pain.

d. Mr. Jensen complained about stomach pain before leaving the office.

5. Parts of a Letter

Identify the 11 key components of a business letter shown on the next page.

1.   7.
2.   8.
3.   9.
4.   10.
5.   11.
6.

Benjamin Matthews, M.D.
999 Oak Road, Suite 313
Middletown, Connecticut 06457
860-344-6000   ①

February 2, 2008   ②

Dr. Adam Meza   ③
Medical Director
Family Practice Associates
134 N. Tater Drive
West Hartford, Connecticut 06157

Re: Ms. Beatrice Suess ④

Dear Doctor Meza: ⑤

Thank you for asking me to evaluate Ms. Suess. I agree with your diagnosis of rheumatoid arthritis. Her prodromal symptoms include vague articular pain and stiffness, weight loss, and general malaise. Ms. Suess states that the joint discomfort is most prominent in the mornings, gradually improving throughout the day.

My physical examination shows a 40-year-old female patient in good health. Heart sounds normal, no murmurs or gallops noted. Lung sounds clear. Enlarged lymph nodes were noted. Abdomen soft, bowel sounds present, and the spleen was not enlarged. Extremities showed subcutaneous nodules and flexion contractures on both hands.

Laboratory findings were indicative of rheumatoid arthritis. See attached laboratory data. I do not feel x-rays are warranted at this time.

My recommendations are to continue Ms. Suess on salicylate therapy, rest, and physical therapy. I suggest that you have Ms. Suess attend physical therapy at the American Rehabilitation Center on Main Street.

Thank you for this interesting consultation.

Yours truly,   ⑦

Benjamin Matthews, MD
Benjamin Matthews, MD   ⑧

BM/es   ⑨

Enc. (2)   ⑩

cc: Dr. Samuel Adams   ⑪

6. The words "Dear Mr. Larson" compose a:

　a. salutation.

　b. closing.

　c. valediction.

　d. letter.

7. The office manager has asked you to compose a letter explaining why the waiting room should be renovated. He hopes your letter will convince the physician to invest in the new waiting room. Of the three organizational formats described in the chapter, which is most appropriate? Why?

_____

_____

8. Of the following, which is an appropriate salutation for a professional letter? Answer *Yes* or *No* in the chart below.

Salutation	Yes	No
a. Dear Denise		
b. To whom it may concern		
c. Dear Mr. Hernandez		
d. Dear Sam Landers		
e. Hi Dr. Kingston		
f. Greetings		
g. Dear Ms. Carter, Mr. Hollings, and Mr. Tan		

9. What will the identification line look like on a letter dictated by Dr. Harriet Unger to her assistant, Byron Coleman?

　a. UNGER/coleman

　b. HU/bc

　c. COLEMAN/unger

　d. HU/BC

10. Dr. Chen asks you to prepare a memorandum for distribution to the entire office. She hands you a note to use as the body. It reads as follows:

> On May 9, Jerry Henderson, a representative of Conrad Insurance, will be visiting the office during the morning. Please extend him the utmost courtesy and introduce yourself if you have not yet met him. Jerry is a wonderful man who has been very helpful to our practice. I will be unavailable during the morning as a result of his visit. Please direct questions to Shelly or Dr. Garcia. Of course, I may be contacted in case of an emergency.

What would be the BEST subject line for the memorandum?

　a. Jerry Henderson is a helpful man

　b. Dr. Chen unavailable in morning on May 9

　c. Introduce yourself to Jerry Henderson

　d. Conrad Insurance person in office May 9

11. What must you do after composing a piece of written communication? Why?

_____

_____

12. A Look at Written Communication

You have been asked to send a summary of a patient's recent visit to a specialist. Review the list of forms of written communication below and place a check mark to indicate whether it is an appropriate means of written communication.

Form	Appropriate	Not Appropriate
a. A formal letter labeled confidential		
b. An e-mail marked urgent		
c. A memorandum		
d. A fax with a confidentiality statement		
e. A memorandum labeled urgent		

13. Every Minute Counts

You always take the minutes at the staff meeting, but you'll be on vacation during the next meeting. Explain to your coworker what information belongs in the minutes.

_____

_____

14. On the Agenda

Why is an agenda useful for meetings?

_____

_____

15. The physician has asked you to prepare an agenda for the November 9, 2008, meeting of the Doctors and Nurses Fraternal Association in Wheaton, Pennsylvania. He asks you to include the following:

- a panel discussion entitled *Improving Health Care Access for Low-Income Families.*
- an introduction to the panel by Dr. Marion Pope.
- announcements.
- adjournment.

Fill in the blanks in the agenda below with the information above.

_____

_____

_____

_____

Meeting Agenda

_____

_____

Call to Order
President
Reading of the Minutes of October Mtg.
Secretary
Introduction of Panel

_____

_____

Panel:

_____

_____

Officers' Reports
Officers

_____

_____

_____

_____

16. The Pony Express

Dr. Epstein is at a week-long conference in another state. She needs a patient's complete history to present to the conference one day from now, but has forgotten it at the office. Name three suitable delivery options.

a. _____

b. _____

c. _____

17. Sorting Mail

Which of the following is/are good practice(s) in regard to handling mail? Place a check mark in the correct box below to answer "Yes" or "No."

	Yes	No
a. handling promotional materials last		
b. opening mail addressed to a physician marked "confidential"		
c. asking a physician or office manager about a piece of mail you are unsure about		
d. leaving patient correspondence in an external mailbox		
e. disposing of a physician's personal mail if he or she is away		
f. informing a covering physician about mail requiring urgent attention		
g. prioritizing patient care related mail over pharmaceutical samples		

18. What three things must be included on every piece of mail before sending it?

a. _____

b. _____

c. _____

19. Match the following key terms to their definitions.

Key Terms

a. agenda _____

b. annotation _____

c. BiCaps/intercaps _____

d. block _____

Definitions

1. an informal intra-office communication, generally used to make brief announcements

2. a typographic style

3. a type of letter format in which the first sentence is indented

4. additional information intended to highlight key points in a document, typically written in margins

e. enclosure _____

f. font _____

g. full block _____

h. margin _____

i. memorandum _____

j. proofread _____

k. salutation _____

l. semiblock _____

m. template _____

n. transcription _____

5. the process of reading a text to check grammatical and factual accuracy

6. a model used to ensure consistent format in writing

7. abbreviations, words, or phrases with unusual capitalization

8. a type of letter format in which all letter components are justified left

9. something that is included with a letter

10. the process of typing a dictated message

11. a brief outline of the topics discussed at a meeting

12. a type of letter format in which the date, subject line, closing, and signatures are justified right, and all other lines are justified left

13. the greeting of a letter

14. the blank space around the edges of a piece of paper that has been written on

20. True or False? Determine whether the following statements are true or false. If false, explain why.

a. You must always use full block formatting when generating business letters.

_____

_____

b. When you are unsure of the gender of the recipient of a letter, your salutation should read "Dear Sir or Madam."

_____

_____

c. Slang and idioms should be avoided when writing business letters.

_____

_____

d. Minutes should include extensive documentation of the discussion surrounding a vote.

_____

_____

APPLICATION

Critical Thinking Practice

1. You are taking minutes at a meeting of several doctors and nurses. They are discussing whether to hold an office holiday party. Doctor Metsoulos expresses the opinion that it is important for office morale, but Doctors Jones and Ramirez think it is an unnecessary expense. Irene, one of the nurses, is concerned that the party will not reflect the religious diversity of the office. Eventually, a vote is held, resulting in a decision not to hold the party. What kind of information should you record in the minutes? Explain your answer.

_____

_____

2. The physician is out of town and has requested that she not be contacted except in the case of emergency. You are inundated with mail. There is a variety of material including several letters addressed to the physician marked "Urgent," "Confidential," and "Personal." Some of the other mail is from patients, but it is not marked in any unusual fashion. Other letters are from insurance companies with which your office is associated. There are also several advertisements and promotional mailings from medical supply companies, pharmaceutical companies, and insurance companies. In addition, there are pieces of mail that do not include a return address. Explain the procedure you would follow in dealing with this mail.

_____

_____

Patient Education

1. The office's policy is to mail a welcome letter to new patients. Make a list of information that should be included in this letter so the patient is prepared for her first visit.

_____

_____

Documentation

1. The physician asks you to send a letter to a patient regarding the results from her Pap smear. The test results came back normal. What should you write in the patient's chart?

_____

_____

Active Learning

1. When writing, it is important to know your audience. The way you write for a physician is different from the way you write for a patient. In the case of a physician, you can assume he or she understands medical terminology, but this is not so of a patient. Do some Internet research to better understand the possible side effects of a common medication like simvastatin (Zocor) or esomeprazole (Nexium). Then, write two letters discussing the side effects, one to a physician and one to a patient. Think about what you must do differently when writing to a patient.

2. On certain occasions, you may need to write on behalf of a physician to a person occupying an important civic function, such as a judge or elected official. Using the Internet or another reference source, determine how such a person is properly addressed and write a brief letter on a relevant subject. For example, the physician may hold an opinion on a bill affecting state funding of health care and wish to express it to a state legislator.

3. Taking dictation can be a difficult task, especially if the speaker is unclear or talks very fast. Practice will help you record dictation rapidly and accurately. Have a friend dictate a letter to you and record the letter as he or she does so. Developing a shorthand system of notes might help you keep up, although it may be less accurate. You must transcribe your notes carefully. Remember, you can always ask the speaker to slow down.

Professional Journal

REFLECT

(Prompts and Ideas: Have you ever received a communication that you felt was not sufficiently professional? How did it make you feel to receive an informal communication when you were expecting a formal one? What does this tell you about the importance of professionalism in communication?)

_____

_____

_____

_____

PONDER AND SOLVE

1. The physician has informed you that he is canceling an appointment with a patient because of a sensitive personal issue (for example, a medical problem, court date, business appointment) and will reschedule as soon as possible. How would you structure a letter to the patient? What information should you tell the patient? What should you withhold? What is an appropriate tone for the letter?

_____

_____

_____

_____

_____

2. One of your coworkers has been tasked with writing an important letter. As he prepares to seal it in an envelope and send it off, you ask whether it has been proofread. He says it has not. What should you do in this situation?

_____

_____

_____

_____

_____

EXPERIENCE

Skills related to this chapter include:

1. Composing a Business Letter (Procedure 7-1).
2. Opening and Sorting Mail (Procedure 7-2).

Record any common mistakes, lessons learned, and/or tips you discovered during your experience of practicing and demonstrating these skills:

_____

_____

_____

_____

_____

Skill Practice

PERFORMANCE OBJECTIVES:

1. Compose a business letter (Procedure 7-1).
2. Open and sort mail (Procedure 7-2).

Name _____   Date _____   Time _____

Procedure 7-1:   COMPOSING A BUSINESS LETTER

EQUIPMENT/SUPPLIES: Computer with word processing software, 8½ × 11 white paper, #10 sized envelope

STANDARDS: Given the needed equipment and a place to work, the student will perform this skill with _____ % accuracy in a total of _____ minutes. (*Your instructor will tell you what the percentage and time limits will be before you begin.*)

KEY: 4 = Satisfactory   0 = Unsatisfactory   NA = This step is not counted

PROCEDURE STEPS	SELF	PARTNER	INSTRUCTOR
1. Move cursor down 2 lines below the letterhead and enter today's date, flush right.	☐	☐	☐
2. Flush left, move cursor down 2 lines and enter the inside address using the name and address of the person to whom you are writing.	☐	☐	☐
3. Double space and type the salutation followed by a colon.	☐	☐	☐
4. Enter a reference line.	☐	☐	☐
5. Double space between paragraphs.	☐	☐	☐
6. Double space and flush right, enter the complimentary close.	☐	☐	☐
7. Move cursor down 4 spaces and enter the sender's name.	☐	☐	☐
8. Double space and enter initials of the sender in all caps.	☐	☐	☐
9. Enter a slash and your initials in lower case letters.	☐	☐	☐
10. Enter c: and names of those who get copies of the letter.	☐	☐	☐
11. Enter Enc: and the number and description of each enclosed sheet.	☐	☐	☐
12. Print on letterhead.	☐	☐	☐
13. Proofread the letter.	☐	☐	☐
14. Attach the letter to the patient's chart.	☐	☐	☐
15. Submit to the sender of the letter for review and signature.	☐	☐	☐
16. Make a copy of the letter for the patient's chart.	☐	☐	☐
17. Address envelopes using all caps and no punctuation.	☐	☐	☐

CALCULATION

Total Possible Points: _____
Total Points Earned: _____ Multiplied by 100 = _____ Divided by Total Possible Points = _____%

Pass   **Fail**
☐   ☐   Comments:

Student's signature _____ Date _____
Partner's signature _____ Date _____
Instructor's signature _____ Date _____

Name_____ Date _____ Time _____

Procedure 7-2:	OPENING AND SORTING INCOMING MAIL

EQUIPMENT/SUPPLIES: Letter opener, paper clips, directional tabs, date stamp

STANDARDS: Given the needed equipment and a place to work, the student will perform this skill with _____ % accuracy in a total of _____ minutes. (*Your instructor will tell you what the percentage and time limits will be before you begin.*)

KEY: 4 = Satisfactory   0 = Unsatisfactory   NA = This step is not counted

PROCEDURE STEPS	SELF	PARTNER	INSTRUCTOR
1. Gather the necessary equipment.	☐	☐	☐
2. Open all letters and check for enclosures.	☐	☐	☐
3. Paper clip enclosures to the letter.	☐	☐	☐
4. Date-stamp each item.	☐	☐	☐
5. Sort the mail into categories and deal with it appropriately. Generally, you should handle the following types of mail as noted: *Correspondence regarding a patient:* **a.** Use a paper clip to attach letters, test results, etc. to the patient's chart. **b.** Place the chart in a pile for the physician to review. *Payments and other checks:* **a.** Record promptly all insurance payments and checks and deposit them according to office policy. **b.** Account for all drug samples and appropriately log them into the sample book.	☐	☐	☐
6. Dispose of miscellaneous advertisements unless otherwise directed.	☐	☐	☐
7. Distribute the mail to the appropriate staff members. For example, mail might be for the physician, nurse manager, office manager, billing clerk, or other personnel.	☐	☐	☐

CALCULATION

Total Possible Points: _____
Total Points Earned: _____ Multiplied by 100 = _____ Divided by Total Possible Points = _____%

Pass   **Fail**
☐   ☐   Comments:

Student's signature _____ Date _____
Partner's signature _____ Date _____
Instructor's signature _____ Date _____

Work Products

Respond to and initiate written communications.

Compose a letter from Dr. Essen Mahlzeit, 321 Gasthaus Lane, Germantown, PA 87641, to Mr. Ligero Delgado, 888 La Sala Boulevard, Germantown, PA 87642.

The letter should inform Mr. Delgado of the following:
• The results of the biopsy taken during his sigmoidoscopy were negative.

• While these initial results are encouraging, his medical complaints need to be investigated further. Dr. Mahlzeit would like to refer Mr. Delgado to a specialist, Dr. Douloureux.

• Dr. Douloureux's practice is in Suite 100 of the Atroce Medical Center, 132 West Broadway, Germantown, PA 87642.

• With Mr. Delgado's consent, his records can be forwarded to Dr. Douloureux and an appointment will be arranged.

Prepare the letter on a sheet of letterhead if available. If this is not available to you, print the letter on a standard 8½ × 11 white paper and attach to this sheet.

Chapter Self-Assessment Quiz

1. In a letter, the word "Enc." indicates the presence of a(n):
   a. summary.
   b. abstract.
   c. enclosure.
   d. review.
   e. invitation.

2. If you are instructed to write using the semiblock format, then you should:
   a. indent the first line of each paragraph.
   b. use left justification for everything.
   c. use right justification for the date only.
   d. write the recipient's full name in the salutation.
   e. indent the first line of the first paragraph.

3. Which of the following items can be abbreviated in an inside address?
   a. City
   b. Town
   c. Recipient's name
   d. Business title
   e. State

4. Which sentence is written correctly?
   a. "We will have to do tests" said Doctor Mathis, "Then we will know what is wrong."
   b. "We will have to do tests" said Doctor Mathis. "Then we will know what is wrong."
   c. "We will have to do tests," said Doctor Mathis "Then we will know what is wrong."
   d. "We will have to do tests", said Doctor Mathis "Then we will know what is wrong."
   e. "We will have to do tests," said Doctor Mathis. "Then we will know what is wrong."

5. Which term should be capitalized?
   a. morphine
   b. fluoxetine
   c. zithromax
   d. antibiotic
   e. catheter

6. If the fax machine is busy when sending a fax, you should:
   a. mail the document instead.
   b. call the recipient and ask him to contact you when the machine is available.
   c. ask a coworker to send the document.
   d. make a note in the patient's chart.
   e. wait with the document until you receive confirmation that it was sent.

7. Which sentence is written correctly?

   a. The patient is 14 years old and is urinating 3 times more than normal.

   b. The patient is 14 years old and is urinating three times more than normal.

   c. The patient is fourteen years old and is urinating 3 times more than normal.

   d. The patient is fourteen years old and is urinating three times more than normal.

   e. The patient is fourteen years old and is urinating three times more than normally.

8. Which of the following always belongs on a fax cover sheet?

   a. The number of pages, not including the cover sheet

   b. The number of pages, including the cover sheet

   c. A summary of the content of the message

   d. A summary of the content of the message, less confidential portions

   e. The name of the patient discussed in the message

9. The USPS permit imprint program:

   a. guarantees overnight delivery.

   b. provides receipt of delivery.

   c. offers physicians cheaper postage.

   d. deducts the postage charges from a prepaid account.

   e. addresses envelopes for no additional charge.

10. Which USPS service will allow you to send a parcel overnight?

   a. Registered mail

   b. First-class mail

   c. Presorted mail

   d. Priority mail

   e. Express mail

11. Which is the best way to highlight a list of key points in a business letter?

   a. Use boldface text.

   b. Use a larger font.

   c. Use bulleted text.

   d. Use a highlighter.

   e. Use italicized test.

Scenario: You are tasked with writing a letter to a patient on the basis of a chart from his last visit. Most important is a diagnosis listed as "HBV infection."

12. Which is an appropriate course of action?

   a. Including the words "HBV infection" in the letter

   b. Consulting the physician on the meaning of the term

   c. Omitting the diagnosis from the otherwise complete letter

   d. Guessing the meaning of the term and writing about that

   e. Asking the office manager what to do about the letter

13. Having learned that HBV means hepatitis B virus, you should:

   a. research HBV infection.

   b. give the patient your condolences.

   c. write a letter based on the physician's instructions.

   d. immediately schedule an appointment for the patient.

   e. ask the patient to visit the office to learn his or her condition.

End Scenario

14. Who might receive a memorandum you have written?

   a. A nurse in your office

   b. A drug sales representative

   c. An insurance agent

   d. An outside specialist

   e. A recently admitted patient

15. Which closing is written correctly?

   a. Best Regards

   b. Sincerely Yours,

   c. Best regards,

   d. Sincerely yours

   e. Best Regards,

16. The purpose of an agenda is to:

   a. summarize the opinions expressed at a meeting.

   b. provide a brief outline for topics to be discussed at a meeting.

   c. inform participants of any changes since the last meeting.

   d. remind group members about an upcoming meeting.

   e. communicate key issues that should be addressed at future meetings.

17. Correspondence that contains information about a patient should be marked:

   a. personal.

   b. confidential.

   c. urgent.

   d. classified.

   e. top secret.

18. Which of these should be included in minutes?

   a. Individuals' statements

   b. Your opinion of the vote

   c. Names of those voting against

   d. Names of those voting in favor

   e. Date and time of the next meeting

19. Which type of mail provides the greatest protection for valuables?

   a. Certified mail

   b. International mail

   c. Registered mail

   d. Standard mail

   e. First class mail

20. Among these, which type of mail should be handled first?

   a. Medication samples

   b. Professional journals

   c. Insurance information

   d. Patient correspondence

   e. Waiting room magazines

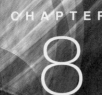

Health Information Management: Electronic and Manual

Chapter Checklist

☐ Read textbook chapter and take notes within the Chapter Notes outline. Answer the Learning Objectives as you reach them in the content, and then check them off.

☐ Work the Content Review questions—both Foundational Knowledge and Application.

☐ Perform the Active Learning exercise(s).

☐ Complete Professional Journal entries.

☐ Complete Skill Practice Activity(s) using Competency Evaluation Forms and Work Products, when appropriate.

☐ Take the Chapter Self-Assessment Quiz.

☐ Insert all appropriate pages into your Portfolio.

Learning Objectives

1. Spell and define the key terms.

2. Explain the requirements of the Health Insurance Portability and Accountability Act relating to the sharing and saving of personal and protected health information.

3. Describe standard and electronic health record systems.

4. Explain the process for releasing medical records to third-party payers and individual patients.

5. List and explain the EHR guidelines established to protect computerized records.

6. List the standard information included in medical records.

7. Identify and describe the types of formats used for documenting patient information in outpatient settings.

8. Explain how to make an entry in a patient's medical record, using abbreviations when appropriate.

9. Explain how to make a correction in a standard and electronic health record.

10. Compare and contrast the differences between alphabetic and numeric filing systems and give an example of each.

11. Identify the various ways medical records can be classified for storage.

12. Explain the guidelines of sound policies for record retention.

Chapter Notes

Note: Bold-faced headings are the major headings in the text chapter; headings in regular font are lower-level headings (i.e., the content is subordinate to, or falls "under," the major headings). Make sure you understand the key terms used in the chapter, as well as the concepts presented as Key Points.

TEXT SUBHEADINGS	NOTES

Introduction _____

_____

Key Points:
- A thorough and accurate medical record furnishes documented evidence of the patient's evaluation, treatment, change in condition, and communication with the physician and staff.
- In 1996, HIPAA was enacted to provide consumers with greater access to health care insurance, to protect the privacy of health care data, and to promote more standardization and efficiency in the health care industry.

☐ **LEARNING OBJECTIVE 1:** Spell and define the key terms.

The Health Insurance Portability and Accountability Act of 1996 _____

_____

Key Point:
- In addition to these issues addressed by HIPAA, the rapid advancement of technology in medical information maintenance caused the need for strict regulations to keep electronically-transmitted and stored protected health information (PHI) safe from unauthorized release.

Covered Entities _____

_____

Key Terms: covered entity; clearinghouses; electronic health record (EHR)
Key Point:
- Covered entities are subject to individual state laws, but if a state and federal law are different, you must follow the strictest laws.

Administrative Simplification _____

_____

_____

The HIPAA Officer _____

_____

Key Points:
- In most cases, as long as reasonable care is taken to comply with the intent of the ruling and that effort is documented, providers are considered compliant with HIPAA.
- HIPAA requires that at least one employee be designated as the HIPAA Officer and one as Privacy Officer.

☐ **LEARNING OBJECTIVE 2:** Explain the requirements of the Health Insurance Portability and Accountability Act relating to the sharing and saving of personal and protected health information.

Releasing Medical Records _____

Key Point:
• Any release of records must first be authorized by the patient or the patient's legal guardian.

HIPAA's Privacy Rule _____

Releasing Records to Patients _____

Proper Authorization _____

Key Point:
• Patients may release only information relating to a specific disorder, or they may specify a time limit. They may not, however, ask that the physician leave out information pertinent to the situation.

Legally Required Disclosures _____

Key Point:
• Certain information is crucial to the patient, needed for the protection of the public, or involves criminal activity, and is released without the patient's permission.

☐ **LEARNING OBJECTIVE 3:** Describe standard and electronic health record systems.

Adopting Electronic Health Records Technology _____

Making the Transition _____

Features and Capabilities of Electronic Health Records _____

_____

Key Term: demographic data

_____

Billing and Coding Using Electronic Health Records _____

_____

_____

The Medical Assistant's Role _____

_____

_____

Electronic Health Record Security _____

_____

Key Point:
• The physician should take care in keeping a personal data system, just as he or she protects the prescription pad.

_____

☐ **LEARNING OBJECTIVE 4:** Explain the process for releasing medical records to third-party payers and individual patients.

Standard Medical Records _____

_____

_____

Contents of the Medical Record _____

_____

_____

☐ **LEARNING OBJECTIVE 5:** List and explain the EHR guidelines established to protect computerized records.

Medical Record Organization _____

_____

Key Term: reverse chronological order

_____

Provider Encounters _____

_____

_____

Narrative Format _____

_____

                  Key Term: narrative

_____

SOAP Format _____

_____

                  Key Point:
                  • SOAP (subjective-objective-assessment-plan)

_____

POMR Format _____

_____

                  Key Term: problem-oriented medical record (POMR)

_____

☐ **LEARNING OBJECTIVE 6:** List the standard information included in medical records.

_____

Electronic Health Records _____

_____

_____

☐ **LEARNING OBJECTIVE 7:** Identify and describe the types of formats used for documenting patient information in outpatient settings.

_____

Documentation Forms _____

_____

_____

Medical History Forms _____

_____

                  Key Term: medical history forms
                  Key Point:
                  • Whether the patient brings the completed form or fills out the history form in the office, you will review the information with the patient to clarify any questions and add additional information gathered in the interview.

_____

Flow Sheets _____

_____

                  Key Term: flow sheet

_____

Progress Notes _____

_____

Key Point:
• This immediate availability makes patient care more efficient and convenient for the physician and the patient.

_____

Medical Record Entries _____

_____

Key Point:
• If the documentation is accurate, timely, and legible, it can
help win a lawsuit or prevent one altogether.

_____

☐ **LEARNING OBJECTIVE 8:** Explain how to make an entry in a patient's medical record, using abbreviations when appropriate.

_____

Charting Communications with Patients _____

_____

Key Term: chronological order
Key Point:
• Dates that are out of order and gaps between entries may
confuse the reader and give the appearance of poor service. For this reason, entries should be made immediately
after communications with the patient.

_____

Additions to Medical Records _____

_____

Key Point:
• All additions to the medical record (e.g., laboratory results,
radiographic reports, consultation reports) should be read
and initialed by the physician before you put them in the
chart.

_____

☐ **LEARNING OBJECTIVE 9:** Explain how to make a correction in a standard and electronic health record.

_____

Workers' Compensation Records _____

_____

Key Term: workers' compensation

_____

Storing Medical Records _____

_____

_____

Medical Record Preparation _____
_____
_____

Filing Procedures _____
_____
_____

Filing Systems _____
_____
_____

Alphabetic Filing _____
_____

Key Term: alphabetic filing
_____

Numeric Filing _____
_____

Key Terms: numeric filing; cross-reference
_____

Other Filing Systems _____
_____

Key Term: subject filing
Key Point:
• A well-kept, complete, and accurate medical record and the ability to quickly retrieve information are reflections of the quality and efficiency of the medical facility in which they are generated.

☐ **LEARNING OBJECTIVE 10:** Compare and contrast the differences between alphabetic and numeric filing systems and give an example of each.

Storing Health Information _____
_____
_____

Electronic Data Storage _____
_____

Key Point:
• The speed of computer technology promises changes and new practices. In order to optimize efficiency, you must keep abreast of these new technologies.

Storage of Standard Medical Records _____

_____

_____

Classification of Records _____

_____

Key Terms: microfilm; microfiche
Key Point:
• You will still keep these records in the office, but they do not have to be as accessible as the active files.

☐ **LEARNING OBJECTIVE 11:** Identify the various ways medical records can be classified for storage.

Record Retention _____

_____

Key Points:
• You must observe the statute of limitations in your particular state to know how long medical and business records should be kept in storage.
• At the least, every reasonable attempt should be made to notify patients and disseminate the information maintained by the retiring or deceased physician.

☐ **LEARNING OBJECTIVE 12:** Explain the guidelines of sound policies for record retention.

Content Review

FOUNDATIONAL KNOWLEDGE

Upholding Patients' Rights

1. HIPAA is the law for the health care industry. Those who must abide by HIPAA are called "covered entities." List the three groups that are considered covered entities.

   a. _____

   b. _____

   c. _____

2. HIPAA has privacy rules that protect your personal health information. Under HIPAA, covered entities must take certain safety measures to protect patients' information. Read the paragraph below. For each blank, there are two choices. Circle the correct word or phrase for each sentence.

   Covered entities must designate a ___(a)___ to keep track of who has access to health information (HIPAA officer, privacy officer). They must also adopt written ___(b)___ procedures (privacy, health care). Under HIPAA, patients have the right to decide if they provide ___(c)___ before their health information can be used or shared for certain purposes (permission, marketing). They also have the right to get a ___(d)___ on when and why their health care information was shared for certain purposes (narrative, report).

It's Electric

3. Describe the difference between standard and electronic health record systems.

_____

_____

4. Making the transition from a paper-based office environment to one using advanced technology has advantages and disadvantages. Complete the chart below with two more advantages and disadvantages of the electronic health care system. The first box has been completed for you.

ELECTRONIC HEALTH CARE SYSTEM	
Advantages	**Disadvantages**
a. **Point-of-care charting**	a. **Cost**
b.	b.
c.	c.

Record Release Party!

5. Sharing information can be fun; but, not so fast: do you know who you can share it with? And who will see it? Releasing medical records to patients and others shouldn't be like a gossip chain. The rules for releasing medical records and authorization are meant to protect patients' privacy rights. Read the questions below regarding the release of medical records and circle "Yes" or "No" for each question.

a. May an 18-year-old patient get copies of his own medical records?	**Yes**	**No**
b. May all minors seek treatment for STDs and birth control without parental knowledge or consent?	**Yes**	**No**
c. When a patient requests copies of her own records, does the doctor make the decision about what to copy?	**Yes**	**No**
d. Must the authorization form give the patient the opportunity to limit the information released?	**Yes**	**No**
e. When a patient authorizes the release of information, may he request that the physician leave out information pertinent to the situation?	**Yes**	**No**

Securing the System

6. HIPAA requirements provide guidelines and suggestions for safe computer practices when storing or transferring patient information. The following is a list of guidelines that medical facilities are urged to follow. Complete each sentence with the appropriate word from the word bank below.

a. Store _____ in a bank safe-deposit box.

b. Change log-in _____ and passwords every 30 days.

c. Turn _____ away from areas where information may be seen by patients.

d. Use _____ with _____ other than letters.

e. Prepare a back-up _____ for use when the computer system is down.

Word Bank

characters	plan	disks	information
codes	passwords	template	terminals

*Note: Not all words will be used.

Piles of Files

7. A standard medical record in an outpatient facility, known as a chart or file, contains clinical information as well as billing and insurance information. In the clinical section of the file, you will often find certain types of information. In the chart below, match the clinical type of information with its correct description.

Name of Clinical Information	Description
a. Chief complaint	**1.** Documentation of each patient encounter
b. Family and personal history	**2.** Provider's opinion of the patient's problem
c. Progress notes	**3.** Symptoms that led the patient to seek the physician's care
d. Diagnosis or medical impression	**4.** Letters or memos generated in the facility and sent out
e. Correspondence pertaining to patient	**5.** Review of major illnesses of family members

Documentation

8. Every medical office may use a different documentation format, depending on physician preference and type of patient (e.g., established, new). As a medical assistant, you should be familiar with the three most common formats. Read the chart below and match the format name with its description.

Format Name	Description
1. Narrative	**a.** A paragraph indicating the contact with the patient, what was done for the patient, and the outcome of any action
2. SOAP	**b.** Lists each problem of the patient, and references each problem with a number throughout the folder
3. POMR	**c.** Has a subjective and an objective component

9. POMR documents are divided into four components. List them below.

a. _____

b. _____

c. _____

d. _____

To Document, or Not to Document?

10. Documentation is a large part of your job as a medical assistant. Legible, correct, and thorough documentation is necessary. List three instances, other than patient visits, when documentation is required.

a. _____

b. _____

c. _____

11. When documenting in a medical record or file, why should you use caution when using abbreviations? Explain.

_____

_____

12. Fill in the chart below to explain how to make a correction in a standard and electronic health record.

Corrections in Standard Health Record	Corrections in Electronic Health Record

13. How does a numeric filing system help a medical office meet HIPAA's privacy requirements?

_____

_____

14. Your medical office uses an alphabetic filing system. Place the following names in the correct order to show how you would place each record in a filing system.

Brandon P. Snow	Kristen F. Darian-Lewes	Shante L. Dawes	Emil S. Faqir, Jr.
Shaunice L. DeBlase	Juan R. Ortiz	Kim Soo	Fernando P. Vasquez, D.O.

a. _____

b. _____

c. _____

d. _____

e. _____

f. _____

g. _____

h. _____

Filing Frenzy

15. List the four steps you should take to ensure that files are filed and retrieved quickly and efficiently.

a. _____

b. _____

c. _____

d. _____

16. For the Record. . .

For the purpose of storing records, they may be classified in three categories. In the chart below, match the type of record with its patient description.

Type of Record	Patient Description
a. Active	**1.** Mr. Arnold hasn't been seen by the physician in the last six years.
b. Inactive	**2.** Mrs. Lin was seen last month by the physician.
c. Closed	**3.** Mr. Angelos has passed away.

17. When a health care provider's practice ends, either from retirement or death, what happens to the records?

_____

_____

18. Organizational Hierarchy

Though there are some exceptions, most information in the paper medical record is placed in a standard order. Do you know the general order of information? Complete the graphic organizer below.

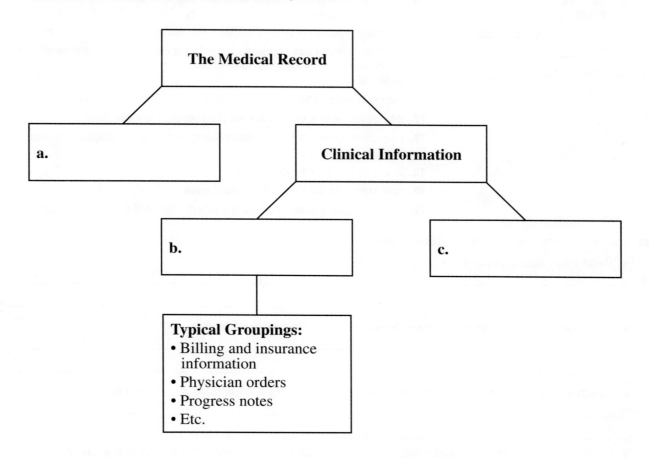

The Medical Record

a.

Clinical Information

b.

c.

Typical Groupings:
• Billing and insurance information
• Physician orders
• Progress notes
• Etc.

19. Match the following key terms to their definitions.

Key Terms

a. alphabetic filing _____

b. chief complaint _____

c. chronological order _____

d. clearinghouse _____

e. covered entity _____

f. cross-reference _____

g. demographic data _____

h. electronic health records (EHR) _____

i. flow sheet _____

j. medical history forms _____

k. microfiche _____

Definitions

1. information about patients that is recorded and stored on computer

2. photographs of records in a reduced size

3. a paragraph indicating the contact with the patient, what was done for the patient, and the outcome of any action

4. a specific account of the chief complaint, including time frames and characteristics

5. a common method of compiling information that lists each problem of the patient, usually at the beginning of the folder, and references each problem with a number throughout the folder

6. notation in a file indicating that a record is stored elsewhere and giving the reference; verification to another source; checking the tabular list against the alphabetic list in ICD-9 coding

7. entity that takes claims and other electronic data from providers and verifies the information and forwards the proper forms to the payors for physicians

l. microfilm _____

m. narrative _____

n. numeric filing _____

o. protected health information (PHI) _____

p. present illness _____

q. problem-oriented medical record (POMR) _____

r. reverse chronological order _____

s. SOAP _____

t. subject filing _____

u. workers' compensation _____

8. employer insurance for treatment of an employee's injury or illness related to the job

9. any information that can be linked to a specific person

10. items placed with oldest first

11. sheets of microfilm

12. arranging files according to their title, grouping similar subjects together

13. a style of charting that includes subjective, objective, assessment, and planning notes

14. arranging of names or titles according to the sequence of letters in the alphabet

15. health plan; health care clearinghouse; or health care provider who transmits any health information in electronic form in connection with a transaction covered under HIPAA

16. placing in order of time; usually the most recent is placed foremost

17. information relating to the statistical characteristics of populations

18. color-coded sheets that allow information to be recorded in graphic or tabular form for easy retrieval

19. arranging files by a numbered order

20. main reason for the visit to the medical office

21. record containing information about a patient's past and present health status

20. True or False? Determine whether the following statements are true or false. If false, explain why.

a. HIPAA allows patients to ask to see and get a copy of their health records.

_____

_____

b. To maintain secure files, you should change log-in codes and passwords every ten days.

_____

_____

c. Medical history forms are commonly used to gather information from the patient before the visit with the physician.

_____

_____

d. Before treating a patient for a possible workers' compensation case, you must first obtain verification from the employer unless the situation is life-threatening.

_____

_____

APPLICATION

Critical Thinking Practice

1. A mother is accused of physically abusing her 16-year-old daughter, a patient with your facility. A police officer who has been asked to investigate visits the medical office and asks for the patient's medical records. What should you do?

_____

_____

2. You're in the medical office and you suddenly realize that you've forgotten to document a telephone conversation you had with a patient 2 days ago. What should you do?

_____

_____

Patient Education

1. Dr. Minato is retiring and will be closing her practice. Write a letter to her patients explaining what they should do about their medical records.

_____

_____

Documentation

1. Maria Juaneza comes to the physician's office complaining of chest congestion and a deep cough. The physician examines the patient and notes that she is straining to breathe. The physician also notes that the patient's throat is red and irritated. The physician suspects that the patient has bronchitis, but he also wants Mrs. Juaneza to have a chest x-ray to rule out pneumonia. He prescribes an antibiotic and tells the patient to take an over-the-counter cough medicine. He also tells Mrs. Juaneza to call the office if her symptoms worsen and come back for a recheck if the symptoms are not cleared up by the end of the week. Use the SOAP method to document this interaction in the patient's chart.

_____

_____

Active Learning

1. If you were opening a new medical facility, consider whether you would want staff members using abbreviations in patient records. Then create a list of acceptable abbreviations that may be used in your new facility. Then create a "Do Not Use" list for abbreviations that may be confusing and should not be included in records. Visit the website for the JCAHO at www.jcaho.gov and include all of those abbreviations in addition to five other abbreviations of your own choice.

2. Choose a filing system that you learned about in this chapter (e.g., chronological, alphabetical, etc.) and practice it using household items. For example, you might organize your music collection or clothing drawers.

3. Make a KWL chart about Patients' Privacy Rights. Fill out the "What I Know" and "What I Would Like To Know" columns first. Then visit HIPAA's website at: http://www.hhs.gov/ocr/hipaa/. Click on "Fact Sheets" at the top, and then "Your Health Information Privacy Rights." Read the sheet and fill out the "What I Learned" column of your chart. Think about how you will apply this new information when you record, retrieve, and store patient health information.

Professional Journal

REFLECT

(Prompts and Ideas: Are you concerned about the prospect of transitioning from a paper-based medical facility to an electronic health record system? How will you make the transition smooth and efficient for yourself and your coworkers? Are there any advantages or disadvantages to using electronic health records that seem especially important to you? Explain.)

_____

_____

_____

_____

_____

_____

PONDER AND SOLVE

1. The golden rule in documentation is, "If it is not documented, it was not done." Explain what this means in regard to a potential malpractice suit.

_____

_____

_____

_____

_____

_____

2. Should a medical facility keep paper health records during the transition to electronic health records? Why or why not?

_____

_____

_____

_____

_____

_____

EXPERIENCE

Skills related to this chapter include:

1. Establishing, Organizing, and Maintaining a Medical File (Procedure 8-1).

2. Filing a Medical Record (Procedure 8-2).

Record any common mistakes, lessons learned, and/or tips you discovered during your experience of practicing and demonstrating these skills:

_____

_____

_____

_____

_____

_____

_____

Skill Practice

PERFORMANCE OBJECTIVES:

1. Establish, organize, and maintain a patient's medical record (Procedure 8-1).
2. File a medical record (Procedure 8-2).

Name _____ Date _____ Time _____

Procedure 8-1:	ESTABLISHING, ORGANIZING AND MAINTAINING A MEDICAL FILE

EQUIPMENT/SUPPLIES: File folder; metal fasteners; hole punch; five divider sheets with tabs, title, year, and alphabetic or numeric labels

STANDARDS: Given the needed equipment and a place to work the student will perform this skill with _____% accuracy in a total of _____ minutes. (*Your instructor will tell you what the percentage and time limits will be before you begin.*)

KEY: 4 = Satisfactory   0 = Unsatisfactory   NA = This step is not counted

PROCEDURE STEPS	SELF	PARTNER	INSTRUCTOR
1. Place the label along the tabbed edge of the folder so that the title extends out beyond the folder itself. (Tabs can be either the length of the folder or tabbed in various positions, such as left, center, and right.)	☐	☐	☐
2. Place a year label along the top edge of the tab before the label with the title. This will be changed each year the patient has been seen. *Note:* Do not automatically replace these labels at the start of a new year; remove the old year and replace with a new one only when the patient comes in for the first visit of the new year.	☐	☐	☐
3. Place the appropriate alphabetic or numeric labels below the title.	☐	☐	☐
4. Apply any additional labels that your office may decide to use.	☐	☐	☐
5. Punch holes and insert demographic and financial information on the left side of the chart using top fasteners across the top.	☐	☐	☐
6. Make tabs for: Ex. H&P, Progress Notes, Medication Log, Correspondence, and Test Results.	☐	☐	☐
7. Place pages behind appropriate tabs.	☐	☐	☐

CALCULATION

Total Possible Points: _____
Total Points Earned: _____ Multiplied by 100 = _____ Divided by Total Possible Points = _____%

Pass   **Fail**
☐   ☐   Comments:

Student's signature _____ Date _____
Partner's signature _____ Date _____
Instructor's signature _____ Date _____

Name _____   Date _____   Time _____

| Procedure 8-2: | **FILING MEDICAL RECORDS** |

EQUIPMENT/SUPPLIES: Simulated patient file folder, several single sheets to be filed in the chart, file cabinet with other files

STANDARDS: Given the needed equipment and a place to work the student will perform this skill with _____% accuracy in a total of _____ minutes. (*Your instructor will tell you what the percentage and time limits will be before you begin.*)

KEY: 4 = Satisfactory   0 = Unsatisfactory   NA = This step is not counted

PROCEDURE STEPS	SELF	PARTNER	INSTRUCTOR
1. Double check spelling of names on the chart and any single sheets to be placed in the folder.	☐	☐	☐
2. Condition any single sheets, etc.	☐	☐	☐
3. Place sheets behind proper tab in the chart.	☐	☐	☐
4. Remove outguide.	☐	☐	☐
5. Place the folder between the two appropriate existing folders, taking care to place the folder between the two charts.	☐	☐	☐
6. Scan color coding to ensure none of the charts in that section are out of order.	☐	☐	☐

CALCULATION

Total Possible Points: _____
Total Points Earned: _____ Multiplied by 100 = _____ Divided by Total Possible Points = _____%

Pass   **Fail**
☐   ☐   Comments:

Student's signature _____ Date _____
Partner's signature _____ Date _____
Instructor's signature _____ Date _____

Chapter Self-Assessment Quiz

1. Who coordinates and oversees the various aspects of HIPAA compliance in a medical office?
   a. Medicaid and Medicare
   b. HIPAA officer
   c. Privacy officer
   d. Office manager
   e. Law enforcement

2. A release of records request must contain the patient's:
   a. next of kin.
   b. home phone number.
   c. original signature.
   d. medical history.
   e. date of birth.

3. Which is an example of protected health information?
   a. Published statistics by a credible source
   b. Insurance company's mailing address
   c. Physician's pager number
   d. First and last name associated with a diagnosis
   e. Poll published in a medical journal

4. If patients believe their rights have been denied or their health information isn't being protected, they can file a complaint with the:
   a. Journal of American Medical Assistants.
   b. American Medical Association.
   c. provider or insurer.
   d. medical assistant.
   e. state's attorney.

5. The only time an original record should be released is when the:
   a. patient asks for the record.
   b. patient is in critical condition.
   c. record is subpoenaed by the court of law.
   d. physician is being sued.
   e. patient terminates the relationship with the physician.

6. Do medical records have the same content if they are on paper or a computer disk?
   a. Yes
   b. No
   c. Sometimes
   d. Most of the time
   e. Never

7. Documentation of each patient encounter is called:
   a. consultation reports.
   b. medication administration.
   c. correspondence.
   d. narrative.
   e. progress notes.

8. Improved medication management is a feature of:
   a. SOAP.
   b. electronic health records.
   c. clearinghouses.
   d. protected health information.
   e. workers' compensation.

9. To maintain security, a facility should:
   a. design a written confidentiality policy for employees to sign.
   b. provide public access to medical records.
   c. keep a record of all passwords and give a copy to each employee.
   d. keep doors unlocked during the evening hours only.
   e. have employees hide patient information from other coworkers.

10. Under source-oriented records, the most recent documents are placed on top of previous sheets. This is called:
    a. chronological order.
    b. reverse chronological order.
    c. alphabetical order.
    d. subject order.
    e. numeric order.

11. The acronym "SOAP" stands for:
    a. subjective-objective-adjustment-plan.
    b. subjective-objective-accounting-plan.
    c. subjective-objective-assessment-plan.
    d. subjective-objective-accounting-problem.
    e. subjective-objective-assessment-problem.

12. The acronym "POMR" stands for:
    a. presentation-oriented medical record.
    b. protection-oriented medical record.
    c. performance-oriented medical record.
    d. professional-oriented medical record.
    e. problem-oriented medical record.

13. Which of the following is contained in a POMR database?

   a. Marketing tools

   b. Field of interest

   c. Job description

   d. Review of systems

   e. Accounting review

14. Which of the following will reflect each encounter with the patient chronologically, whether by phone, by e-mail, or in person?

   a. Microfilm

   b. Narrative

   c. Progress notes

   d. Subject filing

   e. Flow sheet

15. Shingling is:

   a. printing replies to a patient's e-mail.

   b. recording laboratory results in the patient's chart.

   c. telephone or electronic communications with patients.

   d. taping the paper across the top to a regular-size sheet.

   e. filing records in chronological order.

16. How long are workers' compensation cases kept open after the last date of treatment for any follow-up care that may be required?

   a. 6 months

   b. 1 year

   c. 2 years

   d. 5 years

   e. 10 years

17. A cross-reference in numeric filing is called a(n):

   a. open file.

   b. locked file.

   c. straight digit file.

   d. master patient index.

   e. duplication index.

18. Security experts advise storing backup disks:

   a. in the office.

   b. off-site.

   c. at the physician's home.

   d. on every computer.

   e. at the library.

19. Drawer files are a type of:

   a. filing cabinet.

   b. storage container.

   c. computer system.

   d. shelving unit.

   e. subject filing.

20. The statute of limitations is:

   a. the end of a provider's ability to legally practice.

   b. the record retention system.

   c. a miniature photographic system.

   d. the legal time limit set for filing suit against an alleged wrongdoer.

   e. the number of records a storage system is able to hold.

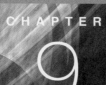

CHAPTER

9

Computer Applications in the Medical Office

Chapter Checklist

- [ ] Read textbook chapter and take notes within the Chapter Notes outline. Answer the Learning Objectives as you reach them in the content, and then check them off.
- [ ] Work the Content Review questions—both Foundational Knowledge and Application.
- [ ] Perform the Active Learning exercise(s).

- [ ] Complete Professional Journal entries.
- [ ] Complete Skill Practice Activity(s) using Competency Evaluation Forms and Work Products, when appropriate.
- [ ] Take the Chapter Self-Assessment Quiz.
- [ ] Insert all appropriate pages into your Portfolio.

Learning Objectives

1. Spell and define the key words.
2. Identify the basic computer components.
3. Explain the basics of connecting to the Internet.
4. Discuss the safety concerns for online searching.
5. Describe how to use a search engine.
6. List sites that can be used by professionals and sites geared for patients.
7. Describe the benefits of an intranet and explain how it differs from the Internet.

8. Describe the various types of clinical software that might be used in a physician's office.
9. Describe the various types of administrative software that might be used in a physician's office.
10. Describe the benefits of a handheld computer.
11. Describe the considerations for purchasing a computer.
12. Describe various training options.
13. Discuss the ethics related to computer access.

Chapter Notes

Note: Bold-faced headings are the major headings in the text chapter; headings in regular font are lower-level headings (i.e., the content is subordinate to, or falls "under," the major headings). Make sure you understand the key terms used in the chapter, as well as the concepts presented as Key Points.

TEXT SUBHEADINGS   **NOTES**

Introduction _____

_____

Key Point:
- You will need excellent computer skills to work as a medical assistant.

☐ **LEARNING OBJECTIVE 1:** Spell and define the key words.

The Computer _____

_____

Hardware _____

_____

Key Points:
- These cells read, analyze, and process data, and instruct the computer how to operate a given program.
- Keep in mind that you need to adhere to copyright laws.

Peripherals _____

_____

Key Term: Ethernet

☐ **LEARNING OBJECTIVE 2:** Identify the basic computer components.

Care and Maintenance of the System and Equipment _____

_____

Key Point:
- As with any piece of equipment in the medical office, it is necessary to maintain your computer on a regular basis.

Internet Basics _____

_____

Key Term: Internet

Getting Started and Connected _____

_____

□ **LEARNING OBJECTIVE 3:** Explain the basics of connecting to the Internet.

Security of Electronically-Shared Health Information

Key Point:
• The HIPAA legislation mandates that when a health care provider and health plan transmit and receive PHI (personal health information) electronically, the transmission must comply with certain standards.

Internet Security

Key Term: cookies
Key Point:
• By examining your cookies, a website can learn what sites you have visited, products for which you have been searching, and files that you have downloaded.

Viruses

Key Term: virus

□ **LEARNING OBJECTIVE 4:** Discuss the safety concerns for online searching.

Downloading Information

Key Term: downloading

Working Offline

Key Point:
• Remember, Web pages are regularly updated, and a page that you have saved to view off-line may not be the latest version.

Electronic Mail

Key Term: encryption

Access _____
_____
_____

Composing Messages _____
_____
_____

Address Books _____
_____
_____

Attachments _____
_____
_____

Opening Electronic Mail _____
_____
_____

Medical Applications of the Internet _____
_____

Key Term: surfing
Key Point:
• Besides e-mail, the Internet offers the World Wide Web, which provides health care professionals with great resources and information.

Search Engines _____
_____

Key Term: search engine

☐ **LEARNING OBJECTIVE 5:** Describe how to use a search engine.

Professional Medical Sites _____
_____

Key Point:
• The Internet can help you communicate with patients who speak a foreign language.

☐ **LEARNING OBJECTIVE 6:** List sites that can be used by professionals and sites geared for patients.

Literary Searches _____

_____

Key Term: literary search
Key Point:
• Your local hospital librarian is often available to assist you with literary searches and may be able to get the article for free.

Health-Related Calculators _____

_____

_____

Insurance-Related Sites _____

_____

_____

Patient Teaching Issues Regarding the Internet _____

_____

Key Point:
• Keep in mind that patients often turn to the Internet when they feel confused or hopeless about their disease or anger about the medical profession.

Buying Medications Online _____

_____

Key Point:
• A good Internet pharmacy will provide information on what the medication is used for, possible side effects, dosage recommendation, and safety concerns.

Financial Assistance for Medications _____

_____

_____

Medical Records _____

_____

_____

Medical Records Forms _____

_____

Key Point:
• Advance directives and legal forms for medical power of attorney are also available online.

Injury Prevention _____

_____

_____

Intranet _____

_____

Key Term: intranet
Key Point:
• The only people with access to an intranet home page are people with an affiliation to the practice.

☐ **LEARNING OBJECTIVE 7:** Describe the benefits of an intranet and explain how it differs from the Internet.

Medical Software Applications _____

_____

Clinical Applications _____

_____

Key Term: virtual
Key Points:
• Clinical software is designed to help the physician, nurse, medical assistant, or other health care professional provide the most efficient, safest, and most reliable health care available.
• A good program that focuses on pharmaceutical information will decrease medication errors, increase patient satisfaction, and provide better patient care; and it can be financially beneficial to the patient and to the practice.

☐ **LEARNING OBJECTIVE 8:** Describe the various types of clinical software that might be used in a physician's office.

Administrative Applications _____

_____

Key Point:
• Again, programs must aim to comply with HIPAA's Privacy Rule; these programs allow you to document your adherence to these rules and regulations.

Paging System Software _____

_____

PowerPoint _____

_____

_____

Meeting Maker _____

_____

_____

☐ **LEARNING OBJECTIVE 9:** Describe the various types of administrative software that might be used in a physician's office.

Handheld Computers _____

_____

Key Point:
• A handheld device can do almost anything that your desktop computer can do.

☐ **LEARNING OBJECTIVE 10:** Describe the benefits of a handheld computer.

Purchasing A Computer _____

_____

Key Point:
• All key members of the staff should be consulted prior to such a purchase and should be actively involved in selecting the hardware and software.

☐ **LEARNING OBJECTIVE 11:** Describe the considerations for purchasing a computer.

Training Options _____

_____

☐ **LEARNING OBJECTIVE 12:** Describe various training options.

Computer Ethics _____

_____

Key Point:
• Its capabilities are endless. It can, however, lead to an invasion of patients' privacy and unethical behavior.

☐ **LEARNING OBJECTIVE 13:** Discuss the ethics related to computer access.

Content Review

FOUNDATIONAL KNOWLEDGE

Computer Basics

1. A computer system is divided into two areas: hardware and peripherals. Take a look at the chart and decide which category each component fits into. Place a check mark in the appropriate box.

Name of component	Hardware	Peripheral
a. Keyboard		
b. Modem		
c. Central processing unit		
d. Printer		
e. Mouse		
f. Monitor		

2. Match these methods of connecting to the Internet with the statements below them.

Method of Connecting to Internet

a. ISP

b. cable television company

c. DSL

Description

1. This is the fastest connection, but it is the most expensive and it is not available in all areas.
2. This is a subscriber system that provides a faster connection than dial-up.
3. This system connects your computer's modem to the Internet through the phone line and is the slowest, but cheapest service.

3. Your office has started converting many of your paper files into digital online files to save time. Recently, you have realized that accessing these records through your ISP is taking a very long time. Check the box next to the solutions to this problem.

Solution

a. Upgrade your office's ISP to cable.	
b. Switch your Web browser.	
c. Switch your search engine.	
d. Upgrade your printer.	
e. Eliminate viruses with a virus scan.	
f. Upgrade your monitor.	
g. Upgrade your office's ISP to DSL.	

4. It is your first week working at a physician's office. You notice that the computer is clean and out of the sunlight. Disks are in a neat pile next to the uncovered computer. What steps would you take to maintain this computer?

a. _____

b. _____

c. _____

Surfing the Web

5. A patient has asked you for information on how she can lower her cholesterol. You have decided to surf the Internet to find the latest information. Place a check in the "Yes" column for those key words that would lead to a faster, more efficient search. Place a check in the "No" column for those key words that would lead to a slower, less efficient search.

Key Words	Yes	No
a. cholesterol		
b. lowering cholesterol		
c. cholesterol diet		
d. How do people lower their cholesterol?		
e. cholesterol reduction		

6. A diabetic patient has been researching information on the disease. He has asked you to review a list of websites he has been reading. Place a check in the "Patient" box for sites that are more useful for patients. Place a check in the "Professional" box for sites that are more useful to physicians and medical assistants.

Websites	Patient	Professional
a. www.mywebmd.com		
b. www.lancet.org		
c. www.jama.com		
d. www.healthfinder.gov		
e. www.tifaq.com		

7. A patient has expressed an interest in learning more about her food allergies on the Internet. You decide to give her advice on what to look out for when surfing. Place a check in the "Yes" column indicating that the statement is good advice. Place a check in the "No" column indicating that the statement is bad advice.

Key Words	Yes	No
a. Almost all testimonials can be trusted.		
b. Don't trust sites that claim to have secret formulas, medical miracles, or breakthroughs.		
c. Some treatments found online are best to not tell your physician about.		
d. No matter how professional the website, you cannot learn lifesaving skills on the Internet.		

8. A patient has told you of his decision to start buying prescription medication on the Internet. What warnings/information should you give to him?

a. _____

b. _____

c. _____

9. What are four benefits of an intranet compared to the Internet?

a. _____

b. _____

c. _____

d. _____

The Best Application

10. Mr. Jones requires special treatment that uses a laser machine. He makes an appointment for Thursday morning and takes time off work to attend. When he arrives at the facility, he is told that the machine is only available on Mondays and that the new receptionist was unaware of this fact when she made his appointment. How could an administrative software program have helped to prevent this situation?

_____

_____

11. Your office manager is taking suggestions for new programs to buy for the office computer. List three benefits of having scheduling software in the office.

a. _____

b. _____

c. _____

12. When shopping for prescription management software, what is the minimum that a physician should be able to do with the program? Circle the correct answer.

a. Find a patient name in a database, write the prescription, and download it to the pharmacy.

b. Find a patient name in a database, check the prescription for contraindication, and download it to the pharmacy.

c. Find a patient name in a database, write the prescription, and print it out for the patient.

d. Find a medication in a database, write the prescription, and download the data to a handheld computer.

e. Find a patient name in a database, write the prescription, download it to the pharmacy, and check that the medication is covered by insurance.

13. What are three benefits of using virtual documents, such as virtual patient charts?

a. _____

b. _____

c. _____

14. What are the benefits of using a handheld computer?

_____

_____

15. Who should be consulted when deciding what type of new computer to purchase?

_____

_____

16. You were out of the office on Monday, and on Tuesday a coworker describes a situation that happened on the previous day. He explains that he received a personal e-mail from a relative requesting that your coworker check a recent lab report of the relative's neighbor, who is a patient at the office. Your coworker tells you that when he tried to check the record, he needed a password to access the lab's database. Now he is asking you to share your password with him. What computer-related ethics issues would you try to explain to your coworker?

a. _____

b. _____

c. _____

Good Training

17. You have been asked to train new employees on how to use an administrative application. However, you do not have a lot of time or extra funding to spend on training. Circle the best option for training the new employees.

a. Have them read the user manual.

b. Have them call the help desk.

c. Have them ask another colleague.

d. Have them take a tutorial on the program.

e. Hire experts from the software company.

18. A physician asks you to place some helpful posters around the office about healthy living. You decide to download some information from the Internet. What do you need to take into consideration before you display this information in the office?

_____

_____

19. Match the following key terms to their definitions.

Key Terms	Definitions
a. cookies _____	**1.** a system that allows the computer to be connected to a cable or DSL system
b. downloading _____	**2.** a private network of computers that share data
c. encryption _____	**3.** a global system used to connect one computer to another
d. Ethernet _____	**4.** tiny files left on your computer's hard drive by a website without your permission
e. Internet _____	**5.** a dangerous invader that enters your computer through a source and can destroy your files, software programs, and possibly even the hard drive
f. intranet _____	**6.** transferring information from an outside location to your computer's hard drive
g. literary search _____	**7.** the process of scrambling e-mail messages so that they cannot be read until they reach the recipient
h. search engine _____	**8.** the process of navigating websites
i. surfing _____	**9.** a program that allows you to find information on the Web related to specific terms
j. virus _____	**10.** a search that involves finding journal articles that present new facts or data about a given topic
k. virtual _____	**11.** simulated by your computer

20. True or False? Determine whether the following statements are true or false. If false, explain why.

a. The advanced search feature of a search engine should return more results. _____

b. Internal job postings are often found on the Internet. _____

c. The most popular program used to write presentations is PowerPoint. _____

d. A computer system is divided into three areas: hardware, peripherals, and software. _____

APPLICATION

Critical Thinking Practice

1. You perform most of the administrative tasks in a physician's office, and have been asked for your input concerning a new office computer. The physician asks you which administrative features you would find helpful in a new computer. List three administrative software programs that you would find useful and explain what functions they perform.

   _____

   _____

2. A physician asks you to perform a literary search to find new information about treatments for bone cancer. He tells you to use the OVID website. Explain the steps you would take to obtain the most useful information as efficiently as possible.

   _____

   _____

Patient Education

1. A patient tells you that her medicine has not been working properly and that she is thinking of researching alternative treatments on the Internet. Write an informational leaflet for the patient, giving her advice about using the Internet for this purpose and advising her when to use caution.

   _____

   _____

Documentation

1. You receive an e-mail from Mr. Stiller saying that his medication is working out well and is not causing any side effects. He will be in for his appointment next Tuesday. How do you document this information in Mr. Stiller's medical record?

   _____

   _____

Active Learning

1. Perform research using the Internet to find information about a disease and possible treatments. Try using different key words to see which ones produce the most useful results. Make a list of the websites you have used and observe whether each one has the logo of a verification program such as the HON (Health on the Net) seal.

2. Use the PowerPoint program on the computer to turn your Internet research about a common disease into a presentation. Use the program to make handouts of your presentation for quick office reference. You can use the tutorial feature on the software if you are unsure how to perform certain functions.

3. Visit the Medicare website at www.medicare.gov. Find the part of the website that addresses FAQ, or frequently asked questions. Choose five of these questions that might be relevant to your patients and print the questions and answers. Then use presentation software to highlight these five questions in a presentation that you will give to your class.

Professional Journal

REFLECT

(Prompts and Ideas: Are you comfortable with computer technology, or do you find it intimidating? Do you currently use any specialized software? Was it difficult to learn how to use that software? Have you found that computer technology has made your life simpler or more complicated?)

_____

_____

_____

_____

_____

_____

_____

PONDER AND SOLVE

1. One of your coworkers has a habit of getting up from her computer and leaving confidential patient information visible on the screen. She says that she sits too far away from patients for them to read anything on the screen, but you have seen several patients near the computer while your coworker is away from her desk. What do you say to her?

_____

_____

_____

_____

_____

_____

2. A patient tells you that she has found a miracle medical cure for her child's cancer on the Internet. She is extremely excited about the treatment and tells you the website address. When you take a look, you notice that the information looks suspicious and is not endorsed by any medical professional. Explain what actions you would take and what you would say to the patient.

_____

_____

_____

_____

_____

_____

EXPERIENCE

Skills related to this chapter include:

1. Care For and Maintain Computer Hardware (Procedure 9-1).

2. Searching on the Internet (Procedure 9-2).

Record any common mistakes, lessons learned, and/or tips you discovered during your experience of practicing and demonstrating these skills:

_____

_____

_____

_____

_____

_____

_____

Skill Practice

PERFORMANCE OBJECTIVES:

1. Care for and maintain computer hardware (Procedure 9-1).

2. Search a given topic on the Internet (Procedure 9-2).

Name _____ Date _____ Time _____

Procedure 9-1:	CARE FOR AND MAINTAIN COMPUTER HARDWARE

EQUIPMENT/SUPPLIES: Computer CPU, monitor, keyboard, mouse, printer, duster, simulated warranties

STANDARDS: Given the needed equipment and a place to work, the student will perform this skill with _____% accuracy in a total of _____ minutes. (*Your instructor will tell you what the percentage and time limits will be before you begin.*)

KEY: 4 = Satisfactory   0 = Unsatisfactory   NA = This step is not counted

PROCEDURE STEPS	SELF	PARTNER	INSTRUCTOR
1. Place the monitor, keyboard, and printer in a cool, dry area out of direct sunlight.	☐	☐	☐
2. Place the computer desk on an antistatic floor mat or carpet.	☐	☐	☐
3. Clean the monitor screen with antistatic wipes.	☐	☐	☐
4. Use dust covers for the keyboard and the monitor when they were not in use.	☐	☐	☐
5. Lock the hard drive when moving the computer.	☐	☐	☐
6. Keep keyboard and mouse free of debris and liquids; dust and/or vacuum the keyboard.	☐	☐	☐
7. Create a file for maintenance and warranty contracts for the computer system.	☐	☐	☐
8. Handle data storage disks with special care.	☐	☐	☐

CALCULATION

Total Possible Points: _____
Total Points Earned: _____ Multiplied by 100 = _____ Divided by Total Possible Points = _____%

Pass   **Fail**
  ☐   ☐

Comments:

Student's signature _____ Date _____
Partner's signature _____ Date _____
Instructor's signature _____ Date _____

Name _____ Date _____ Time _____

Procedure 9-2:   SEARCHING ON THE INTERNET

PURPOSE: To quickly and effectively search the Internet as necessary for good time management.

EQUIPMENT/SUPPLIES: Computer with Web browser software, modem, active Internet connection account

STANDARDS: Given the needed equipment and a place to work, the student will perform this skill with _____% accuracy in a total of _____ minutes. (*Your instructor will tell you what the percentage and time limits will be before you begin.*)

KEY: 4 = Satisfactory   0 = Unsatisfactory   NA = This step is not counted

PROCEDURE STEPS	SELF	PARTNER	INSTRUCTOR
1. Connect computer to the Internet.	☐	☐	☐
2. Locate a search engine.	☐	☐	☐
3. Select two or three key words and type them at the appropriate place on the Web page.	☐	☐	☐
4. View the number of search results. If no sites are found, check spelling and retype or choose new key words.	☐	☐	☐
5. If the search produces a long list, do an advanced search and refine key words.	☐	☐	☐
6. Select an appropriate site and open its home page.	☐	☐	☐
7. If satisfied with the site's information, either download the material or bookmark the page. If unsatisfied with its information, either visit a site listed on the results page or return to the search engine.	☐	☐	☐

CALCULATION

Total Possible Points: _____
Total Points Earned: _____ Multiplied by 100 = _____ Divided by Total Possible Points = _____%

Pass   **Fail**
☐   ☐   Comments:

Student's signature _____ Date _____
Partner's signature _____ Date _____
Instructor's signature _____ Date _____

Work Product

Perform routine maintenance of administrative and clinical equipment.

Clean the monitor, keyboard, and mouse of a computer in your office, school, or home. If you are currently working in a medical office, use a maintenance log sheet from your office. If this is not available to you, use the sample maintenance log below. Document cleaning the specific computer parts on the maintenance log.

Computer Maintenance Log

Model No: _____

Date Purchased: _____

Manufacturer: _____

_____

Telephone: _____

Warranty: _____ **Expiration Date** _____

Technical Service Representative _____

Cleaning Log

Date	Initials	Action Taken	Comments

Chapter Self-Assessment Quiz

1. Another name for a central processing unit is a:

   a. silicon chip.

   b. USB port.

   c. modem.

   d. microprocessor.

   e. handheld computer.

2. The purpose of a zip drive in a computer is to:

   a. scan information.

   b. delete information.

   c. store information.

   d. research information.

   e. translate information.

3. The acronym *DSL* stands for:

   a. data storage location.

   b. digital subscriber line.

   c. digital storage link.

   d. data saved/lost.

   e. digital software link.

4. In a physician's practice, the HIPAA officer:

   a. checks for security threats or gaps in electronic information.

   b. purchases new technological equipment.

   c. maintains computer equipment and fixes problems.

   d. trains staff in how to use computer equipment.

   e. monitors staff who may be misusing computer equipment.

Scenario: A parent approaches you and asks how he can keep his 9-year-old daughter safe on the Internet.

5. Which of these actions would you recommend to the parent?

   a. Don't allow the daughter on the Internet after 7 PM

   b. Stand behind the daughter the entire time she is using the Internet.

   c. Don't permit the daughter to use the Internet until she is ten years old.

   d. Add a filter to the daughter's computer to only allow safe sites as decided by the parent.

   e. Ask other parents for advice.

6. Which of these websites might be helpful to the parent?

   a. www.skyscape.com

   b. www.pdacortec.com

   c. www.ezclaim.com

   d. www.cyberpatrol.com

   e. www.nextgen.com

End Scenario

7. To protect your computer from a virus, you should:

   a. make sure that your computer is correctly shut down every time you use it.

   b. avoid opening any attachments from unknown websites.

   c. only download material from government websites.

   d. consult a computer technician before you use new software.

   e. only open one website at a time.

8. What is the advantage of encrypting an e-mail?

   a. It makes the e-mail arrive at its intended destination faster.

   b. It marks the e-mail as urgent.

   c. It scrambles the e-mail so that it cannot be read until it reaches the recipient.

   d. It translates the e-mail into another language.

   e. It informs the sender when the e-mail has been read by the recipient.

9. Which of these is an example of an inappropriate e-mail?

   a. "There will be a staff meeting on Wednesday at 9 AM."

   b. "Please return Mrs. Jay's call: her number is 608-223-3444."

   c. "If anyone has seen a lost pair of sunglasses, please return them to reception."

   d. "Mr. Orkley thinks he is having a stroke. Please advise."

   e. "Mrs. Jones called to confirm her appointment."

10. Which of the following is a peripheral?

   a. Zip drive

   b. Monitor

   c. Keyboard

   d. Internet

   e. Modem

11. Which of these would you most likely find on an intranet?

   a. Advice about health insurance

   b. Minutes from staff meetings

   c. Information about Medicare

   d. Descriptions of alternative treatments

   e. National guidelines on medical ethics

12. What is the difference between clinical and administrative software packages?

   a. Clinical software helps provide good medical care, while administrative software keeps the office efficient.

   b. Administrative software is designed to be used by medical assistants, while clinical software is used by physicians.

   c. Clinical software is cheaper than administrative software because it offers fewer technical features.

   d. Administrative software lasts longer than clinical software because it is of higher quality.

   e. Clinical software does not allow users to access it without a password, while anyone can use administrative software.

13. Which of these should you remember to do when paging a physician?

    a. Follow up the page with a phone call to make sure the physician got the message.

    b. Keep track of what time the message is sent and re-page if there is no response.

    c. Document the fact that you sent a page to the physician.

    d. Contact the person who left the message to let them know you have paged the physician.

    e. E-mail the physician with a copy of the paged message.

14. You can use the Meeting Maker software program to:

    a. contact patients about appointment changes.

    b. coordinate internal meetings and calendars.

    c. print patient reminders for annual checkups.

    d. create slideshow presentations for meetings.

    e. page office staff when a meeting is about to start.

15. Which of these is an important consideration when purchasing a new computer for the office?

    a. Whether the computer's programs are HIPAA compliant

    b. Whether the computer will be delivered to the office

    c. The number of people who will be using the computer

    d. The amount of space the computer will take up in the office

    e. Which is the best-selling computer on the market

16. When assigning computer log-in passwords to staff, a physician should:

    a. make sure that everyone has the code for the hospital computers.

    b. give staff two log-in passwords: one for professional use and one for personal use.

    c. issue all new employees with their own password.

    d. make sure that everyone has access to his or her e-mails, in case he or she is out of the office.

    e. use a standard log-in password for all the office computers.

17. It is a good idea to lock the hard drive when you are moving a computer to:

    a. prevent the zip drive from falling out.

    b. make sure that no information is erased.

    c. stop viruses from attacking the computer.

    d. protect the CPU and disk drives.

    e. avoid damaging the keyboard.

18. A modem is a(n):

    a. communication device that connects a computer to other computers, including the Internet.

    b. piece of software that enables the user to perform advanced administrative functions.

    c. name for the Internet.

    d. method of storing data on the computer.

    e. type of networking technology for local area networks.

19. Which of the following is true of an abstract found during a literary search?

    a. Abstracts are only found on government websites.

    b. Only physicians can access an abstract during a literary search.

    c. An abstract is a summary of a journal article.

    d. Most medical offices cannot afford to download an abstract.

    e. Abstracts can only be printed at a hospital library.

20. If a computer is exposed to static electricity, there is the potential risk of:

    a. electrical fire.

    b. memory loss.

    c. dust accumulation.

    d. slow Internet connection.

    e. viruses.

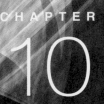

CHAPTER 10

Management of the Medical Office

Chapter Checklist

☐ Read textbook chapter and take notes within the Chapter Notes outline. Answer the Learning Objectives as you reach them in the content, and then check them off.

☐ Work the Content Review questions—both Foundational Knowledge and Application.

☐ Perform the Active Learning exercise(s).

☐ Complete Professional Journal entries.

☐ Complete Skill Practice Activity(s) using Competency Evaluation Forms and Work Products, when appropriate.

☐ Take the Chapter Self-Assessment Quiz.

☐ Insert all appropriate pages into your Portfolio.

Learning Objectives

1. Spell and define the key terms.
2. Describe what is meant by organizational structure.
3. List seven responsibilities of the medical office manager.
4. Explain the five staffing issues that a medical office manager will be responsible for handling.
5. List the types of policies and procedures that should be included in a medical office's policy and procedures manual.
6. List five types of promotional materials that a medical office may distribute.
7. Discuss financial concerns that the medical office manager must be capable of addressing.
8. Describe the duties regarding office maintenance, inventory, and service contracts.
9. Discuss the need for continuing education.

10. Discuss the need for general liability and medical malpractice insurance. List three services provided by most medical malpractice companies.
11. List six guidelines for completing incident reports.
12. List four regulatory agencies that require medical offices to have quality improvement programs.
13. Describe the accreditation process of the Joint Commission on Accreditation of Healthcare Organizations.
14. Describe the steps to developing a quality improvement program.
15. Explain how quality improvement programs and risk management work together in a medical office to improve overall patient care and employee needs.

Chapter Notes

Note: Bold-faced headings are the major headings in the text chapter; headings in regular font are lower-level headings (i.e., the content is subordinate to, or falls "under," the major headings). Make sure you understand the key terms used in the chapter, as well as the concepts presented as Key Points.

TEXT SUBHEADINGS	NOTES

Introduction _____

_____

☐ **LEARNING OBJECTIVE 1:** Spell and define the key terms.

Overview of Medical Office Management _____

_____

_____

Organizational Structure _____

_____

Key Term: organizational chart
Key Point:
- The medical office's organizational structure, or chain of command, is depicted in an **organizational chart**, a flow sheet that allows the manager and employees to identify their team members and to see where they fit into the team.

☐ **LEARNING OBJECTIVE 2:** Describe what is meant by organizational structure.

The Medical Office Manager _____

_____

Key Point:
- The medical office manager must be multiskilled, multitalented, and able to prioritize a variety of issues, juggle responsibilities, and communicate effectively with patients, staff, and physicians. In some settings, the medical office manager may be referred to as the business manager.

☐ **LEARNING OBJECTIVE 3:** List seven responsibilities of the medical office manager.

Responsibilities of the Medical Office Manager _____

_____

Communication _____

_____

Key Point:
- You must be a good listener, have good interpersonal skills, and be aware of your own nonverbal language.

Communicating with Patients _____

_____

Key Point:
• Your goal should be to correct the problem in a timely and professional manner and to alleviate any negative feelings the patient may have.

Communicating with Staff _____

_____

Key Term: job description
Key Point:
• To be an effective manager, you should communicate not only bad news but also positive messages to your employees.

Staffing Issues _____

_____

_____

Writing Job Descriptions _____

_____

Key Point:
• Each employee should receive a copy of his or her job description at the time of hiring and after any revisions to the description are made.

Hiring and Interviewing Employees _____

_____

Key Point:
• Any employee application form should be reviewed by legal counsel prior to its use.

Evaluating Employees _____

_____

Key Point:
• Employee evaluations must be fair, accurate, and objective.

Taking Disciplinary Action _____

_____

> **Key Point:**
> • Determine whether the employee's credentialing agency should be notified of serious infractions.

Terminating Employees _____

_____

_____

Scheduling _____

_____

☐ **LEARNING OBJECTIVE 4:** Explain the five staffing issues that a medical office manager will be responsible for handling.

Policy and Procedures Manuals _____

_____

> **Key Terms:** policy; procedure; mission statement; quality improvement; compliance officer
> **Key Points:**
> • Every business needs written rules and regulations to ensure that its practices are within legal and ethical boundaries.
> • A **mission statement** describes the goals of the practice and whom it serves.

☐ **LEARNING OBJECTIVE 5:** List the types of policies and procedures that should be included in a medical office's policy and procedures manual.

Developing Promotional Materials _____

_____

> **Key Point:**
> • The medical office manager is often responsible for developing and distributing promotional literature for the practice.

☐ **LEARNING OBJECTIVE 6:** List five types of promotional materials that a medical office may distribute.

Financial Concerns _____

_____

_____

Budgets _____
_____

Key Term: budget

Payroll _____
_____

☐ **LEARNING OBJECTIVE 7:** Discuss financial concerns that the medical office manager must be capable of addressing.

Office Maintenance _____
_____

Management of Inventory and Supplies _____
_____

Service Contracts _____
_____

☐ **LEARNING OBJECTIVE 8:** Describe the duties regarding office maintenance, inventory, and service contracts.

Education _____
_____

Staff Education _____
_____

Patient Education _____
_____

Manager Education _____
_____

☐ **LEARNING OBJECTIVE 9:** Discuss the need for continuing education.

Risk Management

Key Point:
• Risk management is an internal process geared to identifying potential problems before they cause injury to patients or employees.

Liability Insurance

☐ **LEARNING OBJECTIVE 10:** Discuss the need for general liability and medical malpractice insurance. List three services provided by most medical malpractice companies.

Incident Reports

Key Term: incident reports
Key Point:
• **Incident reports,** sometimes referred to as occurrence reports, are written accounts of untoward (negative) patient, visitor, or staff events.

When to Complete an Incident Report

Key Point:
• The rule of thumb is, when in doubt, always complete an incident report.

Information Included on an Incident Report

Guidelines for Completing an Incident Report

Key Point:
• State only the facts. Do not draw conclusions or summarize the event.

☐ **LEARNING OBJECTIVE 11:** List six guidelines for completing incident reports.

Trending Incident Reports

Quality Improvement Programs _____

_____

_____

Regulatory Agencies _____

_____

_____

Occupational Safety and Health Administration _____

_____

Key Point:
• OSHA's mission is to save lives, prevent injuries, and protect the health of America's workers.

Joint Commission on Accreditation of Healthcare Organizations (JCAHO) _____

_____

Key Term: sentinel event
Key Points:
• JCAHO is a private agency that sets health care standards and evaluates an organization's implementation of these standards for health care settings.
• Participation in JCAHO is voluntary for health care organizations; without accreditation, however, the health care organization may not be eligible to participate in particular federal and state funding programs, such as Medicare and Medicaid.
• A sentinel event is an unexpected death or serious physical or psychological injury to a patient.

☐ **LEARNING OBJECTIVE 12:** List four regulatory agencies that require medical offices to have quality improvement programs.

Centers for Medicare & Medicaid Services _____

_____

_____

State Health Departments _____

_____

_____

☐ **LEARNING OBJECTIVE 13:** Describe the accreditation process of the Joint Commission on Accreditation of Healthcare Organizations.

Developing a Quality Improvement Program _____

_____

_____

Seven Steps for a Successful Program

Key Terms: task force; expected threshold

Key Points:

- Problems given top priority are those that are high risk (most likely to occur) and those that are most likely to cause injury to patients, family members, or employees.
- A **task force** is a group of employees with different roles within the organization brought together to solve a given problem.
- Thresholds must be realistic and achievable.
- After implementation, the solution must be evaluated to determine whether it worked and if so, how well.

☐ **LEARNING OBJECTIVE 14:** Describe the steps to developing a quality improvement program.

Putting It All Together: A Case Review

☐ **LEARNING OBJECTIVE 15:** Explain how quality improvement programs and risk management work together in a medical office to improve overall patient care and employee needs.

Content Review

FOUNDATIONAL KNOWLEDGE

1. Organizational Structure

Circle every item that would be an appropriate part of a medical organizational chart.

Salaries	Job titles	Who supervises whom
Employees' names	Physicians' names	Social security numbers

2. A Day in the Life of a Medical Office Manager

Circle all the following tasks that are the responsibility of the medical office manager.

a. scheduling staff

b. ordering supplies

c. writing the budget

d. keeping up to date on legal issues

e. assisting with medical procedures

f. cleaning the office and waiting room

g. revising policy and procedures manuals

h. presenting continuing education seminars

i. developing HIPAA and OSHA regulations

j. developing promotional pamphlets or newsletters

Writing Job Descriptions

3. List six of the elements that should be included in any job description.

a. _____

b. _____

c. _____

d. _____

e. _____

f. _____

4. In addition to writing job descriptions and managing employee evaluations, what are three other staffing issues that are the responsibility of the medical office manager?

a. _____

b. _____

c. _____

5. Employee Evaluations

Answer "Yes," "No," or "Yes But" to the following questions about evaluating employees. If you answer "No" or "Yes But," be able to explain why.

	Yes	No	Yes But. . .
a. Are employee evaluations your responsibility as a medical office manager?			
b. Should new employees be evaluated annually?			
c. Should you coach new employees about how to do their jobs well?			
d. Can annual performance appraisals be done orally?			
e. Should you communicate with employees about performance problems when one of the physicians asks you to?			
f. Should you inform a good employee yearly that she or he is doing a good job?			

Office Policies

6. Indicate by a check mark in the "Yes" or "No" column whether an item should be included in a medical office's policy and procedures manual.

	Yes	No
a. a chain of command chart		
b. a list of employee benefits		
c. infection control guidelines		
d. the office operating budget		
e. annual employee evaluations		
f. procedures for bill collections		
g. copies of completed incident reports		
h. a description of the goals of the practice		
i. responsibilities and procedures for ordering supplies		
j. a list of responsibilities for the last employee to leave the office each day		

7. List five types of promotional materials that a medical office might use.

a. _____

b. _____

c. _____

d. _____

e. _____

8. Why might a medical office manager outsource payroll?

_____

_____

9. Service Contracts

a. List three types of service contractors a medical office is likely to use.

_____

_____

_____

_____

_____

b. List three responsibilities of the office manager regarding service contractors.

_____

_____

_____

_____

_____

10. On Budget

Medical offices usually have an operating budget and a capital budget. Separate the following items into the two categories by checking the column for operating budget or capital budget.

Budget Item	Operating Budget	Capital Budget
a. payroll		
b. medical equipment		
c. office supplies		
d. Internet service		
e. medical supplies		
f. building maintenance		
g. telephone service		
h. electricity		
i. expensive furniture		
j. patient materials		
k. continuing education		

11. **Controlling Inventory**

    Inventory control is the responsibility of the office manager. On the checklist below, put an **M** beside the inventory tasks the manager should do and an **A** beside the things an assistant or other office staff member can do.

    _____ Receive supplies

    _____ Initial the packing slip

    _____ Develop a system to keep track of supplies

    _____ Determine the procedures for ordering supplies

    _____ Transfer supplies from packing boxes to supply shelves

    _____ Check the packing slip against the actual supply contents

    _____ Keep receipts or packing slips in a bills-pending file for payment

    _____ Develop a process to check that deliveries of supplies are complete and accurate

12. **Continuing Education**

    Give a practical reason, a psychological reason, and a professional reason for off-site seminars and other continuing education activities for medical office staff.

    a. **PRACTICAL:**

    _____

    _____

    b. **PSYCHOLOGICAL:**

    _____

    _____

    c. **PROFESSIONAL:**

    _____

    _____

Avoiding Malpractice Suits

13. List three services provided by most medical malpractice companies.

    a. _____

    b. _____

    c. _____

14. General liability and medical malpractice insurance is needed:

    a. only by employees in offices that use new medical procedures.

    b. by physicians sued for malpractice, but not by nurses or office personnel.

    c. to protect medical professionals from financial loss due to lawsuits or settlements.

    d. because visitors who are hurt in the waiting room can sue unless an incident report is completed.

15. Each of the following statements about incident reports is <u>false or incomplete</u>. Rewrite each statement to make it true and complete.

    a. You should write up an incident report as the event was reported to you.

    _____

    _____

b. The witness should summarize and explain the event.

_____

_____

c. You should remain anonymous when you fill out a report.

_____

_____

d. The form should be completed within 48 hours of the event.

_____

_____

e. If a particular section of the report does not apply, it should be left blank.

_____

_____

f. Keep a copy of the incident report for your own personal record.

_____

_____

g. If the incident happened to a patient, put a copy of the report in the patient's chart.

_____

_____

h. The report should be reviewed by a supervisor to make sure the office is not liable.

_____

_____

i. Incident reports are written when negative events happen to patients or visitors.

_____

_____

16. **Which Agency?**

Below is a list of four regulatory agencies that require medical offices to have quality improvement programs.
Match the regulatory agency with its description.

Agencies

a. CMS

b. OSHA

c. JCAHO

d. state health department

Descriptions

1. federal agency that regulates and runs Medicare and Medicaid
2. nonfederal agency to license and monitor health care organizations and enforce regulations
3. federal agency that enforces regulations to protect the health and welfare of patients and employees
4. agency that sets voluntary health care standards and evaluates a health care organization's implementation of those standards

Quality Improvement

17. Below is a list of the steps for creating a quality improvement plan. Put the steps in logical order. Then explain the reason for each step.

Steps

Assign an expected threshold.

Document the entire process.

Establish a monitoring plan.

Explore the problem and propose solutions.

Form a task force.

Identify the problem.

Implement the solution.

Obtain feedback.

Step	Reason
1.	
2.	
3.	
4.	
5.	
6.	
7.	
8.	

18. Explain how QI programs and risk management work together in a medical office.

_____

_____

19. Match the following key terms to their definitions.

Key Terms

a. budget _____

b. compliance officer _____

c. expected threshold _____

d. incident report _____

e. job description _____

f. mission statement _____

g. organizational chart _____

h. policy _____

i. procedure _____

j. sentinel event _____

k. quality improvement _____

l. task force _____

Definitions

1. numerical goal for a given problem

2. statement of work-related responsibilities

3. series of steps required to perform a given task

4. written account of untoward patient, visitor, or staff event

5. description of the goals of the practice and whom it serves

6. statement regarding the organization's rules on a given topic

7. unexpected death or serious physical or psychological injury to a patient

8. financial planning tool used to estimate anticipated expenditures and revenues

9. staff member who ensures compliance with the rules and regulations of the office

10. implementation of practices that will help ensure high-quality patient care and service

11. flow sheet that allows staff to identify team members and see where they fit into the team

12. group of employees with different roles brought together to solve a problem

20. True or False? Determine whether the following statements are true or false. If false, explain why.

    a. Health care organizations are required to follow the regulations of the Joint Commission on Accreditation of Healthcare Organizations (JCAHO).

    _____

    _____

    b. Accreditation by JCAHO is valid for 5 years.

    _____

    _____

    c. If JCAHO's initial site review identifies unsatisfactory areas, the health care organization may later prove that corrections have been made by passing a focus survey.

    _____

    _____

    d. The health care organization should prepare for the JCAHO survey by assessing its compliance with OSHA standards.

    _____

    _____

APPLICATION

Critical Thinking Practice

1. As you enter the office on the first day of your new job as the medical office manager, you notice a thick layer of dust on the plastic plants in the waiting room and see that the magazines are old and tattered. The staff greets you with enthusiasm, saying you are just what they need to deal with the patients' complaints about spending too much time waiting to be seen. Someone has left the incident report file on your desk. You look through it right away and learn that a needlestick has been reported almost every Wednesday evening for a month. What should you do first, and why?

_____

_____

2. Your assistant is moving across the country and you need to find a replacement. The office policy and procedures manual contains a job interview questionnaire that has questions relating to gender, race, age, marital status, education, and experience. You think it's important to find out more about a potential employee's personality and how the job is likely to affect his or her other responsibilities, and vice versa. Which of these questions should you not ask, and why?

_____

_____

Patient Education

1. Influenza incidence is predicted to be high this year, and flu season is coming. You find an outdated flu prevention poster in storage but no other patient education materials about flu. Make a plan for this year's flu education effort. Describe the educational materials you want and how you want to use them. Explain any research you should and or any input you will need.

_____

_____

Documentation

1. The office is still running out of medium-sized examination gloves, even though you increased their number last time you ordered them from the supplier. How will better documentation help you solve this problem?

_____

_____

Active Learning

1. When you complete your program of study, you would like to find a job as a medical office manager. Write the job description for your ideal job. Be sure to include all the essential elements, including a position summary, hours, location, and duties.

2. Get a head start on outsourcing services for your office. Search the Internet for service contractors (such as payroll, biohazard collection, office machine maintenance), and compare and contrast the services you find. Prepare a list of questions you would want answered by any service contractor before you decided whether to do business with them.

3. Working together with a partner, search the local classified ads for an open job as a medical office manager. Then prepare to role-play the interview process with your partner, taking turns acting as the interviewer and the interviewee. Make a list of questions that you would ask as both the interviewer and the interviewee. Switch places so you both get to experience the job interview process from each perspective.

Professional Journal

REFLECT

(Prompts and Ideas: Have you ever gone on a job interview before? How did you prepare? Were you nervous beforehand, and, if so, what did you do to calm yourself down? Have you ever started a new job? What kind of information did you get the first week on the job [e.g., policy manual, handbook]? Could your supervisor have done anything else to make you feel more prepared and comfortable in your new position?)

_____

_____

_____

_____

_____

_____

_____

PONDER AND SOLVE

1. Mrs. Hadley, who is blind and walks with a cane, slipped on the wet floor near a leaky water cooler and fell, cutting her forearm. One of the nurses examined and treated her wound and apologized. Mrs. Hadley said it was no problem and left the office. The nurse told you she wasn't going to file an incident report because the wound was minor and Mrs. Hadley had accepted her apology. As the medical office manager, what should you do?

_____

_____

_____

_____

_____

_____

_____

2. One member of the office staff consistently uses all her sick days but she always does a great job when she does come to work. Most of the staff members come in even when they are sick; they brag about it and apparently disapprove of taking sick days. Is this a problem? As the medical office manager, what should your goal be and which staff members should you talk with to meet your goal?

_____

_____

_____

_____

_____

_____

_____

EXPERIENCE

Skills related to this chapter include:

1. Creating a Procedures Manual (Procedure 10-1).

2. Creating a Quality Improvement Plan (Procedure 10-2).

Record any common mistakes, lessons learned, and/or tips you discovered during your experience of practicing and demonstrating these skills.

_____

_____

_____

_____

_____

_____

_____

Skill Practice

PERFORMANCE OBJECTIVES:

1. Create a policy and procedures manual (Procedure 10-1).

2. Create a quality improvement plan (Procedure 10-2).

Name_____ Date_____ Time_____

Procedure 10-1:	CREATING A PROCEDURES MANUAL

EQUIPMENT/SUPPLIES:

STANDARDS: Given the needed equipment and a place to work, the student will perform this skill with _____% accuracy in a total of _____ minutes. (*Your instructor will tell you what the percentage and time limits will be before you begin.*)

KEY: 4 = Satisfactory   0 = Unsatisfactory   NA = This step is not counted

PROCEDURE STEPS	SELF	PARTNER	INSTRUCTOR
1. Check the latest information from key governmental agencies, local and state health departments, and health care organizations, such as OSHA, CDC, JCAHO, etc. to make sure that the policies and procedures being written comply with federal and state legislation and regulations.	☐	☐	☐
2. Gather product information; consult government agencies, if needed. Secure educational pamphlets.	☐	☐	☐
3. Title the procedure properly.	☐	☐	☐
4. Number the procedure appropriately.	☐	☐	☐
5. Define the overall purpose of the procedure in a sentence or two explaining the intent of the procedure.	☐	☐	☐
6. List all necessary equipment and forms. Include everything needed to complete the task.	☐	☐	☐
7. List each step with its rationale.	☐	☐	☐
8. Provide spaces for signatures.	☐	☐	☐
9. Record the date the procedure was written.	☐	☐	☐

CALCULATION

Total Possible Points: _____
Total Points Earned: _____ Multiplied by 100 = _____ Divided by Total Possible Points = _____%

Pass   **Fail**
☐   ☐   Comments:

Student's signature _____ Date _____
Partner's signature _____ Date _____
Instructor's signature _____ Date _____

Name _____   Date _____   Time _____

Procedure 10-2:	CREATE A QUALITY IMPROVEMENT PLAN

EQUIPMENT/SUPPLIES:

STANDARDS: Given the needed equipment and a place to work, the student will perform this skill with _____% accuracy in a total of _____ minutes. (*Your instructor will tell you what the percentage and time limits will be before you begin.*)

KEY: 4 = Satisfactory   0 = Unsatisfactory   NA = This step is not counted

PROCEDURE STEPS	SELF	PARTNER	INSTRUCTOR
1. Identify the problem or potential problem.	☐	☐	☐
2. Form a task force from group of students.	☐	☐	☐
3. Explore the problem and proposed solutions.	☐	☐	☐
4. Assign an expected threshold using measurable, realistic goals.	☐	☐	☐
5. Implement the solution and write a memorandum to the employees with instructions for the implementation.	☐	☐	☐
6. Establish a QI monitoring plan by listing the source, frequency, and person responsible for collecting data.	☐	☐	☐
7. Obtained feedback. Review data collected in the monitoring process.	☐	☐	☐
8. Document the entire process.	☐	☐	☐

CALCULATION

Total Possible Points: _____
Total Points Earned: _____ Multiplied by 100 = _____ Divided by Total Possible Points = _____%

Pass   **Fail**
☐   ☐   Comments:

Student's signature _____ Date _____
Partner's signature _____ Date _____
Instructor's signature _____ Date _____

Work Product 1

Use methods of quality control.

Louise Baggins, a 55-year-old patient, was visiting the physician for a physical exam. While waiting for her appointment, she asked you to direct her to the restroom. On her way into the restroom, she slipped and fell on a magazine that had fallen on the floor in the reception area. You did not see her fall, but she yelled out in pain after she fell. She was able to get up on her own, but injured her wrist. Her wrist was immediately red, swollen, and painful to touch. Dr. Mikuski looked at her wrist and suggested she go to the hospital emergency room to have x-rays. You called an ambulance to transfer Mrs. Baggins to the hospital.

 Fill in the incident report below to document this event.

Workplace Requirements Program for Safety and Health

SUPERVISOR'S ACCIDENT REPORT FORM

This form is to be completed by the supervisor and forwarded to the Payroll Coordinator along with a copy of the North Carolina Industrial Commission Form 19 (Workers Compensation Form) within five days of the accident. All accidents involving serious bodily injury or death must be reported to the safety and health officer immediately.

ACCIDENT DATA

1. NAME OF EMPLOYEE:
or Patient

2. ADDRESS AND PHONE NO:

3. WORK DEPT. OR DIVISION: 4. SEX: ☐ MALE ☐ FEMALE   5. DATE AND TIME OF INJURY:

6. NATURE OF INJURY: 7. PART OF BODY INJURED:

8. CAUSE OF INJURY: 9. LOCATION OF ACCIDENT:

10. OCCUPATION AND ACTIVITY OF PERSON AT TIME OF ACCIDENT: 11. STATUS OF JOB OR ACTIVITY: (CHOOSE ONE) Halted

12. NAME AND PHONE NO. OF ACCIDENT WITNESS:

13. LIST UNSAFE ACT, IF ANY:

14. LIST UNSAFE PHYSICAL OR MECHANICAL CONDITION, IF ANY:

15. UNSAFE PERSONAL FACTOR:

16. LIST HAZARD CONTROLS IN EFFECT AT TIME OF INJURY DESIGNED TO PREVENT INJURY:

17. PERSONAL PROTECTIVE EQUIPMENT BEING USED AT TIME OF ACCIDENT:
GLOVES, SAFETY GLASSES, GOGGLES, FACE SHIELD, OTHER

18. BRIEF DESCRIPTION OF ACCIDENT:

19. CORRECTIVE ACTION TAKEN OR RECOMMENDED TO DEPARTMENT SAFETY COMMITTEE:

TREATMENT DATA

20. WAS INJURED TAKEN TO (CHOOSE ONE): Hospital

21. DIAGNOSIS AND TREATMENT, IF KNOWN:

22. ESTIMATED LOST WORKDAYS: _____ (EXCLUDING DAY OF ACCIDENT)   23. DATE OF REPORT: Month | Day | Year

24. REPORT PREPARED BY:

25. SIGNATURE OF SUPERVISOR:

26. SIGNATURE OF AGENCY SAFETY AND HEALTH OFFICER:

Work Product 2

Use methods of quality control.

After Mrs. Baggins fell in the reception area (see Work Product 1), your supervisor asks you to review any other injuries in the reception area in the past 6 months. There are seven incident reports involving patient falls, and all of those occurred in some part of the reception area. Three patients slipped by the doorway on rainy days. Two more tripped on the corner of the doormat. The last two patients fell in the main lobby—one tripped over a children's toy and the other slipped on a magazine, just like Mrs. Baggins did. You are named to represent the medical assistants on a task force addressing these complaints. Assign an expected threshold using measurable, realistic goals. Explore the problem and propose solutions. Establish a QI monitoring plan explaining how data will be collected. Document the entire process and print the information to attach to this sheet. Using the blank memorandum below, write a memo to the staff with instructions to implement the solutions.

Memo

To:

From:

Date:

Re:

Chapter Self-Assessment Quiz

Scenario: It's your first day on the job as the medical office manager, so there's a lot you don't know yet about this office.

1. You want to know who's responsible for what in the office. Where is the best place to find that information?
   a. Payroll records
   b. The work schedule
   c. The chain of command chart
   d. The recent employee evaluations
   e. The bulletin board

2. You know the office is running low on paper and syringes. You're most likely to find out how to order supplies in:
   a. the QI plan.
   b. the service contracts folder.
   c. the operating budget.
   d. the policy and procedures manual.
   e. the communication notebook.

3. What is the first thing you should do about employee evaluations once you have located the file?
   a. Commit them to memory.
   b. Schedule counseling sessions with the employees.
   c. Check that employee evaluations are all on schedule.
   d. See whether there are any incident reports in the files.
   e. Reorganize the evaluations so they are at the front of the file.

4. The office keeps running out of tongue depressors. Which action should you take first?
   a. Establish a recycling program.
   b. Determine whether someone is stealing supplies.
   c. Review the system for keeping track of supplies.
   d. Tell the physicians not to use so many tongue depressors.
   e. Borrow some tongue depressors from the nearest medical office.

End Scenario

5. Which item should be in any job description?
   a. Age requirements
   b. Salary or hourly pay
   c. Physical requirements
   d. The preferred gender of the applicant
   e. Medical and dental benefits

6. Which task should you be expected to perform as medical office manager?
   a. Clean the waiting room
   b. Assign someone to make coffee
   c. Develop promotional pamphlets
   d. Assist with simple medical procedures
   e. Sign prescription refills

7. Which of the following is a medical office manager's responsibility?
   a. Completing all incident reports
   b. Teaching CPR
   c. Evaluating the physicians
   d. Hiring and firing employees
   e. Teach employees about malpractice insurance

8. Which statement is true of an incident report about a patient?
   a. It should go in the patient's file.
   b. It should be written by a physician.
   c. It should be written within 24 hours of the incident.
   d. It should be written from the patient's point of view.
   e. It should be kept in the medical office.

9. Which action should be taken if an employee is stuck by a patient's needle?
   a. The patient should be informed.
   b. The physician should take disciplinary action against the employee.
   c. The employee should write an incident report.
   d. The employee should be kept away from patients.
   e. The employee should sign a form admitting liability.

10. Which of the following categories is part of a capital budget?
    a. Payroll
    b. Medical supplies
    c. Building maintenance
    d. Heating and air conditioning
    e. Electricity

11. Which item should be part of any medical office budget?

a. Merit bonuses

b. Billing service

c. Continuing education

d. Magazine subscriptions

e. Children's play facility

12. Which agency licenses and monitors health care organizations and enforces regulations?

a. CMS

b. State health department

c. JCAHO

d. OSHA

e. HCFA

13. General liability and medical malpractice insurance is for:

a. all medical professionals.

b. all physicians.

c. physicians who perform risky procedures.

d. medical professionals with high risk profiles.

e. physicians and nurses.

14. The first step in creating a quality improvement plan is to:

a. form a task force.

b. identify the problem.

c. establish a monitoring plan.

d. assign an expected threshold.

e. explore the problem.

15. A QI program is most likely to be begun because of:

a. two needlesticks.

b. five missed cases of nail fungus.

c. two mislabeled biopsy specimens.

d. four complaints about waiting time.

e. a patient falling over in the waiting area.

16. If you fill out an incident report, you should:

a. keep a copy of the report.

b. have a supervisor review it.

c. give your title but not your name.

d. fill out only the sections that apply.

e. summarize what happened in the report.

17. A sentinel event is a(n):

a. untoward staff event.

b. step required to perform a given task.

c. unexpected death or serious injury to a patient.

d. action taken to ensure high-quality patient care and service.

e. annual performance review.

18. Which of the following is used to estimate expenditures and revenues?

a. Budget

b. Tracking file

c. Expected threshold

d. Financial statement

e. Previous expenditures

19. Risk management is a(n):

a. process begun only after a sentinel event.

b. process intended to identify potential problems.

c. external process that deals with OSHA violations.

d. internal process that deals with recurring problems.

e. process undertaken by managers to reduce annual expenditure.

20. Which of the following is true of an expected threshold for a quality improvement program?

a. It is the expected percentage reduction in risk.

b. It is a way to measure the success of the program.

c. It should be set higher for more dangerous problems.

d. It should be set lower than you think you can achieve.

e. It should only be used for particularly severe problems.

Managing the Finances in the Practice

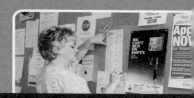

11

Credit and Collections

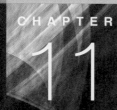

Chapter Checklist

☐ Read textbook chapter and take notes within the Chapter Notes outline. Answer the Learning Objectives as you reach them in the content, and then check them off.

☐ Work the Content Review questions—both Foundational Knowledge and Application.

☐ Perform the Active Learning exercise(s).

☐ Complete Professional Journal entries.

☐ Complete Skill Practice Activity(s) using Competency Evaluation Forms and Work Products, when appropriate.

☐ Take the Chapter Self-Assessment Quiz.

☐ Insert all appropriate pages into your Portfolio.

Learning Objectives

1. Spell and define the key terms.
2. Explain the physician fee schedule.
3. Discuss forms of payment.
4. Explain the legal considerations in extending credit.

5. Discuss the legal implications of credit collection.
6. Describe three methods of debt collection.

Chapter Notes

Note: Bold-faced headings are the major headings in the text chapter; headings in regular font are lower-level headings (i.e., the content is subordinate to, or falls "under," the major headings). Make sure you understand the key terms used in the chapter, as well as the concepts presented as Key Points.

TEXT SUBHEADINGS   **NOTES**

Introduction _____

_____

_____

☐ **LEARNING OBJECTIVE 1:** Spell and define the key terms.

Fees _____

_____

_____

_____

Fee Schedules _____

_____

Key Term: participating providers

_____

☐ **LEARNING OBJECTIVE 2:** Explain the physician fee schedule.

_____

Discussing Fees in Advance _____

_____

Key Term: patient co-payment
Key Points:
- It is always a good policy to discuss fees with patients in advance.
- Ideally you should collect the entire amount due from a new patient on the first visit.

Forms of Payment _____

_____

_____

☐ **LEARNING OBJECTIVE 3:** Discuss forms of payment.

_____

Payment by Insurance Companies _____

_____

Key Point:
- Remember, always make a copy of both sides of the patient's insurance card and place it in the appropriate section of the chart for billing reference.

_____

Adjusting Fees _____

_____

Key Terms: adjustments; professional courtesy; write-off

_____

Credit _____

_____

_____

Extending Credit _____

_____

Key Term: credit

Legal Considerations _____

_____

☐ **LEARNING OBJECTIVE 4:** Explain the legal considerations in extending credit.

Collections _____

_____

_____

Legal Considerations _____

_____

☐ **LEARNING OBJECTIVE 5:** Discuss the legal implications of credit collection.

Collecting a Debt _____

_____

Monthly Billing _____

_____

Key Term: installment
Key Point:
• If your facility changes a billing cycle, you are legally required to notify patients of the change 3 months before the
change takes effect.

Aging Accounts _____

_____

Key Term: aging schedule

Collecting Overdue Accounts _____

_____

☐ **LEARNING OBJECTIVE 6:** Describe three methods of debt collection.

Collection Alternatives _____

_____

Key Term: collections

_____

Content Review

FOUNDATIONAL KNOWLEDGE

1. Office visit fees are usually based on the UCR system. Match the letters in "UCR" with their explanations.

Fees

U (usual) _____
C (customary) _____
R (reasonable) _____

Explanations

a. The fee is a good balance between cost and the clients' expectations.
b. The fee is based on the actual value of the service being provided.
c. The fee is competitive with fees charged by other local practices.

2. Fee setting also considers RBRVS, by which fees are adjusted for geographical differences. What does RBRVS stand for?

_____

_____

3. There should be a sign posted in the office, where patients can see it, giving information about procedure fees. What should be on the sign?

_____

_____

4. Which third-party payers affect fee schedules if the physicians in your office are participating providers, and how many fee schedules might there be?

_____

_____

5. Fill in the missing parts with the things you should do to improve the success of fee collection.

What	When	Why
a. _____	Before any procedure is done	To ensure that patients are aware of the charges
Collect the entire co-pay or other amount due from a new patient.	**b.** _____	To lower your accounts receivable and improve cash flow
Get a picture identification and complete contact information from a new patient, including the names, numbers, and relationships of contacts who can give you information about the patient's location.	On the first visit	**c.** _____

6. Patients are usually allowed to pay for services with cash, a personal check, debit card, or credit card.

   a. If a new patient is paying by check, what should you do?

_____

_____

   b. The office pays a credit card company a percentage. Why is it still sometimes cost effective to accept payment by credit card?

_____

_____

7. How often should you ask the patient for his insurance card, and what should you do with it when you get it?

_____

_____

8. Compare and contrast fee adjustments and fee write-offs in the diagram below.

Professional Courtesy Fees	**Both**	**Fee Write-offs**
• _____	• result in reduced income	• _____
	• _____	

Cash or Credit?

9. Fill out the following 5W chart about extending credit.

Extending Credit

Who	For patients
What	
Where	
Why	
Watch out	

Collection Time

10. Your office employs a billing cycle based on patients' last names. Here is when patients are billed:
- A-H on the 1st of the month
- I-P on the 15th of the month
- Q-Z on the 22nd of the month

Organize the patients below in the chart to determine when you should send their bills in October.

October 1	October 15	October 22

Sanquetta Jones	Taylor Harris	Kim Dewar	Taneesha Rockfield
Imani Wilson	Haywood Barry	Valerie Angeles	Isabelle Smith
Tisha Matthews	Mekhi Currant	So Yin	Seth Noh

11. All the statements below are false or inaccurate. Rewrite each statement so that it accurately reflects the consumer protection laws regarding credit collection.

a. You cannot contact a patient directly about an unpaid bill.

_____

_____

b. You should not try to contact a debtor before 9:00 a.m. or after 5:00 p.m.

_____

_____

c. You have every right to call debtors at work.

_____

_____

d. You should keep calling a patient about a debt after turning the case over to a collection agency, in order to increase your chances of recovering the money.

_____

_____

e. It's okay to use abusive language to intimidate a debtor, as long as you don't give false or misleading information.

_____

_____

f. If a patient dies and the estate can't meet all her debts, the probate court will pay the medical bills first.

_____

_____

12. The three most common ways of collecting overdue accounts are:

a. _____

b. _____

c. _____

13. List three situations in which calling a patient to collect an overdue payment may be least helpful.

a. _____

b. _____

c. _____

14. What should be in a mailing that asks a patient to settle an overdue account?

_____

_____

15. What is a good way to use a patient's visit as an opportunity to try to collect payment on an overdue bill?

_____

_____

16. What should you say and not say if you call a patient to collect on a bill and you are asked to leave a message?

_____

_____

17. For each line in the box below, put an **X** in the "Office" column and/or the "Collection Agency" column to indicate who can take the action.

Action	Office	Collection Agency
Send overdue notices.		
Call patients who have overdue bills.		
Remind patients of bills during office visits.		
Sue in small claims court.		
List debtors with credit bureaus.		

18. How many times should you contact patients asking them to pay overdue bills? Why?

_____

_____

19. Match the following key terms to their definitions.

Key Terms

a. adjustment _____

b. aging schedule _____

c. collections _____

d. credit _____

e. installment _____

f. participating provider _____

g. patient co-payment _____

h. professional courtesy _____

i. write-off _____

Definitions

1. a change in a posted account

2. a total bill being paid off over time

3. process of seeking payment for overdue bills

4. arrangement for a patient to pay on an installment plan

5. charging other health care professionals a reduced rate

6. cancellation of an unpaid debt, usually claimed on the practice's federal taxes

7. a certain share of the bill that a managed care company usually requires the patient to pay

8. physician who agrees to participate with managed care companies and other third-party payers

9. record of a patient's name, balance, payments made, time of outstanding debt, and relevant comments

20. True of False? Determine whether the following statements are true or false. If false, explain why.

a. A physician's fee schedule takes into consideration the costs of operating the office, such as rent, utilities, malpractice insurance, and salaries.

_____

_____

b. If a patient has insurance, you must charge him the insurance carrier's allowed fee for a procedure.

_____

_____

c. To maintain good relations with patients, you should be vague and polite when you ask them to pay their bills.

_____

_____

d. You should monitor the activity on a patient's credit account in order to keep the collection ratio low.

_____

_____

APPLICATION

Critical Thinking Practice

1. What are some of the negative aspects of extending credit to patients? Consider costs, patient attitudes, and legal requirements in your answer.

_____

_____

2. You have several patients who have long-outstanding debts. They don't come into the office anymore, and they don't respond to your telephone calls or letters. The physicians in the practice are absolutely against using a collection agency. What avenues are open to you to help you collect the debts?

_____

_____

Patient Education

1. Mrs. Sanchez is seeing Dr. Roland for the first time and has asked you to explain the physician's fees. Explain to Mrs. Sanchez how Dr. Roland establishes the fees he charges his patients.

_____

_____

Documentation

1. If your office has a computerized billing system, it will automatically document any overdue notices you send to patients to collect fees. However, you have the options of calling patients and speaking to them while they're in the office. Those events won't be automatically input into the computer records, but it's very important that you keep track of them. How could you do that?

_____

_____

Active Learning

1. Use the Internet to research the three major credit bureaus and find out how to check a new patient's credit history. Specifically, find out what's available to help you decide how to handle payment from people without traditional credit histories. This group includes college students, young adults, recent immigrants, traditional housewives, and people who choose not to use credit cards.

2. Many people feel uncomfortable asking other people for money. However, you need to feel comfortable discussing finance and account information with patients. Working with a partner, role-play a scenario in which a patient has an overdue account that the medical assistant must address. Take turns playing the parts of the medical assistant and the patient to understand both perspectives.

3. In recent years, the government has called into question the practice of professional courtesy extended to other health care professionals. Perform research online or talk to health care professionals to find out more about the issues surrounding professional courtesy. Then write a viewpoint paper arguing for or against the practice of professional courtesy.

Professional Journal

REFLECT

(Prompts and Ideas: Have you or a loved one ever been unable to pay a bill right away or been in deep debt? How were you treated, or how do you wish you had been treated? How do you think you may be able to handle debt collections with the right amount of sensitivity toward your patients?)

_____

_____

_____

_____

_____

_____

PONDER AND SOLVE

1. Mr. Green has been a patient with your practice for more than 20 years and has always paid his co-payment or bill before he left the office. Recently, however, he has not been paying anything at all, and his outstanding bill is 60 days past due. You have called his home and left several phone messages, but you still haven't heard from him. What should you do?

_____

_____

_____

_____

_____

2. You outsourced your overdue billing to a collections agency in order to give yourself time to devise a better inventory system, but a few of your long-time patients have told you that they have been very upset by the "nastiness" of the collections people who contacted them. You spoke with a collections agency representative who assured you his employees were doing nothing illegal or inappropriate. However, a week later, another patient apologized for being late on a bill and confided to you that the unnerving call from the collector had gravely upset her. What should you do?

_____

_____

_____

_____

EXPERIENCE

Skills related to this chapter include:

1. Evaluating and Managing a Patient Account (Procedure 11-1).

2. Composing a Collection Letter (Procedure 11-2).

Record any common mistakes, lessons learned, and/or tips you discovered during your experience of practicing and demonstrating these skills.

_____

_____

_____

_____

_____

_____

_____

Skill Practice

PERFORMANCE OBJECTIVES:

1. Evaluate and manage a patient account (Procedure 11-1).
2. Write a collection letter (Procedure 11-2).

Name _____ Date _____ Time _____

Procedure 11-1:	**EVALUATE AND MANAGE A PATIENT'S ACCOUNT**

EQUIPMENT: Simulation including scenario; sample patient ledger card with transactions; yellow, blue, and red stickers (yellow for accounts 30 days past due; blue for accounts 60 days past due; red for accounts 90 days past due)

STANDARDS: Given the needed equipment and a place to work the student will perform this skill with _____% accuracy in a total of _____ minutes. (*Your instructor will tell you what the percentage and time limits will be before you begin.*)

KEY: 4 = Satisfactory   0 = Unsatisfactory   NA = This step is not counted

PROCEDURE STEPS	SELF	PARTNER	INSTRUCTOR
1. Review the patient's account history to determine the "age" of the account. If payment has not been made between 30 and 59 days from today's date, the account is 40 days past due, and so on.	☐	☐	☐
2. Flag the account for appropriate action. Place a yellow flag (sticker) on accounts that are 30 days old. Place a blue flag on accounts that are 60 days old. Place a red flag on accounts that are 90 days old.	☐	☐	☐
3. Set aside accounts that have had no payment in 91 days or longer.	☐	☐	☐
4. Make copies of the ledger cards.	☐	☐	☐
5. Sort the copies by category: 30, 60, 90 days.	☐	☐	☐
6. Write or stamp the copies with the appropriate message.	☐	☐	☐
7. Mail the statements to the patients.	☐	☐	☐
8. Follow through with the collection process by continually reviewing past due accounts.	☐	☐	☐

CALCULATION

Total Possible Points: _____
Total Points Earned: _____ Multiplied by 100 = _____ Divided by Total Possible Points = _____%

Pass   **Fail**
☐   ☐   Comments:

Student's signature _____ Date _____
Partner's signature _____ Date _____
Instructor's signature _____ Date _____

Name_____ Date_____ Time_____

Procedure 11-2:	COMPOSING A COLLECTION LETTER

EQUIPMENT: Ledger cards generated in Procedure 11-1, word processor, stationery with letterhead

STANDARDS: Given the needed equipment and a place to work the student will perform this skill with _____% accuracy in a total of _____ minutes. (*Your instructor will tell you what the percentage and time limits will be before you begin.*)

KEY: 4 = Satisfactory   0 = Unsatisfactory   NA = This step is not counted

PROCEDURE STEPS	SELF	PARTNER	INSTRUCTOR
1. Review the patients' accounts and sort the accounts by age.	☐	☐	☐
2. Design a rough draft of a form letter that can be used for collections.	☐	☐	☐
3. In the first paragraph, tell the patient why you are writing.	☐	☐	☐
4. Inform the patient of the action you expect. For example: "To avoid further action, please pay $50.00 on this account by Friday, May 1, 20__."	☐	☐	☐
5. Proofread the rough draft for errors, clarity, accuracy, and retype.	☐	☐	☐
6. Take the collection letter to a supervisor or physician for approval.	☐	☐	☐
7. Fill in the appropriate amounts and dates on each letter. Ask for at least half of the account balance within a two-week period.	☐	☐	☐
8. Print, sign, and mail the letter.	☐	☐	☐

CALCULATION

Total Possible Points: _____
Total Points Earned: _____ Multiplied by 100 = _____ Divided by Total Possible Points = _____%

Pass   **Fail**
☐   ☐ | Comments: |

Student's signature _____ Date _____
Partner's signature _____ Date _____
Instructor's signature _____ Date _____

Work Product 1

Perform Accounts Receivable Procedures.

Your office's billing cycle posts bills on the first of every month. Review the list of outstanding payments and organize in the Aging of Accounts Receivable Report below.

- Oliver Santino visited the office on April 27 for a physical and blood work. The bill was $250.
- Warren Gates visited the office on May 8. His bill was $55.
- Tamara Jones visited the office on June 18 for a physical. The cost for the physical was $125, with an additional $55 for lab work.
- Amir Shell visited the office on June 25 for a physical exam and chest x-rays. The bill was $315.
- Nora Stevenson visited the office on July 9 to have a wound sutured. The bill was $100.

Below is an aging schedule as of August 30, 2008. Please fill in the information for these patients. Please enter an account number of 000-00-0000 for all patients.

Aging of Accounts Receivable Report: August 30, 2008

Patient Name	Account Number	Due Date	Amount

Accounts 30 Days Past Due:

_____ _____   _____   _____
_____ _____   _____   _____
_____ _____   _____   _____
_____ _____   _____   _____
_____ _____   _____   _____

Accounts 60 Days Past Due:

_____ _____   _____   _____
_____ _____   _____   _____
_____ _____   _____   _____
_____ _____   _____   _____
_____ _____   _____   _____

Accounts 90 Days Past Due:

_____ _____   _____   _____
_____ _____   _____   _____
_____ _____   _____   _____
_____ _____   _____   _____

Accounts 120 Days or More Past Due:

_____ _____   _____   _____
_____ _____   _____   _____
_____ _____   _____   _____
_____ _____   _____   _____
_____ _____   _____   _____

Total Overdue Accounts Receivable   _____

Work Product 2

Perform Billing and Collection Procedures.

Caroline Cusick has an outstanding balance of $415 due to the medical office Pediatric Associates, 1415 San Juan Way, Santa Cruz, CA 95060. Write a collection letter to the patient to tell her about her overdue account. Her contact information is as follows: Caroline Cusick, 24 Beach Street, Santa Cruz, CA 95060. Print the letter and attach to this sheet.

Chapter Self-Assessment Quiz

1. The total of all the charges posted to patients' accounts for the month of May is $16,000. The revenues the practice received for May total $12,000. What is the collection percentage for May?

   a. 5 percent
   b. 25 percent
   c. 75 percent
   d. 80 percent
   e. 133 percent

2. Interest that may be charged to a patient account is determined by:

   a. the physician.
   b. the patient.
   c. the insurance company.
   d. the law.
   e. the state.

3. In the UCR concept, the letters stand for:

   a. user, customer, and regulation.
   b. usual, competitive, and regular.
   c. usage, consumption, and return.
   d. usual, customary, and reasonable.
   e. usage, complaint, and rationale.

4. When credit cards are accepted by a medical practice, the medical practice generally agrees to pay the credit card company:

   a. 5.2 percent.
   b. 1.8 percent.
   c. 15 percent.
   d. 3.1 percent.
   e. 25 percent.

5. Federal regulations require each medical office to describe its services and procedures and to give the procedure codes and prices by:

   a. giving a list to each patient at check in.
   b. offering the list to each patient at payment.
   c. posting a sign stating that a list is available.
   d. answering a patient's questions about billing.
   e. placing an ad in the newspaper describing the fees.

6. Physicians who chose to become participating providers with third-party payers usually do so in order to:

   a. charge higher fees.
   b. simplify fee schedules.
   c. build a solid patient base.
   d. reduce the time before payment.
   e. share a patient load with another physician.

7. It is a good and ethical business practice to:

   a. take payment in cash only.
   b. accept only patients who have insurance.
   c. refuse patients who have third-party payment plans.
   d. discuss fees with patients before they see a physician or nurse.
   e. charge the patient a small fee for paying with a credit card.

8. When dealing with a new patient, you should avoid:

   a. taking cash.
   b. taking a partial payment.
   c. taking a check with two picture IDs.
   d. taking co-payment with an insurance card.
   e. taking a payment by credit card.

9. Most fees for medical services:

   a. are paid by insurance companies.

   b. are paid by Medicare and Medicaid.

   c. are paid by patients who are private payers.

   d. are written off on the practice's federal taxes.

   e. are paid to the physician late.

10. When an insurance adjustment is made to a fee:

   a. the patient is charged less than the normal rate.

   b. the medical office receives more than its normal rate.

   c. the insurance carrier pays the adjustment rate.

   d. the insurance carrier's explanation of benefits shows how much the office may collect for the service.

   e. the difference between the physician's normal fee and the insurance carrier's allowed fee is written off.

11. Why would a medical office extend credit to a patient?

   a. To save money

   b. To accommodate the patient

   c. To postpone paying income tax

   d. To charge interest

   e. To make billing more cost effective

12. Why do many medical offices outsource their credit and billing functions?

   a. They don't want to ask their patients for money directly.

   b. They are not licensed to manage credit card transactions.

   c. Creating their own installment plans is too complicated legally.

   d. Managing patient accounts themselves costs about $5 per month per patient.

   e. Billing companies can manage the accounts more cost effectively.

13. It is illegal for a medical office to

   a. use a collection agency.

   b. disclose fee information to patients who have insurance.

   c. deny credit to patients because they receive public assistance.

   d. charge patients interest, finance charges, or late fees on unpaid balances.

   e. change their established billing cycle

14. If you are attempting to collect a debt from a patient, you must:

   a. use reasonable self-restraint.

   b. call the patient only at home.

   c. hire a licensed bill collection agency.

   d. first take the patient to small claims court.

   e. wait one year before you can ask for payment.

15. When first attempting to collect a debt by telephone, you should:

   a. ask the patient to come in for a checkup.

   b. contact the patient before 8:00 AM or after 9:00 PM

   c. contact the patient only at his place of employment.

   d. leave a message explaining the situation on the answering machine.

   e. speak only to the patient or leave only your first name and number.

16. When you are collecting a debt from an estate, it is best to:

   a. send a final bill to the estate's executor.

   b. take the matter directly to small claims court.

   c. try to collect within a week of the patient's death.

   d. allow the family a month to mourn before asking for payment.

   e. ask a collection agency to contact the family.

17. If a billing cycle is to be changed, you are legally required to notify patients:

   a. one month before their payment is due.

   b. before the next scheduled appointment.

   c. three months prior to the billing change.

   d. after you approve the change with the insurance company.

   e. only if they have outstanding payments.

18. When you age an account, you:

   a. write off debts that have been outstanding longer than 120 days.

   b. send bills first to the patients who had the most recent procedures.

   c. organize patient accounts by how long they have been seeing the physician.

   d. calculate the time between the last bill and the date of the last payment.

   e. determine the time between the procedure and the date of the last payment.

19. A cancellation of an unpaid debt is called a(n):

   a. professional courtesy.

   b. co-payment.

   c. write-off.

   d. adjustment.

   e. credit.

20. Which collections method takes the least staff time?

   a. Using a collection agency

   b. Going to small claims court

   c. Billing the patient monthly until paid

   d. Scheduling all payments on the first of the month

   e. Reporting patients to the credit bureaus

Accounting Responsibilities

☐ Read textbook chapter and take notes within the Chapter Notes outline. Answer the Learning Objectives as you reach them in the content, and then check them off.

☐ Work the Content Review questions—both Foundational Knowledge and Application.

☐ Perform the Active Learning exercise(s).

☐ Complete Professional Journal entries.

☐ Complete Skill Practice Activity(s) using Competency Evaluation Forms and Work Products, when appropriate.

☐ Take the Chapter Self-Assessment Quiz.

☐ Insert all appropriate pages into your Portfolio.

1. Spell and define the key terms.
2. Explain the concept of the pegboard book-keeping system.
3. Describe the components of the pegboard system.
4. Identify and discuss the special features of the pegboard day sheet.
5. Describe the functions of a computer accounting system.
6. List the uses and components of computer accounting reports.
7. Explain banking services, including types of accounts and fees.
8. Describe the accounting cycle.
9. Describe the components of a record-keeping system.
10. Explain the process of ordering supplies and paying invoices.

Note: Bold-faced headings are the major headings in the text chapter; headings in regular font are lower-level headings (i.e., the content is subordinate to, or falls "under," the major headings). Make sure you understand the key terms used in the chapter, as well as the concepts presented as Key Points.

TEXT SUBHEADINGS

NOTES

Introduction _____

_____

_____

☐ **LEARNING OBJECTIVE 1:** Spell and define the key terms.

Accounts Receivable and Daily Bookkeeping _____

_____

Key Terms: bookkeeping; balance; debit; credit
Key Point:
• Because the two sides of the accounting equation must always **balance** (be equal), each transaction requires a **debit** (charge) on one side of the equation and a **credit** (payment) on the other side of the equation; the amount of the debit and credit must be equal.

Manual Accounting _____

_____

_____

Pegboard Bookkeeping System _____

_____

Key Terms: day sheet; ledger card; charge slip
Key Point:
• At the end of the day, all of the transactions are added.

☐ **LEARNING OBJECTIVE 2:** Explain the concept of the pegboard bookkeeping system.

☐ **LEARNING OBJECTIVE 3:** Describe the components of the pegboard system.

Day Sheet _____

_____

Key Terms: posting; adjustment
Key Points:
• The day sheet keeps track of daily patient transactions, such as charges for services to patients, payments received from patients and insurance carriers, and adjustments to patient accounts.
• You should perform a trial balance at the end of each month.

☐ **LEARNING OBJECTIVE 4:** Identify and discuss the special features of the pegboard day sheet.

Ledger Cards _____

_____

Key Term: ledger card
Key Point:
• The ledger card is a legal document and should be kept for the same length of time as the patient's medical record.

Encounter Forms and Charge Slips _____

Key Term: encounter form

Posting a Charge _____

Key Point:
• The charge column of the day sheet is for original charges incurred for services received by the patient from the physician or staff on a specific date.

Posting a Payment _____

Processing a Credit Balance _____

Key Point:
• Brackets indicate the opposite of the column's usual meaning.

Processing Refunds _____

Posting a Credit Adjustment _____

Posting a Debit Adjustment _____

Posting to Cash-Paid-Out Section of Day Sheet _____

Computerized Accounting _____

☐ **LEARNING OBJECTIVE 5:** Describe the functions of a computer accounting system.

Posting to Computer Accounts _____

_____

Key Point:
- If you understand the fundamentals of accounting and how to post entries manually, you will be able to use a computer system with ease.

Computer Accounting Reports _____

_____

☐ **LEARNING OBJECTIVE 6:** List the uses and components of computer accounting reports.

Banks and Their Services _____

_____

Types of Accounts _____

_____

Checking Accounts _____

_____

Key Point:
- A checking account allows you to write checks for funds that are deposited in the account.

Savings Accounts _____

_____

Money Market Accounts _____

_____

Bank Fees _____

_____

Monthly Service Fees _____

_____

Key Term: service charge

Overdraft Protection _____

_____

_____

Returned Check Fee _____

_____

Key Term: returned check fee

☐ **LEARNING OBJECTIVE 7:** Explain banking services, including types of accounts and fees.

Types of Checks _____

_____

_____

Banking Responsibilities _____

_____

_____

Writing Checks for Accounts Payable _____

_____

Key Point:
• Banks require signature cards for each person authorized to sign checks.

Receiving Checks and Making Deposits _____

_____

Key Point:
• This way, if the payments are lost or stolen, no one else can cash them.

Reconciling Bank Statements _____

_____

Key Point:
• This bank statement must be reconciled, or compared for accuracy, with your records each month.

Petty Cash _____

_____

Key Point:
• The value of the petty cash account should always remain the same.

Overview of Accounting _____

_____

_____

Accounting Cycle _____

_____

> **Key Terms:** accounting cycle; Internal Revenue Service (IRS); audit

☐ **LEARNING OBJECTIVE 8:** Describe the accounting cycle.

Record-Keeping Components _____

_____

> **Key Terms:** payroll; liabilities; check register; summation reports; profit-and-loss statement
> **Key Points:**
> - The practice's financial records should include a running record of income, accounts receivable, and total expenditures, including **payroll** (employee salaries), cash on hand, and **liabilities** (amounts the practice owes).
> - Software packages offer the most sophisticated way to maintain financial records, not just for the categorization of expenses but also for the rapid formation of financial reports.
> - If financial data are entered diligently into the bookkeeping system, preparing monthly, quarterly, or yearly reports should not be a daunting task.

☐ **LEARNING OBJECTIVE 9:** Describe the components of a record-keeping system.

Accounts Payable _____

_____

_____

Ordering Goods and Services _____

_____

> **Key Term:** purchase order

Receiving Supplies _____

_____

> **Key Terms:** packing slip; invoice

Paying Invoices _____

_____

_____

Manual Payment _____

_____

Key Term: check stub
Key Point:
• Memos or notations on **check stubs** can be referenced later if a question arises concerning payment by a particular check.

Pegboard Payment _____

_____

Key Term: check register

Computer Payment _____

_____

☐ **LEARNING OBJECTIVE 10:** Explain the process of ordering supplies and paying invoices.

Preparation of Reports _____

_____

_____

Assisting With Audits _____

_____

Key Term: audit

Content Review

FOUNDATIONAL KNOWLEDGE

Features of the Pegboard

1. What is the concept of the pegboard bookkeeping system?

_____

_____

2. A new assistant unfamiliar with the pegboard bookkeeping has asked you to explain the system to her. Briefly describe each component to her.

Component	Description
a. day sheet	
b. ledger card	
c. charge slip	
d. ledger tray	

3. Match the feature of the pegboard day sheet with the proper description.

Feature of Pegboard Day Sheet

a. deposit slip _____

b. distribution columns _____

c. payments _____

d. adjustments _____

e. posting proofs _____

Description

1. used to assign charges for various services

2. the section where you allow for reductions in fees, adding credit to an account, or reinstating charges when a check is returned

3. used to deposit all payments received from patients in the bank

4. the section where you enter the day's totals and balance the sheet

5. the section where you record all payments received

Computerized Accounting Functions

4. There are several advantages of a computerized system over a manual system. Read the selection below, and circle the functions that are computerized accounting functions only.

  a. Entries are recorded in a patient's file

  b. Quickly create invoices and receipts

  c. Calculation of each transaction is made, as well as a total at the end of the day

  d. Performs bookkeeping, making appointments, and generating office reports

  e. Daily activities are recorded

  f. Bill reminders are placed to keep track of expenses

5. The office you are working in has recently updated its bookkeeping system from pegboard to computer. Now, the physician wants to utilize all the capabilities the new system offers. One particular function that interests her is the computer accounting reports. List the different types of reports and briefly describe their uses.

  a. _____

  b. _____

  c. _____

Banking Ins and Outs

6. What are banking services?

_____

_____

7. A medical office is just starting up, and one of the first things the bookkeeper needs to do is find a bank. Fill in the chart below with descriptions of checking, savings, and money market accounts.

Checking Account	Savings Account	Money Market Account

8. What is a returned check fee?

_____

_____

9. The office you are working in has an accounting cycle that begins in June. Describe what the accounting cycle is, and what kind of year your office follows.

_____

_____

10. The office manager ordered a new endorsement stamp from the bank. In the meantime, you need to deposit a check for Rinku Banjere, MD, into account number 123-4567-890. Endorse the check below for deposit.

ENDORSE HERE

_____

_____

_____

DO NOT SIGN/WRITE/STAMP BELOW THIS LINE
FOR FINANCIAL INSTITUTION USE ONLY*

11. List four items that should be readily available in case your office is audited.

a. _____

b. _____

c. _____

d. _____

12. When is it unnecessary to use a charge slip?

_____

_____

13. Why is correction fluid not used in a medical office, and what is the proper procedure to correct a mistake?

_____

_____

14. Why might you run a trial daily report before you run a final daily report?

_____

_____

15. When a patient's check has been returned for insufficient funds, what do you do if the patient asks you to send it back through the bank?

_____

_____

Taking Stock of Supplies and Inventory

16. What are four steps you can take if an item you ordered was not delivered?

a. _____

b. _____

c. _____

d. _____

17. Explain the process of ordering supplies and paying invoices.

_____

_____

18. Where can you find the order number to confirm that an item has been shipped?

_____

_____

19. Match the following key terms to their definitions.

Key Terms	**Definitions**
a. accounting cycle _____	**1.** a preprinted three-part form that can be placed on a day sheet to record the patient's charges and payments along with other information in an encounter form
b. accounts payable _____	
c. adjustment _____	**2.** a charge or money owed to an account
d. audit _____	**3.** a record of all money owed to the business
e. balance _____	**4.** a document that accompanies a supply order and lists the enclosed items
f. bookkeeping _____	**5.** any report that provides a summary of activities, such as a payroll report or profit-and-loss statement
g. charge slip _____	
h. check register _____	**6.** a daily business record of charges and payments
i. check stub _____	**7.** a statement of income and expenditures; shows whether in a given period a business made or lost money and how much
j. credit _____	
k. day sheet _____	**8.** statement of debt owed; a bill
l. debit _____	**9.** a review of an account
m. encounter form _____	**10.** a consecutive 12-month period for financial record keeping following either a fiscal year or the calendar year
n. Internal Revenue Service (IRS) _____	
o. invoice _____	**11.** a balance in one's favor on an account; a promise to pay a bill at a later date; record of payment received

p. liabilities _____

q. ledger card _____

r. packing slip _____

s. posting _____

t. profit-and-loss statement _____

u. purchase order _____

v. returned check fee _____

w. service charge _____

x. summation report _____

12. listing financial transactions in a ledger

13. a continuous record of business transactions with debits and credits

14. change in a posted account

15. a federal agency that regulates and enforces various taxes

16. amount of money a bank or business charges for a check written on an account with insufficient funds

17. amounts of money the practice owes

18. organized and accurate record-keeping system of financial transactions

19. a document that lists required items to be purchased

20. preprinted patient statement that lists codes for basic office charges and has sections to record charges incurred in an office visit, the patient's current balance, and next appointment

21. that which is left over after the additions and subtractions have been made to an account

22. piece of paper that indicates to whom a check was issued, in what amount, and on what date

23. a document used to record the checks that have been written

24. a charge by a bank for various services

20. True or False? Determine whether the following statements are true or false. If false, explain why.

a. Once you have entered a patient transaction on the day sheet, you give the ledger to the patient as a receipt.

_____

_____

b. As long as your bookkeeping records are accurate and the figures balance, you do not need to save receipts.

_____

_____

c. You should always compare the prices and quality of office supplies when you are placing an order.

_____

_____

d. Audits are performed in the office yearly by the IRS.

_____

_____

APPLICATION

Critical Thinking Practice

1. During a staff meeting, the issue of ordering supplies comes up. The office has been buying small quantities of all supplies, causing some items to quickly run out, while others are stockpiled in disuse. The head physician wants to figure out a way to spend the budget more efficiently, and asks you to be in charge of the next order. What steps can you take to determine which items you will order in the office's next purchase? How can you further improve the office's expenditure?

_____

_____

2. Your office currently is using a checking account at a local bank. However, the physician you work for is thinking about changing over to a money market account, because he has heard the interest is much better in a money market account. He knows about an offer through another bank that will waive the minimum balance of $500 for 3 months. What important information should you look into before you give him your opinion? Discuss the differences between a checking account and a money market account, and include the advantages and disadvantages to switching accounts.

_____

_____

Patient Education

1. Your patient is a young woman who does not understand what happens to the difference between what a physician charges and what her insurance company will pay. In her case, the physician's charge is $100, but insurance only allows for $80. The insurance company will pay for 75% of the cost. How much will the patient pay? Explain to her how this works, and how the charge is determined.

_____

_____

Documentation
1. A patient comes in for an office visit, which costs $60. When he comes to pay his bill, he gives you his insurance information. The insurance company will pay for 60% of the procedure. How would you document this on his ledger and on the day sheet?

_____

_____

Active Learning

1. One of the most important aspects of maintaining an orderly office is making sure that the supplies are fully stocked and up to standards. You have been put in charge of ordering new supplies for the office, and you need to see what options are available to you. Go online and compare prices of two different medical suppliers. Make a note of how many units are sold per order, if there is a minimum purchase limit, how long shipping will take, and what shipping might cost. Select five items that you will order for your office, and fill out a purchasing order for those items.

2. Budgeting for new supplies and keeping track of the office budget is another important part of your job. However, this skill can be used in your own life to assess your spending habits. Whenever you go shopping for food or for other items, or whenever you pay the bills, you must take into account your own budget and need for that item. Over the next few weeks, keep track of your spending habits. List each item you buy, as well as the price of that item. Make a note if it was on sale, or if you paid full price for it. After you have made at least four separate entries, examine your results. Which items on the list were most important? Which items would you forgo if you were on a tighter budget? How would you change your spending habits?

3. Working with a fellow student, go through the process of using a pegboard system. Make sure you fill out the day sheet completely, and go through each step from start to finish. Take turns being the patient and the office assistant. Be sure to practice dealing with credit, debit, and returned check charges, and change methods of payment with each turn.

Professional Journal

REFLECT

(Prompts and Ideas: Do you have a natural talent and/or interest in working with numbers and accounting tasks? If so, what do you like about it? If not, what can you do to increase your comfort level?)

_____

_____

_____

_____

_____

_____

PONDER AND SOLVE

1. A patient whose checks have repeatedly bounced has come in for some minor surgery. The physician at your office does not want to perform the surgery without guarantee of payment. What do you say to both patient and physician in this instance? What steps can you take to prevent future situations similar to this?

_____

_____

_____

_____

_____

2. Another assistant in your office is responsible for maintaining the books and financial records in your office. One of her responsibilities is keeping track of the petty cash. You have noticed that recently she has been borrowing money from the petty cash to buy lunch. She always returns the money within the next few days, but you know that this is not standard office policy. How would you address this issue?

_____

_____

_____

_____

_____

_____

EXPERIENCE

Skills related to this chapter include:

1. Posting Charges on a Daysheet (Procedure 12-1).
2. Posting Payments on a Daysheet (Procedure 12-2).
3. Processing a Credit Balance (Procedure 12-3).
4. Processing Refunds (Procedure 12-4).
5. Posting Adjustments (Procedure 12-5).
6. Posting Collection Agency Payments (Procedure 12-6).
7. Posting NSF Checks (Procedure 12-7).
8. Balancing a Daysheet (Procedure 12-8).
9. Completing a Bank Deposit Slip and Make a Deposit (Procedure 12-9).
10. Reconciling a Bank Statement (Procedure 12-10).
11. Maintaining a Petty Cash Account (Procedure 12-11).
12. Ordering Supplies (Procedure 12-12).
13. Writing a Check (Procedure 12-13).

Record any common mistakes, lessons learned, and/or tips you discovered during your experience of practicing and demonstrating these skills:

_____
_____
_____
_____
_____
_____
_____

Skill Practice

PERFORMANCE OBJECTIVES:

1. Post charges on a daysheet (Procedure 12-1).
2. Post payments on a daysheet (Procedure 12-2).
3. Process a credit balance (Procedure 12-3).
4. Process refunds (Procedure 12-4).
5. Post adjustments (Procedure 12-5).
6. Post collection agency payments (Procedure 12-6).
7. Post NSF checks (Procedure 12-7).
8. Balance a daysheet (Procedure 12-8).
9. Complete a bank deposit slip and make a deposit (Procedure 12-9).
10. Reconcile a bank statement (Procedure 12-10).
11. Maintain a petty cash account (Procedure 12-11).
12. Order supplies (Procedure 12-12).
13. Write a check (Procedure 12-13).

Name_____ Date _____ Time _____

Procedure 12-1:	**POST CHARGES ON A DAYSHEET**

EQUIPMENT/SUPPLIES: Pen, pegboard, calculator, daysheet, encounter forms, ledger cards, previous day's balance, list of patients and charges, fee schedule

STANDARDS: Given the needed equipment and a place to work the student will perform this skill with _____% accuracy in a total of _____ minutes. (*Your instructor will tell you what the percentage and time limits will be before you begin.*)

KEY: 4 = Satisfactory   0 = Unsatisfactory   NA = This step is not counted

PROCEDURE STEPS	SELF	PARTNER	INSTRUCTOR
1. Place a new daysheet on the pegboard and record the totals from the previous daysheet.	☐	☐	☐
2. Align the patient's ledger card with the first available line on the daysheet.	☐	☐	☐
3. Place the receipt to align with the appropriate line on the ledger card.	☐	☐	☐
4. Record the number of the receipt in the appropriate column.	☐	☐	☐
5. Write the patient's name on the receipt.	☐	☐	☐
6. Record any existing balance the patient owes in the previous balance column of the daysheet.	☐	☐	☐
7. Record a brief description of the charge in the description line.	☐	☐	☐
8. Record the total charges in the charge column. Press hard so that the marks go through to the ledger card and the daysheet.	☐	☐	☐
9. Add the total charges to the previous balance and record in the current balance column.	☐	☐	☐
10. Return the ledger card to appropriate storage.	☐	☐	☐

CALCULATION

Total Possible Points: _____
Total Points Earned: _____ Multiplied by 100 = _____ Divided by Total Possible Points = _____%

Pass   **Fail**
☐   ☐   Comments:

Student's signature _____ Date _____
Partner's signature _____ Date _____
Instructor's signature _____ Date _____

Name_____ Date_____ Time_____

Procedure 12-2:	POST PAYMENTS ON A DAYSHEET

EQUIPMENT/SUPPLIES: Pen, pegboard, calculator, daysheet, encounter forms, ledger cards, previous day's balance, list of patients and charges, fee schedule

COMPUTER AND MEDICAL OFFICE SOFTWARE: Follow the software requirements for posting credits to patient accounts.

STANDARDS: Given the needed equipment and a place to work the student will perform this skill with _____% accuracy in a total of _____ minutes. (*Your instructor will tell you what the percentage and time limits will be before you begin.*)

KEY: 4 = Satisfactory   0 = Unsatisfactory   NA = This step is not counted

PROCEDURE STEPS	SELF	PARTNER	INSTRUCTOR
1. Place a new daysheet on the pegboard and record the totals from the previous daysheet.	☐	☐	☐
2. Align the patient's ledger card with the first available line on the daysheet.	☐	☐	☐
3. Place receipt to align with the appropriate line on the ledger card.	☐	☐	☐
4. Record the number of the receipt in the appropriate column.	☐	☐	☐
5. Write the patient's name on the receipt.	☐	☐	☐
6. Record any existing balance the patient owes in the previous balance column of the daysheet.	☐	☐	☐
7. Record the source and type of the payment in the description line.	☐	☐	☐
8. Record appropriate adjustments in adjustment column.	☐	☐	☐
9. Record the total payment in the payment column. Press hard so that marks go through to the ledger card and the daysheet.	☐	☐	☐
10. Subtract the payment and adjustments from the outstanding/previous balance, and record the current balance.	☐	☐	☐
11. Return the ledger card to appropriate storage.	☐	☐	☐

CALCULATION

Total Possible Points: _____
Total Points Earned: _____ Multiplied by 100 = _____ Divided by Total Possible Points = _____%

Pass   **Fail**
  ☐   ☐   Comments:

Student's signature _____ Date _____
Partner's signature _____ Date _____
Instructor's signature _____ Date _____

Name _____ Date _____ Time _____

Procedure 12-3:	**PROCESS A CREDIT BALANCE**

EQUIPMENT/SUPPLIES: Pen, pegboard, calculator, daysheet, ledger card

STANDARDS: Given the needed equipment and a place to work the student will perform this skill with _____% accuracy in a total of _____ minutes. (*Your instructor will tell you what the percentage and time limits will be before you begin.*)

KEY: 4 = Satisfactory   0 = Unsatisfactory   NA = This step is not counted

PROCEDURE STEPS	SELF	PARTNER	INSTRUCTOR
1. Determine the reason for the credit balance.	☐	☐	☐
2. Place brackets around the balance indicating that it is a negative number.	☐	☐	☐
3. Write a refund check and follow the steps in Procedure 12-7.	☐	☐	☐

CALCULATION

Total Possible Points: _____
Total Points Earned: _____ Multiplied by 100 = _____ Divided by Total Possible Points = _____%

Pass   **Fail**
☐   ☐   Comments:

Student's signature _____ Date _____
Partner's signature _____ Date _____
Instructor's signature _____ Date _____

Name_____ Date_____ Time_____

Procedure 12-4:　　**PROCESS REFUNDS**

EQUIPMENT/SUPPLIES: Pen, pegboard, calculator, daysheet, ledger card, checkbook, check register, word processor letterhead, envelope, postage, copy machine, patient's chart, refund file

STANDARDS: Given the needed equipment and a place to work the student will perform this skill with _____% accuracy in a total of _____ minutes. (*Your instructor will tell you what the percentage and time limits will be before you begin.*)

KEY:　　4 = Satisfactory　　　0 = Unsatisfactory　　　NA = This step is not counted

PROCEDURE STEPS	SELF	PARTNER	INSTRUCTOR
1. Determine who gets the refund, the patient or the insurance company.	☐	☐	☐
2. Pull patient's ledger card and place on current daysheet aligned with the first available line.	☐	☐	☐
3. Post the amount of the refund in the adjustment column in brackets indicating it is a debit, not a credit, adjustment.	☐	☐	☐
4. Write "Refund to Patient" or "Refund to _____" (name of insurance company) in the description column.	☐	☐	☐
5. Write a check for the credit amount made out to the appropriate party.	☐	☐	☐
6. Record the amount and name of payee in the check register.	☐	☐	☐
6. Mail check with letter of explanation to patient or insurance company.	☐	☐	☐
8. Place copy of check and copy of letter in the patient's record or in refund file.	☐	☐	☐
9. Return the patient's ledger card to its storage area.	☐	☐	☐

CALCULATION

Total Possible Points: _____
Total Points Earned: _____ Multiplied by 100 = _____ Divided by Total Possible Points = _____%

Pass　　**Fail**
　☐　　　☐　　| Comments:

Student's signature _____ Date _____
Partner's signature _____ Date _____
Instructor's signature _____ Date _____

Name _____ Date _____ Time _____

Procedure 12-5:   POST ADJUSTMENTS

EQUIPMENT/SUPPLIES: Pen, pegboard, calculator, daysheet, encounter forms, ledger cards, previous day's balance, list of patients and charges, fee schedule

COMPUTER AND MEDICAL OFFICE SOFTWARE: Follow the software requirements for posting credits to patient accounts.

STANDARDS: Given the needed equipment and a place to work the student will perform this skill with _____% accuracy in a total of _____ minutes. (*Your instructor will tell you what the percentage and time limits will be before you begin.*)

KEY: 4 = Satisfactory   0 = Unsatisfactory   NA = This step is not counted

PROCEDURE STEPS	SELF	PARTNER	INSTRUCTOR
1. Pull patient's ledger card and place on current daysheet aligned with the first available line.	☐	☐	☐
2. Post the amount to be written off in the adjustment column in brackets indicating it is a debit, not a credit, adjustment.	☐	☐	☐
3. Subtract the adjustment from the outstanding/previous balance, and record in the current balance column.	☐	☐	☐
4. Return the ledger card to appropriate storage.	☐	☐	☐

CALCULATION

Total Possible Points: _____
Total Points Earned: _____ Multiplied by 100 = _____ Divided by Total Possible Points = _____%

Pass   **Fail**
☐   ☐   Comments:

Student's signature _____ Date _____
Partner's signature _____ Date _____
Instructor's signature _____ Date _____

Name_____   Date _____   Time _____

Procedure 12-6:	POST COLLECTION AGENCY PAYMENTS

EQUIPMENT/SUPPLIES: Pen, pegboard, calculator, daysheet, patient's ledger card

STANDARDS: Given the needed equipment and a place to work the student will perform this skill with _____% accuracy in a total of _____ minutes. (*Your instructor will tell you what the percentage and time limits will be before you begin.*)

KEY: 4 = Satisfactory   0 = Unsatisfactory   NA = This step is not counted

PROCEDURE STEPS	SELF	PARTNER	INSTRUCTOR
1. Review check stub or report from the collection agency explaining the amounts to be applied to the accounts.	☐	☐	☐
2. Pull the patients' ledger cards.	☐	☐	☐
3. Post the amount to be applied in the payment column for each patient.	☐	☐	☐
4. Adjust off the amount representing the percentage of the payment charged by the collection agency.	☐	☐	☐

CALCULATION

Total Possible Points: _____
Total Points Earned: _____ Multiplied by 100 = _____ Divided by Total Possible Points = _____%

Pass   **Fail**
☐   ☐   Comments:

Student's signature _____ Date _____
Partner's signature _____ Date _____
Instructor's signature _____ Date _____

Name _____ Date _____ Time _____

Procedure 12-7:	POST NSF CHECKS

EQUIPMENT/SUPPLIES: Pen, pegboard, calculator, daysheet, patient's ledger card

STANDARDS: Given the needed equipment and a place to work the student will perform this skill with _____% accuracy in a total of _____ minutes. (*Your instructor will tell you what the percentage and time limits will be before you begin.*)

KEY: 4 = Satisfactory   0 = Unsatisfactory   NA = This step is not counted

PROCEDURE STEPS	SELF	PARTNER	INSTRUCTOR
1. Pull patient's ledger card and place on current daysheet aligned with the first available line.	☐	☐	☐
2. Write the amount of the check in the payment column in brackets indicating it is a debit, not a credit, adjustment.	☐	☐	☐
3. Write "Check Returned For Nonsufficient Funds" in the description column.	☐	☐	☐
4. Post a returned check charge with an appropriate explanation in the charge column.	☐	☐	☐
5. Write "Bank Fee for Returned Check" in the description column.	☐	☐	☐
6. Call the patient to advise him of the returned check and the fee.	☐	☐	☐
7. Construct a proper letter of explanation and a copy of the ledger card and mail to patient.	☐	☐	☐
8. Place a copy of the letter and the check in the patient's file.	☐	☐	☐
9. Make arrangements for the patient to pay cash.	☐	☐	☐
10. Flag the patient's account as a credit risk for future transactions.	☐	☐	☐
11. Return the patient's ledger card to its storage area.	☐	☐	☐

CALCULATION

Total Possible Points: _____
Total Points Earned: _____ Multiplied by 100 = _____ Divided by Total Possible Points = _____%

Pass   **Fail**
☐   ☐   Comments:

Student's signature _____ Date _____
Partner's signature _____ Date _____
Instructor's signature _____ Date _____

Name_____ Date_____ Time_____

Procedure 12-8:   BALANCE A DAYSHEET

EQUIPMENT/SUPPLIES: Daysheet with totals brought forward, simulated exercise, calculator, pen

STANDARDS: Given the needed equipment and a place to work the student will perform this skill with _____% accuracy in a total of _____ minutes. (*Your instructor will tell you what the percentage and time limits will be before you begin.*)

KEY: 4 = Satisfactory   0 = Unsatisfactory   NA = This step is not counted

PROCEDURE STEPS	SELF	PARTNER	INSTRUCTOR
1. Be sure the totals from the previous daysheet are recorded in the column for previous totals.	☐	☐	☐
2. Total the charge column and place that number in the proper blank.	☐	☐	☐
3. Total the payment column and place that number in the proper blank.	☐	☐	☐
4. Total the adjustment column and place that number in the proper blank.	☐	☐	☐
5. Total the current balance column and place that number in the proper blank.	☐	☐	☐
6. Total the previous balance column and place that number in the proper blank.	☐	☐	☐
7. Add today's totals to the previous totals.	☐	☐	☐
8. Take the grand total of the previous balances, add the grand total of the charges, and subtract the grand total of the payments and adjustments. This number must equal the grand total of the current balance.	☐	☐	☐
9. If the numbers do not match, calculate your totals again, and continue looking for errors until the numbers match. This will prove that the daysheet is balanced, and there are no errors.	☐	☐	☐
10. Record the totals of the columns in the proper space on the next daysheet. You will be prepared for balancing the new daysheet.	☐	☐	☐

CALCULATION

Total Possible Points: _____
Total Points Earned: _____ Multiplied by 100 = _____ Divided by Total Possible Points = _____%

Pass   **Fail**
☐   ☐   Comments:

Student's signature _____ Date _____
Partner's signature _____ Date _____
Instructor's signature _____ Date _____

Name _____ Date _____ Time _____

Procedure 12-9:	COMPLETE A BANK DEPOSIT SLIP AND MAKE A DEPOSIT

EQUIPMENT/SUPPLIES: Calculator with tape, currency, coins, checks for deposit, deposit slip, endorsement stamp, deposit envelope

STANDARDS: Given the needed equipment and a place to work the student will perform this skill with _____% accuracy in a total of _____ minutes. (*Your instructor will tell you what the percentage and time limits will be before you begin.*)

KEY: 4 = Satisfactory   0 = Unsatisfactory   NA = This step is not counted

PROCEDURE STEPS	SELF	PARTNER	INSTRUCTOR
1. Arrange bills face up and sort with the largest denomination on top.	☐	☐	☐
2. Record the total in the cash block on the deposit slip.	☐	☐	☐
3. Endorse the back of each check with "For Deposit Only."	☐	☐	☐
4. Record the amount of each check beside an identifying number on the deposit slip.	☐	☐	☐
5. Total and record the amounts of checks in the total of checks line on the deposit slip.	☐	☐	☐
6. Total and record the amount of cash and the amount of checks.	☐	☐	☐
7. Record the total amount of the deposit in the office checkbook register.	☐	☐	☐
8. Make a copy of both sides of the deposit slip for office records.	☐	☐	☐
9. Place the cash, checks, and the completed deposit slip in an envelope or bank bag for transporting to the bank for deposit.	☐	☐	☐

CALCULATION

Total Possible Points: _____
Total Points Earned: _____ Multiplied by 100 = _____ Divided by Total Possible Points = _____%

Pass	Fail	
☐	☐	Comments:

Student's signature _____ Date _____
Partner's signature _____ Date _____
Instructor's signature _____ Date _____

Name _____ Date _____ Time _____

Procedure 12-10:   RECONCILE A BANK STATEMENT

EQUIPMENT/SUPPLIES: Simulated bank statement, reconciliation worksheet, calculator, pen

STANDARDS: Given the needed equipment and a place to work the student will perform this skill with _____% accuracy in a total of _____ minutes. (*Your instructor will tell you what the percentage and time limits will be before you begin.*)

KEY: 4 = Satisfactory   0 = Unsatisfactory   NA = This step is not counted

PROCEDURE STEPS	SELF	PARTNER	INSTRUCTOR
1. Compare the opening balance on the new statement with the closing balance on the previous statement.	☐	☐	☐
2. List the bank balance in the appropriate space on the reconciliation worksheet.	☐	☐	☐
3. Compare the check entries on the statement with the entries in the check register.	☐	☐	☐
4. Determine if there are any outstanding checks.	☐	☐	☐
5. Total outstanding checks.	☐	☐	☐
6. Subtract from the checkbook balance items such as withdrawals, automatic payments, or service charges that appeared on the statement but not in the checkbook.	☐	☐	☐
7. Add to the bank statement balance any deposits not shown on the bank statement.	☐	☐	☐
8. Make sure balance in the checkbook and the bank statement agree.	☐	☐	☐

CALCULATION

Total Possible Points: _____
Total Points Earned: _____ Multiplied by 100 = _____ Divided by Total Possible Points = _____%

Pass   **Fail**
☐   ☐   Comments:

Student's signature _____ Date _____
Partner's signature _____ Date _____
Instructor's signature _____ Date _____

Name_____   Date _____   Time _____

Procedure 12-11:	**MAINTAIN A PETTY CASH ACCOUNT**

EQUIPMENT/SUPPLIES: Cash box, play money, checkbook, simulated receipts, and/or vouchers representing expenditures

STANDARDS: Given the needed equipment and a place to work the student will perform this skill with _____% accuracy in a total of _____ minutes. (*Your instructor will tell you what the percentage and time limits will be before you begin.*)

KEY: 4 = Satisfactory   0 = Unsatisfactory   NA = This step is not counted

PROCEDURE STEPS	SELF	PARTNER	INSTRUCTOR
1. Count the money remaining in the box.	☐	☐	☐
2. Total the amounts of all vouchers in the petty cash box and determine the amount of expenditures.	☐	☐	☐
3. Subtract the amount of receipts from the original amount in petty cash, to equal the amount of cash remaining in the box.	☐	☐	☐
4. Balance the cash against the receipts.	☐	☐	☐
5. Write a check only for the amount that was used.	☐	☐	☐
6. Record totals on memo line of check stub.	☐	☐	☐
7. Sort and record all vouchers to the appropriate accounts.	☐	☐	☐
8. File the list of vouchers and attached receipts.	☐	☐	☐
9. Place cash in petty cash fund.	☐	☐	☐

CALCULATION

Total Possible Points: _____
Total Points Earned: _____ Multiplied by 100 = _____ Divided by Total Possible Points = _____%

Pass   **Fail**
☐   ☐ | Comments: |

Student's signature _____ Date _____
Partner's signature _____ Date _____
Instructor's signature _____ Date _____

Name_____ Date _____ Time _____

Procedure 12-12:	ORDERING SUPPLIES

EQUIPMENT/SUPPLIES: 5×7 index cards, file box with divider cards, computer with Internet (optional), medical supply catalogues

STANDARDS: Given the needed equipment and a place to work the student will perform this skill with _____% accuracy in a total of _____ minutes. (*Your instructor will tell you what the percentage and time limits will be before you begin.*)

KEY: 4 = Satisfactory   0 = Unsatisfactory   NA = This step is not counted

PROCEDURE STEPS	SELF	PARTNER	INSTRUCTOR
1. Create a list of supplies to be ordered that is based on inventory done by employees.	☐	☐	☐
2. Create an index card for each supply on the list including the name of the supply in the top left corner, the name and contact information of vendor(s), and product identification number.	☐	☐	☐
3. File the index cards in the file box with divider cards alphabetically or by product type.	☐	☐	☐
4. Record the current price of the item and how the item is supplied.	☐	☐	☐
5. Record the reorder point.	☐	☐	☐

CALCULATION

Total Possible Points: _____

Total Points Earned: _____ Multiplied by 100 = _____ Divided by Total Possible Points = _____%

Pass   **Fail**
☐   ☐   Comments:

Student's signature _____ Date _____
Partner's signature _____ Date _____
Instructor's signature _____ Date _____

Name _____ Date _____ Time _____

Procedure 12-13:　**WRITE A CHECK**

EQUIPMENT/SUPPLIES: Simulated page of checks from checkbook, scenario giving amount of check, check register

STANDARDS: Given the needed equipment and a place to work the student will perform this skill with _____% accuracy in a total of _____ minutes. (*Your instructor will tell you what the percentage and time limits will be before you begin.*)

KEY:　4 = Satisfactory　　0 = Unsatisfactory　　NA = This step is not counted

PROCEDURE STEPS	SELF	PARTNER	INSTRUCTOR
1. Fill out the check register with the following information: 　**a.** check number 　**b.** date 　**c.** payee information 　**d.** amount 　**e.** previous balance 　**f.** new balance	☐	☐	☐
2. Enter date on check.	☐	☐	☐
3. Enter payee on check.	☐	☐	☐
4. Enter the amount of check using numerals.	☐	☐	☐
5. Write out the amount of the check beginning as far left as possible and make a straight line to fill in space between dollars and cents.	☐	☐	☐
6. Record cents as a fraction with 100 as the denominator.	☐	☐	☐
7. Obtain appropriate signature(s).	☐	☐	☐
8. Proofread for accuracy.	☐	☐	☐

CALCULATION

Total Possible Points: _____
Total Points Earned: _____ Multiplied by 100 = _____ Divided by Total Possible Points = _____%

Pass　　**Fail**
☐　　　☐　　Comments:

Student's signature _____ Date _____
Partner's signature _____ Date _____
Instructor's signature _____ Date _____

Work Product 1

Perform an inventory of supplies.

When you are working in a medical office, you may need to keep an inventory of all supplies. The inventory will help you decide when to order new supplies. It will also help you calculate how much money you will need to spend on supplies. Supplies are those items that are consumed quickly and need to be reordered on a regular basis.

If you are currently working in a medical office, use the form below to take an inventory of the supplies in the office. If you do not have access to a medical office, complete an inventory of the supplies in your kitchen or bathroom at home.

**Third Street
Physician's Office, Inc.**
123 Main Street
Baltimore, MD 21201
410-895-6214

Supply Inventory

Item Description	Item Number or Code	Number Needed in Stock	Number Currently in Stock	Date Ordered	Number Ordered	Unit Price	Total	Actual Delivery Date

Work Product 2

Perform an inventory of equipment.

When you are working in a medical office, you may need to keep an inventory of all equipment. The inventory will help you decide when to order new equipment. It will also help you calculate how much money you will need to spend on new equipment. Equipment includes items that can be used over and over and generally last many years.

If you are currently working in a medical office, use the form below to take an inventory of the equipment in the office. If you do not have access to a medical office, complete an inventory of the equipment in your kitchen or bathroom at home.

Third Street
Physician's Office, Inc.
123 Main Street
Baltimore, MD 21201
410-895-6214

Equipment Inventory

Item Description	Item Number or Code	Purchase Date	Condition	Comments	Expected New Purchase Date	Cost if Purchased This Year

Work Product 3

Post entries on a day sheet.

You will need to keep track of charges, payments, and adjustments throughout the day. One way to keep track is by using a day sheet. Fill out the day sheet with the transactions described below.

- Marco Rodriguez arrived at 8:00 AM complaining of a sharp pain in his knee. Mr. Rodriguez was examined by the physician and then x-rayed. Mr. Rodriguez has MedCo Insurance, with a co-pay of $35, which he paid using a credit card.
- Dominica Johnson had a general physical examination at 8:30 AM. In addition to normal examination, she received a tetanus booster shot. Ms. Johnson does not have health insurance. She paid in full by check.
- At 9:30 AM, John Ericksen came in with a sore throat. After examination, he was given a throat culture. Mr. Ericksen has HealthEez insurance. He has a co-pay of $20, which he was unable to pay today.

Physician Fees
Sick visit: $55
General physical: $125
X-ray: $225
Throat culture: $45
Immunization – tetanus: $30
Adjustments for MedCo Insurance: 20%
Adjustments for HeathEez insurance: 25%

Day Sheet

Date	Description	Charges	Payments	Adjustments	Current Balance	Previous Balance	Name

Totals This Page
Totals Previous Page
Month-To-Date Totals

Work Product 4

Process a credit balance.

Mr. Rodriguez has switched to a different insurance company. His co-pay with his old carrier was $35 per visit. His new co-pay is $20 per visit. However, there was a billing oversight and Mr. Rodriguez paid his old co-pay. Process Mr. Rodriguez's credit balance on his ledger card.

DATE	DESCRIPTION	CHARGES	CREDITS PYMNTS.	ADJ.	BALANCE
	BALANCE FORWARD ➝				

FORM MR 10   PLEASE PAY LAST AMOUNT IN BALANCE COLUMN ⬐

Work Product 5

Process a refund.

Mr. Rodriguez has a credit balance of $15 on his account. You need to mail him a refund check. Fill out the patient's ledger card and write a short letter of explanation to Mr. Rodriguez. Print the letter and attach it to this page.

DATE	DESCRIPTION	CHARGES	CREDITS PYMNTS.	ADJ.	BALANCE
	BALANCE FORWARD ➝				

FORM MR 10   PLEASE PAY LAST AMOUNT IN BALANCE COLUMN ⬐

Work Product 6

Post adjustments.

Mr. Rodriguez visits your office for an x-ray of his knee. Your office normally charges $225 for a knee x-ray. However, Mr. Rodriguez's insurance carrier pays your office only $175 for a knee x-ray. Post the proper adjustment on the day sheet.

Day Sheet

Date	Description	Charges	Payments	Adjustments	Current Balance	Previous Balance	Name

Totals This Page					
Totals Previous Page					
Month-To-Date Totals					

Work Product 7

Post NSF checks.

You have just received a check that was returned for nonsufficient funds. The check was written by Martha Montgomery for $750. Post the proper information in the ledger card.

DATE	DESCRIPTION	CHARGES	CREDITS PYMNTS.	ADJ.	BALANCE
	BALANCE FORWARD →				

FORM MR 10   PLEASE PAY LAST AMOUNT IN BALANCE COLUMN ⌐→

Work Product 8

Post collection agency payments.

You receive a check for $787.50 and the following statement from your collection agency.

Jones & Jones Collections
Account: D. Larsen, MD

Debtor	Amount Collected	Fee	Balance
Martha Montgomery	$750.00	$187.50	$562.50
Johan Johansen	$300.00	$75.00	$225.00
		Total	$787.50

Post the payments to the day sheet.

Day Sheet

Date	Description	Charges	Payments	Adjustments	Current Balance	Previous Balance	Name

Totals This Page
Totals Previous Page
Month-To-Date Totals

Work Product 9

Prepare a bank deposit.

Prepare a bank deposit for the following:

- check for $750 from Martin Montgomery
- check for $35 from Rita Gonzalez
- $125 cash

Newtown Bank, N.A. **DEPOSIT**	ITEMS DEPOSITED	DOLLARS	CENTS
	Currency		.
	Coin		.
Name and account number will be verified when presented.	Checks 1		.
Name / Date	2		.
Address	3		.
	4		.
	Sub Total		.
Signature Sign here only if cash is received from deposit	Less Cash		.
Store Number (Commercial Accounts Only) Account Number (For CAP Accounts, use 10-digit number.)	Total Deposit		
* ☐☐☐☐☐☐☐ * ☐☐☐☐☐☐☐☐☐☐☐☐☐ $	☐☐☐☐☐ . ☐☐		

Chapter Self-Assessment Quiz

1. The best place to put petty cash is:

   a. in the same drawer as the other cash and checks.

   b. in a separate, secured drawer.

   c. in an envelope stored in the staff room.

   d. in the physician's office.

   e. in a locked supply cabinet.

2. Which of the following information is found on a patient's ledger card?

   a. Date of birth

   b. Social Security number

   c. Blood type

   d. Insurance information

   e. Marital status

3. The purpose of the posting proofs section is to:

   a. enter the day's totals and balance the day sheet.

   b. update and maintain a patient's financial record.

   c. make note of any credit the patient has on file.

   d. make note of any debit the patient has on file.

   e. allow for any adjustments that need to be made.

4. Which of the following might you purchase using petty cash?

   a. Cotton swabs

   b. Thermometer covers

   c. Office supplies

   d. Non-latex gloves

   e. New x-ray machine

Scenario: A new patient comes in and gives you his insurance card. The patient's insurance allows $60 for a routine checkup. Of this, insurance will pay 75% of his bill. The actual price of the checkup is $60.

5. How much will the patient need to pay?

   a. $0

   b. $15

   c. $30

   d. $45

   e. $60

6. How much of a difference will remain?

   a. $0

   b. $5

   c. $10

   d. $15

   e. $60

End Scenario

7. A check register is used to:

   a. hold checks until they are ready for deposit.

   b. create a checklist of daily office duties.

   c. make a list of payments the office is still owed.

   d. record all checks that go in and out of the office.

   e. remind patients when their payment is due.

8. Ideally, if you are using a pegboard accounting system, what is the best way to organize your ledgers?

   a. File all ledgers alphabetically in a single tray.

   b. Alphabetically file paid ledgers in one tray, and ledgers with outstanding balances in another.

   c. Numerically file paid ledgers in the front of the tray, and ledgers with outstanding balances in the back.

   d. Alphabetically file paid ledgers into patients' folders, and ledgers with outstanding balances in a tray.

   e. File all ledgers into patients' folders.

9. Accounts receivable is:

   a. a record of all monies due to the practice.

   b. the people the practice owes money to.

   c. the transactions transferred from a different office.

   d. any outstanding inventory bills.

   e. a list of patients who have paid in the last month.

10. It is unsafe to use credit card account numbers on purchases made:

   a. over the phone.

   b. by fax.

   c. through e-mail.

   d. from a catalog.

   e. in person.

11. When you have a deposit that includes cash, what is the only way you should get it to the bank?

    a. Deliver it by hand.

    b. Deliver it into a depository.

    c. Send it by mail with enough postage.

    d. Deliver checks by mail and cash by hand.

    e. Do not accept cash as payment.

12. Which of the following is a benefit of paying bills by computer?

    a. You do not need to keep a record of paying your bills.

    b. Entering data into the computer is quick and easy.

    c. Information can be "memorized" and stored.

    d. You can divide columns into groups of expenses (rent, paychecks, etc.).

    e. You can easily correct any errors.

13. Most medical offices generally use:

    a. standard business checks.

    b. certified checks.

    c. traveler's checks.

    d. money orders.

    e. cash deposits.

14. What is a quick way to find order numbers when making a purchase?

    a. Check the packing slip of a previous order.

    b. Find a previous bill for any item numbers.

    c. Check past purchase orders for their order numbers.

    d. Call the supplier for a list of item numbers.

    e. Look at the supplier's website.

15. Summation reports are:

    a. lists of all the clients who entered the office.

    b. reports that track all expenses and income.

    c. computer reports that compile all daily totals.

    d. lists that analyze an office's activities.

    e. reports the IRS sends an office being audited.

16. Why is the adjustment column so important?

    a. It assists you in deciding the discount percentage.

    b. It records all transactions a patient has made in your office.

    c. It allows you to add discounts and credit to change the total.

    d. It keeps track of any changes a patient has in health care.

    e. It keeps track of bounced checks.

17. Which of the following is the correct order in which you use a ledger?

    a. Place ledger over day sheet and charge slip; file ledger in ledger tray; make entry on ledger card; give patient a copy of ledger as a receipt.

    b. Make entry on ledger card; give patient copy of ledger as receipt; place ledger over day sheet and charge slip; file ledger in ledger tray.

    c. Make entry on ledger card; place ledger over day sheet and charge slip; file ledger in ledger tray; give patient copy of ledger as receipt.

    d. Give patient copy of ledger as receipt; place ledger over day sheet and charge slip; make entry on ledger card; file ledger in ledger tray.

    e. Place ledger over day sheet and charge slip; make entry on ledger card; give patient copy of ledger as receipt; file ledger in ledger tray.

18. In a bookkeeping system, things of value relating to the practice are called:

    a. assets.

    b. liabilities.

    c. debits.

    d. credits.

    e. audits.

19. The amount of capital the physician has invested in the practice is referred to as:

    a. assets.

    b. credits.

    c. equity.

    d. liabilities.

    e. invoices.

20. Overpayments under $5 are generally:

    a. sent back to the patient.

    b. placed in petty cash.

    c. left on the account as a credit.

    d. deposited in a special overpayment account.

    e. mailed to the insurance company.

Chapter Checklist

☐ Read textbook chapter and take notes within the Chapter Notes outline. Answer the Learning Objectives as you reach them in the content, and then check them off.

☐ Work the Content Review questions—both Foundational Knowledge and Application.

☐ Perform the Active Learning exercise(s).

☐ Complete Professional Journal entries.

☐ Complete Skill Practice Activity(s) using Competency Evaluation Forms and Work Products, when appropriate.

☐ Take the Chapter Self-Assessment Quiz.

☐ Insert all appropriate pages into your Portfolio.

Learning Objectives

1. Spell and define the key terms.
2. Describe group, individual, and government-sponsored (public) health benefits and explain the differences between them.
3. Explain the differences between Medicare and Medicaid.
4. Explain how managed care programs work.

5. Explain the differences between health maintenance organizations, preferred provider organizations, and physician hospital organizations.
6. List the information required on a medical claim form and explain why each piece of information is needed.
7. Name two legal issues affecting claims submissions.

Chapter Notes

Note: Bold-faced headings are the major headings in the text chapter; headings in regular font are lower-level headings (i.e., the content is subordinate to, or falls "under," the major headings). Make sure you understand the key terms used in the chapter, as well as the concepts presented as Key Points.

TEXT SUBHEADINGS	NOTES
Introduction	
	Key Term: health insurance **Key Point:** • You must keep abreast of changes as you are notified.
☐ **LEARNING OBJECTIVE 1:** Spell and define the key terms.	

Health Benefits Plans _____

_____

_____

_____

Group Health Benefits _____

_____

_____

Key Terms: employee; group member; eligibility; insured; claims; third-party administrator; dependent; claims administrator

Key Points:

- Group health benefits are sponsored by an organization, such as an employer, a union, or an association.
- To confirm a patient's eligibility, check the back of the patient's identification (ID) card (Fig. 13-2) for a web address or phone number to contact the **claims administrator** for the health benefits plan.

Health Care Savings Accounts _____

_____

_____

Key Term: Health Care Savings Accounts (HSAs)

Individual Health Benefits _____

_____

_____

_____

Government-Sponsored (Public) Health Benefits _____

_____

_____

_____

Medicare _____

_____

_____

Key Terms: deductible; crossover claim

Key Point:

- Medicare Part B pays for physician fees, both inpatient and outpatient; diagnostic testing; certain immunizations (influenza and pneumonia); and specific screening tests (PSA, mammograms, Pap smears, bone density testing, colorectal screening).

Medicaid _____

_____

_____

Key Point:

- Medicaid is governed by both federal and state statutes and rules, and then implemented on a state and local level.

TRICARE/CHAMPVA

Key Point:
• Once admitted to the CHAMPVA program, patients select their own physician; this allows them the same benefits as private insurance.

☐ **LEARNING OBJECTIVE 2:** Describe group, individual, and government-sponsored (public) health benefits and explain the differences between them.

☐ **LEARNING OBJECTIVE 3:** Explain the differences between Medicare and Medicaid.

Managed Care

Key Terms: managed care; peer review organization; health maintenance organization (HMO); balance billing
Key Points:
• The contract usually establishes what prices will be charged for each service and the conditions under which a service would be covered.
• Failure to comply with the precertification requirements results in a financial penalty for the patient and possibly also for the physician and the hospital.

☐ **LEARNING OBJECTIVE 4:** Explain how managed care programs work.

Health Maintenance Organizations

Key Terms: deductible; coinsurance; fee-for-service; capitation; independent practice association (IPA); fee schedule
Key Points:
• In this respect, the HMO acts as both an insurer and a provider of service.
• Often, a portion of any reimbursement is withheld by the HMO and paid only if the HMO's total medical expense is within budget; this encourages the physician to be cost conscious in caring for patients.

Preferred Provider Organizations

Key Term: preferred provider organization (PPO)
Key Points:
- Whereas HMOs promise to provide services and have a financial risk in their relationships with subscribers, a **preferred provider organization (PPO)** is a type of health benefit program whose purpose is simply to contract with providers, then lease this network of contracted providers to health care plans.
- The physician agrees to accept the reimbursement by the claims administrator as payment in full, and agrees not to bill the patient for any difference between the physician's usual charge and the PPO-negotiated charge for the service.

Physician Hospital Organizations

Other Managed Care Programs

Key Point:
- The physician must complete and submit a referral form or call the claims administrator for approval of the referral. (See Box 13-2.)

☐ **LEARNING OBJECTIVE 5:** Explain the differences between health maintenance organizations, preferred provider organizations, and physician hospital organizations.

Workers' Compensation

Key Point:
- Workers' compensation benefits were developed to cover the expenses resulting from a work-related illness or injury.

Filing Claims

Key Terms: coordination of benefits; birthday rule; pre-existing condition
Key Point:
- The patient's ID card is a source of information necessary for complete and accurate claims submission.

☐ **LEARNING OBJECTIVE 6:** List the information required on a medical claim form and explain why each piece of information is needed.

Electronic Claims Submission _____

Key Point:
• Remember, HIPAA requires covered entities to submit electronic information safely and confidentially.

☐ **LEARNING OBJECTIVE 7:** Name two legal issues affecting claims submissions.

Explanation of Benefits _____

Key Point:
• You must check the EOB to be sure that all payments made to the physician are for the appropriate procedures and in the correct amounts.

Policies in the Practice _____

Key Terms: usual, customary, and reasonable (UCR); plan maximum
Key Point:
• Managed care plans require physicians to accept assignment, although many physicians do not accept assignment for non–managed care patients.

Content Review

FOUNDATIONAL KNOWLEDGE

The ABCs of Health Care

1. Elaine is 22 years old and is still eligible as a dependent. What could be a possible reason for this?

_____

_____

2. Read each person's health insurance scenario and then match it with the correct type of health insurance plan.

   Scenario

   a. Sandra was recently let go from her job and is unemployed. _____

   b. Thomas has a plan that has less generous coverage and may limit or eliminate benefits for certain illnesses or injuries. _____

   c. Mario just started a new job and signed up for health insurance at work. _____

   Health Insurance Plan

   1. Group
   2. Individual
   3. Government

3. Jim works for a company that offers an employee benefit whereby money is taken out of his paycheck and put toward medical care expenses. What is the name of this practice?

_____

_____

Name That Health Coverage

4. Determine which of the following are characteristics of Medicare or Medicaid. Place a check mark in the appropriate column below.

	Medicare	Medicaid
a. Provides coverage for low-income or indigent persons of all ages		
b. In a crossover claim, this is the primary coverage		
c. Implemented on a state or local level		
d. Physician reimbursement is considerably less than other insurances		
e. Patients receive a new ID card each month		
f. Program is broken down into part A and part B		
g. Provides coverage for persons suffering from end-stage renal disease		

5. Circle the services and procedures below that Medicaid may provide coverage for.

Dentistry

Inpatient hospital care

Cosmetic surgery

Outpatient treatment and services

Diagnostic services

Family planning

Mammograms

Wellness center fees

Alternative medicine

6. Which is true about how a managed care system is different from a traditional insurance coverage system?

    a. They usually are less costly.

    b. They cost more but have more benefits.

    c. They cost the same but have more benefits.

    d. You can only use network physicians.

7. Why do managed care programs require approved referrals?

_____

_____

8. Circle the type of insurance each characteristic matches.

    a. Tom can visit any provider he chooses, but some will be more expensive than others depending on if they are "in" or "out" of network.

HMO	PPO	PHO

b. This plan provides covered services rather than pays for them.

HMO	PPO	PHO

c. This plan does not typically use deductibles or co-insurance.

HMO	PPO	PHO

d. Participating providers, in some cases, assume responsibility for the overall medical budget and in others do not.

HMO	PPO	PHO

e. The purpose of this plan is to contract with providers.

HMO	PPO	PHO

f. This plan uses predetermined co-payments.

HMO	PPO	PHO

g. This plan includes a coalition of physicians and a hospital contracting with large employers, insurance carriers, etc.

HMO	PPO	PHO

9. What does a gatekeeper physician do?

_____

_____

10. A new patient comes to your office, and he hands you his insurance card. What information can you find on the back of his identification card?

_____

_____

Filing Claims Trouble-Free

11. What form do you fill out to submit an insurance claim?

_____

_____

12. When is a physician required to file a patient's claim or to extend credit?

_____

_____

13. Claims are sometimes denied, and it is your responsibility to take corrective actions. Read the scenarios below, and briefly state what action you should take.

a. Services are not covered by the plan. _____

b. Coding is deemed inappropriate for services provided. _____

c. Data is incomplete. _____

d. Patient cannot be identified as a covered person. _____

e. The patient is no longer covered by the plan. _____

14. Kairi is a dependent, and both of her parents have health care plans. There are no specific instructions about which plan is primary, so how do you choose which plan to use?

_____

_____

15. Mandy's primary care physician is included under her health plan. However, she has recently been experiencing chest pains, and her physician refers her to a cardiologist. What steps must you take to determine whether or not the cardiologist's visit will be covered?

_____

_____

16. Describe the main characteristics of primary and secondary insurance below.

Primary Insurance	**Secondary Insurance**
•	•

17. Why is it important to check the Explanation of Benefits?

_____

_____

18. There are some legal issues that affect claims submissions. What is a preexisting condition and how does it affect claim submission?

_____

_____

19. Match the following key terms to their definitions.

Key Terms

a. assignment of benefits _____

b. balance billing _____

c. capitation _____

d. carrier _____

e. claims administrator _____

f. co-insurance _____

g. coordination of benefits _____

h. co-payments _____

i. crossover claim _____

j. deductible _____

k. dependent _____

l. eligibility _____

m. explanation of benefits (EOB) _____

n. fee-for-service _____

o. fee schedule _____

p. group member _____

q. Healthcare Savings Account _____

r. health maintenance organization (HMO) _____

Definitions

1. an individual who manages the third-party reimbursement policies for a medical practice

2. the part of the payment for a service that a patient must pay

3. the determination of an insured's right to receive benefits from a third-party payer based on criteria such as payment of premiums

4. spouse, children, and sometimes other individuals designated by the insured who are covered under a health care plan

5. the transfer of the patient's legal right to collect third-party benefits to the provider of the services

6. a company that assumes the risk of an insurance company

7. a group of physicians and specialists that conducts a review of a disputed case and makes a final recommendation

8. an organization that provides a wide range of services through a contract with a specified group at a predetermined payment

9. billing the patients for the difference between the physician's charges and the Medicare-approved charges

10. an organization of nongroup physicians developed to allow independent physicians to compete with prepaid group practices

11. a coalition of physicians and a hospital contracting with large employers, insurance carriers, and other benefits groups to provide discounted health services

12. an established set of fees charged for specific services and paid by the patient or insurance carrier

s. independent practice association (IPA) _____

t. managed care _____

u. Medicare _____

v. peer review organization _____

w. physician hospital organization _____

x. preferred provider organization (PPO) _____

y. usual, customary, and reasonable (UCR) _____

z. utilization review _____

13. the practice of third-party payers to control costs by requiring physicians to adhere to specific rules as a condition of payment

14. the method of designating the order in multiple-carriers pay benefits to avoid duplication of payment

15. a statement from an insurance carrier that outlines which services are being paid

16. a government-sponsored health benefits package that provides insurance for the elderly

17. a claim that moves over automatically from one coverage to another for payment

18. a policyholder who is covered by a group insurance carrier

19. a type of health benefit program whose purpose is to contract with providers, then lease this network of contracted providers to health care plans

20. an employee benefit that allows individuals to save money through payroll deduction to accounts that can be used only for medical care

21. a list of preestablished fee allowances set for specific services performed by a provider

22. a managed care plan that pays a certain amount to a provider over a specific time for caring for the patients in the plan, regardless of what or how many services are performed

23. the basis of a physician's fee schedule for the normal cost of the same service or procedure in a similar geographic area and under the same or similar circumstances

24. the agreed-upon amount paid to the provider by a policyholder

25. an analysis of individual cases by a committee to make sure services and procedures being billed to a third-party payer are medically necessary

26. the amount paid by the patient before the carrier begins paying

20. True or False? Determine if the statements below are true or false. If false, explain why.

a. Approximately 80% of Americans are enrolled in health benefits plans of one sort or another.

_____

_____

b. A network of providers that make up the PHO may have no financial obligation to subscribers.

_____

_____

c. In managed care, a patient is not usually required to use network providers to receive full coverage.

_____

_____

d. An HMO requires the patient to pay the provider directly, then reimburses the patient.

_____

_____

APPLICATION

Critical Thinking Practice

1. Explain how managed care programs work.

_____

_____

2. A patient may be covered by more than one health plan. For example, the patient may have coverage through an employer while being a dependent on a spouse's plan. Identify the primary plan in this situation and explain coordination of benefits.

_____

_____

Patient Education

1. Mrs. Smith is moving out of the area and is seeing Dr. Jones, her private-practice physician, for the last time. After the move, Mrs. Smith will have to choose a new physician. Mrs. Smith has the choice of an HMO or a PPO. Mrs. Smith asks you to explain the difference. How can you teach Mrs. Smith about the differences between an HMO and a PPO?

_____

_____

Documentation

1. Isabelle Windels brings her 18-month-old daughter to the physician's office for an ear infection. This is the child's fourth ear infection in 3 months and she is no longer responding to antibiotics. The physician refers the patient to an ear, nose, and throat specialist. Mrs. Windels belongs to an HMO. Document this encounter in her chart and then explain any other paperwork you must fill out.

_____

_____

Active Learning

1. Interview three people about their health insurance. Ask them what they like about their service. What do they dislike? Compile a list of their comments to discuss with the class.

2. Visit the website for Medicare at www.medicare.gov. Locate their Frequently Asked Questions page. Read over the questions, and choose five that you believe are the most likely to be asked in a medical office. Design a pamphlet for your office that addresses these five questions.

3. Although a large percentage of Americans have some sort of health insurance, there are still many people who go without. Research online and in medical journals to see what solutions the government and health care companies are devising to reduce the number of uninsured Americans, and to provide better, cheaper, and more widespread health care. Choose one solution, and write a letter to the editor of a local newspaper explaining your position.

Professional Journal

REFLECT

(Prompts and Ideas: Do you currently have health insurance or have you had health insurance in the past? What did you like about it? What did you not like about it?)

_____

_____

_____

_____

PONDER AND SOLVE

1. A Medicare patient feels overwhelmed by the costs of the services. What information can you offer to help?

_____

_____

_____

_____

_____

_____

_____

2. A patient started coverage under a new insurance company and did not tell the medical office that there was any change at her last appointment. When you submitted the paperwork to the old insurance company, you found out that she no longer had coverage. What can you do?

_____

_____

_____

EXPERIENCE

Skills related to this chapter include:

1. Completing a CMS-1500 Claim Form (Procedure 13-1).

Record any common mistakes, lessons learned, and/or tips you discovered during your experience of practicing and demonstrating these skills:

_____
_____
_____
_____
_____
_____
_____
_____

Skill Practice

PERFORMANCE OBJECTIVES:

1. Complete a CMS-1500 claim form (Procedure 13-1).

Name_____ Date _____ Time _____

Procedure 13-1:	**COMPLETING A CMS-1500 CLAIM FORM**

EQUIPMENT: Case scenario, completed encounter form, blank CMS-1500 Claim Form, pen

STANDARDS: Given the needed equipment and a place to work the student will perform this skill with _____% accuracy in a total of _____ minutes. (*Your instructor will tell you what the percentage and time limits will be before you begin.*)

KEY: 4 = Satisfactory   0 = Unsatisfactory   NA = This step is not counted

PROCEDURE STEPS	SELF	PARTNER	INSTRUCTOR
1. Using the information provided in the case scenario, complete the demographic information in lines 1 through 11d.	☐	☐	☐
2. Insert "SOF" (signature on file) on lines 12 and 13. Check to be sure there is a current signature on file in the chart and that it is specifically for the third-party payer being filed.	☐	☐	☐
3. If the services being filed are for a hospital stay, insert information in lines 16, 18, and 32.	☐	☐	☐
4. If the services are related to an injury, insert the date of the accident in line 14.	☐	☐	☐
5. Insert dates of service.	☐	☐	☐
6. Using the encounter form, place the CPT code listed for each service and procedure checked off in column D of lines 21-24 on the form.	☐	☐	☐
7. Place the diagnostic codes indicated on the encounter form in lines 21 (1-4). List the reason for the encounter on line 21.1 and any other diagnoses listed on the encounter form that relate to the services or procedures.	☐	☐	☐
8. Reference the codes placed in lines 21 (1-4) to each line listing a different CPT code by placing the corresponding one-digit in line 24, column E.	☐	☐	☐

Calculation

Total Possible Points: _____
Total Points Earned: _____ Multiplied by 100 = _____ Divided by Total Possible Points = _____%

Pass   **Fail**
☐   ☐   Comments:

Student's signature _____ Date _____
Partner's signature _____ Date _____
Instructor's signature _____ Date _____

Work Products

Complete insurance claim forms.

Jackson Dishman is a 58-year-old man who is seen in the office for acute abdominal pain. Complete the CMS-1500 form using the information provided below:

297-01-2222
Jackson W. Dishman   Group #68735
123 Smith Avenue
Winston-Salem NC 27103   Date of Birth: 06-01-49

He is charged for an office visit which carries the CPT code 99213 and costs $150.00. The doctor has the CMA do a Radiologic Examination, abdomen; complete acute abdomen series (the CPT code 774022); and the charge for the x-rays is $250.00. The x-rays are normal. He pays nothing today. The physician sends Mr. Dishman home with a diagnosis of acute abdominal pain which (IDC-9 code is 789.0). He is to return in 2 days unless the pain becomes unbearable.

PLEASE
DO NOT
STAPLE
IN THIS
AREA

CARRIER

HEALTH INSURANCE CLAIM FORM

PICA   PICA

1. MEDICARE	MEDICAID	CHAMPUS	CHAMPVA	GROUP HEALTH PLAN	FECA BLK LUNG	OTHER	1a. INSURED'S I.D. NUMBER	(FOR PROGRAM IN ITEM 1)
(Medicare #)	(Medicaid #)	(Sponsor's SSN)	(VA File #)	(SSN or ID)	(SSN)	(ID)		

2. PATIENT'S NAME (Last Name, First Name, Middle Initial)

3. PATIENT'S BIRTH DATE   MM | DD | YY   SEX   M   F

4. INSURED'S NAME (Last Name, First Name, Middle Initial)

5. PATIENT'S ADDRESS (No., Street)

6. PATIENT RELATIONSHIP TO INSURED   Self   Spouse   Child   Other

7. INSURED'S ADDRESS (No., Street)

CITY   STATE

8. PATIENT STATUS   Single   Married   Other   Employed   Full-Time Student   Part-Time Student

CITY   STATE

ZIP CODE   TELEPHONE (Include Area Code)   ( )

ZIP CODE   TELEPHONE (INCLUDE AREA CODE)   ( )

9. OTHER INSURED'S NAME (Last Name, First Name, Middle Initial)

10. IS PATIENT'S CONDITION RELATED TO:

11. INSURED'S POLICY GROUP OR FECA NUMBER

a. OTHER INSURED'S POLICY OR GROUP NUMBER

a. EMPLOYMENT? (CURRENT OR PREVIOUS)   YES   NO

a. INSURED'S DATE OF BIRTH   MM | DD | YY   SEX   M   F

b. OTHER INSURED'S DATE OF BIRTH   MM | DD | YY   SEX   M   F

b. AUTO ACCIDENT?   PLACE (State)   YES   NO

b. EMPLOYER'S NAME OR SCHOOL NAME

c. EMPLOYER'S NAME OR SCHOOL NAME

c. OTHER ACCIDENT?   YES   NO

c. INSURANCE PLAN NAME OR PROGRAM NAME

d. INSURANCE PLAN NAME OR PROGRAM NAME

10d. RESERVED FOR LOCAL USE

d. IS THERE ANOTHER HEALTH BENEFIT PLAN?   YES   NO   *If yes,* return to and complete item 9 a-d.

READ BACK OF FORM BEFORE COMPLETING & SIGNING THIS FORM.

12. PATIENT'S OR AUTHORIZED PERSON'S SIGNATURE I authorize the release of any medical or other information necessary to process this claim. I also request payment of government benefits either to myself or to the party who accepts assignment below.

SIGNED _____ DATE _____

13. INSURED'S OR AUTHORIZED PERSON'S SIGNATURE I authorize payment of medical benefits to the undersigned physician or supplier for services described below.

SIGNED _____

PATIENT AND INSURED INFORMATION

14. DATE OF CURRENT: ◄ ILLNESS (First symptom) OR INJURY (Accident) OR PREGNANCY(LMP)   MM | DD | YY

15. IF PATIENT HAS HAD SAME OR SIMILAR ILLNESS. GIVE FIRST DATE   MM | DD | YY

16. DATES PATIENT UNABLE TO WORK IN CURRENT OCCUPATION   MM | DD | YY   FROM   TO   MM | DD | YY

17. NAME OF REFERRING PHYSICIAN OR OTHER SOURCE

17a. I.D. NUMBER OF REFERRING PHYSICIAN

18. HOSPITALIZATION DATES RELATED TO CURRENT SERVICES   MM | DD | YY   FROM   TO   MM | DD | YY

19. RESERVED FOR LOCAL USE

20. OUTSIDE LAB?   YES   NO $ CHARGES

21. DIAGNOSIS OR NATURE OF ILLNESS OR INJURY. (RELATE ITEMS 1,2,3 OR 4 TO ITEM 24E BY LINE)

1. L___ . __   3. L___ . __

2. L___ . __   4. L___ . __

22. MEDICAID RESUBMISSION CODE   ORIGINAL REF. NO.

23. PRIOR AUTHORIZATION NUMBER

24. A DATE(S) OF SERVICE						B Place of Service	C Type of Service	D PROCEDURES, SERVICES, OR SUPPLIES (Explain Unusual Circumstances) CPT/HCPCS	MODIFIER	E DIAGNOSIS CODE	F $ CHARGES	G DAYS OR UNITS	H EPSDT Family Plan	I EMG	J COB	K RESERVED FOR LOCAL USE
From MM	DD	YY	To MM	DD	YY											
1																
2																
3																
4																
5																
6																

25. FEDERAL TAX I.D. NUMBER   SSN EIN

26. PATIENT'S ACCOUNT NO.

27. ACCEPT ASSIGNMENT? (For govt. claims, see back)   YES   NO

28. TOTAL CHARGE $

29. AMOUNT PAID $

30. BALANCE DUE $

31. SIGNATURE OF PHYSICIAN OR SUPPLIER INCLUDING DEGREES OR CREDENTIALS (I certify that the statements on the reverse apply to this bill and are made a part thereof.)

SIGNED _____ DATE _____

32. NAME AND ADDRESS OF FACILITY WHERE SERVICES WERE RENDERED (If other than home or office)

33. PHYSICIAN'S, SUPPLIER'S BILLING NAME, ADDRESS, ZIP CODE & PHONE #

PIN#   GRP#

PHYSICIAN OR SUPPLIER INFORMATION

(APPROVED BY AMA COUNCIL ON MEDICAL SERVICE 8/88)   **PLEASE PRINT OR TYPE**   APPROVED OMB-0938-0008 FORM CMS-1500 (12-90), FORM RRB-1500, APPROVED OMB-1215-0055 FORM OWCP-1500,   APPROVED OMB-0720-0001 (CHAMPUS)

Chapter
Self-Assessment
Quiz

1. Which of the following is frequently not covered in group health benefits packages?
   a. Birth control
   b. Childhood immunizations
   c. Routine diagnostic care
   d. Treatment for substance abuse
   e. Regular physical examinations

2. Any payment for medical services that is not paid by the patient or physician is said to be paid by a(n)
   a. second-party payer.
   b. first-party payer.
   c. insurance party payer.
   d. third-party payer.
   e. health care party payer.

3. The criteria a patient must meet for a group benefit plan to provide coverage are called:
   a. eligibility requirements.
   b. patient requirements.
   c. benefit plan requirements.
   d. physical requirements.
   e. insurance requirements.

4. Eligibility for a dependent requires that he is:
   a. unmarried.
   b. employed.
   c. living with the employee.
   d. younger than 18.
   e. an excellent student.

5. Whom should you contact about the eligibility of a patient for the health benefits plan?
   a. Claims administrator
   b. Claims investigator
   c. Insurance salesperson
   d. Insurance reviewer
   e. Claims insurer

Scenario: Aziz pays premiums directly to the insurance company, and the insurance company reimburses him for eligible medical expenses.

6. What type of insurance does Aziz have?
   a. Individual health benefits
   b. Public health benefits
   c. Managed care
   d. Preferred Provider Organization
   e. Health Maintenance Organization

7. Which of the following is likely true of Aziz's insurance?
   a. The insurance is provided by his employer.
   b. Money can be put aside into accounts used for medical expenses.
   c. There are certain restrictions for some illnesses and injuries.
   d. All providers are under contract with the insurer.
   e. There are two levels of benefits in the health plan.

End Scenario

8. An optional health benefits program offered to persons signing up for Social Security benefits is:
   a. Medicare Part A.
   b. Medicare Part B.
   c. Medicaid.
   d. TRICARE/CHAMPVA.
   e. HMO.

9. After the deductible has been met, what percentage of the approved charges does Medicare reimburse to the physician?
   a. 0
   b. 20
   c. 75
   d. 80
   e. 100

10. Which benefits program bases eligibility on a patient's eligibility for other state programs, such as welfare assistance?
    a. Workers' Compensation
    b. Medicare
    c. Medicaid
    d. TRICARE/CHAMPVA
    e. Social Security

11. Which of the following is a medical expense that Medicaid provides 100% coverage for?

    a. Family planning

    b. Colorectal screening

    c. Bone density testing

    d. Pap smears

    e. Mammograms

12. In a traditional insurance plan:

    a. the covered patient may seek care from any provider.

    b. the insurer has no relationship with the provider.

    c. a patient can be admitted to a hospital only if that admission has been certified by the insurer.

    d. there is no third-party payer.

    e. the patient cannot be billed for the deductible.

13. Which of the following is a plan typically developed by hospitals and physicians to attract patients?

    a. HMO

    b. PPO

    c. HSA

    d. TPA

    e. UCR

14. Which of the following is true about both HMOs and PPOs?

    a. Both allow patients to see any physician of their choice and receive benefits.

    b. Both contract directly with participating providers, hospitals, and physicians.

    c. Both offer benefits at two levels, commonly referred to as in-network and out-network.

    d. Both are not risk bearing and do not have any financial involvement in the health plan.

    e. Both incorporate independent practice associations.

15. Which of the following is a government-sponsored health benefits plan?

    a. TRICARE/CHAMPVA

    b. HMO

    c. HSA

    d. PPO

    e. PHO

16. If a provider is unethical, you should:

    a. correct the issue yourself.

    b. immediately stop working for the provider.

    c. comply with all requests to misrepresent medical records but report the physician.

    d. do whatever the physician asks to avoid confrontation.

    e. explain that you are legally bound to truthful billing, and report the physician.

17. A patient's ID card:

    a. contains the information needed to file a claim on it.

    b. should be updated at least once every 2 years.

    c. must be cleared before an emergency can be treated.

    d. is updated and sent to Medicaid patients bi-monthly.

    e. is not useful for determining if the patient is a dependent.

18. What information is needed to fill out a CMS-1500 claim form?

    a. A copy of the patient's chart

    b. Location where patient will be recovering

    c. Diagnostic codes from encounter form

    d. Copies of hospitalization paperwork

    e. Physician's record and degree

19. Claims that are submitted electronically:

    a. violate HIPAA standards.

    b. contain fewer errors than those that are mailed.

    c. require approval from the patient.

    d. increase costs for Medicare patients.

    e. reduce the reimbursement cycle.

20. Normally, coverage has an amount below which services are not reimbursable. This is referred to as the:

    a. deductible.

    b. coinsurance.

    c. balance billing.

    d. benefits.

    e. claim.

14 Diagnostic Coding

Chapter Checklist

☐ Read textbook chapter and take notes within the Chapter Notes outline. Answer the Learning Objectives as you reach them in the content, and then check them off.

☐ Work the Content Review questions—both Foundational Knowledge and Application.

☐ Perform the Active Learning exercise(s).

☐ Complete Professional Journal entries.

☐ Complete Skill Practice Activity(s) using Competency Evaluation Forms and Work Products, when appropriate.

☐ Take the Chapter Self-Assessment Quiz.

☐ Insert all appropriate pages into your Portfolio.

Learning Objectives

1. Spell and define the key terms.
2. Describe the relationship between coding and reimbursement.
3. Name and describe the coding system used to describe diseases, injuries, and other reasons for encounters with a medical provider.
4. Explain the format of the ICD-9-CM.
5. Give four examples of ways E-codes are used.
6. List the steps in locating a proper code.
7. Explain common diagnostic coding guidelines.

Chapter Notes

Note: Bold-faced headings are the major headings in the text chapter; headings in regular font are lower-level headings (i.e., the content is subordinate to, or falls "under," the major headings). Make sure you understand the key terms used in the chapter, as well as the concepts presented as Key Points.

TEXT SUBHEADINGS   **NOTES**

Introduction _____

_____

Key Terms: *International Classification of Diseases, Ninth Revision, Clinical Modification*; medical necessity; advance beneficiary notice

Key Point:

• Coding is a way to standardize medical information for purposes such as collecting health care statistics, performing a medical care review, and indexing medical records. It is also used for health insurance claims processing (see Chapter 13). Because coding is the basis for reimbursement, it is imperative that you code patient visits accurately and precisely.

☐ **LEARNING OBJECTIVE 1:** Spell and define the key terms.

☐ **LEARNING OBJECTIVE 2:** Describe the relationship between coding and reimbursement.

Diagnostic Coding _____

Key Term: *International Classification of Diseases, Ninth Revision, Clinical Modification*
Key Point:
• ***International Classification of Diseases, Ninth Revision, Clinical Modification*** (ICD-9-CM) is a statistical classification system based on the *International Classification of Diseases, Ninth Revision* (ICD-9), developed by the World Health Organization (WHO).

Inpatient Versus Outpatient Coding _____

Key Terms: service; outpatient; inpatient

☐ **LEARNING OBJECTIVE 3:** Name and describe the coding system used to describe diseases, injuries, and other reasons for encounters with a medical provider.

ICD-9-CM: The Code Book _____

Key Point:
• You must update codes on superbills (preprinted bills listing a variety of procedures) or any other forms you use.

Tabular List of Diseases _____

Key Term: etiology

☐ **LEARNING OBJECTIVE 4:** Explain the format of the ICD-9-CM.

Supplementary Classifications _____

Key Terms: V-codes; E-codes

☐ **LEARNING OBJECTIVE 5:** Give four examples of ways E-codes are used.

Volume 2: Alphabetic Index to Diseases _____

_____

Key Terms: main terms; cross-reference
Key Points:
- Always check all indentations in the index under the condition to ensure that you have the one most appropriate to the diagnosis you intend to code.
- Never code directly from the alphabetic index.

Volume 3: Inpatient Coding _____

_____

Locating the Appropriate Code _____

_____

Using the ICD-9-CM Conventions _____

_____

Key Term: conventions
Key Point:
- They direct and guide the coder to the appropriate code and should be strictly adhered to.

Main Term _____

_____

Key Term: eponym
Key Point:
- Find the condition, not the location.

Fourth and Fifth Digits _____

Key Term: specificity

☐ **LEARNING OBJECTIVE 6:** List the steps in locating a proper code.

Primary Codes _____

_____

Key Term: primary diagnosis

When More Than One Code Is Used _____

_____

Key Point:
- When patients have more than one diagnosis, it is necessary to convey an accurate picture of the patient's total condition.

Late Effects _____

_____

Key Term: late effects

Coding Suspected Conditions _____

_____

Key Point:
- In the inpatient setting, coders list conditions after the patient's testing is complete.

Documentation Requirements _____

_____

Key Term: audit

☐ **LEARNING OBJECTIVE 7:** Explain common diagnostic coding guidelines.

The Future of Diagnostic Coding: *International Classification of Diseases, Tenth Revision* _____

_____

_____

Content Review

FOUNDATIONAL KNOWLEDGE

Who's Who?

1. Many different organizations are involved in developing and maintaining the ICD-9-CM. Match the organization with its role in maintaining the ICD-9-CM. Note: Some organizations may have more than one correct answer.

Organizations

a. Center for Medicare & Medicaid Services _____

b. National Center for Health Statistics _____

c. World Health Organization _____

Tasks

1. Approves changes made to the ICD-9-CM before publication

2. Maintains Volume 1

3. Maintains Volume 2

4. Maintains Volume 3

A Matter of Medical Necessity

2. A reasonable and capable physician believes that a patient needs a chest x-ray to rule out pneumonia. Does the procedure meet the grounds for medical necessity? Why? Why not?

_____

_____

3. A patient comes in complaining of chest pain. When you enter the codes for this patient encounter, you code that the patient has "acute myocardial infarction." Why would it be better to code this encounter "chest pain rule out myocardial infarction"?

_____

_____

4. Review the list of circumstances below and place a check mark to indicate whether a patient would be forced, given the circumstance, to sign an ABN. All of the patients below are covered by Medicare.

Circumstance	ABN	No ABN
a. The patient wishes to receive an immunization not covered by Medicare.		
b. The patient is undergoing a regularly scheduled checkup.		
c. The patient demands to be tested for an illness that the physician considers an impossibility.		
d. The patient has a badly sprained ankle and wishes to be treated.		
e. The patient is undergoing x-ray imaging per order of a physician.		

Coding Cues

5. When it comes to coding, it makes a difference if the patient is seen in an inpatient or outpatient facility. Review the list of places below. Place an _I_ next to those places that are considered "Inpatient" and an _O_ next to those places that are considered "Outpatient."

a. _____ Hospital clinic

b. _____ Health care provider's office

c. _____ Hospital for less than 24 hours

d. _____ Hospital for 24 hours or more

e. _____ Hospital emergency room

6. Why is the third volume of the ICD-9-CM not used at a hospital's emergency department?

_____

_____

7. What is the difference in information used to code in the outpatient and inpatient settings?

_____

_____

8. You are reading a patient's chart and notice that it is marked with an E-code. However, the patient has experienced no physical injuries. Why might an E-code be used in this situation?

_____

_____

9. You ask a veteran medical assistant for advice on coding, especially how to go about finding a diagnosis with more than one word. Her response is, "Find the condition, not the location." What does she mean by this?

_____

_____

Cracking the CMS-1500

10. What is listed first on the CMS-1500? What does it represent?

_____

_____

11. Which of these is an unethical act? Explain why.

   a. Coding multiple conditions on the same CMS-1500

   b. Coding an unsupported diagnosis in order to make a service appear medically necessary

   c. Using a V-code to better explain the reason for a patient's visit

   d. Using ICD-9-CM search software to more easily access the codes contained in the ICD-9-CM

_____

_____

Mind Your Es and Vs

12. If a construction worker falls from a ladder and suffers an ankle fracture, what supplemental code is used?

_____

_____

13. When would you use the V-code for laboratory examination?

_____

_____

Troubleshooting Common Coding Problems

14. What should you do after finding a seemingly appropriate code in the alphabetic listing of volume 1 of the ICD-9-CM?

_____

_____

15. If you do not know the medical terminology for a diagnosis for a common problem, what would be a good first plan of action?

_____

_____

16. Determine the main term for the following multiple-word diagnoses.

Diagnosis	Main Term
a. chronic fatigue syndrome	
b. severe acute respiratory syndrome	
c. hemmorhagic encephalitis	
d. acute fulminating multiple sclerosis	
e. fractured left tibia	
f. breast cyst	

17. What is the purpose of the fourth and fifth digits often appended to categories?

_____

_____

18. Circle the main terms where you will find obstetric conditions.

delivery   *fetus*   *pregnancy*   *labor*

baby   *obstetrics*   *puerperal*   *gestational*

19. Match the following key terms to their definitions.

Key Terms

a. advance beneficiary notice _____

b. audits _____

c. conventions _____

d. cross-reference _____

e. E-codes _____

f. eponym _____

g. etiology _____

h. inpatient _____

i. *International Classification of Diseases, Ninth Revision, Clinical Modification* _____

j. late effects _____

k. main terms _____

l. medical necessity _____

m. outpatient _____

n. primary diagnosis _____

o. service _____

p. specificity _____

q. V-codes _____

Definitions

1. codes indicating the external causes of injuries and poisoning

2. conditions that result from another condition

3. general notes, symbols, typeface, format, and punctuation that direct and guide a coder to the most accurate ICD-9 code

4. the condition or chief complaint that brings a person to a medical facility for treatment

5. a procedure or service that would have been performed by any reasonable physician under the same or similar circumstances

6. a document that informs covered patients that Medicare may not cover a certain service and the patient will be responsible for the bill

7. a word based on or derived from a person's name

8. codes assigned to patients who receive service but have no illness, injury, or disorder

9. the billable tasks performed by a physician

10. refers to a medical setting in which patients are admitted for diagnostic, radiographic, or treatment purposes

11. an investigation performed by government, managed health care companies, and health care organizations to determine compliance and to detect fraud

12. a system for transforming verbal descriptions of disease, injuries, conditions, and procedures to numeric codes

13. refers to the cause of disease

14. refers to a medical setting in which patients receive care but are not admitted

15. verification against another source

16. relating to a definite result

17. words in a multiple-word diagnosis that a coder should locate in the alphabetic listing

20. Code the following diagnoses:

1. sick sinus syndrome
2. congestive heart failure with malignant hypertension
3. bilateral stenosis of carotid artery
4. aspiration pneumonia
5. gynecomastia

6. nephrosis due to diabetes
7. hematemesis
8. portal thrombophlebitis
9. acute viral conjunctivitis with hemorrhage
10. *E. coli* intestinal infection

21. True or False? Determine whether the following statements are true or false. If false, explain why.

a. Only the first three numbers of a code are necessary. _____

b. One should never code directly from the alphabetic index. _____

c. The main term describes a condition, not an aspect of anatomy. _____

d. In the outpatient setting, coders list conditions after the patient's testing is complete. _____

APPLICATION

Critical Thinking Practice

1. A patient entered the office complaining of chest pains. After examination, the physician decided to send him to a specialist in order to rule out the possibility of angina pectoris. Which code should be placed on the CMA-1500 first as the primary diagnosis or reason for the visit? Why?

_____

_____

2. What might result from improper medical coding?

_____

_____

Patient Education

1. After looking at the CMS-1500 for her visit, a patient asks why there is an alphanumeric string instead of a diagnosis. Explain as you would to a patient what the code represents.

_____

_____

Documentation

1. The physician has informed you that the diagnosis for your patient is "atrial septal defect as current complication following acute myocardial infarction." How would you code this diagnosis?

_____

_____

Active Learning

1. Find the ICD-9-CM codes for the following diseases:
- Acute gastric ulcer with hemorrhage and perforation without obstruction
- Meningococcal pericarditis
- Impetigo
- Benign essential hypertension

2. Determine the diseases associated with the following ICD-9-CM codes:
   - 431
   - 558.3
   - 758.0
   - 299.11

3. Determine the E-codes for the following:
   - Inhalation and ingestion of other object causing obstruction of respiratory tract or suffocation
   - Insulins and antidiabetic agents causing adverse effects in therapeutic use
   - Burning caused by conflagration in private dwelling

Professional Journal

REFLECT

(Prompts and Ideas: Digital editions of the ICD-9-CM have changed the way medical coders practice their craft. Reflect on the nature of this change and how digital tools can make your job as a medical coder easier.)

_____

_____

_____

_____

_____

_____

PONDER AND SOLVE

1. In the ICD-9-CM, burns are listed in the range 940–949, a subset of 800–999 — Injury and Poisoning. However, if you look for the code for sunburn, you will not find it there. Find the code for sunburn and explain why it does not belong in the range 940–949. You do not need to know exactly why, but consider the diagnoses that appear in 940–949 and how sunburn compares with them.

_____

_____

_____

_____

_____

2. A patient is concerned that her insurance provider will not cover her visit because the diagnosis is for a very minor ailment. She requests that you mark her CMA-1500 with a more severe disorder that demands similar treatment. How would you deal with this situation? What would you tell the patient? How might you involve the physician?

_____

_____

_____

_____

_____

EXPERIENCE

Skills related to this chapter include:

1. Locating a Diagnostic Code (Procedure 14-1).

Record any common mistakes, lessons learned, and/or tips you discovered during your experience of practicing and demonstrating these skills:

_____

_____

_____

_____

_____

_____

_____

Skill Practice

PERFORMANCE OBJECTIVE:

1. Locate an appropriate ICD-9-CM code (Procedure 14-1).

Name _____   Date _____   Time _____

Procedure 14-1:   LOCATING A DIAGNOSTIC CODE

EQUIPMENT: Diagnosis, ICD-9-CM, Volumes 1 and 2 code book, medical dictionary

STANDARDS: Given the needed equipment and a place to work the student will perform this skill with _____% accuracy in a total of _____ minutes. (*Your instructor will tell you what the percentage and time limits will be before you begin.*)

KEY: 4 = Satisfactory   0 = Unsatisfactory   NA = This step is not counted

PROCEDURE STEPS	SELF	PARTNER	INSTRUCTOR
1. Using the diagnosis "chronic rheumatoid arthritis," choose the main term within the diagnostic statement. If necessary, look up the word(s) in your dictionary.	☐	☐	☐
2. Locate the main term in Volume 2.	☐	☐	☐
3. Refer to all notes and conventions under the main term.	☐	☐	☐
4. Find the appropriate indented subordinate term.	☐	☐	☐
5. Follow any relevant instructions, such as "see also."	☐	☐	☐
6. Confirm the selected code by cross-referencing to Volume 1. Make sure you have added any fourth or fifth digits necessary.	☐	☐	☐
7. Assign the code.	☐	☐	☐

CALCULATION

Total Possible Points: _____
Total Points Earned: _____ Multiplied by 100 = _____ Divided by Total Possible Points = _____%

Pass   **Fail**
☐   ☐   Comments:

Student's signature _____ Date _____
Partner's signature _____ Date _____
Instructor's signature _____ Date _____

Work Product

Perform diagnostic coding.

Kayla Tawes, age 38, has just completed a general physical. Her examination consisted of the following:

- an EKG to monitor a previously diagnosed arrhythmia
- urine collection to test for diabetes
- blood sampling to test cholesterol levels

Because Ms. Tawes is a breast cancer survivor, in addition to the routine examination, she was given a mammogram. Her physician prescribed a tetanus booster as well, because she has been renovating an old stable and has suffered several small skin punctures over the past few weeks.

Complete the CMS-1500 form with the proper diagnostic coding for the patient's visit. Create fictional personal patient information where necessary to fill in all essential details when completing the CMS-1500.

PLEASE
DO NOT
STAPLE
IN THIS
AREA

CARRIER →

HEALTH INSURANCE CLAIM FORM

PICA						PICA	

1. MEDICARE (Medicare #) **MEDICAID** (Medicaid #) **CHAMPUS** (Sponsor's SSN) **CHAMPVA** (VA File #) **GROUP HEALTH PLAN** (SSN or ID) **FECA BLK LUNG** (SSN) **OTHER** (ID)

1a. INSURED'S I.D. NUMBER (FOR PROGRAM IN ITEM 1)

2. PATIENT'S NAME (Last Name, First Name, Middle Initial)

3. PATIENT'S BIRTH DATE MM DD YY **SEX** M ☐ F ☐

4. INSURED'S NAME (Last Name, First Name, Middle Initial)

5. PATIENT'S ADDRESS (No., Street)

6. PATIENT RELATIONSHIP TO INSURED Self ☐ Spouse ☐ Child ☐ Other ☐

7. INSURED'S ADDRESS (No., Street)

CITY ‖ STATE

8. PATIENT STATUS Single ☐ Married ☐ Other ☐

CITY ‖ STATE

ZIP CODE ‖ TELEPHONE (Include Area Code) ( )

Employed ☐ Full-Time Student ☐ Part-Time Student ☐

ZIP CODE ‖ TELEPHONE (INCLUDE AREA CODE) ( )

9. OTHER INSURED'S NAME (Last Name, First Name, Middle Initial)

10. IS PATIENT'S CONDITION RELATED TO:

11. INSURED'S POLICY GROUP OR FECA NUMBER

a. OTHER INSURED'S POLICY OR GROUP NUMBER

a. EMPLOYMENT? (CURRENT OR PREVIOUS) ☐ YES ☐ NO

a. INSURED'S DATE OF BIRTH MM DD YY **SEX** M ☐ F ☐

b. OTHER INSURED'S DATE OF BIRTH MM DD YY **SEX** M ☐ F ☐

b. AUTO ACCIDENT? PLACE (State) ☐ YES ☐ NO

b. EMPLOYER'S NAME OR SCHOOL NAME

c. EMPLOYER'S NAME OR SCHOOL NAME

c. OTHER ACCIDENT? ☐ YES ☐ NO

c. INSURANCE PLAN NAME OR PROGRAM NAME

d. INSURANCE PLAN NAME OR PROGRAM NAME

10d. RESERVED FOR LOCAL USE

d. IS THERE ANOTHER HEALTH BENEFIT PLAN? ☐ YES ☐ NO *If yes,* return to and complete item 9 a-d.

READ BACK OF FORM BEFORE COMPLETING & SIGNING THIS FORM.
12. PATIENT'S OR AUTHORIZED PERSON'S SIGNATURE I authorize the release of any medical or other information necessary to process this claim. I also request payment of government benefits either to myself or to the party who accepts assignment below.

SIGNED _____ DATE _____

13. INSURED'S OR AUTHORIZED PERSON'S SIGNATURE I authorize payment of medical benefits to the undersigned physician or supplier for services described below.

SIGNED _____

14. DATE OF CURRENT: MM DD YY ◄ ILLNESS (First symptom) OR INJURY (Accident) OR PREGNANCY(LMP)

15. IF PATIENT HAS HAD SAME OR SIMILAR ILLNESS. GIVE FIRST DATE MM DD YY

16. DATES PATIENT UNABLE TO WORK IN CURRENT OCCUPATION MM DD YY MM DD YY FROM TO

17. NAME OF REFERRING PHYSICIAN OR OTHER SOURCE

17a. I.D. NUMBER OF REFERRING PHYSICIAN

18. HOSPITALIZATION DATES RELATED TO CURRENT SERVICES MM DD YY MM DD YY FROM TO

19. RESERVED FOR LOCAL USE

20. OUTSIDE LAB? ☐ YES ☐ NO $ CHARGES

21. DIAGNOSIS OR NATURE OF ILLNESS OR INJURY. (RELATE ITEMS 1,2,3 OR 4 TO ITEM 24E BY LINE)

1. ‖___.___ 3. ‖___.___
2. ‖___.___ 4. ‖___.___

22. MEDICAID RESUBMISSION CODE ‖ ORIGINAL REF. NO.

23. PRIOR AUTHORIZATION NUMBER

24. A DATE(S) OF SERVICE From MM DD YY To MM DD YY	B Place of Service	C Type of Service	D PROCEDURES, SERVICES, OR SUPPLIES (Explain Unusual Circumstances) CPT/HCPCS | MODIFIER	E DIAGNOSIS CODE	F $ CHARGES	G DAYS OR UNITS	H EPSDT Family Plan	I EMG	J COB	K RESERVED FOR LOCAL USE
1										
2										
3										
4										
5										
6										

25. FEDERAL TAX I.D. NUMBER SSN ☐ EIN ☐

26. PATIENT'S ACCOUNT NO.

27. ACCEPT ASSIGNMENT? (For govt. claims, see back) ☐ YES ☐ NO

28. TOTAL CHARGE $

29. AMOUNT PAID $

30. BALANCE DUE $

31. SIGNATURE OF PHYSICIAN OR SUPPLIER INCLUDING DEGREES OR CREDENTIALS (I certify that the statements on the reverse apply to this bill and are made a part thereof.)

SIGNED _____ DATE _____

32. NAME AND ADDRESS OF FACILITY WHERE SERVICES WERE RENDERED (If other than home or office)

33. PHYSICIAN'S, SUPPLIER'S BILLING NAME, ADDRESS, ZIP CODE & PHONE #

PIN# ‖ GRP#

(APPROVED BY AMA COUNCIL ON MEDICAL SERVICE 8/88) **PLEASE PRINT OR TYPE** APPROVED OMB-0938-0008 FORM CMS-1500 (12-90), FORM RRB-1500, APPROVED OMB-1215-0055 FORM OWCP-1500, APPROVED OMB-0720-0001 (CHAMPUS)

PATIENT AND INSURED INFORMATION →

PHYSICIAN OR SUPPLIER INFORMATION →

Chapter Self-Assessment Quiz

1. Which most accurately states the purpose of coding?

   a. Coding assists patients in accessing insurance databases.

   b. Coding determines the reimbursement of medical fees.

   c. Coding is used to track a physician's payments.

   d. Coding is used to index patients' claims forms.

   e. Coding identifies patients in a database.

2. A patient signs an advance beneficiary notice (ABN) to:

   a. consent to medically necessary procedures.

   b. assign payment to Medicare.

   c. accept responsibility for payment.

   d. assign responsibility for payment to a beneficiary.

   e. consent to a medically unnecessary procedure.

3. The content of the ICD-9-CM is a(n):

   a. classification of diseases and list of procedures.

   b. statistical grouping of trends in diseases.

   c. clinical modification of codes used by hospitals.

   d. ninth volume in an index of diseases.

   e. international document for monitoring coding.

4. Which is true of Volume 3 of the ICD-9-CM?

   a. It is organized by location on the patient's body.

   b. It is used to code mostly outpatient procedures.

   c. It is an alphabetical listing of diseases.

   d. It is used by hospitals to report procedures and services.

   e. It is an index of Volumes 1 and 2.

5. Physician's services are reported:

   a. on the UB-92.

   b. on the CMS-1500.

   c. on the uniform bill.

   d. on the advance beneficiary notice.

   e. on bills from health institutions.

6. Which of these would be considered inpatient coding?

   a. Hospital same-day surgery

   b. Hour-long testing in a hospital CAT scan

   c. Treatment in the emergency room

   d. Observation status in a hospital

   e. Meals and testing during a hospital stay

7. In Volume 1 of the ICD-9-CM, chapters are grouped:

   a. by alphabetic ordering of diseases and injuries.

   b. alphabetically by eponym.

   c. by location in the body.

   d. by etiology and anatomic system.

   e. by surgical specialty.

8. The fourth and fifth digits in a code indicate the:

   a. anatomical location where a procedure was performed.

   b. number of times a test was executed.

   c. higher definitions of a code.

   d. code for the patient's general disease.

   e. traumatic origins of a disease (i.e., injury, deliberate violence).

9. A V-code might indicate a(n):

   a. immunization.

   b. poisoning.

   c. accident.

   d. diagnosis.

   e. treatment.

10. V-codes are used:

    a. for outpatient coding.

    b. when reimbursement is not needed.

    c. when a patient is not sick.

    d. to indicate testing for HIV.

    e. for infectious diseases.

11. What is the purpose of E-codes?

    a. They code for immunizations and other preventive procedures.

    b. They are used to code medical testing before a diagnosis.

    c. They assist insurance companies in making reimbursements.

    d. They indicate why a patient has an injury or poisoning.

    e. They indicate if a procedure was inpatient or outpatient.

12. Which of the following agencies are *least* interested in E-codes?

a. Insurance underwriters

b. Insurance claim providers

c. National safety programs

d. Public health agencies

e. Workers' compensation lawyers

13. How is Volume 2 of the ICD-9-CM different from Volume 1?

a. Volume 2 contains diagnostic terms that are not used in Volume 1.

b. Volume 2 is organized into 17 chapters rather than 3 sections.

c. Volume 2 does not contain E-codes, but Volume 1 does.

d. Volume 2 contains hospital coding to cross-reference with Volume 1.

e. Volume 2 provides information about the fourth and fifth digits of a code.

14. After finding a code in Volume 2, you should:

a. record the code on the CMS-1500.

b. consult Volume 3 for subordinate terms.

c. cross-reference the code with Volume 1.

d. indicate if the code is inpatient or outpatient.

e. record the code on the UB-92.

15. Volume 3 of the ICD-9-CM is organized:

a. by disease.

b. by anatomy.

c. into 17 chapters.

d. into three sections.

e. by surgical specialty.

16. One example of an eponym is:

a. Crohn disease.

b. bacterial meningitis.

c. influenza virus.

d. pruritus.

e. pneumonia.

17. What is the first step to locating a diagnostic code?

a. Determine where the diagnosis occurs in the body.

b. Choose the main term within the diagnostic statement.

c. Begin looking up the diagnosis in Volume 1 of the ICD-9-CM.

d. Consult the CMS-1500 for reimbursement codes.

e. Use Volume 3 of the ICD-9-CM to find the disease.

18. Which code is listed first on a CMS-1500?

a. A reasonable second opinion

b. Relevant laboratory work

c. Diagnostic tests

d. The symptoms of an illness

e. The primary diagnosis

19. How do you code for late effects?

a. Code for the treatment of the disease that causes late effects.

b. Code for the disease that is causing the current condition.

c. First code for the current condition, and then list the cause.

d. Only code for the current condition.

e. Only code for the cause of the current condition.

20. You should not code for a brain tumor:

a. when the patient comes in for an MRI.

b. after the tumor is confirmed on an MRI.

c. when the diagnosed patient comes in for treatment.

d. any time after the patient has been diagnosed.

e. when the patient seeks specialist care.

Chapter Checklist

☐ Read textbook chapter and take notes within the Chapter Notes outline. Answer the Learning Objectives as you reach them in the content, and then check them off.

☐ Work the Content Review questions—both Foundational Knowledge and Application.

☐ Perform the Active Learning exercise(s).

☐ Complete Professional Journal entries.

☐ Complete Skill Practice Activity(s) using Competency Evaluation Forms and Work Products, when appropriate.

☐ Take the Chapter Self-Assessment Quiz.

☐ Insert all appropriate pages into your Portfolio.

Learning Objectives

1. Spell and define the key terms.
2. Explain the Healthcare Common Procedure Coding System (HCPCS), levels I and II.
3. Explain the format of level I, Current Procedural Terminology (CPT-4) and its use.
4. Explain what diagnostic related groups (DRGs) are and how they are used to determine Medicare payments.
5. Discuss the goals of resource-based relative value system (RBRVS).
6. Describe the relationship between coding and reimbursement.

Chapter Notes

Note: Bold-faced headings are the major headings in the text chapter; headings in regular font are lower-level headings (i.e., the content is subordinate to, or falls "under," the major headings). Make sure you understand the key terms used in the chapter, as well as the concepts presented as Key Points.

TEXT SUBHEADINGS   **NOTES**

Introduction _____

_____

_____

☐ **LEARNING OBJECTIVE 1:** Spell and define the key terms.

_____

Health Care Procedural Coding System _____

_____

Key Term: Healthcare Common Procedure Coding System

☐ **LEARNING OBJECTIVE 2:** Explain the Healthcare Common Procedure Coding System (HCPCS), levels I and II.

Physician's Current Procedural Terminology (CPT) _____

_____

Key Term: Current Procedural Terminology
Key Point:
• HCPCS level I codes or the Physician's **Current Procedural Terminology (CPT)** is a comprehensive listing of medical terms and codes for the uniform coding of procedures and services provided by physicians.

Performing Procedural Coding _____

_____

Key Term: procedure

The Layout of CPT-4 _____

_____

The Alphabetic Index _____

_____

Reading Descriptors _____

_____

Key Term: descriptor

Place of Service _____

_____

_____

Section Guidelines _____

_____

_____

Unlisted Procedures and Special Reports _____

_____

_____

☐ **LEARNING OBJECTIVE 3:** Explain the format of level I, Current Procedural Terminology (CPT-4) and its use.

_____

Evaluation and Management Codes _____

_____

> **Key Point:**
> • E/M codes describe various patient histories, examinations, and decisions physicians must make in evaluating and treating patients in various settings (e.g., office, outpatient, hospital).

Key Components _____

_____

> **Key Term:** key components
> **Key Point:**
> • History, physical examination, and medical decision making are three **key components** for a visit.

History _____

_____

_____

Examination _____

_____

_____

Medical Decision Making _____

_____

_____

Time _____

_____

> **Key Point:**
> • When time spent with the patient is more than 50% of the typical time for the visit, time becomes the deciding factor in choosing an E/M code.

Other Categories of Evaluation and Management Codes _____

_____

_____

Anesthesia Section _____

_____

Key Term: modifiers

Surgery Section _____

_____

_____

Content of the Surgery Section _____

_____

_____

Radiology Section _____

_____

_____

Pathology and Laboratory Section _____

_____

_____

Medicine Section _____

_____

_____

CPT-4 Modifiers _____

_____

_____

Key Point:
• Failure to use an appropriate modifier causes database and reimbursement errors.

Reimbursement _____

_____

_____

Diagnostic Related Groups _____

_____

Key Terms: diagnostic related groups; outlier
Key Point:
• **Diagnostic related groups** (DRGs) are categories into which inpatients are placed according to the similarity of their diagnoses, treatment, and length of hospital stay.

☐ **LEARNING OBJECTIVE 4:** Explain what diagnostic related groups (DRGs) are and how they are used to determine Medicare payments.

Resource-Based Relative Value Scale _____

_____

Key Term: resource-based relative value scale
Key Point:
• The goal of RBRVS is to reduce Medicare Part B costs and to establish national standards for payment based on CPT-4 codes.

☐ **LEARNING OBJECTIVE 5:** Discuss the goals of resource-based relative value system (RBRVS).

Fraud and Coding _____

_____

Key Term: upcoding

☐ **LEARNING OBJECTIVE 6:** Describe the relationship between coding and reimbursement.

Content Review

FOUNDATIONAL KNOWLEDGE

Understanding the CPT-4

1. Fill in the chart below to show the difference between Level I HPCS and Level II.

Level I	Level II

2. What are the six major sections of the CPT-4?

a. _____

b. _____

c. _____

d. _____

e. _____

f. _____

3. How is the CPT alphabetic index used in the medical office?

_____

_____

Understanding E/M Codes

4. Define the seven components of the E/M codes.

Component	Definition
a. history	
b. physician examination	
c. medical decision making	
d. counseling	
e. coordination of care	
f. nature of presenting problem	
g. time	

5. How many numbers do E/M codes have?

    a. Two

    b. Five

    c. Seven

    d. Ten

6. Read the scenario below. Then, highlight or underline the medical decision making section.

Anikka was seen today for a follow-up on her broken wrist. The cast was removed 2 weeks ago, and she said she is still unable to achieve full range of movement in her wrist without pain. On exam, her wrist appeared swollen, and she mentioned tenderness. X-ray revealed slight fracture in carpals. Dr. Levy splinted the wrist, and referred her to an orthopedic surgeon for possible surgery. I spoke with Anikka, instructing her to avoid exerting her wrist and to keep it splinted until she has seen the surgeon. Dr. Levy suggested aspirin for pain.

7. Now, read the same scenario again. Then, highlight or underline the history section.

Anikka was seen today for a follow-up on her broken wrist. The cast was removed 2 weeks ago, and she said she is still unable to achieve full range of movement in her wrist without pain. On exam, her wrist appeared swollen, and she mentioned tenderness. X-ray revealed slight fracture in carpals. Dr. Levy splinted the wrist, and referred her to an orthopedic surgeon for possible surgery. I spoke with Anikka, instructing her to avoid exerting her wrist and to keep it splinted until she has seen the surgeon. Dr. Levy suggested aspirin for pain.

8. Read the scenario below.

Mr. Ekko presents today for removal of stitches from calf wound. Upon inspection, wound seems to have healed well, but scar tissue is still slightly inflamed. I prescribed antibacterial cream for him to apply twice a day, and instructed him to still keep the area bandaged. I told him to let us know if the swelling has not gone down within a week, and to come in if it gets any worse.

Circle the correct level of medical decision making involved.

Straightforward   Low complexity

Moderate complexity   High complexity

9. Why is it important to check the constitution of a surgery package with a third-party payer?

_____

_____

10. A patient experiences complications after an appendectomy and has to be hospitalized for several days. Will the time spent in the hospital be coded as part of a surgery package or separately?

_____

_____

11. Fill in the medical terminology chart below about the CPT subcategory on repair, revision, or reconstruction.

Suffix	Meaning
-pexy	
	surgical repair
-rrhaphy	

12. Name four factors that go into radiology coding.

a. _____

b. _____

c. _____

d. _____

13. What role do modifiers play in coding?

_____

_____

14. When would you use 99 as the first numbers in your modifier?

_____

_____

Reimbursement

15. What is the goal of the resource-based relative value scale (RBRVS)?

_____

_____

16. How does coding play a part in reimbursement?

_____

_____

17. What are DRGs, and how are they used to determine Medicare payments?

_____

_____

18. Medicare is often a target for upcoding and fraud. What can Medicare do to protect itself from this?

_____

_____

19. Match the following key terms to their definitions.

Key Terms	Definitions
a. Current Procedural Terminology _____	1. a patient whose hospital stay is longer than amount allowed by the DRG
b. descriptor _____	2. categories used to determine hospital and physician reimbursement for Medicare patients' inpatient services

c. Diagnostic Related Group _____

d. Health Care Common Procedure Coding System _____

e. key component _____

f. modifiers _____

g. outlier _____

h. procedure _____

i. Resource-Based Relative Value Scale _____

j. upcoding _____

3. a value scale designed to decrease Medicare Part B costs and establish national standards for coding and payment

4. billing more than the proper fee for a service by selecting a code that is higher on the coding scale

5. description of a service listed with its code number

6. numbers or letters added to a code to clarify the service or procedure provided

7. a comprehensive listing of medical terms and codes for the uniform coding of procedures and services that are provided by physicians

8. a medical service or test that is coded for reimbursement

9. a standardized coding system that is used primarily to identify products, supplies, and services

10. the criteria or factors on which the selection of CPT-4 evaluation and management is based

20. Assign the appropriate CPT code for the following:

a. occult blood in stool, two simultaneous guaiac tests

b. blood ethanol levels

c. transurethral resection of prostate

d. flexible sigmoidoscopy for biopsy

e. radiation therapy requiring general anesthesia

f. hair transplant, 21 punch grafts

g. breast reduction, left

h. open repair of left Dupuytren's contracture

i. partial removal left turbinate

j. newborn clamp circumcision

21. True or False? Determine whether the following statements are true or false. If false, explain why.

a. It is permissible to leave out modifiers if a note is made on the patient's sheet.

_____

_____

b. When time spent with a patient is more than 50% of the typical time for the visit, time becomes the deciding factor in choosing a code.

_____

_____

c. The number of tests you perform is the final number in the coding.

_____

_____

d. The amount of time a physician spends with a patient has no effect on the coding for that exam.

_____

_____

APPLICATION

Critical Thinking Practice

1. A patient undergoes surgery to remove her gallbladder, and she needs to stay in the hospital overnight. Her insurance company labels this sort of operation as an outpatient surgery. What can you do to code this information on the claim form?

_____

_____

2. What are some ways to reduce the likelihood of a Medicare audit of your office?

_____

_____

Patient Education

1. A patient has a recurring skin rash, and the physician suggests that she see a dermatologist. The patient doesn't understand the difference between a referral and a consultation. How would you explain this to her?

_____

_____

Documentation

1. An 18-year-old patient visits a gynecologist for the first time. She needs a Pap smear and a breast examination, as well as consultation regarding contraceptives. Write a detailed note in her chart that can be used for coding purposes.

_____

_____

_____

Active Learning

1. Read the scenario below.

A young teen comes in for a routine check. He is weighed and measured, and blood is drawn for diagnosis. The physician comes in and spends approximately 15 minutes of a 25-minute visit discussing how the teen recently became a vegetarian. The physician offers advice on ways to supplement his diet to keep him healthy. Blood tests come back with a low iron count, so the physician prescribes iron tablets.

Look online or go through a HCPCS book to find the correct coding for the teen's chart. Be sure to get all the information on his chart, but avoid upcoding and adding modifiers for services not mentioned.

2. Create five different medical scenarios that would require coding, and write them down on a sheet of paper. Then, after you have coded each scenario on a separate piece of paper, switch with a partner. When you are both done, compare notes. Check for any discrepancies between your answers by going through an HCPCS book.

3. It is important to familiarize yourself with the code book so that when you are coding for billing, you know how and where to search for a specific code. Using a copy of both the CPT-4 book and the ICD-9-CM book, flip through and find codes for common office procedures such as taking blood samples, testing reflexes, counseling, and testing blood pressure. Then, look through and make a list of codes for a less common task, like mole removal or splinting a fractured ankle. Be sure to list the steps you took to find your code (e.g., looking up _splint, fractures, ankle_). Also make a note of what types of codes you would use from the ICD-9 book, and jot down a few codes you might be likely to use.

Professional Journal

REFLECT

(Prompts and Ideas: Sometimes upcoding is accidental; however, many times this is not the case. What would motivate someone to upcode deliberately? How can it happen accidentally?)

_____

_____

_____

PONDER AND SOLVE

1. For 20 minutes of a 30-minute exam, the physician was talking with the patient. Most of this time was spent talking about getting more exercise and keeping in shape; however, almost ten minutes of the time was spent discussing non-health-related issues. The physician marked the patient's chart as having talked for 20 minutes. How would you code this? Do you still write in 20 minutes, because they were talking, or do you code it as 10 minutes, which is the amount of time they talked about health-related things? Why?

_____

_____

_____

_____

_____

_____

2. A patient complains that she is getting charged too much, and you check over her chart. You find that the physician has been up-coding regularly on this patient's chart. How do you react to this situation? How do you deal with the patient, and how would you confront the physician?

_____

_____

_____

_____

_____

_____

_____

EXPERIENCE

Skills related to this chapter include:

1. Locating a CPT Code (Procedure 15-1).

Record any common mistakes, lessons learned, and/or tips you discovered during your experience of practicing and demonstrating these skills:

_____

_____

_____

_____

_____

_____

_____

Skill Practice

PERFORMANCE OBJECTIVES:

1. Perform procedural coding (Procedure 15-1).

Name_____ Date _____ Time _____

Procedure 15-1:   LOCATING A CPT CODE

EQUIPMENT: CPT-4 code book, patient chart, scenario

STANDARDS: Given the needed equipment and a place to work the student will perform this skill with _____% accuracy in a total of _____ minutes. (*Your instructor will tell you what the percentage and time limits will be before you begin.*)

KEY: 4 = Satisfactory   0 = Unsatisfactory   NA = This step is not counted

PROCEDURE STEPS	SELF	PARTNER	INSTRUCTOR
1. Identify the exact procedure performed.	☐	☐	☐
2. Obtain the documentation of the procedure in the patient's chart.	☐	☐	☐
3. Choose the proper code book.	☐	☐	☐
4. Using the alphabetic index, locate the procedure.	☐	☐	☐
5. Locate the code or range of codes given in the tabular section.	☐	☐	☐
6. Read the descriptors to find the one that most closely describes the procedure.	☐	☐	☐
7. Check the section guidelines for any special circumstances.	☐	☐	☐
8. Review the documentation to be sure it justifies the code.	☐	☐	☐
9. Determine if any modifiers are needed.	☐	☐	☐
10. Select the code and place it in the appropriate field of the CMS-1500 form.	☐	☐	☐

CALCULATION

Total Possible Points: _____
Total Points Earned: _____ Multiplied by 100 = _____ Divided by Total Possible Points = _____%

Pass   **Fail**
☐   ☐   Comments:

Student's signature _____ Date _____
Partner's signature _____ Date _____
Instructor's signature _____ Date _____

Work Product 1

Perform procedural coding.

Kayla Tawes, age 38, has just completed a general physical. Her examination consisted of the following:

- an EKG to monitor a previously diagnosed arrhythmia
- urine collection to test for diabetes
- blood sampling to test cholesterol levels

Because Ms. Tawes is a breast cancer survivor, in addition to the routine examination, she was given a mammogram. Her physician prescribed a tetanus booster as well, because she has been renovating an old stable and has suffered several small skin punctures over the past few weeks.

Complete the CMS-1500 form with the proper procedural coding for the patient's visit. Use the same personal patient information you used for Work Product 1 in Chapter 14 to fill in all essential details when completing the CMS-1500.

PLEASE
DO NOT
STAPLE
IN THIS
AREA

CARRIER

HEALTH INSURANCE CLAIM FORM

PICA | | | | PICA | |

1. MEDICARE MEDICAID CHAMPUS CHAMPVA GROUP HEALTH PLAN FECA BLK LUNG OTHER | 1a. INSURED'S I.D. NUMBER (FOR PROGRAM IN ITEM 1)

☐ (Medicare #) ☐ (Medicaid #) ☐ (Sponsor's SSN) ☐ (VA File #) ☐ (SSN or ID) ☐ (SSN) ☐ (ID)

2. PATIENT'S NAME (Last Name, First Name, Middle Initial) | 3. PATIENT'S BIRTH DATE MM DD YY SEX M ☐ F ☐ | 4. INSURED'S NAME (Last Name, First Name, Middle Initial)

5. PATIENT'S ADDRESS (No., Street) | 6. PATIENT RELATIONSHIP TO INSURED Self ☐ Spouse ☐ Child ☐ Other ☐ | 7. INSURED'S ADDRESS (No., Street)

CITY | STATE | 8. PATIENT STATUS Single ☐ Married ☐ Other ☐ | CITY | STATE

ZIP CODE | TELEPHONE (Include Area Code) ( ) | Employed ☐ Full-Time Student ☐ Part-Time Student ☐ | ZIP CODE | TELEPHONE (INCLUDE AREA CODE) ( )

9. OTHER INSURED'S NAME (Last Name, First Name, Middle Initial) | 10. IS PATIENT'S CONDITION RELATED TO: | 11. INSURED'S POLICY GROUP OR FECA NUMBER

a. OTHER INSURED'S POLICY OR GROUP NUMBER | a. EMPLOYMENT? (CURRENT OR PREVIOUS) ☐ YES ☐ NO | a. INSURED'S DATE OF BIRTH MM DD YY SEX M ☐ F ☐

b. OTHER INSURED'S DATE OF BIRTH MM DD YY SEX M ☐ F ☐ | b. AUTO ACCIDENT? PLACE (State) ☐ YES ☐ NO | b. EMPLOYER'S NAME OR SCHOOL NAME

c. EMPLOYER'S NAME OR SCHOOL NAME | c. OTHER ACCIDENT? ☐ YES ☐ NO | c. INSURANCE PLAN NAME OR PROGRAM NAME

d. INSURANCE PLAN NAME OR PROGRAM NAME | 10d. RESERVED FOR LOCAL USE | d. IS THERE ANOTHER HEALTH BENEFIT PLAN? ☐ YES ☐ NO *If yes*, return to and complete item 9 a-d.

READ BACK OF FORM BEFORE COMPLETING & SIGNING THIS FORM.
12. PATIENT'S OR AUTHORIZED PERSON'S SIGNATURE I authorize the release of any medical or other information necessary to process this claim. I also request payment of government benefits either to myself or to the party who accepts assignment below.

SIGNED _____ DATE _____

13. INSURED'S OR AUTHORIZED PERSON'S SIGNATURE I authorize payment of medical benefits to the undersigned physician or supplier for services described below.

SIGNED _____

PATIENT AND INSURED INFORMATION

14. DATE OF CURRENT: ◄ ILLNESS (First symptom) OR INJURY (Accident) OR PREGNANCY(LMP) MM DD YY | 15. IF PATIENT HAS HAD SAME OR SIMILAR ILLNESS. GIVE FIRST DATE MM DD YY | 16. DATES PATIENT UNABLE TO WORK IN CURRENT OCCUPATION MM DD YY FROM TO MM DD YY

17. NAME OF REFERRING PHYSICIAN OR OTHER SOURCE | 17a. I.D. NUMBER OF REFERRING PHYSICIAN | 18. HOSPITALIZATION DATES RELATED TO CURRENT SERVICES MM DD YY FROM TO MM DD YY

19. RESERVED FOR LOCAL USE | 20. OUTSIDE LAB? ☐ YES ☐ NO $ CHARGES

21. DIAGNOSIS OR NATURE OF ILLNESS OR INJURY. (RELATE ITEMS 1,2,3 OR 4 TO ITEM 24E BY LINE) | 22. MEDICAID RESUBMISSION CODE ORIGINAL REF. NO.

1. _____ . _____   3. _____ . _____ | 23. PRIOR AUTHORIZATION NUMBER

2. _____ . _____   4. _____ . _____

24. A DATE(S) OF SERVICE From MM DD YY To MM DD YY	B Place of Service	C Type of Service	D PROCEDURES, SERVICES, OR SUPPLIES (Explain Unusual Circumstances) CPT/HCPCS	MODIFIER	E DIAGNOSIS CODE	F $ CHARGES	G DAYS OR UNITS	H EPSDT Family Plan	I EMG	J COB	K RESERVED FOR LOCAL USE
1											
2											
3											
4											
5											
6											

25. FEDERAL TAX I.D. NUMBER SSN ☐ EIN ☐ | 26. PATIENT'S ACCOUNT NO. | 27. ACCEPT ASSIGNMENT? (For govt. claims, see back) ☐ YES ☐ NO | 28. TOTAL CHARGE $ | 29. AMOUNT PAID $ | 30. BALANCE DUE $

31. SIGNATURE OF PHYSICIAN OR SUPPLIER INCLUDING DEGREES OR CREDENTIALS (I certify that the statements on the reverse apply to this bill and are made a part thereof.)

SIGNED _____ DATE _____

32. NAME AND ADDRESS OF FACILITY WHERE SERVICES WERE RENDERED (If other than home or office)

33. PHYSICIAN'S, SUPPLIER'S BILLING NAME, ADDRESS, ZIP CODE & PHONE #

PIN# | GRP#

PHYSICIAN OR SUPPLIER INFORMATION

(APPROVED BY AMA COUNCIL ON MEDICAL SERVICE 8/88) *PLEASE PRINT OR TYPE* APPROVED OMB-0938-0008 FORM CMS-1500 (12-90), FORM RRB-1500, APPROVED OMB-1215-0055 FORM OWCP-1500, APPROVED OMB-0720-0001 (CHAMPUS)

Chapter Self-Assessment Quiz

1. In the case of an unlisted code, the medical assistant should:

   a. notify the AMA so that a new code is issued.

   b. submit a copy of the procedure report with the claim.

   c. obtain authorization from the AMA to proceed with the procedure.

   d. include the code that fits the most and add a note to explain the differences.

   e. not charge the patient for the procedure.

2. Which kind of information appears in a special report?

   a. Type of medicine prescribed

   b. Patient history

   c. Allergic reactions

   d. Possible procedural risks

   e. Equipment necessary for the treatment

3. On a medical record, the key components contained in E/M codes indicate:

   a. the scope and result of a medical visit.

   b. the duties of a physician toward his patients.

   c. the definition and description of a performed procedure.

   d. the services that a medical assistant may perform.

   e. the charges that are owed to the insurance company.

4. Time becomes a key component in a medical record when:

   a. the visit lasts more than one hour.

   b. more than half of the visit is spent counseling.

   c. the physician decides for a series of regular visits.

   d. the visit lasts longer than it was initially established.

   e. the patient is constantly late for his or her appointments.

5. When assigning a level of medical decision making, you should consider the:

   a. medication the patient is on.

   b. available coding for the procedure.

   c. patient's symptoms during the visit.

   d. insurance coverage allowed to the patient.

   e. patient's medical history.

6. In the anesthesia section, the physical status modifier indicates the patient's:

   a. medical history.

   b. conditions after surgery.

   c. good health before surgery.

   d. reactions to past anesthesia.

   e. condition prior to the administration of anesthesia.

7. Which of the following is included in a surgical package?

   a. General anesthesia

   b. Hospitalization time

   c. Complications related to the surgery

   d. Prescriptions given after the operation

   e. Uncomplicated follow-up care

8. How are procedures organized in the subsections of the surgery section of the CPT-4?

   a. By invasiveness

   b. By location and type

   c. In alphabetical order

   d. In order of difficulty of procedure

   e. By average recurrence of procedure

9. Which is the first digit that appears on radiology codes?

   a. 1

   b. 6

   c. 7

   d. 8

   e. 9

10. Diagnostic related groups (DRGs) are a group of:

   a. codes pertaining to one particular treatment.

   b. inpatients sharing a similar medical history.

   c. modifiers attached to a single procedural form.

   d. physicians agreeing on a procedure for a particular medical condition.

   e. inpatients sharing similar diagnoses, treatment, and length of hospital stay.

11. The resource-based relative value scale (RBRVS) gives information on the:

    a. difficulty level of a particular surgical operation.

    b. maximum fee that physicians can charge for a procedure.

    c. reimbursement given to physicians for Medicare services.

    d. average fee asked by physicians for emergency procedures.

    e. mminimum amount of time the physician should spend with a patient.

12. The Medicare allowed charge is calculated by:

    a. adding the RVU and the national conversion factor.

    b. dividing the RVU by the national conversion factor.

    c. multiplying the RVU by the national conversion factor.

    d. subtracting the RVU from the national conversion factor.

    e. finding the average between the RVU and the national conversion factor.

13. Upcoding is:

    a. billing more than the proper fee for a service.

    b. correcting an erroneous code in medical records.

    c. auditing claims retroactively for suspected fraud.

    d. comparing the documentation in the record with the codes received.

    e. researching new codes online.

14. Who has jurisdiction over a fraudulent medical practice?

    a. CMS

    b. AMA

    c. Medicare

    d. U.S. Attorney General

    e. State's supreme court

15. The purpose of the Level II HCPCS codes is to:

    a. decode different types of code modifiers.

    b. attribute a code to every step of a medical procedure.

    c. list the practices eligible for reimbursement by Medicare.

    d. identify services, supplies, and equipment not identified by CPT codes.

    e. provide coding information for various types of anesthesia.

16. Which of these sections is included in the HCPCS Level I code listing?

    a. Orthotics

    b. Injections

    c. Vision care

    d. Dental services

    e. Pathology and laboratory

17. How is a consultation different from a referral?

    a. A consultation is needed when the patient wants to change physicians.

    b. A consultation is needed when the physician asks for the opinion of another provider.

    c. A consultation is needed when the patient is transferred to another physician for treatment.

    d. A consultation is needed when the physician needs a team of doctors to carry out a procedure.

    e. A consultation is needed before the physician can submit insurance claims.

18. Which of the following is contained in Appendix B in the CPT-4?

    a. Legislation against medical fraud

    b. Detailed explanation of the modifiers

    c. Revisions made since the last editions

    d. Explanation on how to file for reimbursement

    e. Examples concerning the Evaluation and Management sections

19. Drug screening is considered quantitative when checking:

    a. for the amount of illegal drugs in the blood.

    b. for the presence of illegal drugs in the blood.

    c. for the proper level of therapeutic drug in the blood.

    d. that the therapeutic drug is not interacting with other medications.

    e. that the drug is not causing an allergic reaction.

20. Which place requires the use of an emergency department service code?

    a. Private clinic

    b. Nursing home

    c. Physician's office

    d. 24-hour pharmacy

    e. Mental health center

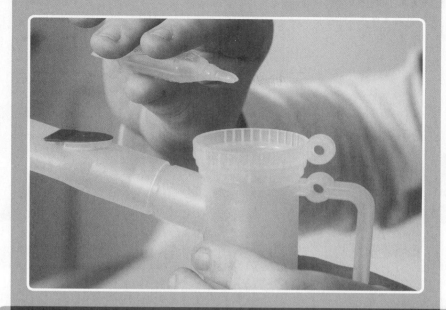

PART

III

The Clinical Medical Assistant

Fundamentals of Clinical Medical Assisting

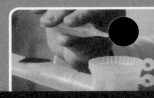

16 Nutrition and Wellness

Chapter Checklist

☐ Read textbook chapter and take notes within the Chapter Notes outline. Answer the Learning Objectives as you reach them in the content, and then check them off.

☐ Work the Content Review questions—both Foundational Knowledge and Application.

☐ Perform the Active Learning exercise(s).

☐ Complete Professional Journal entries.

☐ Complete Skill Practice Activity(s) using Competency Evaluation Forms and Work Products, when appropriate.

☐ Take the Chapter Self-Assessment Quiz.

☐ Insert all appropriate pages into your Portfolio.

Learning Objectives

1. Spell and define the key terms.
2. Name all of the essential nutrients.
3. Describe the body's digestion and metabolism of these nutrients.
4. Discuss the body's metabolism and its importance in weight.
5. Understand how to use the food guide pyramid, MyPyramid.
6. Read and explain the information on food labels.

7. Describe special therapeutic diets and the patients who need them.
8. Describe the components of physical fitness.
9. Discuss weight management and the elements involved in changing weight.
10. List suggestions for living a healthy lifestyle.
11. Explain the importance of disease prevention.
12. Recognize the dangers of substance abuse.
13. List and describe the effects of the substances most commonly abused.

Chapter Notes

Note: Bold-faced headings are the major headings in the text chapter; headings in regular font are lower-level headings (i.e., the content is subordinate to, or falls "under," the major headings). Make sure you understand the key terms used in the chapter, as well as the concepts presented as Key Points.

TEXT SUBHEADINGS	NOTES

Introduction _____

_____

Key Point:
• You will have opportunities to teach patients the essentials of good health, and, in the process, you will learn how to stay healthy, happy, and productive.

☐ **LEARNING OBJECTIVE 1:** Spell and define the key terms.

Essentials of Nutrition _____

_____

Key Term: homeostasis

Nutrients _____

_____

_____

Carbohydrates _____

_____

Key Point:
• Refined sugars have a high caloric value but no nutritious value and should be kept to a minimum.

Proteins _____

_____

Key Term: essential amino acids
Key Point:
• Proteins contain amino acids, provide energy, help to build and repair tissue, and assist with antibody production.

Fats _____

_____

Key Term: catabolize

Vitamins _____

_____

Key Terms: spina bifida; anencephaly
Key Point:
• Too much of these vitamins should be avoided because the body stores these vitamins and an excess can result in serious illness.

Minerals _____

_____

Key Term: minerals

Cholesterol _____

_____

_____

Lipoproteins _____

_____

_____

Fiber _____

_____

_____

☐ **LEARNING OBJECTIVE 2:** Name all of the essential nutrients.

Digestion _____

_____

Key Point:
• Digestion consists of both the physical and chemical breakdown of complex food into simpler substances that the body can use.

Metabolism _____

_____

Key Terms: metabolism; anabolism; calories

☐ **LEARNING OBJECTIVE 3:** Describe the body's digestion and metabolism of these nutrients.

☐ **LEARNING OBJECTIVE 4:** Discuss the body's metabolism and its importance in weight.

Nutritional Guidelines _____
_____
_____

MyPyramid _____
_____

Key Point:
• By following these dietary guidelines, you and your patients will have the best chance of fighting disease and staying healthy.

Grains _____
_____
_____

Vegetables _____
_____
_____

Fruits _____
_____
_____

Milk _____
_____
_____

Meat and Beans _____
_____
_____

Oils _____
_____
_____

☐ **LEARNING OBJECTIVE 5:** Understand how to use the food guide pyramid, MyPyramid.

Understanding Food Labels _____
_____
_____

☐ **LEARNING OBJECTIVE 6:** Read and explain the information on food labels.

Therapeutic Nutrition _____

_____

Key Point:
- The purposes of these therapeutic diets are to facilitate the healing process, promote healthy weight, assist with chewing and swallowing, or influence the components found in blood, such as cholesterol.

☐ **LEARNING OBJECTIVE 7:** Describe special therapeutic diets and the patients who need them.

Physical Fitness _____

_____

Key Terms: endorphins; euphoria
Key Point:
- Physical movement helps maintain a healthy musculoskeletal system, a normal weight, and a positive mental attitude.

Components of Physical Fitness _____

_____

_____

☐ **LEARNING OBJECTIVE 8:** Describe the components of physical fitness.

Weight Management _____

_____

Key Points:
- During this period of time, the obesity rate has doubled among children and tripled among adolescents.
- Even losing a small amount of weight (e.g., 10 pounds) can benefit a person's health and help prevent future weight gain.

Physiological Issues _____

_____

_____

Basal Metabolic Rate _____

_____

Key Term: basal metabolic rate

Level of Physical Activity _____

_____

_____

Calories _____

_____

_____

Body Mass Index _____

_____

Key Term: Body Mass Index

_____

Sociological and Psychological Issues _____

_____

Key Point:
• Instead of facing the stresses of everyday life, emotional eaters use food to cope.

☐ **LEARNING OBJECTIVE 9:** Discuss weight management and the elements involved in changing weight.

Staying Well _____

_____

Key Point:
• With some planning and determination, though, you can make even subtle changes to improve your health and quality of life.

Stress _____

_____

Key Terms: predisposed; guided imagery
Key Point:
• Although a certain amount of good stress is needed to function and thrive in everyday life, too much stress can be harmful.

Pollution _____

_____

Seat Belt Use and Airbags _____

_____

Key Points:
• Thankfully, proper seat belt use can prevent up to half of these deaths.
• When air bags are used in addition to lap belts and shoulder restraints, the risk of injury to the head is greatly reduced.

Dental Health _____

_____

Key Term: dental cavities

Positive Mental Outlook _____

_____

Key Point:
• Having a positive mental outlook can benefit your health and well-being.

Genetics _____

_____

Key Point:
• In other words, good genes can be negated by bad health habits.

Infectious Disease Prevention _____

_____

Key Point:
• Wearing personal protective equipment when handling body fluids will protect you in the workplace.

☐ **LEARNING OBJECTIVE 10:** List suggestions for living a healthy lifestyle.

☐ **LEARNING OBJECTIVE 11:** Explain the importance of disease prevention.

Substance Abuse _____

_____

_____

Alcohol _____

_____

Key Point:
• Others are prone to addiction, which is an illness, and should be treated as such.

Drugs _____

_____

Smoking Cessation _____

_____

_____

☐ **LEARNING OBJECTIVE 12:** Recognize the dangers of substance abuse.

☐ **LEARNING OBJECTIVE 13:** List and describe the effects of the substances most commonly abused.

Content Review

FOUNDATIONAL KNOWLEDGE

Healthy Eating

1. What is homeostasis?

_____

_____

2. Match each essential nutrient with its description.

Nutrient	**Description**
a. carbohydrates _____	**1.** cushion and protect body organs and sustain normal body temperature
b. proteins _____	**2.** chemical substances that provide the body with energy
c. fats _____	**3.** inorganic substances used in the formation of hard and soft body tissue
d. vitamins _____	**4.** organic substances that enhance the breakdown of other nutrients in the body
e. minerals _____	**5.** substances that contain amino acids and help to build and repair tissue

3. Identify the following vitamins as fat soluble or water soluble. Write **FS** on the line if the vitamin is fat soluble or **WS** if the vitamin is water soluble.

a. _____ Vitamin A

b. _____ Vitamin B-complex

c. _____ Vitamin C

d. _____ Vitamin D

e. _____ Vitamin E

f. _____ Vitamin K

g. _____ Thiamin

h. _____ Riboflavin

i. _____ Niacin

j. _____ Folic Acid

Metabolism and Weight Gain

4. There are two phases in the process of metabolism: anabolism and catabolism. Review the statements about metabolism below and place a check mark to indicate if it describes anabolism or catabolism.

Metabolism	Anabolism	Catabolism
a. Constructive phase		
b. Amino acids are converted into proteins		
c. Destructive phase		
d. Smaller molecules are converted into larger molecules		
e. Larger molecules are converted into smaller molecules		
f. Breakdown fats to use it for energy		
g. Complex carbohydrates, such as starch, are converted into simple sugars		

5. While conducting a patient interview, the patient complains about gaining weight. She says she eats the same foods as her roommate but her roommate does not gain weight and she does. Her roommate told her she does not have a fast metabolism rate. The patient asks you to explain what metabolism is and what it has to do with weight. How will you answer her?

_____

_____

A Healthy Pyramid

6. Review the food pyramid in Figure 16.2 in your textbook. Then answer the following questions below about the food pyramid based on a 2,000-calorie diet.

   a. How much food from the grains category should be eaten in a day? _____

   b. How many vegetables should be eaten in a day? _____

   c. How much fruit should be eaten in a day? _____

   d. How much milk should be consumed in a day? _____

   e. How much from the meat and beans category should be consumed in a day? _____

7. Explain the difference between whole grains and refined grains.

Whole Grains	Refined Grains

8. Not all fats are bad. Look at the list of foods and place a check mark in the appropriate box to indicate if it contains good fat or bad fat.

Food	Good Fat	Bad Fat
a. Salmon		
b. Olive oil		
c. Fast food		
d. Margarine		
e. Crackers		
f. Soybean oil		
g. Nuts		
h. Cookies		
i. Meat		
j. Sunflower Oil		
k. Sardines		
l. Canola Oil		

Reading Food Labels

9. Review the food label in Figure 16-4 in your textbook. Then answer the following questions.

   a. How many servings are in this can of vegetables? _____

   b. What is the serving size? _____

   c. How many calories from fat per serving? _____

   d. What is the least amount of sugar you would consume if you ate 1 cup of this vegetable? _____

   e. What is the percentage of sodium in one serving? _____

10. The physician asks you to explain the DASH diet to a patient with high blood pressure. List four basic dietary guidelines for the diet.

   a. _____

   b. _____

   c. _____

   d. _____

Work It Out

11. Dr. Mercer has given Joe, an overweight patient, clearance to start exercising. He told him to include workouts that will target each of the components of physical fitness. Joe feels overwhelmed. Explain the three components of physical fitness and how each one will help his body and health.

   a. _____

   b. _____

   c. _____

12. Calculate the maximum heart rate and target heart rate for the individuals below based on their age and desired intensity.

Person	Age	Maximum Heart Rate	Desired Intensity	Target Heart Rate
a. Tara	25		80%	
b. Yolanda	45		65%	
c. Hilel	37		75%	
d. Marco	18		90%	

13. What is BMI and how is it calculated?

_____

_____

14. Explain the three basic ways the body expends energy.

   a. Basal metabolic rate: _____

   b. Levels of physical activity: _____

   c. Thermic effect of food: _____

Healthy Habits

15. List three techniques that can help lessen stress.

   a. _____

   b. _____

   c. _____

16. What is the best defense against illness?

_____

_____

17. Angelo, a 22-year-old, comes to the office for a checkup. While interviewing him, he tells you that he drinks a lot on the weekends but it's no big deal. Tell Angelo three things that may help him to see that excessive alcohol is a big deal.

   a. _____

   b. _____

   c. _____

18. Drugs can be classified as stimulants or depressants. They each cause different effects on the body. Read each symptom below and place a check in the appropriate column.

Symptom	Depressant	Stimulant	Both
a. Can impair a fetus' health			
b. Increases heart rate			
c. Can cause psychological and physical dependence			
d. Increases pulse rate			
e. Causes respiratory depression			
f. Causes sleeplessness and anxiety			
g. Slows down the activities of the central nervous system			

19. Match the following key terms to their definitions.

Key Terms

a. anabolism _____

b. anencephaly _____

c. basal metabolic rate _____

d. body mass index _____

e. calorie _____

f. catabolism _____

g. dental cavities _____

h. endorphins _____

i. essential amino acids _____

j. euphoria _____

k. homeostasis _____

l. metabolism _____

m. minerals _____

n. spina bifida _____

Definitions

1. inorganic substances used in the formation of hard and soft body tissue

2. a process in which larger molecules break down into smaller molecules

3. a neural tube defect that causes an incomplete closure of a fetus' spine during early pregnancy

4. a neural tube defect that affects the fetus' brain during early pregnancy

5. a good feeling

6. maintaining a constant internal environment by balancing positive and negative feedback

7. a process in which smaller molecules are converted into larger molecules as food is absorbed into the bloodstream

8. the amount of energy used in a unit of time to maintain vital function by a fasting, resting subject

9. the sum of chemical processes that result in growth, energy production, elimination of waste, and body functions performed as digested nutrients are distributed

10. areas of decay in the teeth

11. pain-relieving substance released naturally from the brain

12. an individual's ratio of fat to lean body mass

13. proteins that come from your diet because the body does not produce them

14. the amount of energy used by the body

20. True or False? Determine whether the following statements are true or false. If false, explain why.

a. There is an increased risk for people to develop skin cancer because of the damage to the ozone layer.

_____

_____

b. Air pollution is harmful to the environment, but not people's health.

_____

_____

c. If your car is equipped with an air bag, it is not necessary to wear a seat belt.

_____

_____

d. According to genetics, if there is no history of diabetes or heart disease in your family, you are not susceptible to these diseases.

_____

_____

APPLICATION

Critical Thinking Practice

1. Mr. Consuelo is the president of a large manufacturing company. He is seeing Dr. Smith for frequent headaches. Dr. Smith has diagnosed the headaches as stress induced and has recommended that Mr. Consuelo develop some coping mechanisms to reduce the stress in his life. As Mr. Consuelo leaves the office, he asks you about ways he can comply with Dr. Smith's recommendations. What strategies can you offer this patient?

_____

_____

2. Marco is 53-years-old and has been smoking since he was 13. He says he would like to try and quit smoking, but he doesn't think it's worth it because the damage is probably already done. What would you say to him?

_____

_____

Patient Education

1. Carolyn is working with a nutritionist to improve her health. The nutritionist told her it is okay to take vitamins C and B every day. However, she should not take vitamin E every day. Carolyn responds that she thought it was necessary to take all vitamins every day. Explain why the nutritionist instructed Carolyn otherwise.

_____

_____

Documentation

1. A 40-year-old woman comes to talk to the physician because she would like to start a new exercise routine and change her diet to lose 15 pounds. She is currently 25 pounds overweight, so this is a great idea and a good move toward healthy living. The physician asks you to discuss exercise and diet changes with the patient. Write a narrative patient note describing your interaction with the patient to include in her chart.

_____

_____

Active Learning

1. It is estimated that 16% of children and adolescents are overweight. The pediatrician has asked you to create a presentation about preventing childhood obesity in your office. Perform research using the Internet to identify the risks related to adolescents being overweight. Outline steps adolescents should take to reduce their weight. Create a list of exercises that could help overweight adolescents lose and maintain weight, including the reasons for performing each type of exercise. Then create a presentation on your findings to present to your classmates.

2. The Centers for Disease Control (CDC) offers a body mass calculator on its website. Visit the website www.cdc.gov and search for the BMI calculator. Calculate your own BMI and find out what category you're in. Then write down three things you can do to either maintain your current weight or lose weight if necessary.

3. Many of your patients complain that they don't have the time to eat healthy foods because they are always busy. Working with a partner, create a meal plan for two days that incorporates healthy ingredients and essential nutrients. Each day should include breakfast, lunch, dinner, and one prepared snack. Look in cookbooks or online to find eight healthy and simple recipes that a home cook can easily prepare on a tight schedule, and add them to the meal plan.

Professional Journal

REFLECT

(Prompts and Ideas: Do you struggle finding the time to eat well and exercise on a regular basis? What things do you do for your health that you are proud of? What are some things you would like to change to create a healthier lifestyle?)

_____

_____

_____

_____

_____

_____

_____

PONDER AND SOLVE

1. A patient is upset because he has been placed on a special therapeutic diet because of his high blood pressure. He doesn't understand why he needs to stop eating some of his favorite foods, and he's worried he will not be successful with changing his diet. How can you explain the need for his new diet and encourage him to comply?

_____

_____

_____

_____

_____

_____

2. Your 17-year-old patient comes in to the physician's office because he has a bad cough that seems to indicate bronchitis. This is the second time this winter that he has seen the physician for respiratory problems. When you review the patient's chart, you see that he had asthmatic tendencies when he was younger. You ask the patient if he smokes, and he becomes uncomfortable and says that he does occasionally. He says that he smokes only occasionally with his friends and that he's not "a smoker" because he's not addicted to nicotine. His parents have no idea, so he asks you to not tell them about his new habit. What should you say to this patient?

_____

_____

_____

_____

_____

_____

EXPERIENCE

Skills related to this chapter include:

1. Teaching a Patient to Read a Food Label (Procedure 16-1).

Record any common mistakes, lessons learned, and/or tips you discovered during your experience of practicing and demonstrating these skills.

_____

_____

_____

_____

_____

_____

_____

Skill Practice

PERFORMANCE OBJECTIVES:

1. Teach a patient to read food labels (Procedure 16-1).

Name_____ Date _____ Time _____

Procedure 16-1:	TEACHING A PATIENT TO READ A FOOD LABEL

EQUIPMENT/SUPPLIES: Two boxes of the same item, one low calorie or "lite," the other regular; measuring cup; two bowls

STANDARDS: Given the needed equipment and a place to work the student will perform this skill with _____% accuracy in a total of _____ minutes. (*Your instructor will tell you what the percentage and time limits will be before you begin.*)

KEY: 4 = Satisfactory   0 = Unsatisfactory   NA = This step is not counted

PROCEDURE STEPS	SELF	PARTNER	INSTRUCTOR
1. Identify the patient.	☐	☐	☐
2. Introduce yourself and explain the procedure.	☐	☐	☐
3. Have the patient look at the labels, comparing the two.	☐	☐	☐
4. Ask the patient to pour out a normal serving.	☐	☐	☐
5. Measure the exact serving size printed on the label.	☐	☐	☐
6. Compare the two. Discuss the difference, if any.	☐	☐	☐
7. Explain to the patient the sections of the label: serving size and servings per package.	☐	☐	☐
8. Explain column for amount in serving.	☐	☐	☐
9. Explain column for percent daily value (RDA).	☐	☐	☐
10. Explain calories and calories from fat.	☐	☐	☐
11. Have the patient calculate the percentage of fat calories and compare with label.	☐	☐	☐
12. Read down the label and discuss each nutrient, pointing out the amounts and percentages.	☐	☐	☐
13. Have the patient compare the two labels and tell you how many total carbohydrates are in each label, sugars, protein, etc.	☐	☐	☐
14. Ask the patient if she has any questions.	☐	☐	☐
15. Document the instruction.	☐	☐	☐

CHARTING EXAMPLE:

Per Dr. Dunn, instructed patient in reading a food label using a sample label. The patient's questions were answered, and she states that she understands. The patient states, "I am eager to get started on my weight loss program." Susan Raney, CMA

CALCULATION

Total Possible Points: _____
Total Points Earned: _____ Multiplied by 100 = _____ Divided by Total Possible Points = _____%

Pass   **Fail**

☐   ☐   Comments:

Student's signature _____ Date _____
Partner's signature _____ Date _____
Instructor's signature _____ Date _____

1. The nutrient that cushions and protects body organs and sustains normal body temperature is a:
   a. carbohydrate.
   b. lipid.
   c. mineral.
   d. protein.
   e. vitamin.

2. The purpose of a therapeutic diet is to:
   a. promote healthy weight.
   b. enjoy foods that put a person in a good mood.
   c. experiment with foods not normally allowed on other diets.
   d. eat foods the person likes but only in moderation.
   e. help soothe an upset stomach.

3. Which of the following is true about the effects of drugs or alcohol on a developing fetus?
   a. They have no effect on the developing fetus.
   b. They could cause the baby to be addicted to the substance after birth.
   c. Drugs could cause the brain to stop developing, but alcohol has no effect.
   d. They can harm the fetus only if the mother harms herself while using them.
   e. They could make the fetus hyper in the womb but cause no long-term effects after birth.

4. Which of the following statements about cholesterol is true?
   a. A diet high in cholesterol is a healthy diet.
   b. Cholesterol is found only in animal products.
   c. Cholesterol is found in fresh fruits and vegetables.
   d. Since the body cannot produce cholesterol it must be part of the diet.
   e. Adults should consume at least 350 mg of dietary cholesterol each day.

5. Which of the following would leave a person vulnerable to a disease?
   a. Keeping your immunizations up-to-date
   b. Washing your hands after using the bathroom
   c. Wearing insect repellent when outside in the summer
   d. Using someone else's antibiotics because she didn't finish them
   e. Washing cutting boards with soap and water after cutting uncooked chicken

6. Although alcohol intoxication can give a person a euphoric feeling, alcohol is a depressant. What does that mean?
   a. It gives the person a sad and gloomy feeling.
   b. It causes the person to suffer from depression.
   c. It causes increased heart rate and sleeplessness.
   d. It speeds up the functioning of the central nervous system.
   e. It causes a lack of coordination and impaired brain function.

7. Which of the following statements about exercise is true?
   a. It induces stress.
   b. It suppresses the production of endorphins.
   c. It is most effective if done for at least 40 minutes.
   d. It can reduce the risk of developing certain diseases.
   e. Aerobic activities are most effective before target heart rate is reached.

8. Basal metabolic rate is:
   a. the constructive phase of metabolism.
   b. the destructive phase of metabolism.
   c. the baseline metabolic rate that is considered normal for the average adult.
   d. the amount of energy used in a unit of time to maintain vital functions by a fasting, resting person.
   e. the combination of the calories a person can consume and how long it takes to burn those calories.

9. A person who follows a lacto-ovo-vegetarian diet eats:
   a. vegetables only.
   b. vegetables and milk and cheese.
   c. vegetables and milk, eggs, and cheese.
   d. vegetables and milk, eggs, and poultry.
   e. vegetables and milk, eggs, and seafood.

10. Which of the following foods is a good source of fiber?
    a. Fish
    b. Milk
    c. Butter
    d. Chicken
    e. Vegetables

11. The five basic food groups include:

 a. dairy, vitamins, produce, meat, and grains.

 b. carbohydrates, fiber, vegetables, fruits, and meat.

 c. oils, lipids, refined sugars, whole grains, and dairy.

 d. grains, vegetables, milk, fruits, and meat and beans.

 e. proteins, carbohydrates, lipids, cholesterol, and minerals.

12. An overweight teenager asks you to suggest a cardiovascular exercise. Which of the following could you suggest?

 a. Yoga

 b. Sit-ups

 c. Stretching

 d. Lifting weights

 e. Jumping rope

13. Which vitamin is important for pregnant women because it reduces the risk of neural tube defects?

 a. Calcium

 b. Folate

 c. Mercury

 d. Potassium

 e. Zinc

14. To determine the correct number of daily servings from each food group, you need to know your:

 a. resting heart rate.

 b. height and weight.

 c. age and gender.

 d. waist measurement and target heart rate.

 e. level of physical activity and blood type.

15. How are refined grains different from whole grains?

 a. Refined grains are full of fiber.

 b. Whole grains lack fiber and iron.

 c. Whole grains are made with the entire grain kernel.

 d. Refined grains contain nutrients like carbohydrates and proteins.

 e. Refined grains are darker in color because they have more nutrients.

16. Water-soluble vitamins should be consumed:

 a. once a week.

 b. once a month.

 c. twice a week.

 d. daily.

 e. twice a month.

17. Pregnant women are advised to eat only one can of tuna per week because of its:

 a. iron content.

 b. lead content.

 c. mercury content.

 d. zinc content.

 e. calcium content.

18. How are substances such as cocaine and marijuana different from alcohol and nicotine?

 a. Alcohol and nicotine are legal; marijuana and cocaine are illegal.

 b. Cocaine and marijuana will not cause sudden death; alcohol and nicotine will cause sudden death.

 c. Alcohol and nicotine do not harm the body; marijuana and cocaine do harm the body.

 d. Cocaine and marijuana are used by people with health problems; alcohol and nicotine are not.

 e. Alcohol and nicotine are not additive drugs; marijuana and cocaine are addictive drugs.

19. Which of the following drugs damages blood vessels, decreases heart strength, and causes several types of cancer?

 a. Caffeine

 b. Nicotine

 c. Hashish

 d. Mescaline

 e. Phencyclidine

20. Why does inhaling marijuana smoke cause more damage to a person's body than tobacco smoke?

 a. Marijuana smoke is inhaled as unfiltered smoke, so users take in more cancer-causing agents and do more damage to the respiratory system than with regular filtered tobacco smoke.

 b. Marijuana smoke is thicker and more odorous.

 c. Marijuana smoke is inhaled as filtered smoke, so users take in less cancer-causing agents and do more damage to the respiratory system than with regular filtered tobacco smoke.

 d. Marijuana smoke is inhaled more quickly than tobacco smoke.

 e. Marijuana plants are grown in more toxic environments than tobacco plants.

☐ **LEARNING OBJECTIVE 3:** Explain the components of the infectious process cycle.

Modes of Transmission _____

_____

_____

Direct Transmission _____

_____

Key Point:
• Direct contact between the infected reservoir host and the susceptible host produces direct transmission.

Indirect Transmission _____

_____

Key Terms: vector; viable
Key Point:
• Indirect transmission may occur through contact with a vehicle known as a **vector**.

☐ **LEARNING OBJECTIVE 4:** List the various ways microbes are transmitted.

Sources of Transmission _____

_____

Key Term: asymptomatic
Key Point:
• Human hosts include people who are ill with an infectious disease, people who are carriers of an infectious disease, and people who are incubating an infectious disease but are not exhibiting symptoms.

Principles of Infection Control _____

_____

Key Term: Occupational Safety and Health Administration (OSHA)
Key Point:
• Most transmission of infectious disease in the medical office can be prevented by strict adherence to guidelines issued by the **Occupational Safety and Heath Administration (OSHA)** and the Centers for Disease Control and Prevention (CDC).

Medical Asepsis

Key Points:
- Medical asepsis does not mean that an object or area is free from all microorganisms. It refers to practices that render an object or area free from pathogenic microorganisms.
- Handwashing is the most important medical aseptic technique to prevent the transmission of pathogens.

☐ **LEARNING OBJECTIVE 5:** Explain the concepts of medical asepsis and infection control.

Levels of Infection Control

Key Terms: sterilization; disinfection; germicides; sanitization
Key Point:
- **Sterilization**, the highest level of infection control, destroys all forms of microorganisms, including spores, on inanimate surfaces.

☐ **LEARNING OBJECTIVE 6:** Compare the effectiveness in reducing or destroying microorganisms using the four levels of infection control.

Sanitation

Key Term: sanitation
Key Point:
- **Sanitation** is the maintenance of a healthful, disease-free, and hazard-free environment.

☐ **LEARNING OBJECTIVE 7:** Define sanitation.

Disinfection

Key Term: germicide
Key Points:
- Disinfectants, or **germicides**, inactivate virtually all recognized pathogenic microorganisms but not necessarily all microbial forms, including spores, on inanimate objects.
- High-level disinfection destroys most forms of microbial life except certain bacterial spores.
- Intermediate-level disinfection destroys many viruses, fungi, and some bacteria, including *Mycobacterium tuberculosis* (*M. tuberculosis*), the bacterium that causes tuberculosis.
- Low-level disinfection destroys many bacteria and some viruses, but not *M. tuberculosis* or bacterial spores.

☐ **LEARNING OBJECTIVE 8:** Distinguish between the need for disinfection and sterilization.

Occupational Safety and Health Administration Guidelines for the Medical Office

Key Point:
• OSHA is the federal agency responsible for ensuring the safety of all workers, including those in health care.

Exposure Risk Factors and Exposure Control Plan

Key Terms: exposure risk factor; personal protective equipment (PPE); immunization; exposure control plan; biohazardous; postexposure testing
Key Point:
• Medical offices must provide clear instructions in the policy or infection control manual for preventing employee exposure and reducing the danger of exposure to **biohazardous** materials.

☐ **LEARNING OBJECTIVE 9:** Discuss risk management procedures relative to the Occupational Safety and Health Administration guidelines for the medical office.

☐ **LEARNING OBJECTIVE 10:** List the required components of an exposure control plan.

Standard Precautions

Key Term: standard precautions
Key Point:
• **Standard precautions** are a set of procedures recognized by the CDC to reduce the chance of transmitting infectious microorganisms in any health care setting, including medical offices.

☐ **LEARNING OBJECTIVE 11:** Explain the importance of following Standard Precautions in the medical office.

Personal Protective Equipment

☐ **LEARNING OBJECTIVE 12:** Identify various personal protective equipment (PPE) items.

☐ **LEARNING OBJECTIVE 13:** Describe circumstances when PPE items would be appropriately worn by the medical assistant.

Handling Environmental Contamination _____

_____

Key Point:
- Sanitization is cleaning or washing equipment or surfaces by removing all visible soil.

Disposing of Infectious Waste _____

_____

☐ **LEARNING OBJECTIVE 14:** Describe the procedures for cleaning, handling, and disposing of biohazardous waste in the medical office.

Hepatitis B and Human Immunodeficiency Viruses _____

_____

Key Point:
- HBV is more viable than HIV and may survive in a dried state on clinical equipment and counter surfaces at room temperature for more than a week.

☐ **LEARNING OBJECTIVE 15:** Explain the facts pertaining to the transmission and prevention of the Hepatitis B virus and the Human Immunodeficiency Virus in the medical office.

☐ **LEARNING OBJECTIVE 16:** Describe how to avoid becoming infected with the Hepatitis B and Human Immunodeficiency viruses.

Content Review

FOUNDATIONAL KNOWLEDGE

1. Buggin' Out

We are surrounded by microorganisms. Most are benign, even helpful and important to our bodies. On occasion, it's where the germ resides that makes the germ bad. For each of the microorganisms below, identify whether it is a resident or transient flora.

Organism	Location	Resident	Transient
a. *Escherichia coli (E. coli)*	Large intestine		
b. *Staphylococcus aureus (S. aureus)*	Subcutaneous skin		
c. *Escherichia coli (E. coli)*	Peritoneum		
d. *Staphylococcus aureus (S. aureus)*	On skin surface		
e. *Helicobacter pylori*	Digestive tract		

2. Under Stress

Place a check mark next to any of the following patients who are likely to have a decreased resistance to pathogens.

a. a 40-year-old male patient with HIV	
b. a 40-year-old male patient with a sprained ankle	
c. a 62-year-old female undergoing chemotherapy for breast cancer	
d. a 12-year-old female experiencing menstruation	
e. a 75-year-old male who recently recovered from pneumonia	
f. a newborn baby girl	

3. All's Fair in Love and War

Think about this: Your body is in a constant state of war—battling the pathogens in the outside environment that are intent on getting in to grow and reproduce. Fortunately, your body has a variety of mechanisms to fight off infection. For each of the terms below, explain how it is involved with "germ warfare."

a. Nose cilia:
b. Mucus:
c. Skin:
d. Urination:
e. Tears:
f. Saliva:
g. Stomach:

4. Baking a "Bug Cake"

Imagine that you wanted to "bake" a bug cake full of flourishing microorganisms. You have a cookbook in front of you that tells you how to make such a bug cake. Check any of the following directions that you would expect to find in this odd cookbook. (In other words, which conditions encourage pathogens to grow?)

a. Turn oven on to 99 degrees.	
b. Remove as much moisture from the mix as possible.	
c. Chill in the freezer for 2 hours after baking.	
d. Store in a dark place.	
e. Seal in a vacuum-packed package to maintain freshness.	
f. Add a cup of sugar to make it sweet.	
g. Add vinegar to the mix until it tastes very tart.	

5. Giving It Away: The Infection Cycle

In order for infection to occur, there must be a series of processes that are linked together. You can relate it this way: You are at home when your friend calls you. He would like to borrow your DVD of a popular movie that you both like. Since you were going out to the store anyway, you suggest that you will drop the movie off at his house on the way to the store. He agrees.

Link each of the steps illustrated below in order to complete this task. Then, label each of the steps with the appropriate link of the infection cycle.

- Means of transmission
- New reservoir host
- Susceptible host
- Pathogen leaving host
- Portal of entry

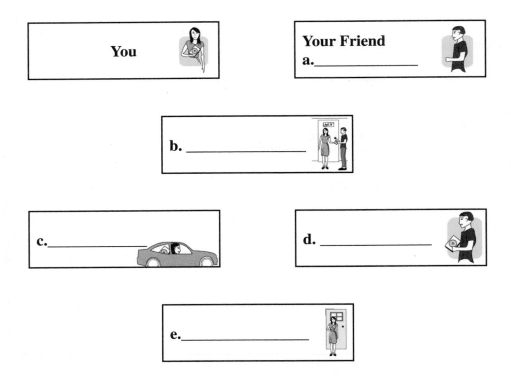

6. Pass It Along

Identify whether the following statements are related to a direct or indirect mode of disease transmission.

	Direct	Indirect
a. "Nice to meet you." (Shake hands with person)		
b. "Wow, now that's a big mosquito bite."		
c. "A blood tube broke on the floor. I'll clean it up."		
d. "Gesundheit."		
e. "I'm thirsty."		

7. We're from the Government

Which of the following federal agencies regulate and provide guidelines for controlling disease transmission?

a. Drug Enforcement Agency

b. Centers for Disease Control

c. Department of Homeland Security

d. Occupational Safety and Health Administration

e. Joint Committee on Accreditation of Hospital Organizations

f. Federal Emergency Management Agency

8. Which of the following is the single most important procedure that reduces pathogen transmission?

   a. Double gloving

   b. Wearing a mask

   c. Handwashing

   d. Not touching patients

9. How Many Times?

Mei Lin is a clinical medical assistant who works in an outpatient clinic. Today she arrives at work with a minor cold. Over the course of an hour, she sees four patients. She draws a blood sample from one patient and retrieves a urine sample from another patient. During the hour she sneezes three times. She is preparing to leave for her lunch break. How many times should she have washed her hands during this time period?

_____

_____

10. Does This Make Me Look Protected?

Personal protective equipment is a must-have for medical assistants. You just can't go wrong with a pair of latex or nitrile gloves; they go with just about any uniform. However, what should medical assistants wear when facing specific types of bodily fluids? Check off each of the types of PPE you would use, based on the patient's presentation.

Patient Presentation	Gloves	Protective Eyewear	Mask	Gown
a. Abdominal pain, vomiting				
b. Abdominal pain				
c. Headache, coughing				
d. Confused, nauseous				
e. Fever, chest pain, nonproductive cough				
f. Generalized weakness				

11. A speculum has just been used by the physician on a patient. After the exam is over and the patient leaves, how do you prepare this equipment for its next use?

_____

_____

12. Name four factors that affect the disinfection process.

   a. _____

   b. _____

   c. _____

   d. _____

13. You have the following instruments to disinfect. Which one(s) will require a high level of disinfection? Circle the correct answer(s).

   a. stethoscope

   b. blood pressure cuff

   c. endoscope

14. Which of the following are medical offices required to maintain and provide per OSHA mandates? (Note: There may be more than one correct answer.)

   a. Infection control plan

   b. Personal protective equipment

    c. A 10-minute rest break during a 4-hour work period

    d. A description of an employee's exposure risk factor

    e. Documentation of patient care

15. You accidentally stick yourself with a bloody needle. After washing the site, you should:

    a. Immediately seek the assistance of a physician.

    b. Ask about the infection status of the patient and report exposure if the patient has an infectious disease.

    c. Report exposure to your supervisor and request the infection status of the source patient.

    d. Make sure you are up-to-date on your immunizations and remain alert for symptoms.

16. What agents cause communicable diseases?

_____

_____

17. Why is the respiratory tract more prone to pathogen invasion than the skin is?

_____

_____

18. Health care providers must use standard precautions:

    a. only during patient contact when the risk of exposure to bodily fluids is high.

    b. only with patients who shows signs of having an infectious disease.

    c. only with patients known to have an identified infectious disease.

    d. with every patient, even those without symptoms of infectious disease.

19. Describe the correct method for removing gloves.

_____

_____

20. Match the following key terms to their definitions.

Key Terms	Definitions
a. aerobe _____	**1.** the killing or rendering inert of most, but not all, pathogenic microorganisms
b. asymptomatic _____	**2.** disease-causing microorganisms
c. disinfection _____	**3.** bacterial life form that resists destruction by heat, drying, or chemicals
d. germicide _____	**4.** highly pathogenic and disease-producing; describes a microorganism
e. immunization _____	**5.** chemical that kills most pathogenic microorganisms; disinfectant
f. microorganisms _____	**6.** maintenance of a healthful, disease-free environment
g. pathogens _____	**7.** microscopic living organisms
h. resistance _____	**8.** usual steps to prevent injury or disease
i. spore _____	**9.** without any symptoms
j. sanitation _____	**10.** body's immune response to prevent infections by invading pathogenic microorganisms
k. standard precautions _____	**11.** microorganism that requires oxygen to live and reproduce
l. virulent _____	**12.** act or process of rendering an individual immune to specific disease

21. True or False? Determine whether the following statements are true or false. If false, explain why.

    a. Adhering to "clean technique," or medical asepsis, ensures that an object or area is free from all microorganisms.

    _____

    _____

    b. Sterilization is the highest level of infection control.

    _____

    _____

    c. Low-level disinfection destroys bacteria, but not viruses.

    _____

    _____

    d. There are three levels of disinfection: minor, moderate, and severe.

    _____

    _____

APPLICATION

Critical Thinking Practice

1. A middle-aged male comes into the medical office with a low-grade fever and productive cough that has lasted several weeks. The physician orders a chest x-ray to aid in diagnosis. After the patient goes to the radiology department, you set out to clean the room for the next patient. What level of disinfection will you use? What product(s) will you use? Provide detailed information about your actions, including dilution instructions, if appropriate.

_____

_____

2. You work in a pediatrician's office and have been working extra hours to save for a new, more reliable vehicle. Between work and school, you are tired and run-down. This morning, you woke up with a sore throat and headache. The last thing you want to do is call in sick, because you need the money, and you want your supervisor to think you are reliable. What should you do? Explain your answer.

_____

_____

Patient Education

1. Your patient is a 24-year-old female who has been diagnosed with bacterial pneumonia. The physician has ordered antibiotic therapy and bedrest, and the patient is heading home. She expresses concern over the fact that she has a 7-month-old baby at home. Type a sheet of instructions that clearly explain to the patient what steps she can take to avoid transmitting her illness to her child.

_____

_____

Documentation

1. Although you always take care to protect yourself from exposure to biohazardous materials, you spill a tube of a patient's blood while performing hematology testing. You have a fresh cut on your hand that came into contact with the blood. Following your office's Exposure Control Plan, you clean up and then document the incident. What information will you make sure to include in your report?

_____

_____

Active Learning

1. You have been asked to select the best hand soap for use throughout the urgent care center where you work.

   • Perform research using the Internet to identify different types of antibacterial agents that are commonly used in hand soaps.

   • Cite any evidence you can find as to the effectiveness of the agents.

   • Determine which soap you believe is best.

   • Write a letter to the office manager that gives your recommendation, clearly explaining why you chose that soap.

2. If you are performing an externship, perform a "white glove" test of sorts in the clinical setting. Look closely at the patient care rooms and lab areas. Observe the safety precautions taken by your co-workers. Do conditions exist that could promote the growth and transmission of microorganisms? Are health care workers wearing the appropriate PPE items? Is the appropriate equipment readily available? Did you identify any areas in which staff training would be helpful? (Hint: Use Box 17-3 in the textbook as a checklist.) Make a list of recommended improvements and share it with your supervisor, if you are comfortable doing so.

3. Locate your vaccination record. Are there any vaccinations you need to protect yourself when you work in a health care setting? If so, make an appointment with your physician to obtain them.

Professional Journal

REFLECT

(Prompts and Ideas: Do you worry about exposure to infectious diseases? If so, what do you have control over in that regard? Do you have a friend or family member with a serious infectious disease? If so, how would you like him or her to be treated by health care professionals when visiting medical offices?)

_____

_____

_____

_____

_____

_____

_____

_____

PONDER AND SOLVE

1. One of your office's regular patients is a 38-year-old female with AIDS. One of your coworkers, Steve, is afraid of interacting with this patient and has made disparaging remarks about her in the back office. You worry that Steve's attitude will affect patient care and decide to talk with him. What points will you make? Should you also talk with your supervisor about Steve? Why, or why not?

_____

_____

_____

_____

_____

2. The test results for 15-year-old Ashley Lewis come in and show that she is positive for Hepatitis C. Her mother phones and asks you for the results. Is it appropriate for you to give her mother Ashley's test results? Why, or why not?

_____

_____

_____

_____

_____

_____

EXPERIENCE

Skills related to this chapter include:

1. Handwashing for Medical Asepsis (Procedure 17-1).
2. Removing Contaminated Gloves (Procedure 17-2).
3. Cleaning Biohazardous Spills (Procedure 17-3).

Record any common mistakes, lessons learned, and/or tips you discovered during your experience of practicing and demonstrating these skills:

_____

_____

_____

_____

_____

_____

Skill Practice

PERFORMANCE OBJECTIVES:

1. Perform a medical aseptic handwashing procedure (Procedure 17-1).
2. Remove and discard contaminated personal protective equipment appropriately (Procedure 17-2).
3. Clean and decontaminate biohazardous spills (Procedure 17-3).

Name _____ Date _____ Time _____

Procedure 17-1:   HANDWASHING FOR MEDICAL ASEPSIS

EQUIPMENT/SUPPLIES: Liquid soap, disposable paper towels, an orangewood manicure stick, a waste can

STANDARDS: Given the needed equipment and a place to work, the student will perform this skill with _____% accuracy in a total of _____ minutes. *(Your instructor will tell you what the percentage and time limits will be before you begin practicing.)*

KEY: 4 = Satisfactory   0 = Unsatisfactory   NA = This step is not counted

PROCEDURE STEPS	SELF	PARTNER	INSTRUCTOR
1. Remove all rings and wristwatch.	☐	☐	☐
2. Stand close to the sink without touching it.	☐	☐	☐
3. Turn on the faucet and adjust the temperature of the water to warm.	☐	☐	☐
4. Wet hands and wrists, apply soap, and work into a lather.	☐	☐	☐
5. Rub palms together and rub soap between your fingers at least 10 times.	☐	☐	☐
6. Scrub one palm with fingertips, work soap under nails, and then reverse hands.	☐	☐	☐
7. Rinse hands and wrists under warm running water.	☐	☐	☐
8. Hold hands lower than elbows and avoid touching the inside of the sink.	☐	☐	☐
9. Using the orangewood stick, clean under each nail on both hands.	☐	☐	☐
10. Reapply liquid soap and rewash hands and wrists.	☐	☐	☐
11. Rinse hands again while holding hands lower than the wrists and elbows.	☐	☐	☐
12. Use a dry paper towel to dry your hands and wrists gently.	☐	☐	☐
13. Use a dry paper towel to turn off the faucets and discard the paper towel.	☐	☐	☐

CALCULATION

Total Possible Points: _____
Total Points Earned: _____ Multiplied by 100 = _____ Divided by Total Possible Points = _____%

Pass   **Fail**
☐   ☐   Comments:

Student's signature _____ Date _____
Partner's signature _____ Date _____
Instructor's signature _____ Date _____

Name_____ Date _____ Time _____

Procedure 17-2:	REMOVING CONTAMINATED GLOVES

EQUIPMENT/SUPPLIES: Clean examination gloves; biohazard waste container

STANDARDS: Given the needed equipment and a place to work, the student will perform this skill with _____% accuracy in a total of _____ minutes. *(Your instructor will tell you what the percentage and time limits will be before you begin practicing.)*

KEY: 4 = Satisfactory   0 = Unsatisfactory   NA = This step is not counted

PROCEDURE STEPS	SELF	PARTNER	INSTRUCTOR
1. Choose the appropriate size gloves and apply one glove to each hand.	☐	☐	☐
2. After "contaminating" gloves, grasp the glove palm of the nondominant hand with fingers of the dominant hand.	☐	☐	☐
3. Pull the glove away from the nondominant hand.	☐	☐	☐
4. Slide the nondominant hand out of the contaminated glove while rolling the contaminated glove into the palm of the gloved dominant hand.	☐	☐	☐

5. Hold the soiled glove in the palm of your gloved hand.
  a. Slip ungloved fingers under the cuff of the gloved hand.
  b. Stretch the glove of the dominant hand up and away from your hand while turning it inside out with the nondominant hand glove balled up inside.
	☐	☐	☐

6. Discard both gloves as one unit into a biohazard waste receptacle.	☐	☐	☐
7. Wash your hands.	☐	☐	☐

CALCULATION

Total Possible Points: _____
Total Points Earned: _____ Multiplied by 100 = _____ Divided by Total Possible Points = _____%

Pass   **Fail**
☐   ☐   Comments:

Student's signature _____ Date _____
Partner's signature _____ Date _____
Instructor's signature _____ Date _____

Name _____ Date _____ Time _____

Procedure 17-3:   CLEANING BIOHAZARDOUS SPILLS

EQUIPMENT/SUPPLIES: Commercially prepared germicide OR 1:10 bleach solution, gloves, disposable towels, chemical absorbent, biohazardous waste bag, protective eyewear (goggles or mask and face shield), disposable shoe coverings, disposable gown or apron made of plastic or other material that is impervious to soaking up contaminated fluids

STANDARDS: Given the needed equipment and a place to work, the student will perform this skill with _____% accuracy in a total of _____ minutes. *(Your instructor will tell you what the percentage and time limits will be before you begin practicing.)*

KEY: 4 = Satisfactory   0 = Unsatisfactory   NA = This step is not counted

PROCEDURE STEPS	SELF	PARTNER	INSTRUCTOR
1. Put on gloves.	☐	☐	☐
2. Wear protective eyewear, gown or apron, and shoe covers if splashing is anticipated.	☐	☐	☐
3. Apply chemical absorbent to the spill.	☐	☐	☐
4. Clean up the spill using disposable paper towels.	☐	☐	☐
5. Dispose of paper towels and absorbent material in a biohazard waste bag.	☐	☐	☐
6. Further decontaminate using a commercial germicide or bleach solution. **a.** Wipe with disposable paper towels. **b.** Discard the towels used for decontamination in a biohazard bag.	☐	☐	☐
7. With gloves on, remove the protective eyewear and discard or disinfect.	☐	☐	☐
8. Remove the gown/apron and shoe coverings and place in biohazard bag.	☐	☐	☐
9. Place the biohazard bag in an appropriate waste receptacle.	☐	☐	☐
10. Remove contaminated gloves and wash hands thoroughly.	☐	☐	☐

CALCULATION

Total Possible Points: _____
Total Points Earned: _____ Multiplied by 100 = _____ Divided by Total Possible Points = _____%

Pass   **Fail**
☐   ☐   Comments:

Student's signature _____ Date _____
Partner's signature _____ Date _____
Instructor's signature _____ Date _____

Chapter Self-Assessment Quiz

Scenario: Susan enters the examination room, where a patient is being seen for flu-type symptoms. While Susan takes the patient's blood pressure, the patient suddenly coughs near her face. Three days later Susan has the same signs and symptoms as the patient.

1. Which of the following terms best describes the patient in the infection cycle?

  a. Reservoir host

  b. Disease portal

  c. Pathogen portal

  d. Susceptible host

  e. Disease transmitter

2. Which of the following procedures could Susan have performed that might have helped to minimize contracting the patient's disease?

  a. Ask the patient to look the other way while coughing.

  b. Put on a face mask before entering the exam room.

  c. Run out of the room right after the patient coughed.

  d. Wash her face right after the coughing episode.

  e. Sterilize the examination room.

3. What type of transmission process occurred during Susan's contact with the patient?

  a. Direct

  b. Vector

  c. Viable

  d. Manual

  e. Indirect

End Scenario

4. *Clostridium tetani* causes tetanus. Because it does not require oxygen to survive, this microbe is an example of an:

  a. anoxic bacteria.

  b. aerobic bacteria.

  c. anaerobic bacteria.

  d. anaerolytic bacteria.

  e. aerosolized bacteria.

5. Which of the following groups of conditions best favors microbial growth?

  a. Cold, light, and dry

  b. Dry, dark, and warm

  c. Dark, moist, and cool

  d. Warm, moist, and light

  e. Moist, warm, and dark

6. *Escherichia coli* is normally found in the intestinal tract. *E. coli* can be transmitted to the urinary tract, causing an infection. When in the urinary tract, *E. coli* is an example of a:

  a. viral flora.

  b. normal flora.

  c. resident flora.

  d. resistant flora.

  e. transient flora.

7. Which of the following practices is most important for maintaining medical asepsis?

  a. Airing out examination rooms after each patient

  b. Receiving all available vaccinations on an annual basis

  c. Wearing gloves before and after handling medical tools

  d. Wearing a gown if you are concerned about bodily fluids

  e. Washing your hands before and after each patient contact

8. To minimize infection, an endoscope should be:

  a. rinsed.

  b. sanitized.

  c. sterilized.

  d. disinfected.

  e. germicided.

9. At which temperature do microorganisms that are most likely to be pathogenic to humans thrive?

  a. Below 32°F

  b. Above 212°F

  c. Around body temperature

  d. Around room temperature

  e. At any temperature

10. What level of disinfection would be appropriate to use when cleaning a speculum?

  a. None

  b. Low

  c. Intermediate

  d. High

  e. Sterilization

11. Which of the following job responsibilities has the highest risk exposure in the group?

    a. Measuring a patient's body temperature

    b. Covering a urine-filled specimen jar

    c. Drawing blood for lab analysis

    d. Auscultating a blood pressure

    e. Sampling cervical cells

12. OSHA is responsible for:

    a. certifying all medical doctors.

    b. vaccinating school-age children.

    c. ensuring the safety of all workers.

    d. analyzing medical laboratory samples.

    e. caring for people with contagious diseases.

13. Jeremy approaches you and says that he just accidentally stuck himself with a needle while drawing a blood sample from a patient. He points to his thumb, where you can see a puncture. There is no bleeding. Which of the following actions should you take first?

    a. Direct Jeremy to wash his hands with soap and water.

    b. Lance the puncture with a scalpel to induce bleeding.

    c. Help him complete an exposure report right away.

    d. Call the physician in the office to ask for advice.

    e. Drive him to an occupational health clinic.

14. One example of personal protective equipment includes:

    a. name tag.

    b. stethoscope.

    c. face shield.

    d. scrub pants.

    e. syringe.

15. A patient arrives at the emergency department complaining of nausea. As you begin to assess her, she begins to vomit bright red blood. Which of the following sets of personal protective equipment (PPE) would be *most* appropriate to wear in this circumstance?

    a. Gown, gloves, and booties

    b. Eyewear, gown, and uniform

    c. Face shield and safety glasses

    d. Gloves, face shield, and gown

    e. Face shield, gown, and booties

16. Which of the following statements is *true* regarding hepatitis B virus (HBV)?

    a. HBV dies quickly outside the host body.

    b. There are no effective treatments for HBV.

    c. There is no vaccine protection against HBV.

    d. HBV is transmitted through blood contact, via needle puncture.

    e. It is easier to contract human immunodeficiency virus (HIV) than HBV.

17. Which of the following is not part of the body's natural defenses against disease?

    a. Plasma in blood

    b. Mucus in the nose

    c. Lysozyme in tears

    d. Saliva in the mouth

    e. Acid in the stomach

18. A vial of blood fell on the floor, glass broke, and the contents spilled on the floor. Proper cleaning of this spill includes:

    a. depositing the blood-soaked towels into a biohazard container.

    b. pouring hot water carefully onto the spill to avoid any splash.

    c. using paper towels to wipe up the blood.

    d. allowing the blood to dry before cleaning.

    e. trying to piece the vial back together.

19. If a biohazard container becomes contaminated on the outside, you should:

    a. fill out a biohazard report form.

    b. immediately wash the surface in a sink.

    c. dispose of the container in a trash facility outside.

    d. place the container inside another approved container.

    e. call the biohazard removal company as soon as possible.

20. You should change your gloves after:

    a. touching a patient's saliva.

    b. measuring a patient's weight.

    c. auscultating a blood pressure.

    d. palpating a patient's abdomen.

    e. taking a patient's temperature.

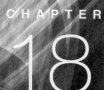
Medical History and Patient Assessment

Chapter Checklist

Chapter Checklist

☐ Read textbook chapter and take notes within the Chapter Notes outline. Answer the Learning Objectives as you reach them in the content, and then check them off.

☐ Work the Content Review questions—both Foundational Knowledge and Application.

☐ Perform the Active Learning exercise(s).

☐ Complete Professional Journal entries.

☐ Complete Skill Practice Activity(s) using Competency Evaluation Forms and Work Products, when appropriate.

☐ Take the Chapter Self-Assessment Quiz.

☐ Insert all appropriate pages into your Portfolio.

Learning Objectives

1. Spell and define the key terms.
2. Give examples of the type of information included in each section of the patient history.
3. Identify guidelines for conducting a patient interview using principles of verbal and nonverbal communication.

4. Explain the difference between a sign and symptom and give examples of each.
5. Discuss open-ended and closed-ended questions and explain when to use each type during the patient interview.

Chapter Notes

Note: Bold-faced headings are the major headings in the text chapter; headings in regular font are lower-level headings (i.e., the content is subordinate to, or falls "under," the major headings). Make sure you understand the key terms used in the chapter, as well as the concepts presented as Key Points.

TEXT SUBHEADINGS

NOTES

Introduction _____

_____

Key Terms: medical history; assessment
Key Point:
• The **medical history** is a record containing information about a patient's past and present health status, the health status of related family members, and relevant information about a patient's social habits.

☐ **LEARNING OBJECTIVE 1:** Spell and define the key terms.

The Medical History _____

_____

_____

Methods of Collecting Information _____

_____

Key Point:
- In some medical practices, medical assistants gather initial patient information by interviewing the patient using a printed list of questions.

Elements of the Medical History _____

_____

Key Terms: HIPAA; demographic; familial; hereditary
Key Point:
- The medical history forms used by the office may vary with the practice specialty, but most forms are composed of these common elements: identifying data (database), past history (PH), review of systems (ROS), family history (FH), and social history.

☐ **LEARNING OBJECTIVE 2:** Give examples of the type of information included in each section of the patient history.

Conducting the Patient Interview _____

_____

_____

Preparing for the Interview _____

_____

Key Points:
- As a medical assistant, your primary goal during a patient interview is to obtain accurate and pertinent information.
- Judgments made about these observations should not be documented in the patient's record, because the terminology used (depressed, abused) may be diagnostic, which is out of the scope of training for the medical assistant.
- Before you start interviewing the patient, make sure you are familiar with the medical history form and any previous medical history provided by the patient.

Introducing Yourself _____

_____

Key Points:
- Always begin the interview with new or established patients by identifying yourself, your title, and the purpose of the interview.
- By developing professional rapport, you will gain the patient's confidence and trust in you, the physician, and the office staff.

Barriers to Communication _____

_____

Key Point:
- As you begin speaking with the patient, you must assess any barriers to communication, such as unfamiliarity with English, hearing impairment, or cognitive impairment.

☐ **LEARNING OBJECTIVE 3:** Identify guidelines for conducting a patient interview using principles of verbal and nonverbal communication.

Assessing the Patient _____

_____

_____

Signs and Symptoms _____

_____

Key Terms: signs; symptoms
Key Points:
- Signs are objective information that can be observed or perceived by someone other than the patient.
- Symptoms, or subjective information, are indications of disease or changes in the body as sensed by the patient.

☐ **LEARNING OBJECTIVE 4:** Explain the difference between a sign and symptom and give examples of each.

Chief Complaint and Present Illness _____

Key Terms: chief complaint; over-the-counter; homeopathic
Key Points:
- Open-ended questions allow the patient to answer with more than one or two words.
- The CC, one statement describing the signs and symptoms that led the patient to seek medical care, is documented in the patient's medical record at each visit.
- Once you have obtained the CC, continue to probe for more details to further define the patient's present illness (PI).

☐ **LEARNING OBJECTIVE 5:** Discuss open-ended and closed-ended questions and explain when to use each type during the patient interview.

Content Review

FOUNDATIONAL KNOWLEDGE

Get to Know Your Patients

1. During a patient interview, you'll ask questions that will help determine the patient's present illness (PI). It is important to avoid questions that are not helpful because they either are closed-ended or suggest symptoms. Review this list of questions and place a check mark to indicate whether the question is helpful or not helpful during a patient assessment.

Question	Helpful	Not Helpful
a. "Do you feel pain?"		
b. "How often does the pain occur?"		
c. "What were you doing when the pain started?"		
d. "Have you taken ibuprofen for the pain?"		
e. "Does lying down lessen the pain you feel?"		

2. What is the purpose of gathering a patient's social history?

_____

_____

3. You are responsible for compiling a complete and accurate assessment during a patient interview. This includes observations of the patient's physical or mental status. Which of the following observations should be documented in the medical record? Circle all that apply.

   a. Patient has redness around the nose and mouth.
   b. Patient is hesitant to answer questions about his or her sexual history.
   c. Patient has trouble recalling his or her telephone number and address.
   d. Patient asks to use the restroom during the interview.
   e. Patient is accompanied by his or her mother, but does not share any physical characteristics with her.
   f. Patient is especially pale.

Assessing Signs and Symptoms

4. List three signs and three symptoms of influenza (flu).

Signs	Symptoms
a.	a.
b.	b.
c.	c.

5. Fill in the blanks with the appropriate term.

a. The section of the patient history that reviews each body system and invites the patient to share any information that he or she may have forgotten to mention earlier is called _____.

b. The _____ section covers the health status of the patient's immediate family members.

c. Information needed for administrative purposes, such as the patient's name, address, and telephone number, is included in the _____ section.

d. Important information about the patient's lifestyle is documented in the _____ section.

e. The section of the patient history that focuses on the patient's prior health status is called _____.

6. Alicia, a medical assistant in Dr. Howard's office, has recorded the following in a patient assessment:

"CC: Pt. c/o fatigue, depressed mood, and inability to stay asleep at night. Has taken Tylenol PM for 2 nights with "no effect" on sleep. Has not eaten for 2 days because of lack of appetite, which is likely caused by his depression. Face pale, skin clammy." What information should Alicia not have included in this assessment?

_____

_____

7. When are closed-ended questions appropriate during a patient interview? Give one example of an appropriate closed-ended question.

_____

_____

Successful Interview Tips

8. During a patient interview, you learn that the patient is an extreme sports enthusiast and works in a coal mine. Where should you record this information in the patient's medical history forms?

_____

_____

9. Why is the reception area a poor place to interview a patient? Name a better location for interviewing a patient.

_____

_____

10. You are interviewing a patient, Mr. Gibson. You learn that Mr. Gibson is a 55-year-old male. He is starting a new job as a child care provider and needs to submit a physical examination to his new place of employment. Mr. Gibson's father died of colon cancer when he was 60 and Mr. Gibson's wife is a smoker. Mr. Gibson says he feels healthy and has not had any health-related problems in the last few years. What should you record as the chief complaint in Mr. Gibson's medical record?

_____

_____

11. During a patient interview, you may learn that a patient has tried a home remedy to treat his or her illness before coming to the medical office. Two types of home remedies are over-the-counter medications and homeopathic medications. Determine whether the items below are over-the-counter or homeopathic medications. Place a check mark in the appropriate column.

	Over-the-counter medication	Homeopathic medication
a. 1000 mg of acetaminophen to relieve the pain of a sprained ankle		
b. a small dose of mercury to treat symptoms similar to mercury poisoning		
c. ingesting ipecacuanha, a root that causes vomiting, in order to treat vomiting		
d. a cooling topical ointment applied to skin afflicted by sunburn		

12. Giles is a medical assistant in Dr. Yardley's office. Giles enters examination room A to interview a patient. Giles notices that the patient is lying on the examination table, holding his abdomen. He is holding a black trash bin which contains a small amount of his vomit. The patient is flushed and sweating. Before even speaking to the patient, Giles has realized some of the patient's signs and symptoms of illness. Explain the significance of signs and symptoms and then fill in this patient's signs and symptoms in the chart below.

Signs: _____   **Symptoms:** _____

a.	**a.**
b.	**b.**
c.	

13. Name two ways in which a patient's medical history is gathered in medical offices.

_____

_____

14. What should you say to the patient when introducing yourself? Why is a thorough introduction important?

_____

_____

15. There are two patients waiting in examination rooms to see the physician. Patient A is a new patient, and Patient B is coming into the office for a complete physical examination. What is one factor to consider when sorting these patients?

_____

_____

16. What are your ethical and legal responsibilities as a medical assistant concerning a patient's medical history records?

_____

_____

17. As a medical assistant, you have many responsibilities. Which of the following will you be responsible for? Place a check mark next to the actions that you will be performing as a medical assistant.

Action

a. Documenting the patient's chief complaint (CC)	
b. Assessing the patient's present illness (PI) during a patient interview	

c. Presenting the patient's medical files to the patient's family and friends	
d. Reviewing the patient's medical history before interviewing the patient	
e. Recording judgments based on the patient's appearance in the patient's record	
f. Advising patient which over-the-counter or homeopathic treatments to use	

18. Name three demographic details about yourself and where you would include this information in your own medical history.

_____

_____

19. Match the following key terms to their definitions.

Key Terms

a. assessment _____
b. chief complaint _____
c. demographic _____
d. familial _____
e. hereditary _____
f. HIPAA _____
g. homeopathic _____
h. medical history _____
i. over-the-counter _____
j. signs _____
k. symptoms _____

Definitions

1. relating to the statistical characteristics of populations
2. a federal law that protects the privacy of patients' health information
3. subjective indications of disease or bodily dysfunction as sensed by the patient
4. process of gathering information about a patient and the presenting condition
5. a record containing information about a patient's past and present health status
6. traits or disorders that are passed from parent to offspring
7. objective indications of disease or bodily dysfunction as observed or measured by the health care professional
8. the main reason for a patient's visit to the medical office
9. medications and natural drugs that are available without a prescription
10. traits that tend to occur often within a particular family
11. describing a type of alternative medicine in which patients are treated with small doses of substances that produce similar symptoms and use the body's own healing abilities

20. True or False? Determine which of the following statements are true or false. If false, explain why.

a. Unlike over-the-counter medications, homeopathic medications are only available by prescription.

_____

_____

b. Nausea is a sign of food poisoning.

_____

_____

c. It is always the patient's responsibility to fill out his medical history completely and accurately.

_____

_____

d. The chief complaint is always a description of a patient's signs and symptoms.

_____

_____

APPLICATION

Critical Thinking Practice

1. Mrs. Frank is a returning patient at Dr. Mohammad's office. She is 89-years-old and needs the assistance of a wheelchair. What are some important considerations that you should make when showing Mrs. Frank to an exam room, gathering her medical history, and performing a patient assessment? How would those considerations change if the patient was a 2-year-old child?

_____

_____

2. Your patient is a 49-year-old female who speaks very little English. She is a returning patient, so her medical history is already on file at the office. You have called a co-worker who can act as a translator, but he will not arrive at the office for an hour. Meanwhile, the patient is clearly uncomfortable. She appears sweaty and lethargic. She leans on you as you escort her to an examination room. Describe how you can determine the patient's chief complaint and present illness so that you and the physician can begin to help her.

_____

_____

Patient Education

1. Your patient is a 17-year-old male. His symptoms are shortness of breath and fatigue. After you interview the patient, you learn that his father and older brother are obese. You also learn that both of his grandfathers died of complications resulting from heart disease. The patient tells you that he does not have time to exercise. The physician is concerned that the patient will become obese. Write a sheet of instructions that clearly outline the changes that the patient needs to make in his lifestyle as well as in his home in order to improve his health. Include suggestions for the members of his family to follow to help their loved one stay healthy.

_____

_____

Documentation

1. You are interviewing a young patient during an assessment when you notice that he has three small burn marks on his arm. The burns are round and less than a centimeter in diameter. When you ask the patient about the burns, he suddenly turns solemn and avoids answering the question. You suspect that the patient has been abused. How should you document this interaction on the patient's chart?

_____

_____

Active Learning

1. Conduct a patient interview with a family member or friend. Use a sample patient history form such as the one found in this chapter. Be sure to perform the interview in person so that you can observe the physical and mental status of your patient. When you are finished, ask your patient for feedback, such as demeanor and professionalism or comfort level of the patient. Use their comments to set one goal for yourself regarding your skills conducting patient interviews.

2. Research your own family history. Select one disease or disorder with familial or hereditary tendencies that appears in your family history. Prepare a one-page patient education handout for other patients with a family history of this disease or disorder that addresses signs, symptoms, and preventative care for the disease or disorder. If you are unable to trace your family history or are unable to uncover any familial or hereditary conditions, prepare a patient education handout on a familial or hereditary condition of your choosing.

3. Speak to five family members or friends about their experiences in a medical office. Ask each person these questions:
   • Have you ever felt uncomfortable in a medical office? Why?

   • Have you ever felt safe and cared for in a medical office? What made you feel this way?

   • Think of one physician or medical assistant that cared for you during your visit to a medical office. What do you remember most about this person? Is your memory negative or positive?

   Using their responses, make a list of the ways that medical office personnel make their patients comfortable and ways that they make their patient uncomfortable. Turn your list into a "do's and don'ts" list for interacting with patients in a medical office.

Professional Journal

REFLECT

(Prompts and Ideas: "If each man or woman could understand that every other human life is as full of sorrows, or joys, or base temptations, of heartaches and of remorse as his own . . . how much kinder, how much gentler he would be." — William Allen White Reflect on this quote. What can you learn from it? How can you apply the idea presented in this quote to your role as a medical assistant?)

_____

_____

_____

_____

_____

_____

_____

_____

PONDER AND SOLVE

1. Ms. Butler, a 20-year-old patient, received a pregnancy test during a visit to the physician's office. A week later, Mr. Gordon, a 25-year-old male, comes into the office demanding to see the results of Ms. Butler's test. He tells you that he is her boyfriend, and that if Ms. Butler is pregnant, he deserves to know. What would you tell Mr. Gordon?

_____

_____

_____

_____

_____

_____

_____

2. On your way to exam room 3, you notice a coworker weighing another patient outside of exam room 1. As the patient steps onto the scale, your coworker moves the weights on the scale and then reads the patient's weight out loud. The patient appears embarrassed to have his weight read out loud. What would you say to your coworker?

_____

_____

_____

_____

_____

_____

_____

EXPERIENCE

Skills related to this chapter include:

1. Interviewing the Patient to Obtain a Medical History (Procedure 18-1).
2. Document a Chief Complaint and Present Illness (Procedure 18-2).

Record any common mistakes, lessons learned, and/or tips you discovered during your experience of practicing and demonstrating these skills:

_____

_____

_____

_____

_____

_____

_____

Skill Practice

PERFORMANCE OBJECTIVES:

1. Obtain and record a patient history using appropriate communication techniques (Procedure 18-1).
2. Accurately document a chief complaint and present illness (Procedure 18-2).

Name_____ Date _____ Time _____

| Procedure 18-1: | **INTERVIEWING THE PATIENT TO OBTAIN A MEDICAL HISTORY** |

EQUIPMENT: Medical history form or questionnaire, black or blue pen

STANDARDS: Given the needed equipment and a place to work the student will perform this skill with _____% accuracy in a total of _____ minutes. (*Your instructor will tell you what the percentage and time limits will be before you begin.*)

KEY: 4 = Satisfactory   0 = Unsatisfactory   NA = This step is not counted

PROCEDURE STEPS	SELF	PARTNER	INSTRUCTOR
1. Gather the supplies.	☐	☐	☐
2. Review the medical history form for completeness.	☐	☐	☐
3. If the form is partially completed or if the patient could not complete any of the form, take the patient to a private area or the examination room and assist them with completing the form.	☐	☐	☐
4. Sit across from the patient at eye level and maintain frequent eye contact.	☐	☐	☐
5. Introduce yourself and explain the purpose of the interview.	☐	☐	☐
6. Ask the appropriate questions and document the patient's responses.	☐	☐	☐
7. Listen actively by looking at the patient from time to time while he or she is speaking.	☐	☐	☐
8. Avoid projecting a judgmental attitude with words or actions.	☐	☐	☐
9. Explain to the patient what to expect during examinations or procedures at that visit.	☐	☐	☐
10. Thank the patient for cooperating during the interview and offer to answer any questions.	☐	☐	☐

CALCULATION

Total Possible Points: _____
Total Points Earned: _____ Multiplied by 100 = _____ Divided by Total Possible Points = _____%

Pass   **Fail**
☐   ☐   Comments:

Student's signature _____ Date _____
Partner's signature _____ Date _____
Instructor's signature _____ Date _____

Name _____   Date _____   Time _____

Procedure 18-2:	DOCUMENT A CHIEF COMPLAINT (CC) AND PRESENT ILLNESS (PI)

EQUIPMENT: Patient medical record including a cumulative problem list or progress notes form, black or blue ink pen

STANDARDS: Given the needed equipment and a place to work the student will perform this skill with _____% accuracy in a total of _____ minutes. (*Your instructor will tell you what the percentage and time limits will be before you begin.*)

KEY: 4 = Satisfactory   0 = Unsatisfactory   NA = This step is not counted

PROCEDURE STEPS	SELF	PARTNER	INSTRUCTOR
1. Gather the supplies, including the medical record containing the cumulative problem list or progress note form.	☐	☐	☐
2. Review new or established patient's medical history form.	☐	☐	☐
3. Greet and identify the patient while escorting him or her to the examination room and close the door.	☐	☐	☐
4. Use open-ended questions to find out why the patient is seeking medical care; maintain eye contact.	☐	☐	☐
5. Determine the PI using open-ended and closed-ended questions.	☐	☐	☐
6. Document the CC and PI correctly on the cumulative problem list or progress report form.	☐	☐	☐
7. Thank the patient for cooperating and explain that the physician will soon be in to examine the patient.	☐	☐	☐

CALCULATION

Total Possible Points: _____
Total Points Earned: _____ Multiplied by 100 = _____ Divided by Total Possible Points = _____%

Pass   **Fail**
☐   ☐   Comments:

Student's signature _____ Date _____
Partner's signature _____ Date _____
Instructor's signature _____ Date _____

Work Product 1

Obtain and record patient history.

Interview a friend or family member in order to complete the patient history form on the following pages. (Note: If your patient prefers, he or she may pretend to be someone else, with a different medical history. Just make sure to ask the right questions and record all information accurately.)

Professional Medical Associates – History Form

NAME: _____ DATE OF BIRTH: _____

What is the main reason for your visit to the doctor? _____

_____

Were you referred? _____ If so, by whom? _____

PAST MEDICAL HISTORY:

Are you allergic to any medication? _____

If so, list medications: _____

List current medications, dosage, and how many times a day you take them:

Medication	Dose	Times A Day

Alcohol Consumption: What type? _____ Amount? _____ How Often? _____

History of Alcoholism? _____

When was your last TB or Tine test? _____

Have you ever had a positive test for tuberculosis? _____

When was your last Tetanus shot? _____

List all surgeries you have had in the past:

Date	Type of Surgery

List all past hospitalizations (not involving surgeries above):

Date	Reason For Hospital Stay

List all past problems with trauma (broken bones, lacerations, etc.):

_____

REVIEW OF SYSTEMS, PAST MEDICAL PROBLEMS:
If you have been told you have any of the problems listed below, or are having any of the problems listed below, please CIRCLE:

1. <u>GENERAL:</u> Weight loss, weight gain, fever, chills, night sweats, hot flashes, tire easily, problems with sleep, crying spells, history of cancer.

2. <u>SKIN:</u> Rash, sores that won't heal, moles that are new or changing, history of skin problems.

3. <u>HEENT:</u> Headache, eye problems, hearing problems, sinus problems, hay fever, dizziness, hoarseness, sores in your mouth that won't heal, dental problems.

   Do you chew tobacco or dip snuff? _____

4. <u>METABOLIC/ENDOCRINE:</u> Thyroid problems, diabetes or sugar problems, high cholesterol.

5. <u>RESPIRATORY:</u> Cough, wheezing, breathing problems, history of asthma, history of lung problems.

   Do you smoke cigarettes or a pipe? _____

   How much? _____ For how long? _____

6. <u>BREAST (WOMEN):</u> Breast lumps, changes in nipples, nipple discharge, breast problems, family history of breast cancer. When was your last mammogram? _____

7. <u>CARDIOVASCULAR:</u> Heart murmur, rheumatic fever, high blood pressure, angina, heart problems, heart attack, abnormal heart rhythm, chest pain, palpitations, leg swelling, history of phlebitis or blood clots.

8. <u>GI:</u> Problems with appetite, swallowing, heartburn, nausea, vomiting, pain in the abdomen, constipation, diarrhea, blood in stool, history of ulcers, liver problems, hepatitis, jaundice, pancreas problems, gallbladder problems, or colon problems.

9. <u>REPRODUCTIVE (WOMEN):</u> Problems with irregular menstrual cycles, abnormal vaginal bleeding or discharge, history of sexually transmitted diseases, sexual problems.

   AGE OF FIRST MENSES (PERIOD) _____ AGE OF MENOPAUSE _____

   LAST PAP SMEAR _____ METHOD OF CONTRACEPTION _____

   Obstetric History (Women)

   NUMBER OF PREGNANCIES _____ PLEASE LIST AS FOLLOWS:

   Delivery Date   Pregnancy Complications   Type Delivery   Baby's Weight

   _____

   _____

   <u>MEN:</u> Problems with genital discharge, history of venereal diseases, sexual problems, prostate problems.

   METHOD OF CONTRACEPTION _____

10. <u>UROLOGIC:</u> Problems with painful urination, urinary frequency, blood in urine, weak urinary stream, history of bladder or kidney infections, or kidney stones.

11. <u>MUSCULOSKELETAL:</u> Arthritis, back pain, cramps in legs.

12. <u>NEUROLOGIC:</u> Seizures, stroke, arm or leg weakness or numbness, black-out spells, memory or thinking problems, depression, anxiety, psychiatric problems.

13. <u>HEMATOLOGIC:</u> Anemia, bleeding problems, enlarged lymph nodes.

HAVE YOU EVER HAD A BLOOD TRANSFUSION? _____ DATE _____

FAMILY HISTORY:

List any medical problems that run in your family and which family members have these problems.

_____

_____

SOCIAL HISTORY:

MARITAL STATUS: _____

OCCUPATION: _____

EDUCATION: _____

HOBBIES: _____

WHAT DO YOU DO FOR ENJOYMENT? _____

Work Product 2

Document appropriately.

Ask a friend or family member to pretend to be your patient. Interview your patient to determine his or her chief complaint and present illness. If you are currently working in a medical office, use a blank paper patient chart from the office. If this is not available to you, use the space below to document this information in the chart.

_____

_____

_____

_____

Chapter Self-Assessment Quiz

1. The best place to interview a patient is:
   a. over the phone.
   b. at the patient's home.
   c. in the reception area.
   d. in an examination room.
   e. in the physician's office.

2. Which of the following would appear in the past history (PH) section of a patient's medical history?
   a. Hospitalizations
   b. Chief complaint
   c. Insurance carrier
   d. Review of systems
   e. Deaths in immediate family

3. You are collecting the medical history of a patient. The patient discloses that her brother, sister, paternal grandfather, and paternal aunt are overweight. For this patient, obesity is considered to be:
   a. familial.
   b. historic.
   c. hereditary.
   d. homeopathic.
   e. demographic.

4. Under HIPAA, who may access a patient's medical records?
   a. Any health care provider
   b. The patient's family and friends
   c. Anyone who fills out the proper forms
   d. Only the patient's primary care physician
   e. Only health care providers directly involved in the patient's care

5. During an interview, your patient tells you that she drinks alcohol four to five times a week. This information should be included in the:
   a. chief complaint.
   b. past history.
   c. present illness.
   d. social history.
   e. family history.

6. Which of the following is included in the patient's present illness (PI)?
   a. Self-care activities
   b. Hereditary diseases
   c. Signs and symptoms
   d. Preventative medicine
   e. Name, address, and phone number

7. Who completes the patient's medical history form?
   a. The patient only
   b. The patient's insurance provider
   c. The patient's immediate family
   d. The patient, the medical assistant, and the physician
   e. The patient's former physician or primary care provider

8. A homeopathic remedy for headache could be a(n):
   a. prescription painkiller.
   b. extended period of rest.
   c. 1000 mg of acetaminophen.
   d. icepack on the forehead for ten minutes.
   e. small dose of an agent that causes headache.

9. An open-ended question is one that:

   a. determines the patient's level of pain.

   b. determines where something happened.

   c. is rhetorical and does not require an answer.

   d. can be answered with a "yes" or a "no" response.

   e. requires the responder to answer using more than one word.

10. One sign of illness might be:

    a. coughing.

    b. headache.

    c. dizziness.

    d. self-care.

    e. muscle pain.

11. Which of the following is a closed-ended question?

    a. "What is the reason for your appointment today?"

    b. "Is there anything you do to make the pain better?"

    c. "Does the pain leave and return throughout the day?"

    d. "How would you describe the pain you are feeling?"

    e. "What have you done to help eliminate the pain?"

12. At the beginning of an interview, you can establish a trusting, professional relationship with the patient by:

    a. thoroughly introducing yourself.

    b. listing the physician's credentials.

    c. observing the patient's signs of illness.

    d. conducting the review of systems (ROS).

    e. disclosing the patient's weight in private.

13. If you suspect that the patient you are assessing is the victim of abuse, you should:

    a. report your suspicions to the local police station.

    b. record your suspicion of abuse in the patient's chief complaint (CC).

    c. ask the patient if he or she is being abused with a closed-ended question.

    d. document the objective signs and notify the physician of your suspicions.

    e. review the patient's medical history for signs of an abusive spouse or parent.

14. Which of the following is included in the identifying database of a patient's medical history?

    a. The patient's emergency contact

    b. The patient's Social Security number

    c. The patient's reason for visiting the office

    d. The patient's signs and symptoms of illness

    e. The patient's family's addresses

15. One example of a symptom of an illness is:

    a. rash.

    b. cough.

    c. nausea.

    d. vomiting.

    e. wheezing.

16. The patient's present illness (PI) includes which of the following:

    a. social history.

    b. family history.

    c. chronology of the illness.

    d. demographic information.

    e. history of hospitalizations.

17. Before you proceed with a patient interview, you should obtain:

    a. signs and symptoms.

    b. social and family history.

    c. the duration of pain and self-treatment information.

    d. the chief complaint and patient's present illness.

    e. the location of pain and self-treatment information.

18. Which of the following is a poor interview technique?

    a. Asking open-ended questions

    b. Noting observable information

    c. Suggesting expected symptoms

    d. Introducing yourself to the patient

    e. Reading through the patient's medical history beforehand

19. You think that a patient has a disease that was passed down from her parents. Where could you look to find information on the patient's parents?

    a. Medical history forms

    b. History of self-treatment

    c. Demographic information

    d. Notes during the patient interview

    e. Chief complaints from previous visits

20. While obtaining a patient's present illness, you need to find out:

    a. where she lives.

    b. the chief complaint.

    c. if she smokes tobacco.

    d. the severity of the pain.

    e. any hereditary disease(s) she has.

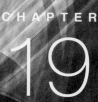

CHAPTER 19

Anthropometric Measurements and Vital Signs

Chapter Checklist

☐ Read textbook chapter and take notes within the Chapter Notes outline. Answer the Learning Objectives as you reach them in the content, and then check them off.

☐ Work the Content Review questions—both Foundational Knowledge and Application.

☐ Perform the Active Learning exercise(s).

☐ Complete Professional Journal entries.

☐ Complete Skill Practice Activity(s) using Competency Evaluation Forms and Work Products, when appropriate.

☐ Take the Chapter Self-Assessment Quiz.

☐ Insert all appropriate pages into your Portfolio.

Learning Objectives

1. Spell and define the key terms.
2. Explain the procedures for measuring a patient's height and weight.
3. List the fever process, including the stages of fever.
4. Identify and describe the types of thermometers.
5. Compare the procedures for measuring a patient's temperature using the oral, rectal, axillary, and tympanic methods.
6. Identify the various sites on the body used for palpating a pulse.
7. Describe the procedures for measuring a patient's pulse and respiratory rates.
8. Define Korotkoff sounds and the five phases of blood pressure.
9. Identify factors that may influence the blood pressure.
10. Explain the factors to consider when choosing the correct blood pressure cuff size.

Chapter Notes

Note: Bold-faced headings are the major headings in the text chapter; headings in regular font are lower-level headings (i.e., the content is subordinate to, or falls "under," the major headings). Make sure you understand the key terms used in the chapter, as well as the concepts presented as Key Points.

TEXT SUBHEADINGS　　　　**NOTES**

Introduction _____

_____

Key Terms: cardinal signs; anthropometric; baseline

☐ **LEARNING OBJECTIVE 1:** Spell and define the key terms.

Anthropometric Measurements _____

_____

_____

Weight _____

_____

Key Point:
- Types of scales used to measure weight include balance beam scales, digital scales, and dial scales.

Height _____

_____

Key Point:
- Height is measured in inches or centimeters, depending upon the physician's preference.

☐ **LEARNING OBJECTIVE 2:** Explain the procedures for measuring a patient's height and weight.

Vital Signs _____

_____

_____

Temperature _____

_____

Key Terms: afebrile; febrile; tympanic
Key Points:
- Body temperature reflects a balance between heat produced and heat lost by the body.
- Thermometers are used to measure body temperature using either the Fahrenheit or Celsius scale.

Fever Processes _____

_____

Key Point:

- Although a patient's temperature is influenced by heat lost or produced by the body, it is regulated by the hypothalamus in the brain.

Stages of Fever _____

_____

Key Terms: pyrexia; hyperpyrexia; sustained; remittent; intermittent; relapsing
Key Point:
• An elevated temperature, or fever, usually results from a disease process, such as a bacterial or viral infection.

☐ **LEARNING OBJECTIVE 3:** List the fever process, including the stages of fever.

Types of Thermometers _____

_____

Glass Mercury Thermometers _____

_____

Key Points:
• Oral, rectal, and axillary temperatures have traditionally been measured using the mercury glass thermometer.
• Before using a glass thermometer, place it in a clear plastic disposable sheath.

Electronic Thermometers _____

_____

Tympanic Thermometers _____

_____

Temporal Artery Thermometer _____

_____

Key Point:
• The temporal artery thermometer measures actual blood temperature by placing the unit on the front of the forehead, depressing the "on/off" button, and sliding the probe scanner over the forehead and down to the temporal artery area of the forehead.

Disposable Thermometers

Key Term: diaphoresis
Key Point:
- Single-use disposable thermometers are fairly accurate but are not considered as reliable as electronic, tympanic, or glass thermometers.

☐ **LEARNING OBJECTIVE 4:** Identify and describe the types of thermometers.

☐ **LEARNING OBJECTIVE 5:** Compare the procedures for measuring a patient's temperature using the oral, rectal, axillary, and tympanic methods.

Pulse

Key Term: palpation
Key Points:
- This expansion and relaxation of the arteries can be felt at various points on the body where you can press an artery against a bone or other underlying firm surface.
- **Palpation** of the pulse is performed by placing the index and middle fingers, the middle and ring fingers, or all three fingers over a pulse point.
- The apical pulse is auscultated using a stethoscope with the bell placed over the apex of the heart.

☐ **LEARNING OBJECTIVE 6:** Identify the various sites on the body used for palpating a pulse.

Pulse Characteristics

Key Points:
- While palpating the pulse, you also assess the rate, rhythm, and volume as the artery wall expands with each heartbeat.
- In healthy adults, the average pulse rate is 60 to 100 beats per minute.
- The *rhythm* is the interval between each heartbeat or the pattern of beats.
- *Volume*, the strength or force of the heartbeat, can be described as soft, bounding, weak, thready, strong, or full.

Factors Affecting Pulse Rates _____

_____

Key Term: cardiac output
Key Point:
- The radial artery is most often used to determine pulse rate because it is convenient for both the medical assistant and the patient.

Respiration _____

_____

Key Point:
- Respiration is the exchange of gases between the atmosphere and the blood in the body.

Respiration Characteristics _____

_____

Key Points:
- The characteristics of respirations include rate, rhythm, and depth.
- Abnormal sounds during inspiration or expiration are usually a sign of a disease process.

Factors Affecting Respiration _____

_____

Key Terms: dyspnea; apnea; hyperpnea; hyperventilation; hypopnea; orthopnea
Key Point:
- In healthy adults, the average respiratory rate is 14 to 20 breaths per minute.

☐ **LEARNING OBJECTIVE 7:** Describe the procedures for measuring a patient's pulse and respiratory rates.

Blood Pressure _____

_____

Key Terms: systole; diastole; cardiac cycle; sphygmomanometer; postural hypotension
Key Points:
- Blood pressure is a measurement of the pressure of the blood in an artery as it is forced against the arterial walls.
- Although only one type actually contains mercury, both types are calibrated and measure blood pressure in millimeters of mercury (mm Hg).

Korotkoff Sounds _____

_____

Key Point:

• Korotkoff sounds can be classified into five phases of sounds heard while auscultating the blood pressure as described by the Russian neurologist Nikolai Korotkoff.

Pulse Pressure _____

_____

Key Point:
• The difference between the systolic and diastolic readings is known as the pulse pressure.

Auscultatory Gap _____

_____

Key Term: hypertension
Key Point:
• An auscultatory gap is the loss of any sounds for a drop of up to 30 mm Hg (sometimes more) during the release of air from the blood pressure cuff after the first sound is heard.

☐ **LEARNING OBJECTIVE 8:** Define Korotkoff sounds and the five phases of blood pressure.

Factors Influencing Blood Pressure _____

_____

☐ **LEARNING OBJECTIVE 9:** Identify factors that may influence the blood pressure.

Blood Pressure Cuff Size _____

_____

Key Point:
• Before beginning to take a patient's blood pressure, assess the size of the patient's arm and choose the correct size accordingly.

☐ **LEARNING OBJECTIVE 10:** Explain the factors to consider when choosing the correct blood pressure cuff size.

Content Review

FOUNDATIONAL KNOWLEDGE

Measurements

1. The table below lists typical office measurements. Place a check mark in the "Anthropometric" column if the measurement is an anthropometric measurement. Similarly, place check marks in the other columns for measurements that are baseline (first visit) measurements, measurements taken at every visit, measurements of cardinal (vital) signs, and measurements typically done by a medical assistant. Many rows will have more than one check mark.

	Anthropometric	Baseline (First Time)	Every Time	Cardinal Sign	Medical Assistant
Blood pressure					
Cardiac output					
Height					
Pulse rate					
Respiratory rate					
Temperature					
Weight					

Weighing Patients

2. What two things should you do <u>before</u> greeting a patient you are going to weigh? Why should you do these two things? Fill in the chart below with your answer.

Before You Greet a Patient You Are Going to Weigh, You Should:	Explanation
a.	
b.	

3. What five things should you do between greeting a patient and assisting the patient onto the scale?

a. _____

b. _____

c. _____

d. _____

e. _____

4. The directions below for measuring weight include parts that are inaccurate or incorrect. Rewrite the directions so that they are completely correct:

Stand on one side of the scale. Ask the patient to step onto the scale facing you. Encourage the patient to hold your hand so you can help him or her balance during the weighing process.

_____

_____

5. The steps for weighing a patient with a balance beam scale are listed below, but they are <u>not</u> in the correct order. Number them so that they are in the right order.

___ Record the weight.

___ Memorize the weight.

___ Help the patient off the scale.

___ Help the patient onto the scale.

___ Be sure the counterweights are both at zero.

___ Be sure the counterweights are both at zero.

___ Slide the larger counterweight toward zero until it rests securely in a notch.

___ Slide the smaller counterweight toward zero until the balance bar is exactly at the midpoint.

___ Slide the larger counterweight away from zero until the balance bar moves below the midpoint.

___ Slide the smaller counterweight away from zero until the balance bar moves below the midpoint.

___ Add the readings from the two counterweight bars, counting each line after the smaller counterweight as 1/4 pound.

Measuring Height

6. For each step in measuring a patient's height, underline the correct choice.

a. Wash your hands if the height is measured at (a different time from/the same time as) the weight.

b. The patient should (remove/wear) shoes.

c. The patient should stand straight with heels (a hand's width apart/together).

d. The patient's eyes should be looking (at the floor/straight ahead).

e. A better measurement is usually taken with the patient's (back/front) to the ruler.

f. Position the measuring bar perpendicular to the (ruler/top of the head).

g. Slowly lower the measuring bar until it touches the patient's (hair/head).

h. Measure at the (point of movement/top of the ruler).

i. A measurement of 66 inches should be recorded as (5 feet, 6 inches/66 inches).

Temperatures and Fevers

7. List the six types of thermometers used in a medical office, and briefly describe how each one is used.

Type of Thermometer	How Is It Used?
a.	
b.	
c.	
d.	
e.	
f.	

8. Hot or Cold?

a. What does the hypothalamus do when it senses that the body is too warm?

_____

_____

b. What happens when the body temperature is too cool?

_____

_____

c. What factors aside from illness affect body temperature?

_____

_____

9. List and describe the three stages of fever. Include the variations in the time and their related terms.

Stage 1	Stage 2	Stage 3

Measuring Pulses

10. The points on the body where you can press an artery against a bone or other underlying firm surface are known as pulse points. Name the pulse point <u>most</u> commonly palpated. Then name all the pulse points commonly palpated, from head to toe.

_____

_____

11. List the three steps you should follow when using a Doppler unit to measure a patient's heartbeat.

a. _____

b. _____

c. _____

Measuring Respirations

12. When should you determine a patient's respiration rate?

_____

_____

13. If the patient has 19 full inspirations and 18 full expirations in 1 minute, what is the patient's respiration rate?

_____

_____

14. In addition to respiration rate, what are four other respiration characteristics you should record in the patient's chart?

a. _____

b. _____

c. _____

d. _____

Measuring Blood Pressure

15. Organize the Korotkoff sounds with the correct phases in the table below.

Phases	Sounds
I	Last sound
II	Soft swishing
III	Soft tapping that becomes faint
IV	Rhythmic, sharp, distinct tapping
V	Faint tapping heard as the cuff deflates

Phase	Sounds
.	

16.

    a. Fill in the blank: Korotkoff sounds are sounds heard while _____.

    b. At which sound is the systolic blood pressure recorded? _____

    c. At which sound is the diastolic blood pressure recorded? _____

17. Place a check mark next to each factor that can affect blood pressure.

Factor	Affect Blood Pressure
Activity	
Age	
Alcohol use	
Arteriosclerosis	
Atherosclerosis	
Body position	
Dietary habits	
Economic status	
Education	
Exercise	
Family history of heart conditions	
Gender	
General health of the patient	
Height	
History of heart conditions	
Medications	
Occupation	
Stress	
Tobacco use	

18. The following statements are incorrect or inaccurate. Rewrite each statement so that it is accurate and correct.

    a. The width of a blood pressure cuff should be 75% to 80% of the circumference of the arm.

_____

_____

b. To determine the correct blood pressure cuff size, wrap the length of the cuff around the forearm.

_____

_____

c. The cuff width should reach not quite three-quarters of the way around the arm.

_____

_____

d. Cuffs are available in widths from about 3 inches for children to 12 inches for adults.

_____

_____

e. Different cuff sizes are used so that patients are not uncomfortable during blood pressure measurements.

_____

_____

19. Match the following key terms to their definitions.

Key Terms	**Definitions**
a. afebrile _____	**1.** profuse sweating
b. anthropometric _____	**2.** fever that is fluctuating
c. apnea _____	**3.** no respiration
d. baseline _____	**4.** fever that is constant
e. calibrated _____	**5.** shallow respirations
f. cardiac cycle _____	**6.** occurring at intervals
g. cardinal signs _____	**7.** elevated blood pressure
h. diastole _____	**8.** pertaining to measurements of the human body
i. diaphoresis _____	**9.** difficult or labored breathing
j. dyspnea _____	**10.** device used to measure blood pressure
k. febrile _____	**11.** abnormally deep, gasping breaths
l. hyperpnea _____	**12.** phase in which the heart contracts
m. hyperpyrexia _____	**13.** having a temperature above normal
n. hypertension _____	**14.** original or initial measure with which other measurements will be compared
o. hyperventilation _____	**15.** having a temperature within normal limits
p. hypopnea _____	**16.** extremely high temperature, from 105° to 106°F
q. intermittent _____	**17.** marked in units of measurement
r. orthopnea _____	**18.** phase in which the heart pauses briefly to rest and refill
s. palpation _____	**19.** fever of 102°F or higher rectally or 101°F or higher orally
t. postural hypotension _____	**20.** act of pressing an artery against an underlying firm surface
u. pyrexia _____	**21.** sudden drop in blood pressure upon standing
v. relapsing fever _____	**22.** fever returning after an extended period of normal readings
w. remittent fever _____	**23.** respiratory rate that greatly exceeds the body's oxygen demand
x. sphygmomanometer _____	**24.** period from the beginning of one heartbeat to the beginning of the next
y. sustained fever _____	**25.** inability to breathe lying down
z. systole _____	**26.** measurements of vital signs

20. True or False? Determine whether the following statements are true or false. If false, explain why.

a. The weight scale should be kept in the waiting room for ease of access.

_____

_____

b. An axillary temperature can be taken with either an oral or a rectal thermometer.

_____

_____

c. In pediatric offices, temperatures are almost always taken rectally.

_____

_____

d. If a glass mercury thermometer breaks, you should soak up the mercury immediately with tissues and put them in the trash before the mercury sinks into any surfaces.

_____

_____

APPLICATION

Critical Thinking Practice

1. Ms. Green arrived at the office late for her appointment, frantic and explaining that her alarm clock had not gone off. She discovered that her car was almost out of gas, and she had to stop to refuel. Once she got to the clinic, she could not find a parking place in the lot and she had to park two blocks away. How would you expect this to affect her vital signs? Explain why.

_____

_____

2. A patient comes into the office complaining of fever and chills. While taking her vital signs, you notice that she feels very warm. When you take her temperature, you find that her oral temperature is 105°F. What should you do, and how quickly?

_____

_____

Patient Education

1. Mr. Juarez, the father of a 6-month-old and a 4-year-old, would like to purchase a thermometer. He is not sure which one to buy and isn't familiar with how to use the different kinds of thermometers. He also isn't aware of the possible variations that may occur in readings. Create a graph to show him the types of thermometers and temperature readings. Include Fahrenheit readings.

Documentation

1. How should you record an axillary temperature, and why is it important to record it differently from other temperatures?

_____

_____

Active Learning

1. With a partner, practice taking body temperature measurements with all the types of thermometers you have access to. For those you can't access, mime the process so that you at least have the steps down the first time you are faced with the real thermometer. For all methods, go through all the steps from picking up the thermometer to returning it to the disinfectant or returning the unit to the charging base.

2. Find and memorize the mathematical formulas for converting from Fahrenheit to Celsius degrees and from Celsius to Fahrenheit. If you know you're not likely to remember the formulas, make a table for yourself listing the temperatures that are most important to remember—in both Fahrenheit and Celsius degrees. For example, list the normal oral, axillary, and rectal temperatures and the Celsius equivalents of 101°F and 105°F.

3. With a partner, practice taking radial pulse, respiration, and blood pressure measurements. Then perform 15 minutes of light exercise, such as walking, and take your rates again to see if there is any difference.

Professional Journal

REFLECT

(Prompts and Ideas: Have you ever been annoyed at the doctor's office when the medical assistant wouldn't tell you your blood pressure or another measurement? Do you know people who really don't want to know their measurements? How will you respond to patients who feel either way? If you're feeling sick, how do you usually take your own temperature? What kind of thermometers do you have at home? Are you comfortable using all of them?)

_____

_____

_____

_____

PONDER AND SOLVE

1. Mrs. Chin has come into the office complaining of pain in her right foot. You take her vital signs, which are normal, and you help her remove her shoes so that the doctor can examine both feet. You notice a difference in appearance between her two feet, and it occurs to you to check her femoral, popliteal, posterior tibial, and dorsalis pedis pulses. What are you looking for, and what should you look for next?

_____

_____

_____

_____

2. You've noticed that whenever you try to take Mr. Kimble's respiration rate, he always breathes in when you do and breathes out when you do. You're concerned that you're not assessing Mr. Kimble's breathing accurately, and you know that he has had asthma on occasion. What can you do to get an accurate reading?

_____

_____

_____

EXPERIENCE

Skills related to this chapter include:

1. Measure and Record a Patient's Weight (Procedure 19-1).

2. Measure and Record a Patient's Height (Procedure 19-2).

3. Measure and Record a Patient's Oral Temperature Using a Glass Mercury Thermometer (Procedure 19-3).

4. Measure and Record a Rectal Temperature (Procedure 19-4).

5. Measure and Record an Axillary Temperature (Procedure 19-5).

6. Measure and Record a Patient's Temperature Using an Electronic Thermometer (Procedure 19-6).

7. Measure and Record a Patient's Temperature Using a Tympanic Thermometer (Procedure 19-7).

8. Measure and Record a Patient's Temperature Using a Temporal Artery Thermometer (Procedure 19-8).

9. Measure and Record a Patient's Radial Pulse (Procedure 19-9).

10. Measure and Record a Patient's Respirations (Procedure 19-10).

11. Measure and Record a Patient's Blood Pressure (Procedure 19-11).

Record any common mistakes, lessons learned, and/or tips you discovered during your experience of practicing and demonstrating these skills.

_____

_____

_____

_____

_____

_____

_____

_____

Skill Practice

PERFORMANCE OBJECTIVES:

1. Measure and record a patient's weight (Procedure 19-1).
2. Measure and record a patient's height (Procedure 19-2).
3. Measure and record a patient's oral temperature using a glass mercury thermometer (Procedure 19-3).
4. Measure and record a patient's rectal temperature (Procedure 19-4).
5. Measure and record a patient's axillary temperature (Procedure 19-5).
6. Measure and record a patient's temperature using an electronic thermometer (Procedure 19-6).
7. Measure and record a patient's temperature using a tympanic thermometer (Procedure 19-7).
8. Measure and record a patient's temperature using a temporal artery thermometer (Procedure 19-8).
9. Measure and record a patient's radial pulse (Procedure 19-9).
10. Measure and record a patient's respirations (Procedure 19-10).
11. Measure and record a patient's blood pressure (Procedure 19-11).

Name_____ Date_____ Time_____

Procedure 19-1:   MEASURE AND RECORD A PATIENT'S WEIGHT

EQUIPMENT/SUPPLIES: Calibrated balance beam scale, digital scale or dial scale; paper towel

STANDARDS: Given the needed equipment and a place to work, the student will perform this skill with _____% accuracy in a total of _____ minutes. *(Your instructor will tell you what the percentage and time limits will be before you begin practicing.)*

KEY: 4 = Satisfactory   0 = Unsatisfactory   NA = This step is not counted

PROCEDURE STEPS	SELF	PARTNER	INSTRUCTOR
1. Wash your hands.	☐	☐	☐
2. Ensure that the scale is properly balanced at zero.	☐	☐	☐
3. Escort the patient to the scale and place a paper towel on the scale.	☐	☐	☐
4. Have the patient remove shoes, heavy coats, or jackets.	☐	☐	☐
5. Assist the patient onto the scale facing forward.	☐	☐	☐
6. Ask patient to stand still, without touching or holding on to anything if possible.	☐	☐	☐
7. Weigh the patient.	☐	☐	☐
8. Return the bars on the top and bottom to zero.	☐	☐	☐
9. Assist the patient from the scale if necessary and discard the paper towel.	☐	☐	☐
10. Record the patient's weight.	☐	☐	☐

CALCULATION

Total Possible Points: _____
Total Points Earned: _____ Multiplied by 100 = _____ Divided by Total Possible Points = _____%

Pass   **Fail**
☐   ☐   Comments:

Student's signature _____ Date _____
Partner's signature _____ Date _____
Instructor's signature _____ Date _____

Name _____ Date _____ Time _____

Procedure 19-2:	MEASURE AND RECORD A PATIENT'S HEIGHT

EQUIPMENT/SUPPLIES: A scale with a ruler

STANDARDS: Given the needed equipment and a place to work, the student will perform this skill with _____% accuracy in a total of _____ minutes. *(Your instructor will tell you what the percentage and time limits will be before you begin practicing.)*

KEY: 4 = Satisfactory   0 = Unsatisfactory   NA = This step is not counted

PROCEDURE STEPS	SELF	PARTNER	INSTRUCTOR
1. Wash your hands.	☐	☐	☐
2. Have the patient remove the shoes and stand straight and erect on the scale, heels together, and eyes straight ahead.	☐	☐	☐
3. With the measuring bar perpendicular to the ruler, slowly lower until it firmly touches patient's head.	☐	☐	☐
4. Read the measurement at the point of movement on the ruler.	☐	☐	☐
5. Assist the patient from the scale.	☐	☐	☐
6. Record the height measurements in the medical record. The height may be recorded with the weight measurement.	☐	☐	☐

CALCULATION

Total Possible Points: _____
Total Points Earned: _____ Multiplied by 100 = _____ Divided by Total Possible Points = _____%

Pass   **Fail**
☐   ☐   Comments:

Student's signature _____ Date _____
Partner's signature _____ Date _____
Instructor's signature _____ Date _____

Name _____ Date _____ Time _____

Procedure 19-3:	MEASURE AND RECORD A PATIENT'S ORAL TEMPERATURE USING A GLASS MERCURY THERMOMETER

EQUIPMENT/SUPPLIES: Glass mercury oral thermometer, tissues or cotton balls, disposable plastic sheath, gloves, biohazard waste container, cool soapy water, disinfectant solution

STANDARDS: Given the needed equipment and a place to work, the student will perform this skill with _____% accuracy in a total of _____ minutes. *(Your instructor will tell you what the percentage and time limits will be before you begin practicing.)*

KEY: 4 = Satisfactory   0 = Unsatisfactory   NA = This step is not counted

PROCEDURE STEPS	SELF	PARTNER	INSTRUCTOR
1. Wash your hands and assemble the necessary supplies.	☐	☐	☐
2. Dry the thermometer if it has been stored in disinfectant.	☐	☐	☐
3. Carefully check the thermometer for chips or cracks.	☐	☐	☐
4. Check the level of the mercury in the thermometer.	☐	☐	☐
5. If the mercury level is above 94°F, carefully shake down.	☐	☐	☐
6. Insert the thermometer into the plastic sheath.	☐	☐	☐
7. Greet and identify the patient.	☐	☐	☐
8. Explain the procedure and ask about any eating, drinking hot or cold fluids, gum chewing, or smoking.	☐	☐	☐
9. Place the thermometer under the patient's tongue.	☐	☐	☐
10. Tell the patient to keep the mouth and lips closed but caution against biting down on the glass stem.	☐	☐	☐
11. Leave the thermometer in place for 3 to 5 minutes.	☐	☐	☐
12. At the appropriate time, remove the thermometer from the patient's mouth while wearing gloves.	☐	☐	☐
13. Remove the sheath by holding the very edge of the sheath with your thumb and forefinger.	☐	☐	☐
14. Discard the sheath into a biohazard waste container.	☐	☐	☐
15. Hold the thermometer horizontal at eye level and note the level of mercury in the column.	☐	☐	☐
16. Record the patient's temperature.	☐	☐	☐

CALCULATION

Total Possible Points: _____
Total Points Earned: _____ Multiplied by 100 = _____ Divided by Total Possible Points = _____%

Pass **Fail**
☐ ☐ Comments:

Student's signature _____ Date _____
Partner's signature _____ Date _____
Instructor's signature _____ Date _____

Name_____ Date_____ Time_____

Procedure 19-4:	**MEASURE AND RECORD A RECTAL TEMPERATURE**

EQUIPMENT/SUPPLIES: Glass mercury rectal thermometer, tissues or cotton balls, disposable plastic sheaths, surgical lubricant, biohazard waste container, cool soapy water, disinfectant solution, gloves

STANDARDS: Given the needed equipment and a place to work, the student will perform this skill with _____% accuracy in a total of _____ minutes. *(Your instructor will tell you what the percentage and time limits will be before you begin practicing.)*

KEY: 4 = Satisfactory   0 = Unsatisfactory   NA = This step is not counted

PROCEDURE STEPS	SELF	PARTNER	INSTRUCTOR
1. Wash your hands and assemble the necessary supplies.	☐	☐	☐
2. Dry the thermometer if it has been stored in disinfectant.	☐	☐	☐
3. Carefully check the thermometer for chips or cracks.	☐	☐	☐
4. Check the level of the mercury in the thermometer.	☐	☐	☐
5. If the mercury level is above 94°F, carefully shake down.	☐	☐	☐
6. Insert the thermometer into the plastic sheath.	☐	☐	☐
7. Spread lubricant onto a tissue and then from the tissue onto the sheath of the thermometer.	☐	☐	☐
8. Greet and identify the patient and explain the procedure.	☐	☐	☐
9. Ensure patient privacy by placing the patient in a side-lying position facing the examination room door. Drape appropriately.	☐	☐	☐
10. Apply gloves and visualize the anus by lifting the top buttock with your nondominant hand.	☐	☐	☐
11. Gently insert thermometer past the sphincter muscle.	☐	☐	☐
12. Release the upper buttock and hold the thermometer in place with your dominant hand for 3 minutes.	☐	☐	☐
13. After 3 minutes, remove the thermometer and the sheath.	☐	☐	☐
14. Discard the sheath into a biohazard waste container.	☐	☐	☐
15. Note the reading with the thermometer horizontal at eye level.	☐	☐	☐
16. Give the patient a tissue to wipe away excess lubricant.	☐	☐	☐
17. Assist with dressing if necessary.	☐	☐	☐
18. Record the procedure and mark the letter *R* next to the reading.	☐	☐	☐

CALCULATION

Total Possible Points: _____
Total Points Earned: _____ Multiplied by 100 = _____ Divided by Total Possible Points = _____%

Pass **Fail**

☐ ☐ Comments:

Student's signature _____ Date _____
Partner's signature _____ Date _____
Instructor's signature _____ Date _____

Name _____   Date _____   Time _____

Procedure 19-5:	MEASURE AND RECORD AN AXILLARY TEMPERATURE

EQUIPMENT/SUPPLIES: Glass mercury (oral or rectal) thermometer, tissues or cotton balls, disposable plastic sheaths, biohazard waste container, cool soapy water, disinfectant solution

STANDARDS: Given the needed equipment and a place to work, the student will perform this skill with _____% accuracy in a total of _____ minutes. *(Your instructor will tell you what the percentage and time limits will be before you begin practicing.)*

KEY: 4 = Satisfactory   0 = Unsatisfactory   NA = This step is not counted

PROCEDURE STEPS	SELF	PARTNER	INSTRUCTOR
1. Wash your hands and assemble the necessary supplies.	☐	☐	☐
2. Dry the thermometer if it has been stored in disinfectant.	☐	☐	☐
3. Carefully check the thermometer for chips or cracks.	☐	☐	☐
4. Check the level of the mercury in the thermometer.	☐	☐	☐
5. If the mercury level is above 94°F, carefully shake down.	☐	☐	☐
6. Insert the thermometer into the plastic sheath.	☐	☐	☐
7. Expose the patient's axilla, exposing as little of upper body as possible.	☐	☐	☐
8. Place the bulb of the thermometer well into the axilla.	☐	☐	☐
9. Bring the patient's arm down, crossing the forearm over the chest.	☐	☐	☐
10. Leave the thermometer in place for 10 minutes.	☐	☐	☐
11. After 10 minutes, remove the thermometer from the patient's axilla.	☐	☐	☐
12. Remove the sheath and discard the sheath into a biohazard waste container.	☐	☐	☐
13. Hold the thermometer horizontal at eye level and note the level of mercury.	☐	☐	☐
14. Record the procedure and mark a letter *A* next to the reading, indicating an axillary temperature.	☐	☐	☐

CALCULATION

Total Possible Points: _____
Total Points Earned: _____ Multiplied by 100 = _____ Divided by Total Possible Points = _____%

Pass   **Fail**
☐   ☐   Comments:

Student's signature _____ Date _____
Partner's signature _____ Date _____
Instructor's signature _____ Date _____

Name _____ Date _____ Time _____

Procedure 19-6:	MEASURE AND RECORD A PATIENT'S TEMPERATURE USING AN ELECTRONIC THERMOMETER

EQUIPMENT/SUPPLIES: Electronic thermometer with oral or rectal probe, lubricant and gloves for rectal temperatures, disposable probe covers, biohazard waste container

STANDARDS: Given the needed equipment and a place to work, the student will perform this skill with _____% accuracy in a total of _____ minutes. *(Your instructor will tell you what the percentage and time limits will be before you begin practicing.)*

KEY: 4 = Satisfactory 0 = Unsatisfactory NA = This step is not counted

PROCEDURE STEPS	SELF	PARTNER	INSTRUCTOR
1. Wash your hands and assemble the necessary supplies.	☐	☐	☐
2. Greet and identify the patient and explain the procedure.	☐	☐	☐
3. Choose the method (oral, axillary, or rectal) most appropriate for the patient.	☐	☐	☐
4. Insert the probe into a probe cover.	☐	☐	☐
5. Position the thermometer.	☐	☐	☐
6. Wait for the electronic thermometer unit to "beep."	☐	☐	☐
7. Remove the probe and note the reading on the digital display screen on the unit.	☐	☐	☐
8. Discard the probe cover into a biohazard waste container.	☐	☐	☐
9. Record the procedure result.	☐	☐	☐
10. Return the unit and probe to the charging base.	☐	☐	☐

CALCULATION

Total Possible Points: _____
Total Points Earned: _____ Multiplied by 100 = _____ Divided by Total Possible Points = _____%

Pass **Fail**
☐ ☐

Comments:

Student's signature _____ Date _____
Partner's signature _____ Date _____
Instructor's signature _____ Date _____

Name _____ Date _____ Time _____

Procedure 19-7:	MEASURE AND RECORD A PATIENT'S TEMPERATURE USING A TYMPANIC THERMOMETER

EQUIPMENT/SUPPLIES: Tympanic thermometer, disposable probe covers, biohazard waste container

STANDARDS: Given the needed equipment and a place to work, the student will perform this skill with _____% accuracy in a total of _____ minutes. *(Your instructor will tell you what the percentage and time limits will be before you begin practicing.)*

KEY: 4 = Satisfactory 0 = Unsatisfactory NA = This step is not counted

PROCEDURE STEPS	SELF	PARTNER	INSTRUCTOR
1. Wash your hands and assemble the necessary supplies.	☐	☐	☐
2. Greet and identify the patient and explain the procedure.	☐	☐	☐
3. Insert the ear probe into a probe cover.	☐	☐	☐
4. Place the end of the ear probe into the patient's ear after retracting the pinna correctly to straighten the ear canal.	☐	☐	☐
5. Press the button on the thermometer. Watch the digital display.	☐	☐	☐
6. Remove the probe at "beep" or other thermometer signal.	☐	☐	☐
7. Discard the probe cover into a biohazard waste container.	☐	☐	☐
8. Record the procedure result.	☐	☐	☐
9. Return the unit and probe to the charging base.	☐	☐	☐

CALCULATION

Total Possible Points: _____
Total Points Earned: _____ Multiplied by 100 = _____ Divided by Total Possible Points = _____%

Pass **Fail**
☐   ☐   Comments:

Student's signature _____ Date _____
Partner's signature _____ Date _____
Instructor's signature _____ Date _____

Name _____ Date _____ Time _____

Procedure 19-8:	MEASURE AND RECORD A PATIENT'S TEMPERATURE USING A TEMPORAL ARTERY THERMOMETER

EQUIPMENT/SUPPLIES: Temporal artery thermometer, antiseptic wipes

STANDARDS: Given the needed equipment and a place to work, the student will perform this skill with _____% accuracy in a total of _____ minutes. *(Your instructor will tell you what the percentage and time limits will be before you begin practicing.)*

KEY: 4 = Satisfactory   0 = Unsatisfactory   NA = This step is not counted

PROCEDURE STEPS	SELF	PARTNER	INSTRUCTOR
1. Wash your hands and assemble the necessary supplies.	☐	☐	☐
2. Greet and identify the patient and explain the procedure.	☐	☐	☐
3. Place the flat end of the tympanic thermometer against the patient's forehead.	☐	☐	☐
4. Depress the "on" button and slide the thermometer across the forehead, stopping at the temporal artery.	☐	☐	☐
5. Release the "on" button and remove the thermometer from the skin.	☐	☐	☐
6. Read the temperature on the digital display screen.	☐	☐	☐
7. Record the procedure result.	☐	☐	☐
8. Return the unit to the charging base.	☐	☐	☐

CALCULATION

Total Possible Points: _____
Total Points Earned: _____ Multiplied by 100 = _____ Divided by Total Possible Points = _____%

Pass   **Fail**
☐   ☐   Comments:

Student's signature _____ Date _____
Partner's signature _____ Date _____
Instructor's signature _____ Date _____

Name _____ Date _____ Time _____

Procedure 19-9:	MEASURE AND RECORD A PATIENT'S RADIAL PULSE

EQUIPMENT/SUPPLIES: A watch with a sweeping second hand

STANDARDS: Given the needed equipment and a place to work, the student will perform this skill with _____% accuracy in a total of _____ minutes. *(Your instructor will tell you what the percentage and time limits will be before you begin practicing.)*

KEY: 4 = Satisfactory   0 = Unsatisfactory   NA = This step is not counted

PROCEDURE STEPS	SELF	PARTNER	INSTRUCTOR
1. Wash your hands.	☐	☐	☐
2. Greet and identify the patient and explain the procedure.	☐	☐	☐
3. Position the patient with the arm relaxed and supported.	☐	☐	☐
4. Locate the radial artery.	☐	☐	☐
5. If the pulse is regular, count the pulse for 30 seconds (irregular, count 60 seconds).	☐	☐	☐
6. Multiply the number of pulsations in 30 seconds by 2 (record pulses in 60 seconds as is).	☐	☐	☐
7. Record the rate in the patient's medical record with the other vital signs.	☐	☐	☐
8. Also, note the rhythm if irregular and the volume if thready or bounding.	☐	☐	☐

CALCULATION

Total Possible Points: _____
Total Points Earned: _____ Multiplied by 100 = _____ Divided by Total Possible Points = _____%

Pass   **Fail**
☐   ☐   Comments:

Student's signature _____ Date _____
Partner's signature _____ Date _____
Instructor's signature _____ Date _____

Name _____ Date _____ Time _____

Procedure 19-10:	MEASURE AND RECORD A PATIENT'S RESPIRATIONS

EQUIPMENT/SUPPLIES: A watch with a sweeping second hand

STANDARDS: Given the needed equipment and a place to work, the student will perform this skill with _____% accuracy in a total of _____ minutes. *(Your instructor will tell you what the percentage and time limits will be before you begin practicing.)*

KEY: 4 = Satisfactory   0 = Unsatisfactory   NA = This step is not counted

PROCEDURE STEPS	SELF	PARTNER	INSTRUCTOR
1. Wash your hands.	☐	☐	☐
2. Greet and identify the patient and explain the procedure.	☐	☐	☐
3. Observe watch second hand and count a rise and fall of the chest as one respiration.	☐	☐	☐
4. For a regular breathing pattern count for 30 seconds and multiply by 2 (irregular for 60 seconds).	☐	☐	☐
5. Record the respiratory rate.	☐	☐	☐
6. Note the rhythm if irregular and any unusual or abnormal sounds such as wheezing.	☐	☐	☐

CALCULATION

Total Possible Points: _____
Total Points Earned: _____ Multiplied by 100 = _____ Divided by Total Possible Points = _____%

Pass   **Fail**
☐   ☐   Comments:

Student's signature _____ Date _____
Partner's signature _____ Date _____
Instructor's signature _____ Date _____

Name_____ Date_____ Time_____

Procedure 19-11:	**MEASURE AND RECORD A PATIENT'S BLOOD PRESSURE**

EQUIPMENT/SUPPLIES: Sphygmomanometer, stethoscope

STANDARDS: Given the needed equipment and a place to work, the student will perform this skill with _____% accuracy in a total of _____ minutes. *(Your instructor will tell you what the percentage and time limits will be before you begin practicing.)*

KEY: 4 = Satisfactory   0 = Unsatisfactory   NA = This step is not counted

PROCEDURE STEPS	SELF	PARTNER	INSTRUCTOR
1. Wash your hands and assemble your equipment.	☐	☐	☐
2. Greet and identify the patient and explain the procedure.	☐	☐	☐
3. Position the patient with upper arm supported and level with the patient's heart.	☐	☐	☐
4. Expose the patient's upper arm.	☐	☐	☐
5. Palpate the brachial pulse in the antecubital area.	☐	☐	☐
6. Center the deflated cuff directly over the brachial artery.	☐	☐	☐
7. Lower edge of the cuff should be 1 to 2 inches above the antecubital area.	☐	☐	☐
8. Wrap the cuff smoothly and snugly around the arm, secure with the Velcro edges.	☐	☐	☐
9. Turn the screw clockwise to tighten. Do not tighten it too tightly for easy release.	☐	☐	☐
10. Palpate the brachial pulse. Inflate the cuff.	☐	☐	☐
11. Note the point or number on the dial or mercury column at which the brachial pulse disappears.	☐	☐	☐
12. Deflate the cuff by turning the valve counterclockwise.	☐	☐	☐
13. Wait at least 30 seconds before reinflating the cuff.	☐	☐	☐
14. Place the stethoscope earpieces into your ear canals with the openings pointed slightly forward.	☐	☐	☐
15. Stand about 3 feet from the manometer with the gauge at eye level.	☐	☐	☐
16. Place the diaphragm of the stethoscope against the brachial artery and hold in place.	☐	☐	☐
17. Close the valve and inflate the cuff.	☐	☐	☐
18. Pump the valve bulb to about 30 mm Hg above the number noted during step 11.	☐	☐	☐
19. Once the cuff is inflated to proper level, release air at a rate of about 2–4 mm Hg per second.	☐	☐	☐
20. Note the point on the gauge at which you hear the first clear tapping sound.	☐	☐	☐
21. Maintaining control of the valve screw, continue to deflate the cuff.	☐	☐	☐

22. When you hear the last sound, note the reading and quickly deflate the cuff.	☐	☐	☐
23. Remove the cuff and press the air from the bladder of the cuff.	☐	☐	☐
24. If this is the first recording or the first time the patient has been into the office, the physician may also want a reading in the other arm or in a position other than sitting.	☐	☐	☐
25. Record the reading with the systolic over the diastolic pressure (note which arm was used or any position other than sitting).	☐	☐	☐

CALCULATION

Total Possible Points: _____
Total Points Earned: _____ Multiplied by 100 = _____ Divided by Total Possible Points = _____%

Pass   **Fail**
☐   ☐   Comments:

Student's signature _____ Date _____
Partner's signature _____ Date _____
Instructor's signature _____ Date _____

Name _____   Date _____   Time _____

Work Product 1

Obtain vital signs.

Use the equipment available to you at a medical office or at school to measure and record the temperature of at least one volunteer or patient. Measure temperature in as many ways as you can. Compare the different measurements to the temperature you take orally, to determine whether your measurements are accurate. Fill in the temperature table below.

TEMPERATURE TABLE

Patient Name	Oral Temp. (glass)	Axillary Temp. (glass)	Rectal Temp. (glass)	Electronic Temp. (oral/ axillary/ rectal)	Temporal Artery Temp.	Tympanic Temp.

Work Product 2

Obtain vital signs.

Use the equipment available to you at a medical office or at school to measure and record the pulse rate of at least one volunteer or patient. Measure as many pulse rates as you can. Fill in the pulse rate table below.

PULSE RATE TABLE

Patient Name	Radial Pulse	Carotid Pulse	Brachial Pulse	Femoral Pulse	Popliteal Pulse	Posterior Tibial Pulse	Dorsalis Pedis Pulse

Work Product 3

Document appropriately.

Measure a patient's respiratory rate. If you are currently working in a medical office, use a blank paper patient chart from the office. If this is not available to you, use the space below to record the information in the chart.

_____

_____

_____

_____

Work Product 4

Document appropriately.

Measure a patient's blood pressure while the patient is sitting and while the patient is standing. If you are currently working in a medical office, use a blank paper patient chart from the office. If this is not available to you, use the space below to record the information in the chart.

_____

_____

_____

_____

Chapter Self-Assessment Quiz

1. Anthropometric measurements:
   a. include vital signs.
   b. include height and weight.
   c. don't include height in adults.
   d. are taken only at the first visit.
   e. are used only as baseline information.

2. What are the cardinal signs?
   a. Height and weight
   b. Baseline measurements
   c. Pulse, respiration, and blood pressure
   d. Pulse, respiration, blood pressure, and temperature
   e. Temperature, pulse, blood pressure, respiration, and cardiac output

3. When you greet a patient, what should you <u>always</u> do before taking any measurements?
   a. Put on gloves.
   b. Identify the patient.
   c. Get a family history.
   d. Get a medical history.
   e. Determine whether the patient speaks English.

4. After getting an accurate weight measurement, what is the <u>next</u> thing you should do?
   a. Remove the paper towel.
   b. Write down the measurement.
   c. Assist the patient off the scale.
   d. Tell the patient his or her weight.
   e. Convert the measurement to kilograms.

5. If the balance bar of a balance beam scale points to the midpoint when the large counterweight is at 100 and the small counterweight is 2 lines to the right of the mark for 30, what is the patient's weight?
   a. 32 pounds
   b. 73 pounds
   c. 128 pounds
   d. 132 pounds
   e. 264 pounds

6. To get an accurate height measurement, you should:
   a. wash your hands and put down a paper towel.
   b. have the patient stand barefoot with heels together.
   c. have the patient face the ruler and look straight ahead.
   d. put the measuring bar on the patient's hair and deduct an inch.
   e. record the measurement before helping the patient off the scale.

7. An axillary temperature would be a good measurement to take when:
   a. the patient is very talkative.
   b. there are no more disposable plastic sheaths.
   c. the office is so full that there is little privacy.
   d. the patient is wearing many layers of clothing.
   e. you need to know the temperature as quickly as possible.

8. One difference between using electronic thermometers and using glass and mercury thermometers is the:

    a. use of gloves for rectal measurements.

    b. use of a disposable cover for the thermometer.

    c. color code for oral and rectal measurements.

    d. wait time before the thermometer is removed.

    e. receptacle for disposable covers after measurements.

9. The three stages of fever are:

    a. abrupt onset, course, and lysis.

    b. onset, various course, and lysis.

    c. onset, sustained fever, and crisis.

    d. abrupt or gradual onset, course, and resolution.

    e. onset, fluctuating course, and abrupt resolution.

10. Which method would you use to take a brachial pulse?

    a. Palpation alone

    b. Auscultation alone

    c. Palpation and/or auscultation

    d. Palpation and/or use of a Doppler unit

    e. Auscultation and/or use of a Doppler unit

11. Which method would you use to take an apical pulse?

    a. Palpation alone

    b. Auscultation alone

    c. Palpation and/or auscultation

    d. Palpation and/or use of a Doppler unit

    e. Auscultation and/or use of a Doppler unit

12. Which statement is true of a respiration rate?

    a. It increases when a patient is lying down.

    b. It is the number of expirations in 60 seconds.

    c. It is the number of complete inspirations per minute.

    d. It should be taken while the patient is not aware of it.

    e. It is the number of inspirations and expirations in 30 seconds.

13. You should document breathing:

    a. that is medium and rhythmic.

    b. that is regular and consistent.

    c. if you can hear air moving in and out.

    d. that is shallow or if you hear wheezing.

    e. if you hear crackles, or breaths are 19 per minute.

14. Hyperpnea is:

    a. no respiration.

    b. shallow respirations.

    c. abnormally deep, gasping breaths.

    d. inability to breathe while lying down.

    e. a respiratory rate that is too high for oxygen demand.

15. The Korotkoff sound that signals systolic blood pressure is:

    a. faint tapping.

    b. soft swishing.

    c. soft tapping that becomes faint.

    d. rhythmic, sharp, distinct tapping.

    e. sharp tapping that becomes soft swishing.

16. Which group of factors are likely to affect blood pressure?

    a. Age, exercise, occupation

    b. Activity, stress, tobacco use

    c. Alcohol, education, prescriptions

    d. Body position, height, history of heart conditions

    e. Dietary habits, wealth, family history of heart disease

17. Which blood pressure cuff is the correct size?

    a. One that has the Velcro in places that match up

    b. One with a length that wraps three times around the arm

    c. One with a width that goes halfway around the upper arm

    d. One with a width that wraps all the way around the lower arm

    e. One with a length that wraps one and a half times around the arm

18. Which measurement is a normal axillary temperature?

    a. 36.4°C

    b. 37.0°C

    c. 37.6°C

    d. 98.6°F

    e. 99.6°F

19. A tympanic thermometer measures temperature:

    a. in the ear.

    b. in the mouth.

    c. under the armpit.

    d. on the temple.

    e. in the rectum.

20. Diaphoresis is:

    a. sweating.

    b. constant fever.

    c. elevated blood pressure.

    d. needing to sit upright to breathe.

    e. blood pressure that drops upon standing.

Assisting with the Physical Examination

Chapter Checklist

☐ Read textbook chapter and take notes within the Chapter Notes outline. Answer the Learning Objectives as you reach them in the content, and then check them off.

☐ Work the Content Review questions—both Foundational Knowledge and Application.

☐ Perform the Active Learning exercise(s).

☐ Complete Professional Journal entries.

☐ Complete Skill Practice Activity(s) using Competency Evaluation Forms and Work Products, when appropriate.

☐ Take the Chapter Self-Assessment Quiz.

☐ Insert all appropriate pages into your Portfolio.

Learning Objectives

1. Spell and define the key terms.
2. Identify and state the use of the basic and specialized instruments and supplies used in the physical examination.
3. Describe the four methods used to examine the patient.
4. State your responsibilities before, during, and after the physical examination.
5. List the basic sequence of the physical examination.

Chapter Notes

Note: Bold-faced headings are the major headings in the text chapter; headings in regular font are lower-level headings (i.e., the content is subordinate to, or falls "under," the major headings). Make sure you understand the key terms used in the chapter, as well as the concepts presented as Key Points.

TEXT SUBHEADINGS

NOTES

Introduction _____

_____

Key Terms: baseline; diagnosis; clinical diagnosis; differential diagnosis
Key Point:
• The purpose of the complete physical examination is to assess the patient's general state of health and detect signs and symptoms of disease.

☐ **LEARNING OBJECTIVE 1:** Spell and define the key terms.

Basic Instruments and Supplies _____

Key Term: applicators
Key Point:
- Instruments used during the physical examination enable the examiner to see, hear, or feel areas of the body being assessed. In most cases, it is the physician who uses these instruments, but you must be familiar with the instruments and supplies.

Percussion Hammer _____

Key Term: Babinski reflex
Key Point:
- The percussion hammer is used to test neurologic reflexes.

Tuning Fork _____

Key Point:
- The tuning fork is used to test hearing.

Nasal Speculum _____

Key Term: speculum
Key Point:
- The nasal **speculum** is a stainless steel instrument that is inserted into the nostril to assist in the visual inspection of the lining of the nose, nasal membranes, and septum.

Otoscope and Audioscope _____

Key Term: tympanic membrane
Key Points:
- The otoscope permits visualization of the ear canal and tympanic membrane.
- The audioscope is used to screen patients for hearing loss.

Ophthalmoscope _____

_____

Key Point:
• The ophthalmoscope is used to examine the interior structures of the eyes.

Examination Light and Gooseneck Lamp _____

_____

_____

Stethoscope _____

_____

Key Point:
• The stethoscope is used for listening to body sounds.

Penlight or Flashlight _____

_____

Key Point:
• A penlight or flashlight provides additional light to a specific area during the examination.

☐ **LEARNING OBJECTIVE 2:** Identify and state the use of the basic and specialized instruments and supplies used in the physical examination.

Instruments and Supplies Used in Specialized Examinations _____

_____

_____

Head Light or Mirror _____

_____

Key Point:
• An ear, nose, and throat specialist (otorhinolaryngologist)
may wear a headlight or head mirror during the examination of these structures.

Laryngeal Mirror and Laryngoscope _____

_____

Key Point:
• The laryngeal mirror is a stainless steel instrument with a
long, slender handle and a small, round mirror.

Vaginal Speculum _____

_____

Key Term: Papanicolaou
Key Point:
- To obtain the cells for a Pap smear, or to visually examine internal female reproductive structures, the vaginal speculum is inserted into the vagina to expand the opening.

Lubricant _____

_____

Key Terms: lubricant; bimanual
Key Point:
- **Lubricant** is a water-soluble gel used to reduce friction and provide easy insertion of an instrument in the physical examination.

Anoscope, Proctoscope, and Sigmoidoscope _____

_____

Key Points:
- The anoscope is a short stainless steel or plastic speculum that is inserted into the rectum to inspect the anal canal.
- The proctoscope is another type of speculum that is used to visualize the rectum and the anus.
- A longer instrument used to visualize the rectum and the sigmoid colon is the sigmoidoscope.

Examination Techniques _____

_____

Key Terms: inspection; palpation; percussion; auscultation

Inspection _____

_____

Key Terms: symmetry; asymmetry
Key Point:
- Inspection is looking at areas of the body to observe physical features.

Palpation _____

_____

Key Terms: manipulation; range of motion
Key Point:
• Palpation is touching or moving body areas with the fingers or hands.

Percussion _____

_____

Key Point:
• Percussion is tapping or striking the body with the hand or an instrument to produce sounds.

Auscultation _____

_____

Key Point:
• Auscultation is listening to the sounds of the body.

☐ **LEARNING OBJECTIVE 3:** Describe the four methods used to examine the patient.

Responsibilities of the Medical Assistant _____

_____

_____

Room Preparation _____

_____

_____

Patient Preparation _____

_____

Key Point:
• It is important that you develop rapport with your patients and practice good interpersonal skills.

Assisting the Physician _____

_____

Key Point:
• Depending on the examination and the physical condition of the patient, you may also assist the patient into an appropriate position and adjust the drape to expose only the body area being examined.

Postexamination Duties

☐ **LEARNING OBJECTIVE 4:** State your responsibilities before, during, and after the physical examination.

Physical Examination Format

Head and Neck

Key Term: bruit
Key Point:
• The patient's skull, scalp, hair, and face are inspected and palpated for size, shape, and symmetry.

Eyes and Ears

Key Terms: sclera; PERRLA; extraocular; peripheral; cerumen
Key Points:
• Normal pupil reaction is recorded as **PERRLA,** which means the *p*upils are *e*qual, *r*ound, and *r*eactive to *l*ight and *a*ccommodation.
• Normally the tympanic membrane is pearly gray and concave.

Nose and Sinuses

Key Terms: nasal septum; transillumination
Key Point:
• The external nose is palpated for abnormalities and inspected using a nasal speculum and light.

Mouth and Throat

Key Point:
• The physician inspects the mucous membranes of the mouth, gums, teeth, tongue, tonsils, and throat using clean gloves, a light source, and a tongue blade.

Chest, Breasts, and Abdomen _____

Key Terms: inguinal; hernia
Key Points:
• The physician observes the general appearance and symmetry of the chest and breast area, the respiratory rate and pattern, and any obvious masses or swelling.
• The tissue subject to breast examination includes not only the breast and nipple, but the tissue extending up to the clavicle, under the axilla, and down to the bottom of the rib cage.

Genitalia and Rectum _____

Key Terms: occult; rectovaginal
Key Points:
• The male genitalia are inspected to note symmetry, lesions, swelling, masses, and hair distribution.
• The female genitalia and rectum are usually examined with the patient in the lithotomy position and with one corner of the drape extending over the genitalia and the other corner covering the patient's chest.

Legs _____

Key Point:
• The legs are inspected and the peripheral pulse sites palpated with the patient supine.

Reflexes _____

Key Point:
• The examiner uses the percussion hammer to test the patient's reflexes by striking the biceps, triceps, patellar, Achilles, and plantar tendons.

Posture, Gait, Coordination, Balance, and Strength _____

Key Term: gait

☐ **LEARNING OBJECTIVE 5:** List the basic sequence of the physical examination.

General Health Guidelines and Checkups _____

Key Points:
- For patients aged 20 to 40 years, physical examinations are scheduled about every 1 to 3 years.
- All patients should have a baseline electrocardiogram (ECG) at age 40 and follow-up ECGs as necessary.

Content Review

FOUNDATIONAL KNOWLEDGE

Tools and Techniques

1. A patient comes into the physician's office complaining of ringing in her ears. Which of the following instruments would the physician be likely to ask for during the patient examination? Circle all that apply.

   a. percussion hammer

   b. tuning fork

   c. laryngeal mirror

   d. otoscope

   e. opthalmoscope

2. Look at the following pictures.

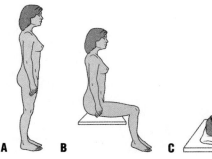

A   B   C

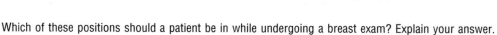

   Which of these positions should a patient be in while undergoing a breast exam? Explain your answer.

   _____

   _____

3. A patient comes into the physician's office with severe stomach pains. Before touching the patient, the physician places a stethoscope to the patient's abdomen. Explain why this is the correct order of examination.

   _____

   _____

4. Listed below are the features inspected in a physical examination. However, they are not listed in the correct order. Review the features and then place a number next to each to show the correct order.

   a. _____ Eyes and Ears

   b. _____ Legs

   c. _____ Head and Neck

   d. _____ Chest, Breasts, and Abdomen

   e. _____ Nose and Sinuses

   f. _____ Reflexes

   g. _____ Posture, Gait, Balance, and Strength

   h. _____ Mouth and Throat

   i. _____ Genitalia and Rectum

5. Which of the following are recognized as early warning signs for cancer? Circle all that apply.

   a. an itchy rash on the arms and legs

   b. a nagging cough or hoarse voice

   c. unusual bleeding or discharge

   d. stiffness in joints

   e. a sore that will not heal

6. A physician uses four basic techniques to gather information about a patient during the examination. Match the name of each technique with the correct definition.

   Technique

   a. inspection _____

   b. palpation _____

   c. percussion _____

   d. auscultation _____

   Definition

   1. touching or moving body areas with fingers or hands

   2. looking at areas of the body to observe physical features

   3. listening to the sounds of the body

   4. tapping the body with the hand or an instrument to produce sounds

7. Take a look at the following picture.

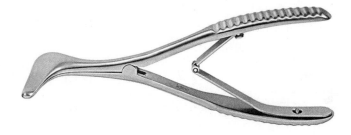

   What would this instrument be used for?

   a. examining the external nose for abnormalities

   b. performing a rectal examination

   c. inspecting the mouth and throat

8. Match the following instruments with their correct definitions.

Instruments	Definitions
a. tuning fork _____	**1.** an instrument used for listening to body sounds and taking blood pressure
b. opthalmoscope _____	**2.** an instrument used to examine the interior structures of the eyes
c. anoscope _____	**3.** an instrument with two prongs used to test hearing
d. stethoscope _____	**4.** a light attached to a headband that provides direct light on the area being examined
e. laryngeal mirror _____	**5.** an instrument used to examine areas of the patient's throat and larynx
f. headlight _____	**6.** a short stainless steel or plastic speculum used to inspect the anal canal

The Medical Assistant's Role and Responsibilities

9. As a medical assistant, you are responsible for checking each examination room at the beginning of the day to make sure that it is ready for patients. List three things that need to be done to ensure that a room is ready.

a.

b.

c.

10. While you are escorting a patient to the front desk, the patient asks you whether an over-the-counter medication will affect her prescribed treatment. You are familiar with both drugs. What is the correct response?

_____

_____

11. You are assisting a physician during a genital and pelvic examination on a female disabled patient who cannot be placed into the lithotomy position. What is the correct course of action?

_____

_____

12. As a medical assistant, you will be required to assist the physician before, during, and after physical examinations. Read the list of tasks in the table below. Then decide whether you would perform the task before, during, or after the examination.

Task	Before	During	After
a. Escort the patient to the front desk.			
b. Obtain a urine specimen from the patient, if required.			
c. Adjust the drape on the patient to expose the necessary body part.			
d. Ask the patient about medication used on a regular basis.			
e. Check the patient's medical record to ensure all the information has been accurately documented.			
f. Place the patient's chart outside the examining room door.			
g. Offer reassurance to the patient and check for signs of anxiety.			

Understanding Patients' Conditions

13. Which factors can increase the risk of prostate cancer in males? Circle all that apply.

a. being under 30

b. having close family affected by the disease

c. living a sedentary lifestyle

d. being African American

e. playing vigorous sports

14. A patient comes into the physician's office with her daughter. She mentions that her child cries continuously, has been vomiting regularly, and stumbles a lot. Which of these do you recommend?

    a. Tell her that it is probably a bug and to keep her child home from school for a couple of days.

    b. Advise that she keep an eye on the child and inform the physician if there is any change.

    c. Tell her to have the child examined immediately.

15. Take a look at the following pictures.

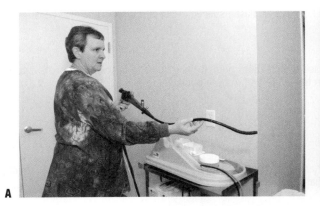
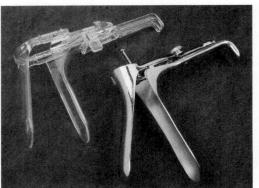

Which of these would be used to perform a rectal examination?

_____

_____

16. Dr. O'Brien tells you that a patient's ear drum is infected. What are the symptoms that could have led Dr. O'Brien to this diagnosis?

_____

_____

17. Which of these can cause a loss in the ability to taste or smell? Check all that apply.

    a. medication _____

    b. sinus infection _____

    c. pregnancy _____

    d. aging _____

    e. tumor _____

18. A patient comes into the physician's office with an open wound. When obtaining the patient's medical records, you discover that he last had a tetanus booster four years ago. What is the correct procedure?

a. Recommend the patient has another tetanus booster.

b. Tell the patient he does not need immunizing for another six years.

c. Tell the patient he should have a booster if he is traveling abroad.

20. Match the following key terms to their definitions.

Key Terms	Definitions
a. auscultation _____	**1.** an instrument used for examining body cavities
b. Babinski reflex _____	**2.** thin, semitransparent membrane in the middle ear that transmits vibrations
c. bimanual _____	**3.** a reflex noted by the extension of the great toe and abduction of the other toes
d. bruit _____	**4.** a test in which cells from the cervix are examined microscopically for abnormalities
e. cerumen _____	**5.** an examination performed with both hands
f. extraocular _____	**6.** the extent of movement in the joints
g. hernia _____	**7.** abnormal sound or murmur in the blood vessels
h. occult _____	**8.** white fibrous tissue covering the eye
i. Papanicolaou (Pap) test _____	**9.** passage of light through body tissues for the purpose of examination
j. PERRLA _____	**10.** blood present in stool that is not visibly apparent
k. range of motion (ROM) _____	**11.** a diagnosis based only on a patient's symptoms
l. sclera _____	**12.** act of listening to the sounds within the body to evaluate the heart, lungs, intestines, or fetal heart tones
m. speculum _____	**13.** an acronym that means pupils are equal, round, and reactive to light and accommodation
n. transillumination _____	**14.** earwax
o. tympanic membrane _____	**15.** a protrusion of an organ through a weakened muscle wall
p. clinical diagnosis _____	**16.** outside of the eye
q. differential diagnosis _____	**17.** a diagnosis made by comparing symptoms of several diseases
r. gait _____	**18.** the passive movement of the joints to determine the extent of movement
s. lubricant _____	**19.** pertaining to the rectum and vagina
t. manipulation _____	**20.** equality in size and shape or position of parts on opposite sides of the body
u. nasal septum _____	**21.** a water-soluble agent that reduces friction
v. rectovaginal _____	**22.** device for applying local treatments and tests
w. peripheral _____	**23.** inequality in size and shape on opposite sides of the body
x. applicator _____	**24.** pertaining to or situated away from the center
y. symmetry _____	**25.** partition dividing the nostrils
z. asymmetry _____	**26.** a manner of walking

20. True or False? Determine whether the following statements are true or false. If false, explain why.

a. A normal tympanic membrane will be light pink and curve slightly outward.

_____

_____

b. Patients should have a baseline electrocardiogram (ECG) when they turn 60.

_____

_____

c. The instruments used to examine the rectum and colon are all one standard size.

_____

_____

d. The medical assistant is responsible for preparing the examination room, preparing the patient, assisting the physician, and cleaning the equipment and examination room.

_____

_____

APPLICATION

Critical Thinking Practice

1. A 19-year-old patient has never had a Pap smear before and does not understand what the test is for, or what is going to happen during the procedure. The physician asks you to explain the process to her in simple terms. List three key aspects of a Pap smear and explain the purpose of the procedure.

_____

_____

2. Alicia is assisting a male physician perform a gynecological examination. Midway through the examination, she is paged to assist another medical procedure. Explain what she should do and why.

_____

_____

Patient Education

1. Your patient is a 35-year-old male who has a long family history of cancer. The patient is terrified of developing cancer and has been to see the physician several times for minor false alarms. Write an information sheet for the patient, explaining the early warning signs of cancer and giving examples of bodily changes that he should look out for.

Documentation

1. A 45-year-old patient comes into the office for a routine physical examination. He has high blood pressure and is considerably overweight. The patient asks you for advice on healthy eating, and you provide him with several pamphlets and advise him to cut down on fatty foods. How would you document this interaction in the patient's chart?

_____

_____

Active Learning

1. Even though the physician is the person who is responsible for using most of the instruments discussed in this chapter, you should still be familiar with how all the instruments are used. Working with a partner, access at least three of the following instruments: tongue depressor, percussion hammer, tuning fork, nasal speculum, otoscope, and stethoscope. If you do not have access to these instruments, ask your teacher if he or she can assist you. Once you have the instruments, identify the main use of those instruments during a physical exam.

2. You overhear a physician talking about how few of her male patients undergo regular prostate exams, and how important it is to detect early warning signs of prostate cancer. Research the subject on the Internet to identify which groups of men are at a high risk of developing prostate cancer. Produce a one-page leaflet to hand out at the office, targeting these men. Explain the symptoms of prostate cancer and explain how it can be detected early on, through regular checkups. Include statistics from your Internet research.

3. Work with a partner to practice the different patient examining positions. Assign one person to be the patient and the other person to be the medical assistant. The patient should think of different physical examinations (breast examination, reflex test etc.), while the medical assistant should help the patient into the correct position. Try three different scenarios and then change places.

Professional Journal

REFLECT

(Prompts and Ideas: Do you have a physical examination on a regular basis? How are you treated by the medical staff at your physician's office? Do they make you feel comfortable? Are all your questions always answered fully? What advice or information would be helpful before your examination?)

_____

_____

_____

PONDER AND SOLVE

1. You are assisting with the physical examination of a 55-year-old male. When the physician begins to prepare for the rectal examination, the patient refuses and says that it is unnecessary and that he is fine. What would you say to the patient to encourage him to complete the physical examination?

_____

_____

_____

2. At the beginning of the day, you are preparing the examination rooms with a fellow medical assistant. You are both in a hurry because the first patients are arriving and the physicians are waiting for you to finish. Your fellow medical assistant suggests that you don't need to check the batteries in the equipment because everything worked well yesterday. What do you say to your co-worker?

_____

_____

_____

EXPERIENCE

Skills related to this chapter include:

1. Assisting with the Adult Physical Examination (Procedure 20-1).

Record any common mistakes, lessons learned, and/or tips you discovered during your experience of practicing and demonstrating these skills:

_____

_____

_____

Skill Practice

PERFORMANCE OBJECTIVES:

1. Assist the physician with a patient's physical examination (Procedure 20-1).

Name _____   Date _____   Time _____

Procedure 20-1:	**ASSISTING WITH THE ADULT PHYSICAL EXAMINATION**

EQUIPMENT/SUPPLIES: A variety of basic instruments and supplies including a stethoscope, ophthalmoscope, otoscope, penlight, tuning fork, nasal speculum, tongue blade, percussion hammer, gloves, and patient gowning and draping supplies

STANDARDS: Given the needed equipment and a place to work, the student will perform this skill with _____% accuracy in a total of _____ minutes. *(Your instructor will tell you what the percentage and time limits will be before you begin practicing.)*

KEY: 4 = Satisfactory   0 = Unsatisfactory   NA = This step is not counted

PROCEDURE STEPS	SELF	PARTNER	INSTRUCTOR
1. Wash your hands.	☐	☐	☐
2. Prepare the examination room and assemble the equipment.	☐	☐	☐
3. Greet the patient by name and escort him or her to the examining room.	☐	☐	☐
4. Explain the procedure.	☐	☐	☐
5. Obtain and record the medical history and chief complaint.	☐	☐	☐
6. Take and record the vital signs, height, weight, and visual acuity.	☐	☐	☐
7. If anticipated, instruct the patient to obtain a urine specimen and escort him or her to the bathroom.	☐	☐	☐
8. When patient has returned, instruct him or her in disrobing. Leave the room unless the patient needs assistance.	☐	☐	☐
9. Assist patient into a sitting position on the edge of the examination table. Cover the lap and legs with a drape.	☐	☐	☐
10. Place the patient's medical record outside the examination room door. Notify the physician that the patient is ready.	☐	☐	☐
11. Assist the physician during the examination by: **a.** handing him or her the instruments needed for the examination. **b.** positioning the patient appropriately.	☐	☐	☐
12. Help the patient return to a sitting position.	☐	☐	☐
13. Perform any follow-up procedures or treatments.	☐	☐	☐
14. Leave the room while the patient dresses unless assistance is needed.	☐	☐	☐
15. Return to the examination room after the patient has dressed to: **a.** answer questions. **b.** reinforce instructions. **c.** provide patient education.	☐	☐	☐
16. Escort the patient to the front desk.	☐	☐	☐
17. Properly clean or dispose of all used equipment and supplies.	☐	☐	☐
18. Clean the room with a disinfectant and prepare for the next patient.	☐	☐	☐

19. Wash your hands.	☐	☐	☐
a. Record any instructions that were ordered for the patient.			
b. Note if any specimens were obtained.			
c. Indicate the results of the test or note the laboratory where the specimens are being sent for testing.			

CALCULATION

Total Possible Points: _____

Total Points Earned: _____ Multiplied by 100 = _____ Divided by Total Possible Points = _____%

Pass   **Fail**

☐   ☐   Comments:

Student's signature _____ Date _____

Partner's signature _____ Date _____

Instructor's signature _____ Date _____

Chapter Self-Assessment Quiz

1. Which of these instruments would a physician use to examine a patient's throat?

   a. Stethoscope

   b. Laryngeal mirror

   c. Percussion hammer

   d. Ayre spatula

   e. Ophthalmoscope

2. The purpose of a regular physical examination is to:

   a. identify a disease or condition.

   b. compare symptoms of several diseases.

   c. look for early warning signs of disease.

   d. maintain the patient's health and prevent disease.

   e. ensure the patient is maintaining a healthy diet and exercise regime.

3. Which of the following tasks would be performed by a medical assistant?

   a. Collecting specimens for diagnostic testing

   b. Diagnosing a patient

   c. Prescribing treatment for a patient

   d. Performing a physical examination

   e. Testing a patient's reflexes

4. Which of the following statements is true about physical examinations?

   a. Patients aged 20–40 should have a physical examination every year.

   b. It is not necessary to have a physical examination until you are over 40.

   c. Women should have physical examinations more frequently than men.

   d. Patients aged 20–40 should have a physical examination every 1–3 years.

   e. Patients over the age of 60 should have a physical examination every 6 months.

5. In which information-gathering technique might a physician use her sense of smell?

   a. Palpation

   b. Percussion

   c. Inspection

   d. Auscultation

   e. Visualization

6. If a physician notices asymmetry in a patient's features, it means that the patient:

   a. is normal and has nothing wrong.

   b. has features that are of unequal size or shape.

   c. has features that are abnormally large.

   d. will need immediate surgery.

   e. has perfectly even features.

7. Which part of the body can be auscultated?

   a. Lungs

   b. Legs

   c. Spine

   d. Feet

   e. Ears

8. The best position in which to place a female patient for a genitalia and rectum examination is the:

   a. Sims' position.

   b. Fowler's position.

   c. lithotomy position.

   d. Trendelenburg position.

   e. prone position.

9. A patient may be asked to walk around during a physical examination in order to:

   a. raise the pulse rate.

   b. observe gait and coordination.

   c. loosen the muscles in the legs.

   d. assess posture.

   e. demonstrate balance.

10. Women over 40 should receive mammograms every:

    a. 6 months.

    b. 2 years.

    c. 5 years.

    d. 1 year.

    e. 3 months.

11. How would you use a tuning fork to test a patient's hearing?

    a. By striking the prongs against the patient's leg and holding the handle in front of the patient's ear

    b. By holding the prongs behind the patient's ear and tapping the handle against their head

    c. By striking the prongs against your hand and holding the handle against the skull near the patient's ear

    d. By repeatedly tapping the prongs against the skull near the patient's ear

    e. By tapping the prongs on the table and inserting the handle into the patient's ear

12. Which of these may be an early warning sign of cancer?

    a. Obvious change in a wart or mole

    b. Dizziness or fainting spells

    c. Loss of appetite

    d. Inability to focus attention

    e. Sudden weight gain

13. How would a physician most likely be able to diagnose a hernia?

    a. Inspection

    b. Percussion

    c. Auscultation

    d. Palpation

    e. Visualization

Scenario: A patient arrives for her physical check-up. While you are obtaining the patient's history, she mentions to you that she is taking several over-the-counter medications.

14. What is the correct procedure?

    a. Tell the physician immediately.

    b. Tell the patient that it will not affect her physical examination.

    c. Make a note of the medications the patient is taking in her medical record.

    d. Ask the patient to reschedule the physical examination when she has stopped taking the medications.

    e. Prepare the necessary materials for a blood test.

15. During the patient's physical examination, the physician asks you to hand her the instruments needed to examine the patient's eyes. You should give her a(n):

    a. otoscope and penlight.

    b. stethoscope and speculum.

    c. opthalmoscope and penlight.

    d. laryngoscope and gloves.

    e. anoscope and speculum.

16. Once the examination is over, you escort the patient to the front desk. After he has left the office, what do you do with his medical record?

    a. Check that the data has been accurately documented and release it to the billing department.

    b. Check that the data has been accurately documented and file the medical report under the patient's name.

    c. Pass the medical report on to the physician to check for any errors.

    d. Give the medical report directly to the billing department to maintain confidentiality.

    e. File the medical report under the patient's name for easy retrieval.

End Scenario

17. What is the difference between an otoscope and an audioscope?

    a. An otoscope is used to screen patients for hearing loss, while an audioscope is used to assess the internal structures of the ear.

    b. An audioscope is used to screen patients for hearing loss, while an otoscope is used to assess the internal structures of the ear.

    c. An otoscope is made of stainless steel, while an audioscope is made of plastic.

    d. An audioscope is made of plastic, while an otoscope is made of stainless steel.

    e. An otoscope is an older version of an audioscope and is not used much anymore.

18. A baseline examination is a(n):

    a. examination to determine the cause of an illness.

    b. full medical examination for people over the age of 50.

    c. initial examination to give physicians information about the patient.

    d. examination based on the patient's symptoms.

    e. examination of the abdominal regions of the patient.

19. Which of the following materials should be stored in a room away from the examination room?

    a. Gloves

    b. Tongue depressors

    c. Tape measure

    d. Cotton tipped applicators

    e. Syringes

20. What does the "P" stand for in PERRLA?

    a. Position

    b. Protrusion

    c. Posture

    d. Pupil

    e. Perception

Sterilization and Surgical Instruments

Chapter Checklist

☐ Read textbook chapter and take notes within the Chapter Notes outline. Answer the Learning Objectives as you reach them in the content, and then check them off.

☐ Work the Content Review questions—both Foundational Knowledge and Application.

☐ Perform the Active Learning exercise(s).

☐ Complete Professional Journal entries.

☐ Complete Skill Practice Activity(s) using Competency Evaluation Forms and Work Products, when appropriate.

☐ Take the Chapter Self-Assessment Quiz.

☐ Insert all appropriate pages into your Portfolio.

Learning Objectives

1. Spell and define the key terms.
2. Describe several methods of sterilization.
3. Categorize surgical instruments based on use and identify each by its characteristics.
4. Identify surgical instruments specific to designated specialties.
5. State the difference between reusable and disposable instruments.
6. Explain how to handle and store instruments, equipment, and supplies.
7. Describe the necessity and steps for maintaining documents and records of maintenance for instruments and equipment.

Chapter Notes

Note: Bold-faced headings are the major headings in the text chapter; headings in regular font are lower-level headings (i.e., the content is subordinate to, or falls "under," the major headings). Make sure you understand the key terms used in the chapter, as well as the concepts presented as Key Points.

TEXT SUBHEADINGS

NOTES

Introduction _____

_____

Key Terms: disinfection; sterilization
Key Points:
- The practice of surgical asepsis, also known as sterile technique, should be used during any office surgical procedure; when handling sterile instruments to be used for incisions and excisions into body tissue; and when changing wound dressings.
- Any break in sterile technique, no matter how small, can lead to infection the body cannot fight.

☐ **LEARNING OBJECTIVE 1:** Spell and define the key terms.

Principles and Practices of Surgical Asepsis _____

Key Point:
- Surgical asepsis requires the absence of microorganisms, infection, and infectious material on instruments, equipment, and supplies.

Sterilization _____

Key Terms: sanitation; sanitize; ethylene oxide

Sterilization Equipment _____

The Autoclave _____

Key Term: autoclave
Key Points:
- The most frequently used piece of equipment for sterilizing instruments today is the **autoclave**.
- Sterilization is required for surgical instruments and equipment that will come into contact with internal body tissues or cavities that are considered sterile.

Sterilization Indicators _____

Key Points:
- Sterilization indicators placed inside the packs register that the proper pressure and temperature were attained for the required time to allow steam to penetrate the inner parts of the pack.
- Although most types of sterilization indicators work well, the best method for determining effectiveness of sterilization is the culture test.

Loading the Autoclave _____

Key Point:
- Load the autoclave loosely to allow steam to circulate.

Operating the Autoclave

Key Points:
- All components of autoclaving—temperature, pressure, steam, and time—must be correct for the items to reach sterility.
- The temperature, pressure, and time required vary with the items being sterilized.
- The timer should not be set until the proper temperature has been attained.
- Do not handle or remove items from the autoclave until they are dry, because bacteria from your hands would be drawn through the moist coverings and contaminate the items inside the wrapping.

☐ **LEARNING OBJECTIVE 2:** Describe several methods of sterilization.

Surgical Instruments

Key Terms: forceps; scissors; scalpel
Key Point:
- A surgical instrument is a tool or device designed to perform a specific function, such as cutting, dissecting, grasping, holding, retracting, or suturing.

Forceps

Key Terms: hemostat; Kelly clamp; sterilizer forceps; needle holder; spring or thumb forceps; serration; ratchet
Key Point:
- Forceps are surgical instruments used to grasp, handle, compress, pull, or join tissue, equipment, or supplies.

Scissors

Key Terms: straight scissors; curved scissors; suture scissors; bandage scissors
Key Point:
- Scissors are used for dissecting superficial, deep, or delicate tissues and for cutting sutures and bandages.

Scalpels and Blades _____

_____

Key Point:
• A scalpel is a small surgical knife with a straight handle and a straight or curved blade.

Towel Clamps _____

_____

Key Point:
• Towel clamps are used to maintain the integrity of the sterile field by holding the sterile drapes in place, allowing exposure of the operative site.

Probes and Directors _____

_____

Key Point:
• A probe shows the angle and depth of the operative area, and a director guides the knife or instrument once the procedure has begun.

Retractors _____

_____

Key Point:
• Retractors hold open layers of tissue, exposing the areas beneath.

☐ **LEARNING OBJECTIVE 3:** Categorize surgical instruments based on use and identify each by its characteristics.

☐ **LEARNING OBJECTIVE 4:** Identify surgical instruments specific to designated specialties.

☐ **LEARNING OBJECTIVE 5:** State the difference between reusable and disposable instruments.

Care and Handling of Surgical Instruments _____

_____

Key Term: OSHA

☐ **LEARNING OBJECTIVE 6:** Explain how to handle and store instruments, equipment, and supplies.

Storage and Record Keeping _____

_____

Key Point:
- Most offices have specific storage or supply areas for keeping sterile and other instruments and equipment.

☐ **LEARNING OBJECTIVE 7:** Describe the necessity of and steps for maintaining documents and records of maintenance for instruments and equipment.

Maintaining Surgical Supplies _____

_____

Key Point:
- As a clinical medical assistant, you should keep an up-to-date master list of all supplies including purchases and replacements.

Content Review

FOUNDATIONAL KNOWLEDGE

Sterilization

1. Describe the process by which an autoclave sterilizes instruments.

_____

_____

2. Complete this table, which describes the most effective method of sterilizing various instruments and materials.

Method of sterilization	Most effective for
a.	minor surgical instruments
	surgical storage trays and containers
	bowls for holding sterile equipment
b.	instruments or equipment subject to water damage
c.	instruments or equipment subject to heat damage

3. Which of the following needs to be sterilized before use? Circle all that apply.

- **a.** forceps
- **b.** scissors
- **c.** scalpels
- **d.** clamps
- **e.** probes and clamps
- **f.** retractors

4. What is the purpose of sterilization indicators? What factors may alter the results of a sterilization indicator?

_____

_____

5. What four components must be properly set in order for the autoclave to work effectively?

a. _____

b. _____

c. _____

d. _____

Surgical Tools and Equipment

6. Complete this table, which identifies four types of scissors and their use.

Type	Use
bandage scissors	a.
b.	dissect superficial and delicate tissues
straight scissors	cut deep or delicate tissues and sutures
suture scissors	c.

7. Match the following tasks with the instrument that should be used to perform the task. Some instruments may have more than one task.

Instrument

1. forceps _____

2. scissors _____

3. scalpels _____

4. clamps _____

5. retractors _____

Task

a. Dissect delicate tissue

b. Hold sterile drapes in place

c. Grasp tissue for dissection

d. Make an incision

e. Transfer sterile supplies

f. Cut off a bandage

g. Excise tissue

h. Hold open layers of tissue

8. A dentist is performing oral surgery on a patient. Before he makes any incisions in the gums, the dentist wants to know the depth and direction of the operative area. Which instrument will the dentist use to perform this task?

_____

_____

A Sterilized and Organized Medical Office

9. Which of the following items are needed in order to maintain a complete and accurate record of sterilized items and equipment? Place a check mark next to the necessary items.

a. Results of the sterilization indicator	
b. Date and time of last procedure in which the load was used	
c. General description of the load	
d. Exposure time and temperature	
e. Date and time of the sterilization cycle	
f. Name or initials of the operator	
g. Location of the load	
h. Expiration date of the load (usually 30 days)	

10. List four guidelines that you should follow when handling and storing sharp instruments.

a. _____

b. _____

c. _____

d. _____

11. What is the purpose of autoclave tape?

_____

_____

12. The physician has just completed a procedure in which he used a scalpel with a reusable handle. How should you dispose of this instrument? What if the physician had used a scalpel with a disposable handle?

_____

_____

Name That Instrument

13. Complete the chart below by identifying one instrument used in each specialty.

Specialty	Instrument
Obstetrics, Gynecology	**a.**
Orthopedics	**b.**
Urology	**c.**
Proctology	**d.**
Otology, Rhinology	**e.**
Ophthalmology	**f.**
Dermatology	**g.**

14. Indicate which type of forceps should be used for each procedure:

    a. a gynecological procedure _____

    b. holding a needle during suturing _____

    c. tissue dissection _____

    d. grasping a blood vessel _____

    e. moving a sterile instrument to a sterile field _____

15. Place a check mark in the appropriate box below to indicate which type of scissors should be used for each procedure.

Task	Bandage Scissors	Curved Scissors	Straight Scissors	Suture Scissors
a. remove a bandage				
b. cut skin tissues				
c. cut deep tissue				
d. cut sutures				

16. Indicate which instrument should be used for each procedure.

    a. hold sterile drapes in place _____

    b. determine the angle and depth of the operative area before operating _____

    c. hold open layers of tissue _____

    d. guide an instrument _____

    e. make an incision _____

17. Which method of sterilization is more effective: boiling water or the autoclave? Why?

_____

_____

18. List four qualities of medical asepsis and surgical asepsis.

Medical Asepsis	Surgical Asepsis
a.	**a.**
b.	**b.**
c.	**c.**
d.	**d.**

19. Match the following key terms to their definitions.

Key Terms	Definitions
a. autoclave _____	**1.** a surgical instrument used to grasp, hold, compress, pull, or join tissue, equipment, or supplies
b. disinfection _____	**2.** a long instrument used to explore or dilate body cavities
c. ethylene oxide _____	**3.** a gas used to sterilize surgical instruments and other supplies
d. forceps _____	**4.** appliance used to sterilize medical instruments with steam under pressure
e. hemostat _____	

f. needle holder _____

g. obturator _____

h. OSHA _____

i. ratchet _____

j. sanitation _____

k. sanitize _____

l. scalpel _____

m. scissors _____

n. serration _____

o. sound _____

p. sterilization _____

5. a surgical instrument with slender jaws that is used to grasp blood vessels

6. groove, either straight or criss-cross, etched or cut into the blade or tip of an instrument to improve its bite or grasp

7. a notched mechanism that clicks into position to maintain tension on the opposing blades or tips of the instrument

8. killing or rendering inert most but not all pathogenic microorganisms

9. to reduce the number of microorganisms on a surface by use of low-level disinfectant practices

10. a sharp instrument composed of two opposing cutting blades, held together by a central pin on which the blades pivot

11. a type of forceps that is used to hold and pass suture through tissue

12. a federal agency that oversees working conditions

13. a small pointed knife with a convex edge for surgical procedures

14. a process, act, or technique for destroying microorganisms using heat, water, chemicals, or gases

15. the maintenance of a healthful, disease-free environment

16. a smooth, rounded, removable inner portion of a hollow tube that allows for easier insertion

20. True or False? Determine whether the following statements are true or false. If false, explain why.

a. Equipment must be sanitized before it is sterilized.

_____

_____

b. Autoclave indicator tape is 100% effective in indicating whether a package is sterile.

_____

_____

c. It is the medical assistant's responsibility to maintain complete and accurate records of sterilized equipment.

_____

_____

d. The handle and blade of a reusable steel scalpel may be reused after being properly sterilized.

_____

_____

APPLICATION

Critical Thinking Practice

1. You are one of two medical assistants working in a small office that specializes in ophthalmology. There is one examination room. The office sees about 50 patients a week, with an average of 3 patients a week needing minor ophthalmologic procedures. The physician has asked you to order new instruments for the office for the next month. What are two of the instruments that you will order? What factors will you need to consider when placing the order?

_____

_____

2. Your medical office has one autoclave along with two pairs of sterilized suture scissors and adequate numbers of other instruments. In the morning, the physician uses one pair of suture scissors to perform a minor procedure. He tosses the scissors into a sink when he is finished, damaging the instrument. At noon, the autoclave suddenly malfunctions, and you put in a service request to repair it. In the afternoon, a patient comes into the office complaining that her sutures are painful. The physician decides that he must remove them right away. Right before the procedure begins, the physician drops the only sterile pair of suture scissors in the office before he can use them. Describe two possible plans of action you can take to help the patient who is still in pain.

_____

_____

Patient Education

1. Your patient is about to undergo a minor office surgery and is concerned. She explains to you that she once received a facial piercing that led to a massive infection because of improperly sterilized instruments. Now, she is worried about the cleanliness of your office. You realize that many patients may be curious about whether your office ensures surgical asepsis. Create a patient education pamphlet that explains the precautions your office takes to ensure that all instruments and equipment are safe and sterile. Answer any questions that your patients may have about the sterilization methods used and their effectiveness. Be sure to use language that a person not accustomed to complex medical terms would understand.

_____

_____

Documentation

1. The autoclave in your office has not been working properly. It takes twice as long for the steam in the autoclave to reach an adequate temperature for sterilization. You realize that this may affect daily procedures within the office and could lead to bigger problems with the autoclave. You decide to have the autoclave serviced by a professional. What documentation will be needed in connection with this service request?

_____

_____

Active Learning

1. Test your skills at keeping accurate and complete records. Select three appliances in your home or office. Create equipment records for these appliances. Maintain the records as carefully as you would a piece of equipment in your medical office. Do not forget to include all of the nine necessary details for each item.

2. Using the library and the Internet, research the instruments and equipment commonly used by the following medical specialties: endocrinology, rheumatology, palliative care, and radiology. Add to the list found in Chapter 21 of your text with the information you find. Include images of some of the instruments and equipment.

3. Work with a partner to practice sterilizing equipment. Each person will follow the instructions for sanitizing an instrument, wrapping it for sterilization, and sterilizing it using the autoclave while the other person watches. Gently interject to remind each other of missed steps or other mistakes. Use simulations and substitutions if you do not have access to the necessary equipment. Then, switch roles and repeat the steps.

Professional Journal

REFLECT

(Prompts and Ideas: Consider the sanitation practices that other businesses use. What do restaurants, hotels, department stores, and beauty shops do to ensure a sanitary environment for their patrons? What would they be risking by not following these procedures? How would you feel if you knew businesses did not follow these procedures? How does this relate to how your patients feel when walking into your medical office?)

_____

_____

_____

PONDER AND SOLVE

1. A package of presterilized disposable scalpels has arrived at your office. You and your coworker look around the office for something to open the package with, but are unable to find the pair of scissors that is usually kept at the reception desk. Your coworker disappears into a storage closet and emerges with a pair of sterilized suture scissors. Should you allow your coworker to use the suture scissors to open the package? What reason would you give your coworker for allowing or not allowing him or her to use the suture scissors?

_____

_____

_____

_____

_____

_____

2. You are using formaldehyde to sterilize an instrument. While transporting the materials you are using, you spill the formaldehyde. What steps should you to take in order to clean the spill safely?

_____

_____

_____

_____

_____

_____

_____

EXPERIENCE

Skills related to this chapter include:

1. Sanitizing Equipment for Disinfection and Sterilization (Procedure 21-1).
2. Wrapping Instruments for Sterilization in an Autoclave (Procedure 21-2).
3. Operating an Autoclave (Procedure 21-3).

Record any common mistakes, lessons learned, and/or tips you discovered during your experience of practicing and demonstrating these skills:

_____

_____

_____

_____

_____

_____

_____

_____

Skill Practice

PERFORMANCE OBJECTIVES:

1. Sanitize equipment and instruments (Procedure 21-1).
2. Properly wrap instruments for autoclaving (Procedure 21-2).
3. Perform sterilization techniques: Operating an autoclave (Procedure 21-3).

Name _____ Date _____ Time _____

Procedure 21-1:	SANITIZING EQUIPMENT FOR DISINFECTION OR STERILIZATION

EQUIPMENT/SUPPLIES: Instruments or equipment to be sanitized, gloves, eye protection, impervious gown, soap and water, small hand-held scrub brush

STANDARDS: Given the needed equipment and a place to work, the student will perform this skill with _____% accuracy in a total of _____ minutes. *(Your instructor will tell you what the percentage and time limits will be before you begin practicing.)*

KEY: 4 = Satisfactory   0 = Unsatisfactory   NA = This step is not counted

PROCEDURE STEPS	SELF	PARTNER	INSTRUCTOR
1. Put on gloves, gown, and eye protection.	☐	☐	☐
2. For equipment that requires assembly, take removable sections apart.	☐	☐	☐
3. Check the operation and integrity of the equipment.	☐	☐	☐
4. Rinse the instrument with cool water.	☐	☐	☐
5. Force streams of soapy water through any tubular or grooved instruments.	☐	☐	☐
6. Use a hot, soapy solution to dissolve fats or lubricants left on the surface.	☐	☐	☐

7. Soak 5 to 10 minutes.
   a. Use friction (brush or gauze) to wipe down the instruments.
   b. Check jaws or scissors/forceps to ensure that all debris has been removed.
	☐	☐	☐

8. Rinse well.	☐	☐	☐
9. Dry well before autoclaving if sterilizing or soaking in disinfecting solution.	☐	☐	☐
10. Items (brushes, gauze, solution) used in sanitation process must be disinfected or discarded.	☐	☐	☐

CALCULATION

Total Possible Points: _____
Total Points Earned: _____ Multiplied by 100 = _____ Divided by Total Possible Points = _____%

Pass   **Fail**
☐   ☐   Comments:

Student's signature _____ Date _____
Partner's signature _____ Date _____
Instructor's signature _____ Date _____

Name_____ Date _____ Time _____

Procedure 21-2:	WRAPPING INSTRUMENTS FOR STERILIZATION IN AN AUTOCLAVE

EQUIPMENT/SUPPLIES: Sanitized and wrapped instruments or equipment, distilled water, autoclave operating manual

STANDARDS: Given the needed equipment and a place to work, the student will perform this skill with _____% accuracy in a total of _____ minutes. *(Your instructor will tell you what the percentage and time limits will be before you begin practicing.)*

KEY: 4 = Satisfactory   0 = Unsatisfactory   NA = This step is not counted

PROCEDURE STEPS	SELF	PARTNER	INSTRUCTOR
1. Assemble the equipment and supplies.	☐	☐	☐
2. Check the instruments being wrapped for working order.	☐	☐	☐
3. Obtain correct material for wrapping instruments to be autoclaved.	☐	☐	☐
4. Tear off 1 to 2 pieces of autoclave tape. On one piece, label the contents of the pack, the date, and your initials.	☐	☐	☐

5. Lay the wrap diagonally on a flat, clean, dry surface.
  a. Place instrument in the center, with ratchets or handles in open position.
  b. Include a sterilization indicator.
	☐	☐	☐

6. Fold the first flap up at the bottom of the diagonal wrap. Fold back the corner to make a tab.	☐	☐	☐
7. Fold left corner of the wrap toward the center. Fold back the corner to make a tab.	☐	☐	☐
8. Fold right corner of the wrap toward the center. Fold back the corner to make a tab.	☐	☐	☐
9. Fold the top corner down, making the tab tuck under the material.	☐	☐	☐
10. Secure the package with labeled autoclave tape.	☐	☐	☐

CALCULATION

Total Possible Points: _____
Total Points Earned: _____ Multiplied by 100 = _____ Divided by Total Possible Points = _____%

Pass   **Fail**
☐   ☐   Comments:

Student's signature _____ Date _____
Partner's signature _____ Date _____
Instructor's signature _____ Date _____

Name_____ Date _____ Time _____

Procedure 21-3:	**OPERATING AN AUTOCLAVE**

EQUIPMENT/SUPPLIES: Sanitized and wrapped instruments or equipment, distilled water, autoclave operating manual

STANDARDS: Given the needed equipment and a place to work, the student will perform this skill with _____% accuracy in a total of _____ minutes. *(Your instructor will tell you what the percentage and time limits will be before you begin practicing.)*

KEY: 4 = Satisfactory   0 = Unsatisfactory   NA = This step is not counted

PROCEDURE STEPS	SELF	PARTNER	INSTRUCTOR
1. Assemble the equipment including the wrapped articles. Refer to the manufacturer's manual for information specific to the model of autocalve.	☐	☐	☐
2. Check the water level of the autoclave reservoir and add more if needed.	☐	☐	☐
3. Add water to the internal chamber of the autoclave to the fill line.	☐	☐	☐
4. Load the autoclave: **a.** Place trays and packs on their sides, 1 to 3 inches from each other. **b.** Put containers on the sides with the lids off. **c.** In mixed loads, place hard objects on bottom shelf and softer packs on top racks.	☐	☐	☐
5. Read the instructions, which should be available and close to the machine. **a.** Close the door and secure or lock it. **b.** Turn the machine on. **c.** When the gauge reaches the temperature required for the contents of the load (usually 250°F), set the timer. **d.** When the timer indicates that the cycle is over, vent the chamber. **e.** After pressure has been released to a safe level, crack the door of autoclave.	☐	☐	☐
6. When the load has cooled, remove the items.	☐	☐	☐
7. Check the separately wrapped sterilization indicator, if used, for proper sterilization.	☐	☐	☐
8. Store the items in a clean, dry, dust-free area for 30 days.	☐	☐	☐
9. Clean the autoclave following the manufacturer's directions.	☐	☐	☐
10. Rinse the machine thoroughly and allow it to dry.	☐	☐	☐

CALCULATION

Total Possible Points: _____
Total Points Earned: _____ Multiplied by 100 = _____ Divided by Total Possible Points = _____%

Pass   **Fail**
☐   ☐   Comments:

Student's signature ⎯⎯⎯⎯⎯⎯⎯⎯⎯⎯⎯⎯⎯⎯⎯⎯⎯⎯⎯⎯⎯⎯⎯⎯⎯ Date ⎯⎯⎯⎯⎯
Partner's signature ⎯⎯⎯⎯⎯⎯⎯⎯⎯⎯⎯⎯⎯⎯⎯⎯⎯⎯⎯⎯⎯⎯⎯⎯⎯ Date ⎯⎯⎯⎯⎯
Instructor's signature ⎯⎯⎯⎯⎯⎯⎯⎯⎯⎯⎯⎯⎯⎯⎯⎯⎯⎯⎯⎯⎯⎯⎯ Date ⎯⎯⎯⎯⎯

Chapter Self-Assessment Quiz

1. A sterile field is defined as an area:
   a. where the autoclave is kept.
   b. that is free of all microorganisms.
   c. where sterilized instruments are stored.
   d. that has been cleaned with boiling water.
   e. in which only sanitized equipment can be used.

2. Instruments that are sterilized in the autoclave maintain their sterility for:
   a. 15 days.
   b. 20 days.
   c. 25 days.
   d. 30 days.
   e. 35 days.

3. Autoclave tape indicates that an object:
   a. has not been sterilized.
   b. contains a specific type of microorganism.
   c. has been exposed to steam in the autoclave.
   d. needs to be placed on its side in the autoclave.
   e. did not reach the proper pressure and temperature in the autoclave.

4. Material used to wrap items that are being sterilized in the autoclave must be:
   a. permeable to steam but not contaminants.
   b. permeable to distilled water but not tap water.
   c. permeable to heat but not formaldehyde.
   d. permeable to ethylene oxide but not pathogens.
   e. permeable to contaminants but not microorganisms.

5. Which of the following should be included in an equipment record?
   a. Expiration date
   b. Date of purchase
   c. Physician's name
   d. The office's address
   e. Date of last sterilization

6. Which of the following should be included in a sterilization record?
   a. Location of the item
   b. Number of items in the load
   c. Method of sterilization used
   d. Reason for the service request
   e. Results of the sterilization indicator

7. One instrument commonly used in urology is a(n):
   a. curet.
   b. tonometer.
   c. urethral sound.
   d. sigmoidoscope.
   e. uterine dilator.

8. Forceps are used to:
   a. cut sutures.
   b. dissect tissue.
   c. make incisions.
   d. guide instruments.
   e. compress or join tissue.

9. All packs containing bowls or containers should be placed in the autoclave:
   a. upright.
   b. under a cloth.
   c. on their sides.
   d. stacked on top of each other.
   e. with their sterilization indicators facing up.

10. Consult the material safety data sheet (MSDS) before:
    a. handling a chemical spill.
    b. reading a sterilization indicator.
    c. sterilizing an instrument in the autoclave.
    d. requesting service for a piece of equipment.
    e. disposing of a disposable scalpel handle and blade.

11. Why does the autoclave use pressure in the sterilization process?
    a. Pathogens and microorganisms thrive in low-pressure environments.
    b. High pressure makes the wrapping permeable to steam and not contaminants.
    c. Pressure must be applied to distilled water in order to release sterilizing agents.
    d. High pressure prevents microorganisms from penetrating the objects being sterilized.
    e. High pressure allows the steam to reach the high temperatures needed for sterilization.

12. Which of the following instruments are used to hold sterile drapes in place during surgical procedures?

    a. Directors

    b. Serrations

    c. Towel clamps

    d. Curved scissors

    e. Alligator biopsies

13. Notched mechanisms that hold the tips of the forceps together tightly are called:

    a. springs.

    b. sutures.

    c. ratchets.

    d. serrations.

    e. clamps.

14. After use, scalpel blades should be:

    a. sterilized in the autoclave.

    b. discarded in a sharps container.

    c. reattached to a scalpel handle.

    d. processed in a laboratory.

    e. wrapped in cotton muslin.

15. The instrument used to hold open layers of tissue to expose the areas underneath during a surgical procedure is a:

    a. retractor.

    b. scalpel.

    c. director.

    d. clamp.

    e. forceps.

16. Ratcheted instruments should be stored:

    a. open.

    b. closed.

    c. hanging.

    d. standing.

    e. upside down.

17. Medical asepsis is intended to prevent the spread of microbes from:

    a. one patient to another.

    b. the autoclave to the patient.

    c. the instruments to the physician.

    d. the inside to the outside of the body.

    e. the physician to the medical assistant.

18. A punch biopsy is used to:

    a. diagnose glaucoma.

    b. dissect delicate tissues.

    c. explore bladder depths.

    d. remove tissue for microscopic study.

    e. guide an instrument during a procedure.

19. The best way to test the effectiveness of an autoclave is to use:

    a. thermometers.

    b. wax pellets.

    c. autoclave tape.

    d. color indicators.

    e. strips with heat-resistant spores.

20. Which is a step in operating the autoclave?

    a. Stacking items on top of each other

    b. Filling the reservoir tank with tap water

    c. Filling the reservoir a little past the fill line

    d. Removing items from the autoclave the moment they are done

    e. Setting the timer after the correct temperature has been reached

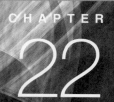

Assisting with Minor Office Surgery

Chapter Checklist

☐ Read textbook chapter and take notes within the Chapter Notes outline. Answer the Learning Objectives as you reach them in the content, and then check them off.

☐ Work the Content Review questions—both Foundational Knowledge and Application.

☐ Perform the Active Learning exercise(s).

☐ Complete Professional Journal entries.

☐ Complete Skill Practice Activity(s) using Competency Evaluation Forms and Work Products, when appropriate.

☐ Take the Chapter Self-Assessment Quiz.

☐ Insert all appropriate pages into your portfolio.

Learning Objectives

1. Spell and define the key terms.
2. List your responsibilities before, during, and after minor office surgery.
3. Identify the guidelines for preparing and maintaining sterility of the field and surgical equipment during a minor office procedure.
4. State your responsibility in relation to informed consent and patient preparation.
5. Explain the purpose of local anesthetics and list three commonly used in the medical office.

6. Describe the types of needles and sutures and the uses of each.
7. Describe the various methods of skin closure used in the medical office.
8. Explain your responsibility during surgical specimen collection.
9. List the types of laser surgery and electrosurgery used in the medical office and explain the precautions for each.
10. Describe the guidelines for applying a sterile dressing.

Chapter Notes

Note: Bold-faced headings are the major headings in the text chapter; headings in regular font are lower-level headings (i.e., the content is subordinate to, or falls "under," the major headings). Make sure you understand the key terms used in the chapter, as well as the concepts presented as Key Points.

TEXT SUBHEADINGS

NOTES

Introduction _____

_____

Key Terms: dressing; bandage

_____

☐ **LEARNING OBJECTIVE 1:** Spell and define the key terms.

☐ **LEARNING OBJECTIVE 2:** List your responsibilities before, during, and after minor office surgery.

Preparing and Maintaining a Sterile Field

Key Point:
• Minor office surgery involves procedures that penetrate the body's normally intact surface.

Sterile Surgical Packs

Key Points:
• Some medical offices prepackage sterile setups in a suitable wrapper and prepare them in the office by autoclave sterilization.
• Disposable surgical packs have become increasingly popular because they are convenient and can contain an almost infinite variety of contents.
• If the surgical pack is opened improperly, the contents will be contaminated and cannot be used.
• Labels on commercially prepared packs list the contents in the pack item by item; site-prepared packs usually only state the type of setup.

Sterile Transfer Forceps

Key Point:
• In the event that sterile items must be manipulated or placed on the sterile field, sterile transfer forceps or sterile gloved hands must be used, because the hands can never be sterilized.

Adding Peel-Back Packages and Pouring Sterile Solutions

Key Points:
• Keep in mind that the inside of the sealed package and the contents are sterile but will be contaminated if touched by anything that is not sterile, such as your fingers, or if talking, coughing, or sneezing occurs as you open it.
• In most cases, items in presterilized peel-back envelopes cannot be sterilized after being opened and must be discarded even if not used.
• Solutions must be added as needed at the time of setup.

☐ **LEARNING OBJECTIVE 3:** Identify the guidelines for preparing and maintaining the sterility of the field and surgical equipment during a minor office procedure.

Preparing the Patient for Minor Office Surgery _____

Patient Instructions and Consent _____

Key Point:
- The informed consent document must state the procedure, its purpose, and expected results along with possible side effects, risks, and complications.

☐ **LEARNING OBJECTIVE 4:** State your responsibility in relation to informed consent and patient preparation.

Positioning and Draping _____

Key Points:
- Expose only the area necessary for the procedure to ensure the patient's privacy.
- Do not make the patient maintain an uncomfortable position, such as the lithotomy or knee-chest, while waiting for the physician.
- When removing contaminated drapes from the patient following a procedure, put on clean examination gloves and carefully roll the items away from the body, keeping the contaminated areas innermost.

Preparing the Patient's Skin _____

Key Terms: vector; viable
Key Point:
- The goal of preoperative skin preparation is to remove as many microorganisms as possible from the skin to decrease the chance of wound contamination.

Assisting the Physician _____

Local Anesthetics

Key Points:
- When office surgery of any kind is performed, the site is first anesthetized (numbed) with a local anesthetic to minimize the pain and discomfort felt by the patient.
- Epinephrine is added to local anesthetics to cause vasoconstriction and to slow absorption by the body and lengthen the anesthetic's effectiveness.

☐ **LEARNING OBJECTIVE 5:** Explain the purpose of local anesthetics and list three commonly used in the medical office.

Wound Closure

Key Term: dehiscence
Key Point:
- Many types of wounds require closure to ensure rapid healing with minimal scarring.

Needles and Sutures

Key Terms: atraumatic; traumatic; swaged needle
Key Points:
- Needles used in minor office surgery are chosen for the type of surgery to be performed.
- Cutting needles are used on tough tissues, such as skin. Round or tapered (noncutting) needles are used on subcutaneous tissue, peritoneum, and muscle.
- Sutures, needles, and suture–needle combinations are contained in peel-apart packages that are sterile on the inside so that they can be added to the sterile field.
- Sutures also come in absorbable and nonabsorbable forms.

☐ **LEARNING OBJECTIVE 6:** Describe the types of needles and sutures and the uses of each.

Skin Staples

Key Point:
- Another form of nonabsorbable suture is the metal skin clip or staple.

Adhesive Skin Closures

Key Term: approximate
Key Points:
- Adhesive skin closures are used to **approximate** the edges of a small wound if sutures are not needed.
- Never pull the strips away from the wound because tension on the wound site may disrupt the healing process.

☐ **LEARNING OBJECTIVE 7:** Describe the various methods of skin closure used in the medical office.

Specimen Collection

Key Term: preservative
Key Points:
- You are responsible for attaching a label to the specimen container with the patient's name and the date written clearly on the label, and you must complete a laboratory request form to send with the specimen.

☐ **LEARNING OBJECTIVE 8:** Explain your responsibility during surgical specimen collection.

Electrosurgery

Key Terms: coagulate; cautery; electrodes
Key Points:
- Electrosurgery uses high-frequency alternating electric current to destroy or cut and remove tissue.
- An advantage of electrical surgery is the **cautery** produced by the electricity that seals small bleeding vessels and **coagulates** surrounding cells to reduce bleeding and loss of cell fluid.
- Because electric current is delivered to the tip by the electrosurgical machine, great care should be exercised to prevent injuries.

Laser Surgery

Key Points:
- Lasers are devices that focus high-intensity light in a narrow beam to create extreme heat and energy.
- Everyone who is in the room during the laser procedure, including the patient, is required to wear goggles for eye protection.

☐ **LEARNING OBJECTIVE 9:** List the types of laser surgery and electrosurgery used in the medical office and explain the precautions for each.

Postsurgical Procedures _____

Sterile Dressings _____

Key Term: purulent
Key Points:
- Sterile dressings are items such as 4 × 4 inch absorbent gauze sponges and nonadhering dressings that have been processed for use on open wounds.
- Dressings should be handled with sterile technique.
- A sterile dressing is considered contaminated if it is damp or outdated, if its wrapper is damaged, or if it is improperly removed from its wrapper.
- When you remove a sterile dressing or change an existing one, always wear clean examination gloves and carefully observe for any drainage or exudates, noting this in the patient's chart.

☐ **LEARNING OBJECTIVE 10:** Describe the guidelines for applying a sterile dressing.

Cleaning the Examination Table and Operative Area _____

Key Point:
- In preparation for the next patient, all used equipment must be discarded properly or transported to the equipment room for sanitizing before sterilization.

Commonly Performed Office Surgical Procedures _____

Key Terms: lentigines; keratoses

Excision of a Lesion _____

Key Terms: cryosurgery; fulgurated

Incision and Drainage _____

_____

Key Point:
• An abscess is a local collection of pus in a cavity surrounded by inflamed tissue.

Assisting with Suture and Staple Removal _____

_____

Key Points:
• Patients should understand that they might feel a pulling sensation during suture removal but should not feel pain.
• Following hospital surgery, some incisions are closed with metal staples rather than sutures.

Content Review

FOUNDATIONAL KNOWLEDGE

Measurements

1. Assisting with Minor Surgery

As a medical assistant, you may be called on to assist a physician with minor office surgery. Review the list of tasks below and determine which tasks you are responsible for as a medical assistant. Place a check in the "Yes" column for those duties you will assist with as a medical assistant, and place a check in the "No" column for those tasks that fall to another member of the health care team.

Task	Yes	No
a. Remind the patient of the physician's pre-surgery instructions, such as fasting.		
b. Prepare the treatment room, including the supplies and equipment.		
c. Obtain the informed consent document from the patient.		
d. Inject the patient with local anesthesia if necessary.		
e. Choose the size of the suture to be used to close the wound.		
f. Apply a dressing or bandage to the wound.		
g. Instruct the patient about postoperative wound care.		
h. Prescribe pain medication for the patient to take at home.		
i. Prepare lab paperwork for any specimens that must be sent out to the lab.		
j. Clean and sterilize the room for the next patient.		

2. Keeping It Sterile

A patient comes into the physician's office with a large wound on his leg. The physician asks you to assist with minor surgery to care for the wound. She reminds you that you must help her maintain a sterile field before and during the procedure. Review this list of actions below and place a check mark to indicate whether sterility was maintained or if there has been any possible contamination.

Action	Sterile	Contaminated
a. The sterile package was moist before the surgery started.		
b. The physician spills a few drops of sterile water onto the sterile field.		
c. You hold the sterile items for the physician above waist level.		
d. The physician rests the sterile items in the middle of the sterile field.		
e. You ask the physician a question over the sterile field.		
f. The physician leaves the room and places a drape over the field.		
g. The physician passes soiled gauze over the sterile field and asks you to dispose of them properly.		

3. Inspecting Sterile Packages

You're responsible for preparing and maintaining sterile packs. You are reviewing the office's inventory and need to determine if the packs are appropriately sterilized or if they need to be repackaged and sterilized again. Place a check mark next to those packages that should be sterilized again because they might be contaminated.

a. No moisture is present on the pack.	
b. The package was sterilized on-site 15 days ago.	
c. The wrapper is ripped down one side.	
d. The sterilization indicator has changed color.	
e. An item from the package fell out onto the floor when you picked it up.	

4. Move It to the Sterile Field

List the three ways in which you may add the contents of peel-back packages to a sterile field.

a. _____

b. _____

c. _____

5. Informed Consent

Which of the following information must be stated on the informed consent document? Circle all that apply.

a. The name of the procedure

b. The tools used in the procedure

c. The purpose of the procedure

d. The expected results

e. The patient's Social Security number

f. Possible side effects

g. The length of the procedure

h. Potential risks and complications

i. The date of the follow-up appointment

Anesthesia Basics

6. Why are local anesthetics used? Name four that are commonly used in a medical office.

    a. _____

    b. _____

    c. _____

    d. _____

7. Dante is a clinical medical assistant who is assisting a physician with minor office surgery. Dr. Yan asks him to prepare the local anesthesia. Dante draws the anesthetic into a syringe and keeps the vial beside the syringe for Dr. Yan's approval. Should Dr. Yan put on sterile gloves before or after she administers the anesthesia? Explain your answer.

    _____

    _____

Needles and Sutures

8. Name three ways in which needles can be classified.

    a. _____

    b. _____

    c. _____

9. A patient comes in with a cut on his face. The physician wants to choose the best size suture to ensure minimal scarring. Which size suture would be better for this procedure—a size 3 suture or a size 23-0 suture? Explain.

    _____

    _____

10. A variety of sutures are available to close wounds and speed up the healing process. In the chart below, decide whether it would be best to use nonabsorbable sutures or skin staples to close wounds.

Location of Surgery/Wound	Nonabsorbable Suture	Skin Staple
a. Hip		
b. Intestines		
c. Abdomen		
d. Heart valves		
e. Bone grafts		
f. Knee		

11. Look at the picture of the small wound below. The physician has determined that sutures are not necessary and will be using adhesive skin closures instead. Draw lines below to represent how the adhesive skin closures should be placed for ideal approximation of the wound.

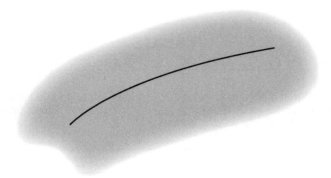

12. The physician just removed a small cyst from a patient's foot. The physician asks you to have the cyst sent to the laboratory. Describe three steps you should take next.

a. _____

b. _____

c. _____

It's Electric!

13. Electrosurgery is increasingly popular in physicians' offices, so it's important that you're aware of the various procedures. Match the name of each procedure below with the correct description.

Procedure Names

a. electrocautery _____

b. electrodesiccation _____

c. electrosection _____

d. fulguration _____

Descriptions

1. destroys tissue with controlled electric sparks

2. causes quick coagulation of small blood vessels with the heat created by the electric current

3. is used for incision or excision of tissue

4. dries and separates tissue with an electric current

14. When assisting during electrosurgery, how should you pass the electrode to the physician?

_____

_____

Keeping Things Sterile

15. When do you use sterile dressings?

_____

_____

16. Ghani is a clinical medical assistant. On Monday, he assisted the physician while she sutured a deep wound on a 7-year-old boy's leg. A few hours after the surgery, the mother brings the boy back to the office because she is concerned the site is infected. When Ghani inspects the sterile dressing, he notes that there is a moderate amount of pink drainage. What does this drainage indicate about the healing process?

_____

_____

17. Listed below are the steps that a medical assistant should take to clean the examination room and prepare it for the next patient. However, they are not listed in the correct order. Review the steps and then place a number next to each step to show the correct order in which they should occur.

    a. _____ Put on gloves.

    b. _____ Remove papers and sheets from the table and discard properly.

    c. _____ Replace the table sheet paper for the next patient.

    d. _____ Wipe down the examination table, surgical stand, sink, counter, and other surfaces used during the procedure with a disinfectant and allow them to dry.

18. A patient comes in with an abscess on his foot. What needs to happen before the abscess can begin to heal?

_____

_____

19. Match the following key terms to their definitions.

Key Terms	Definitions
a. approximate _____	**1.** separation or opening of the edges of a wound
b. atraumatic _____	**2.** a medium for conducting or detecting electrical current
c. bandage _____	**3.** tissue surfaces that are as close together as possible
d. cautery _____	**4.** a covering applied directly to a wound to apply pressure, support, absorb secretions, protect from trauma, slow or stop bleeding, or hide disfigurement
e. coagulate _____	**5.** a means or device that destroys tissue using an electric current, freezing, or burning
f. cryosurgery _____	**6.** causing or relating to tissue damage
g. dehiscence _____	**7.** a swaged type of needle that does not require threading
h. dressing _____	**8.** to destroy tissue by electrodesiccation
i. electrode _____	**9.** a soft material applied to a body part to immobilize the body part or control bleeding
j. fulgurate _____	**10.** to change from a liquid to a solid or semi-solid mass
k. keratosis _____	**11.** brown skin macules occurring after exposure to the sun; freckles
l. lentigines _____	**12.** drainage from a wound that is white, green, or yellow, signaling an infection
m. preservative _____	**13.** a metal needle fused to suture material
n. purulent _____	**14.** a skin condition characterized by overgrowth and thickening
o. swaged needle _____	**15.** a substance that delays decomposition
p. traumatic _____	**16.** surgery in which abnormal tissue is removed by freezing

20. True or False? Determine whether the following statements are true or false. If false, explain why.

    a. Anesthesia with epinephrine is approved for use on the tips of the fingers, toes, nose, and penis.

_____

_____

    b. Atraumatic needles need to be threaded by the physician before they can be used.

_____

_____

    c. Nonabsorbable sutures must be removed after healing.

_____

_____

d. All metal must be removed from a patient before electrosurgery.

APPLICATION

Critical Thinking Practice

1. The physician asks you to position a patient for surgery in the lithotomy position. You know that the physician has to meet with another patient before he will come into the room to perform the surgery. What can you do to keep the patient comfortable before the physician is ready to begin? List three things you can do, and explain why they are important.

---

2. There is a delay in the office, and all of the appointments are running 30 minutes late. The patients are becoming upset, and the office manager said that you should work quickly to try to get back on schedule. You assist the physician with the removal of a small wart from a patient's neck. After the surgery is completed, you need to meet with a new patient to go over the new patient interview and paperwork. But it's also your job to label the specimen and complete the paperwork to send it to the lab. It's almost lunchtime, and you know the lab won't get to it right away. Which task should you complete first—meeting with the patient or preparing the specimen for the lab? Explain your answer.

Patient Education

1. Your patient is a 40-year-old female who has had a cyst excised from her forearm. The cyst is being sent out for pathology to rule out skin cancer. You give her extra bandages so she can change the dressing herself and explain that the physician wants to see her back in the office in one week. Write a sheet of instructions that clearly explains to the patient how to care for the wound and what she should look for in the event of infection.

---

2. Your patient is a 13-year-old boy who received staples for a wound he got in a biking accident. While you are removing the staples, he asks why staples are being used, and not stitches. Explain the difference between sutures and staples, and when it is more appropriate to use each.

Documentation
1. A patient is recovering from a Cesarian section and returns to the office to have her staples removed. The physician asks you to remove the staples and apply adhesive skin closures over the incision site. The patient asks you when the strips should be removed, and you tell her that they should fall off on their own within 10 days. How would you document this interaction in the patient's chart?

Active Learning

1. One of the most common minor surgeries performed in your office is the excision of skin lesions and moles, often related to the possibility of skin cancer. Skin cancer is prevalent today, and you feel that it's important to educate young people on the importance of taking proper precautions to protect skin from harmful sun rays. You have been asked to prepare a one-page patient education handout highlighting the dangers of skin cancer and prevention techniques designed especially for young adults.

   - Perform research using the Internet to identify the leading causes of skin cancer and dangers associated with harmful sun exposure. Gather any statistics that are available from reputable websites.
   - Outline steps that can be taken to protect the skin when outside.
   - Highlight issues that are especially important to teens (for example, summer jobs as lifeguards and outdoor sports practice during the day).
   - Create a one-page handout to be given to teens in the office explaining how to protect their skin from the sun.

2. Perform a skin cancer self-examination to check for any abnormalities in your own skin that should be monitored. Make a list of any irregularities that you should discuss with your physician at your next visit.

3. Laser surgery is replacing traditional office surgery for a variety of procedures. One specific type of laser surgery that has gained popularity in recent years is laser surgery to correct vision problems. Perform research on LASIK surgery and write a paragraph describing the surgery. Are there are any side effects or complications? Think about this procedure and decide if you would undergo laser surgery to correct a vision problem. Justify your answer with facts from your research.

Professional Journal

REFLECT

(Prompts and Ideas: Have you or a loved one ever undergone surgery, minor or major, in a medical office or hospital? What do you wish you had known beforehand? How were you or your loved one treated by medical staff before and after surgery? Did you feel nervous or frightened? Did you receive adequate instructions for self-care after discharge?)

_____

_____

_____

_____

PONDER AND SOLVE

1. A 15-year-old patient has a mole on her face that needs to be removed. She feels anxious about having to wear a large dressing to cover the wound on her face while it heals, and she's nervous about the possibilities of scarring. On top of that, she's worried that the mole is cancerous. What can you say to her to ease her mind before and after the procedure?

_____

_____

_____

_____

2. You are working with another medical assistant to prepare a sterile field for surgery. You are almost finished setting up the sterile field when your coworker sneezes over the sterile field. She says that it's only allergies and that she's not contagious, so the field isn't contaminated. She assures you that you don't need to start your work over again. What would you say to your coworker? What should you do next?

_____

_____

_____

_____

EXPERIENCE

Skills related to this chapter include:

1. Opening Sterile Surgical Packs (Procedure 22-1).
2. Using Sterile Transfer Forceps (Procedure 22-2).
3. Adding Sterile Solution to a Sterile Field (Procedure 22-3).
4. Performing Skin Preparation and Hair Removal (Procedure 22-4).
5. Applying Sterile Gloves (Procedure 22-5).
6. Applying a Sterile Dressing (Procedure 22-6).
7. Changing an Existing Dressing (Procedure 22-7).
8. Assisting with Excisional Surgery (Procedure 22-8).
9. Assisting with Incision and Drainage (Procedure 22-9).
10. Removing Sutures (Procedure 22-10).
11. Removing Staples (Procedure 22-11).

Record any common mistakes, lessons learned, and/or tips you discovered during your experience of practicing and demonstrating these skills.

_____

_____

_____

_____

Skill Practice

PERFORMANCE OBJECTIVES:

1. Open sterile surgical packs (Procedure 22-1).
2. Use sterile transfer forceps (Procedure 22-2).
3. Add sterile solution to a sterile field (Procedure 22-3).
4. Perform skin preparation and hair removal (Procedure 22-4).
5. Apply sterile gloves (Procedure 22-5).
6. Apply a sterile dressing (Procedure 22-6).
7. Change an existing dressing (Procedure 22-7).
8. Assist with excisional surgery (Procedure 22-8).
9. Assist with incision and drainage (Procedure 22-9).
10. Remove sutures (Procedure 22-10).
11. Remove staples (Procedure 22-11).

Name _____ Date _____ Time _____

Procedure 22-1:	**OPENING STERILE SURGICAL PACKS**

EQUIPMENT/SUPPLIES: Surgical pack, surgical or Mayo stand

STANDARDS: Given the needed equipment and a place to work, the student will perform this skill with _____% accuracy in a total of _____ minutes. *(Your instructor will tell you what the percentage and time limits will be before you begin practicing.)*

KEY: 4 = Satisfactory   0 = Unsatisfactory   NA = This step is not counted

PROCEDURE STEPS	SELF	PARTNER	INSTRUCTOR
1. Verify the surgical procedure to be performed and gather supplies.	☐	☐	☐
2. Check the label for contents and the expiration date.	☐	☐	☐
3. Check the package for tears or areas of moisture.	☐	☐	☐
4. Place the package, with the label facing up on Mayo or surgical stand.	☐	☐	☐
5. Wash your hands.	☐	☐	☐
6. Without tearing the wrapper, carefully remove the sealing tape.	☐	☐	☐
7. Open the first flap: pull it up, out, and away; let it fall over the far side of the table.	☐	☐	☐
8. Open the side flaps in a similar manner. Do not touch the sterile inner surface.	☐	☐	☐
9. Pull the remaining flap down and toward you.	☐	☐	☐
10. Repeat steps 4 through 6 for packages with a second or inside wrapper.	☐	☐	☐
11. If you must leave the area after opening the field, cover the tray with a sterile drape.	☐	☐	☐

CALCULATION

Total Possible Points: _____
Total Points Earned: _____ Multiplied by 100 = _____ Divided by Total Possible Points = _____%

Pass   **Fail**
☐   ☐   Comments:

Student's signature _____ Date _____
Partner's signature _____ Date _____
Instructor's signature _____ Date _____

Name _____ Date _____ Time _____

| Procedure 22-2: | **USING STERILE TRANSFER FORCEPS** |

EQUIPMENT/SUPPLIES: Sterile transfer forceps in a container with sterilization solution, sterile field, sterile items to be transferred

STANDARDS: Given the needed equipment and a place to work, the student will perform this skill with _____% accuracy in a total of _____ minutes. *(Your instructor will tell you what the percentage and time limits will be before you begin practicing.)*

KEY: 4 = Satisfactory   0 = Unsatisfactory   NA = This step is not counted

PROCEDURE STEPS	SELF	PARTNER	INSTRUCTOR
1. Slowly lift the forceps straight up and out of the container without touching the inside above the level of the solution or outside of the container.	☐	☐	☐
2. Hold the forceps with the tips down at all times.	☐	☐	☐
3. Keep the forceps above waist level.	☐	☐	☐
4. With the forceps, pick up the articles to be transferred and drop them onto the sterile field, but do not let the forceps come into contact with the sterile field.	☐	☐	☐
5. Carefully place the forceps back into the sterilization solution.	☐	☐	☐

CALCULATION

Total Possible Points: _____
Total Points Earned: _____ Multiplied by 100 = _____ Divided by Total Possible Points = _____%

Pass   **Fail**
☐   ☐   Comments:

Student's signature _____ Date _____
Partner's signature _____ Date _____
Instructor's signature _____ Date _____

Name _____ Date _____ Time _____

Procedure 22-3:   ADDING STERILE SOLUTION TO A STERILE FIELD

EQUIPMENT/SUPPLIES: Sterile setup, container of sterile solution, sterile bowl or cup

STANDARDS: Given the needed equipment and a place to work, the student will perform this skill with _____% accuracy in a total of _____ minutes. *(Your instructor will tell you what the percentage and time limits will be before you begin practicing.)*

KEY: 4 = Satisfactory   0 = Unsatisfactory   NA = This step is not counted

PROCEDURE STEPS	SELF	PARTNER	INSTRUCTOR
1. Identify the correct solution by carefully reading the label.	☐	☐	☐
2. Check the expiration date on the label.	☐	☐	☐
3. If adding medications into the solution, show medication label to the physician.	☐	☐	☐
4. Remove the cap or stopper; avoid contamination of the inside of the cap.	☐	☐	☐
5. If it is necessary to put the cap down, place on side table with opened end facing up.	☐	☐	☐
6. Retain bottle to track amount added to field.	☐	☐	☐
7. Grasp container with label against the palm of your hand.	☐	☐	☐
8. Pour a small amount of the solution into a separate container or waste receptacle.	☐	☐	☐
9. Slowly pour the desired amount of solution into the sterile container.	☐	☐	☐
10. Recheck the label for the contents and expiration date and replace the cap.	☐	☐	☐
11. Return the solution to its proper storage area or discard the container after rechecking the label again.	☐	☐	☐

CALCULATION

Total Possible Points: _____
Total Points Earned: _____ Multiplied by 100 = _____ Divided by Total Possible Points = _____%

Pass   **Fail**
☐   ☐   Comments:

Student's signature _____ Date _____
Partner's signature _____ Date _____
Instructor's signature _____ Date _____

Name_____   Date _____   Time _____

Procedure 22-4:	PERFORMING SKIN PREPARATION AND HAIR REMOVAL

EQUIPMENT/SUPPLIES: Nonsterile gloves; shave cream, lotion, or soap; new disposable razor; gauze or cotton balls; warm water; antiseptic; sponge forceps

STANDARDS: Given the needed equipment and a place to work, the student will perform this skill with _____% accuracy in a total of _____ minutes. *(Your instructor will tell you what the percentage and time limits will be before you begin practicing.)*

KEY: 4 = Satisfactory   0 = Unsatisfactory   NA = This step is not counted

PROCEDURE STEPS	SELF	PARTNER	INSTRUCTOR
1. Wash your hands.	☐	☐	☐
2. Assemble the equipment.	☐	☐	☐
3. Greet and identify the patient; explain the procedure and answer any questions.	☐	☐	☐
4. Put on gloves.	☐	☐	☐
5. Prepare the patient's skin.	☐	☐	☐
6. If the patient's skin is to be shaved, apply shaving cream or soapy lather. **a.** Pull the skin taut and shave in the direction of hair growth. **b.** Rinse and pat the shaved area thoroughly dry using a gauze square.	☐	☐	☐
7. If the patient's skin is not to be shaved, wash with soap and water; rinse well and pat the area thoroughly dry using a gauze square.	☐	☐	☐
8. Apply antiseptic solution to the operative area using sterile gauze sponges. **a.** Wipe skin in circular motions starting at the operative site and working outward. **b.** Discard each sponge after a complete sweep has been made. **c.** If circles are not appropriate, the sponge may be wiped straight outward from the operative site and discarded. **d.** Repeat the procedure until the entire area has been thoroughly cleaned.	☐	☐	☐
9. Instruct the patient not to touch or cover the prepared area.	☐	☐	☐
10. Remove your gloves and wash your hands.	☐	☐	☐
11. Inform the physician that the patient is ready for the surgical procedure.	☐	☐	☐
12. Drape the prepared area with a sterile drape if the physician will be delayed more than 10 or 15 minutes.	☐	☐	☐

CALCULATION

Total Possible Points: _____

Total Points Earned: _____ Multiplied by 100 = _____ Divided by Total Possible Points = _____%

Pass   **Fail**

☐   ☐

Comments:

Student's signature _____ Date _____

Partner's signature _____ Date _____

Instructor's signature _____ Date _____

Name_____ Date _____ Time _____

Procedure 22-5:   APPLYING STERILE GLOVES

EQUIPMENT/SUPPLIES: One package of sterile gloves in the appropriate size

STANDARDS: Given the needed equipment and a place to work, the student will perform this skill with _____% accuracy in a total of _____ minutes. *(Your instructor will tell you what the percentage and time limits will be before you begin practicing.)*

KEY: 4 = Satisfactory   0 = Unsatisfactory   NA = This step is not counted

PROCEDURE STEPS	SELF	PARTNER	INSTRUCTOR
1. Remove rings and other jewelry.	☐	☐	☐
2. Wash your hands.	☐	☐	☐
3. Place prepackaged gloves on a clean, dry, flat surface with the cuffed end toward you. **a.** Pull the outer wrapping apart to expose the sterile inner wrap. **b.** With the cuffs toward you, fold back the inner wrap to expose the gloves.	☐	☐	☐
4. Grasping the edges of the outer paper, open the package out to its fullest.	☐	☐	☐
5. Use your nondominant hand to pick up the dominant hand glove. **a.** Grasp the folded edge of the cuff and lift it up and away from the paper. **b.** Curl your fingers and thumb together and insert them into the glove. **c.** Straighten your fingers and pull the glove on with your nondominant hand still grasping the cuff.	☐	☐	☐
6. Unfold the cuff by pinching the inside surface and pull it toward your wrist.	☐	☐	☐
7. Place the fingers of your gloved hand under the cuff of the remaining glove. **a.** Lift the glove up and away from the wrapper. **b.** Slide your ungloved hand carefully into the glove with your fingers and thumb curled together. **c.** Straighten your fingers and pull the glove up and over your wrist by carefully unfolding the cuff.	☐	☐	☐
8. Settle the gloves comfortably onto your fingers by lacing your fingers together.	☐	☐	☐
9. Remove contaminated sterile gloves and discard them appropriately. Wash your hands.	☐	☐	☐

CALCULATION

Total Possible Points: _____

Total Points Earned: _____ Multiplied by 100 = _____ Divided by Total Possible Points = _____%

Pass   **Fail**

☐   ☐   Comments:

Student's signature _____ Date _____
Partner's signature _____ Date _____
Instructor's signature _____ Date _____

Name _____ Date _____ Time _____

Procedure 22-6:	APPLYING A STERILE DRESSING

EQUIPMENT/SUPPLIES: Sterile gloves, sterile gauze dressings, scissors, bandage tape, any medication to be applied to the dressing if ordered by the physician

STANDARDS: Given the needed equipment and a place to work, the student will perform this skill with _____% accuracy in a total of _____ minutes. *(Your instructor will tell you what the percentage and time limits will be before you begin practicing.)*

KEY: 4 = Satisfactory   0 = Unsatisfactory   NA = This step is not counted

PROCEDURE STEPS	SELF	PARTNER	INSTRUCTOR
1. Wash your hands.	☐	☐	☐
2. Assemble the equipment and supplies.	☐	☐	☐
3. Greet and identify the patient.	☐	☐	☐
4. Ask about any tape allergies before deciding on what type of tape to use.	☐	☐	☐
5. Cut or tear lengths of tape to secure the dressing.	☐	☐	☐
6. Explain the procedure and instruct the patient to remain still; avoid coughing, sneezing, or talking until the procedure is complete.	☐	☐	☐
7. Open the dressing pack to create a sterile field, maintaining sterile asepsis. **a.** If sterile gloves are to be used, open and place near dressing pack. **b.** If using a sterile transfer forceps, place it near the other supplies.	☐	☐	☐
8. Apply topical medication to the sterile dressing that will cover the wound.	☐	☐	☐
9. Apply the number of dressings necessary to properly cover and protect the wound.	☐	☐	☐
10. Apply sufficient cut lengths of tape over the dressing to secure.	☐	☐	☐
11. Remove contaminated gloves and discard in the proper receptacle. Wash your hands.	☐	☐	☐
12. Provide patient education and supplies as appropriate.	☐	☐	☐
13. Clean and sanitize the room and equipment.	☐	☐	☐
14. Record the procedure.	☐	☐	☐

CALCULATION

Total Possible Points: _____
Total Points Earned: _____ Multiplied by 100 = _____ Divided by Total Possible Points = _____%

Pass   **Fail**
☐   ☐   Comments:

Student's signature _____ Date _____
Partner's signature _____ Date _____
Instructor's signature _____ Date _____

Name_____ Date_____ Time_____

Procedure 22-7:	CHANGING AN EXISTING DRESSING

EQUIPMENT/SUPPLIES: Sterile gloves, nonsterile gloves, sterile dressing, prepackaged skin antiseptic swabs (or sterile antiseptic solution poured into a sterile basin and sterile cotton balls or gauze), tape, approved biohazard containers

STANDARDS: Given the needed equipment and a place to work, the student will perform this skill with _____% accuracy in a total of _____ minutes. *(Your instructor will tell you what the percentage and time limits will be before you begin practicing.)*

KEY: 4 = Satisfactory   0 = Unsatisfactory   NA = This step is not counted

PROCEDURE STEPS	SELF	PARTNER	INSTRUCTOR
1. Wash your hands.	☐	☐	☐
2. Assemble the equipment and supplies.	☐	☐	☐
3. Greet and identify the patient; explain the procedure and answer any questions.	☐	☐	☐
4. Prepare a sterile field including opening sterile dressings.	☐	☐	☐
5. Open a sterile basin and use the inside of the wrapper as the sterile field. **a.** Flip the sterile gauze or cotton balls into the basin. **b.** Pour antiseptic solution appropriately into the basin. **c.** If using prepackaged antiseptic swabs, carefully open an adequate number. **d.** Set swabs aside without contaminating them.	☐	☐	☐
6. Instruct the patient not to talk, cough, sneeze, laugh, or move during the procedure.	☐	☐	☐
7. Wear clean gloves and carefully remove tape from the wound dressing by pulling it toward the wound. **a.** Remove the old dressing. **b.** Discard the soiled dressing into a biohazard container.	☐	☐	☐
8. Inspect wound for the degree of healing, amount and type of drainage, and appearance of wound edges.	☐	☐	☐
9. Observing medical asepsis, remove and discard your gloves.	☐	☐	☐
10. Using proper technique, apply sterile gloves.	☐	☐	☐
11. Clean the wound with the antiseptic solution ordered by the physician.	☐	☐	☐
12. Clean in a straight motion with the cotton or gauze or the prepackaged antiseptic swab. Discard the wipe (cotton ball, swab) after each use.	☐	☐	☐
13. Remove your gloves and wash your hands.	☐	☐	☐
14. Change the dressing using the procedure for sterile dressing application (Procedure 22-6) and using sterile gloves (Procedure 22-5) or sterile transfer forceps (Procedure 22-2).	☐	☐	☐
15. Record the procedure.	☐	☐	☐

CALCULATION

Total Possible Points: _____

Total Points Earned: _____ Multiplied by 100 = _____ Divided by Total Possible Points = _____%

Pass **Fail**

☐ ☐ Comments:

Student's signature _____ Date _____

Partner's signature _____ Date _____

Instructor's signature _____ Date _____

Name_____   Date _____   Time _____

Procedure 22-8:	**ASSISTING WITH EXCISIONAL SURGERY**

PURPOSE: Prepare for and assist with excisional surgery while maintaining sterile technique

EQUIPMENT/SUPPLIES: Sterile gloves, local anesthetic, antiseptic wipes, adhesive tape, specimen container with completed laboratory request; *On the field:* basin for solutions, gauze sponges and cotton balls, antiseptic solution, sterile drape, dissecting scissors, disposable scalpel, blade of physician's choice, mosquito forceps, tissue forceps, needle holder, suture and needle of physician's choice

STANDARDS: Given the needed equipment and a place to work, the student will perform this skill with _____% accuracy in a total of _____ minutes. *(Your instructor will tell you what the percentage and time limits will be before you begin practicing.)*

KEY: 4 = Satisfactory   0 = Unsatisfactory   NA = This step is not counted

PROCEDURE STEPS	SELF	PARTNER	INSTRUCTOR
1. Wash your hands.	☐	☐	☐
2. Assemble the equipment appropriate for the procedure and according to physician preference.	☐	☐	☐
3. Greet and identify the patient; explain the procedure and answer any questions.	☐	☐	☐
4. Set up a sterile field on a surgical stand with additional equipment close at hand.	☐	☐	☐
5. Cover the field with a sterile drape until the physician arrives.	☐	☐	☐
6. Position the patient appropriately.	☐	☐	☐
7. Put on sterile gloves (Procedure 22-5) or use sterile transfer forceps (Procedure 22-2) and cleanse the patient's skin (Procedure 22-4).	☐	☐	☐
8. Be ready to assist during the procedure: adding supplies as needed, assisting the physician, and comforting the patient.	☐	☐	☐
9. Assist with collecting tissue specimen in an appropriate container.	☐	☐	☐
10. At the end of the procedure, wash your hands and dress the wound using sterile technique (Procedure 22-6).	☐	☐	☐
11. Thank the patient and give appropriate instructions.	☐	☐	☐
12. Sanitize the examining room in preparation for the next patient.	☐	☐	☐
13. Discard all disposables in the appropriate biohazard containers.	☐	☐	☐
14. Record the procedure.	☐	☐	☐

CALCULATION

Total Possible Points: _____
Total Points Earned: _____ Multiplied by 100 = _____ Divided by Total Possible Points = _____%

Pass   **Fail**
☐   ☐

Comments:

Student's signature _____ Date _____
Partner's signature _____ Date _____
Instructor's signature _____ Date _____

Name_____   Date _____   Time _____

Procedure 22-9:	ASSISTING WITH INCISION AND DRAINAGE (I & D)

EQUIPMENT/SUPPLIES: Sterile gloves, local anesthetic, antiseptic wipes, adhesive tape, sterile dressings, packing gauze, a culture tube if the wound may be cultured; *On the field:* basin for solutions, gauze sponges and cotton balls, antiseptic solution, sterile drape, syringes and needles for local anesthetic, commercial I & D sterile setup OR scalpel, dissecting scissors, hemostats, tissue forceps, 4 × 4 gauze sponges, probe (optional)

STANDARDS: Given the needed equipment and a place to work, the student will perform this skill with _____% accuracy in a total of _____ minutes. *(Your instructor will tell you what the percentage and time limits will be before you begin practicing.)*

KEY: 4 = Satisfactory   0 = Unsatisfactory   NA = This step is not counted

PROCEDURE STEPS	SELF	PARTNER	INSTRUCTOR
1. Wash your hands.	☐	☐	☐
2. Assemble the equipment appropriate for the procedure and according to physician preference.	☐	☐	☐
3. Greet and identify the patient. Explain the procedure and answer any questions.	☐	☐	☐
4. Set up a sterile field on a surgical stand with additional equipment close at hand.	☐	☐	☐
5. Cover the field with a sterile drape until the physician arrives.	☐	☐	☐
6. Position the patient appropriately.	☐	☐	☐
7. Put on sterile gloves (Procedure 22-5) or use sterile transfer forceps (Procedure 22-2) and cleanse the patient's skin (Procedure 22-4).	☐	☐	☐
8. Be ready to assist during the procedure: adding supplies as needed, assisting the physician, comforting the patient.	☐	☐	☐
9. Assist with collecting culturette specimen for culture and sensitivity.	☐	☐	☐
10. At the end of procedure, remove gloves, wash your hands, and dress the wound using sterile technique (Procedure 22-6).	☐	☐	☐
11. Thank the patient and give appropriate instructions.	☐	☐	☐
12. Sanitize the examining room in preparation for the next patient.	☐	☐	☐
13. Discard all disposables in appropriate biohazard containers.	☐	☐	☐
14. Record the procedure.	☐	☐	☐

CALCULATION

Total Possible Points: _____
Total Points Earned: _____ Multiplied by 100 = _____ Divided by Total Possible Points = _____%

Pass   **Fail**
☐   ☐   Comments:

Student's signature _____ Date _____
Partner's signature _____ Date _____
Instructor's signature _____ Date _____

Name _____ Date _____ Time _____

Procedure 22-10:   REMOVING SUTURES

EQUIPMENT/SUPPLIES: Skin antiseptic, sterile gloves, prepackaged suture removal kit OR thumb forceps, suture scissors, gauze

STANDARDS: Given the needed equipment and a place to work, the student will perform this skill with _____% accuracy in a total of _____ minutes. *(Your instructor will tell you what the percentage and time limits will be before you begin practicing.)*

KEY: 4 = Satisfactory   0 = Unsatisfactory   NA = This step is not counted

PROCEDURE STEPS	SELF	PARTNER	INSTRUCTOR
1. Wash your hands and apply clean examination gloves.	☐	☐	☐
2. Assemble the equipment.	☐	☐	☐
3. Greet and identify the patient; explain the procedure and answer any questions.	☐	☐	☐
4. If dressings have not been removed previously, remove them from the wound area. **a.** Properly dispose of the soiled dressings in the biohazard trash container. **b.** Remove your gloves and wash your hands.	☐	☐	☐
5. Put on another pair of clean examination gloves and cleanse the wound with an antiseptic.	☐	☐	☐
6. Open suture removal packet using sterile asepsis.	☐	☐	☐
7. Put on sterile gloves. **a.** With the thumb forceps, grasp the end of the knot closest to the skin surface and lift it slightly and gently up from the skin. **b.** Cut the suture below the knot as close to the skin as possible. **c.** Use the thumb forceps to pull the suture out of the skin with a smooth motion.	☐	☐	☐
8. Place the suture on the gauze sponge; repeat the procedure for each suture to be removed.	☐	☐	☐
9. Clean the site with an antiseptic solution and cover it with a sterile dressing.	☐	☐	☐
10. Thank the patient.	☐	☐	☐
11. Properly dispose of the equipment and supplies.	☐	☐	☐
12. Clean the work area, remove your gloves, and wash your hands.	☐	☐	☐
13. Record the procedure, including the time, location of sutures, the number removed, and the condition of the wound.	☐	☐	☐

CALCULATION

Total Possible Points: _____
Total Points Earned: _____ Multiplied by 100 = _____ Divided by Total Possible Points = _____%

Pass **Fail**
☐ ☐ Comments:

Student's signature _____ Date _____
Partner's signature _____ Date _____
Instructor's signature _____ Date _____

Name_____ Date_____ Time_____

Procedure 22-11:	**REMOVING STAPLES**

EQUIPMENT/SUPPLIES: Antiseptic solution or wipes, gauze squares, sponge forceps, prepackaged sterile staple removal instrument, examination gloves, sterile gloves

STANDARDS: Given the needed equipment and a place to work, the student will perform this skill with _____% accuracy in a total of _____ minutes. *(Your instructor will tell you what the percentage and time limits will be before you begin practicing.)*

KEY: 4 = Satisfactory 0 = Unsatisfactory NA = This step is not counted

PROCEDURE STEPS	SELF	PARTNER	INSTRUCTOR
1. Wash your hands.	☐	☐	☐
2. Assemble the equipment.	☐	☐	☐
3. Greet and identify the patient; explain the procedure and answer any questions.	☐	☐	☐
4. If the dressing has not been removed, put on clean examination gloves and do so.	☐	☐	☐
5. Dispose of the dressing properly in a biohazard container.	☐	☐	☐
6. Clean the incision with antiseptic solution.	☐	☐	☐
7. Pat dry using dry sterile gauze sponges.	☐	☐	☐
8. Put on sterile gloves.	☐	☐	☐
9. Gently slide the end of the staple remover under each staple to be removed; press the handles together to lift the ends of the staple out of the skin and remove the staple.	☐	☐	☐
10. Place each staple on a gauze square as it is removed.	☐	☐	☐
11. When all staples are removed, clean the incision as instructed for all procedures.	☐	☐	☐
12. Pat dry and dress the site if ordered to do so by the physician.	☐	☐	☐
13. Thank the patient and properly care for, or dispose of, all equipment and supplies.	☐	☐	☐
14. Clean the work area, remove your gloves, and wash your hands.	☐	☐	☐
15. Record the procedure.	☐	☐	☐

CALCULATION

Total Possible Points: _____

Total Points Earned: _____ Multiplied by 100 = _____ Divided by Total Possible Points = _____%

Pass   **Fail**

☐   ☐   Comments:

Student's signature _____ Date _____

Partner's signature _____ Date _____

Instructor's signature _____ Date _____

Work Product 1

Document appropriately.

Raphael Dean came to the office for the removal of 15 surgical staples from his left knee on March 17, 2008, at 10:30 AM. The physician was pleased to see that the edges of the surgical incision had healed together well, leaving very little scar tissue, and that there was no longer any drainage or redness in the area. After the staples were removed, no dressing or bandage was applied, and Raphael left with a smile of relief.

If you are currently working in a medical office, use a blank paper patient chart from the office. If this is not available to you, use the space below to record the procedure and outcome.

_____

_____

_____

_____

Chapter Self-Assessment Quiz

1. Which of the following statements is true about working in a sterile field?
   a. Sterile packages should be kept damp.
   b. Your back must be kept to the sterile field at all times.
   c. A 3-inch border around the field is considered contaminated.
   d. All sterile items should be held above waist level.
   e. Cover your mouth when coughing near the sterile field.

2. Why is a fenestrated drape helpful during surgery?
   a. It is made of lightweight fabric.
   b. It has an opening to expose the operative site.
   c. It can be used as a blanket to keep the patient warm.
   d. It does not need to be sterilized before surgery.
   e. It allows for easy cleanup after the surgery.

3. Epinephrine is added to local anesthetics during surgery to:
   a. ensure sterilization.
   b. protect the tips of the fingers.
   c. lengthen the anesthetic's effectiveness.
   d. prevent vasoconstriction.
   e. create rapid absorption.

4. Which needles are used most frequently in the medical office?
   a. Curved swaged needles
   b. Traumatic needles
   c. Straight needles
   d. Domestic needles
   e. Keith needles

5. A preservative is added to specimen containers to be sent to a pathologist to:
   a. help the pathologist see the specimen.
   b. delay decomposition.
   c. identify the patient.
   d. make the specimen grow.
   e. prevent contamination.

6. Which type of electrosurgery destroys tissue with controlled electric sparks?
   a. Electrocautery
   b. Electrodesiccation
   c. Electrosection
   d. Fulguration
   e. Electrophysiology

7. Why is it important to know if a patient has a pacemaker before performing electrosurgery?

   a. Metal implants can become very hot and malfunction during the procedure.

   b. The electrical charge can cause the electrosurgical device to malfunction.

   c. The patient needs to sign a separate consent form if he has any heart problems.

   d. The patient can receive an electrical shock from the equipment.

   e. The implants may counteract the electrosurgery results.

Scenario: A female patient returns to the office to have sutures removed from her forearm. When you remove the dressing, you notice that there is a small amount of clear drainage.

8. The patient's drainage is:

   a. purulent.

   b. sanguineous.

   c. serous.

   d. copious.

   e. serosanguineous.

9. Before you remove the patient's sutures, you should:

   a. apply a local anesthetic to numb the area.

   b. offer the patient pain medication to reduce discomfort.

   c. place an ice pack on the patient's forearm.

   d. advise the patient that she should feel pulling sensation but not pain.

   e. gently tug on the ends of the suture to make sure they are secure.

End Scenario

10. Which of the following is characteristic of healing by primary intention?

   a. Clean incision

   b. Gaping, irregular wound

   c. Increased granulation

   d. Wide scar

   e. Indirect edge joining

11. What happens during Phase II of wound healing?

   a. Fibroblasts build scar tissue to guard the area.

   b. The scab dries and pulls the edges of the wound together.

   c. Circulation increases and brings white blood cells to the area.

   d. Serum and red blood cells form a fibrin to plug the wound.

   e. An antiseptic sterilizes the area from possible contamination.

12. How must the physician care for an abscess in order for it to heal properly?

   a. Drain the infected material from the site.

   b. Suture the site closed.

   c. Cover the site with a sterile dressing.

   d. Perform cryosurgery to remove the site.

   e. Perform a skin graft to cover the site.

13. Which of the following items should be added to the label on a specimen container?

   a. The contents of the container

   b. The office number

   c. The patient's age

   d. The patient's gender

   e. The date

14. Which of the following is true about laser surgery?

   a. The Argon laser is the only laser used for coagulation.

   b. Colored filters allow the physician to see the path of the laser.

   c. Most lasers are used simply as markers for surgery.

   d. Laser incisions generally bleed more than regular incisions.

   e. Everyone in the room must wear goggles to protect his eyes.

15. What is the best way to prepare a patient for surgery?

   a. Remind the patient of procedures by calling a few days before the surgery.

   b. Tell the patient all the instructions on the visit before the surgery.

   c. Send the patient home with written instructions on what to do.

   d. Instruct the patient to call the day of the procedure for instructions.

   e. Have the patient tell a second person about what she needs to do.

16. Which of the following supplies must be added at the time of setup for a surgery?

   a. Liquids in open containers

   b. Sterile transfer forceps

   c. Peel-back envelopes

   d. Sterile gloves

   e. Fenestrated drape

17. Absorbable sutures are most frequently used:

   a. in medical offices for wound sutures.

   b. in hospitals for deep-tissue surgery.

   c. in hospitals for surface-tissue surgery.

   d. when patients are young and heal easily.

   e. whenever a wound needs to be sutured.

18. Which of the following might contaminate a sterile dressing?

   a. A patient accidentally bumps into another person

   b. The wound still has sutures underneath

   c. The weather outside has been rainy and damp

   d. The patient adjusted the dressing at home

   e. The patient has had a cold for the past week

19. A child came in with a slight cut on his leg, but there is little tension on the skin and the cut is clean. The physician believes the wound will heal on its own, with time, and wants to approximate the edges of the wound so that it will heal with minimum scarring. Which of the following would be best used to close the child's wound?

   a. Adhesive skin closures

   b. Fine absorptive sutures

   c. Traumatic sutures

   d. Staples

   e. Nothing

20. The last step in any surgical procedure is to:

   a. assist the patient to leave.

   b. instruct the patient on postoperative procedures.

   c. remove all biohazardous materials.

   d. wash your hands.

   e. record the procedure.

CHAPTER 23

Pharmacology

Chapter Checklist

☐ Read textbook chapter and take notes within the Chapter Notes outline. Answer the Learning Objectives as you reach them in the content, and then check them off.

☐ Work the Content Review questions—both Foundational Knowledge and Application.

☐ Perform the Active Learning exercise(s).

☐ Complete Professional Journal entries.

☐ Complete Skill Practice Activity(s) using Competency Evaluation Forms and Work Products, when appropriate.

☐ Take the Chapter Self-Assessment Quiz.

☐ Insert all appropriate pages into your Portfolio.

Learning Objectives

1. Spell and define the key terms.
2. Describe basic principles of pharmacology.
3. Identify chemical, trade, and generic drug names.
4. Name the legal regulations and branches of government that impact prescription medications and controlled substances.
5. Explain the various drug actions and interactions including pharmacodynamics and pharmacokinetics.
6. Describe the difference between medication side effects and allergies.
7. Name the sources for locating information on pharmacology.

Chapter Notes

Note: Bold-faced headings are the major headings in the text chapter; headings in regular font are lower-level headings (i.e., the content is subordinate to, or falls "under," the major headings). Make sure you understand the key terms used in the chapter, as well as the concepts presented as Key Points.

TEXT SUBHEADINGS   **NOTES**

Introduction _____

_____

Key Terms: pharmacology; drug
Key Point:
• It is important that you acquire knowledge of medications, their uses and potential abuses, range of dosages, methods of administration, and adverse effects.

_____

☐ **LEARNING OBJECTIVE 1:** Spell and define the key terms.

_____

☐ **LEARNING OBJECTIVE 2:** Describe basic principles of pharmacology.

Medication Names _____

_____

> **Key Terms:** chemical name; generic name; trade name
> **Key Point:**
> • When the drug is available for commercial use and distribution by the original manufacturer, it is given a brand, or trade, name.

☐ **LEARNING OBJECTIVE 3:** Identify chemical, trade, and generic drug names.

Legal Regulations _____

_____

_____

Food and Drug Administration _____

_____

_____

Drug Enforcement Agency _____

_____

> **Key Points:**
> • In 1970, the Controlled Substances Act was passed to regulate the manufacture and distribution of drugs whose use may result in dependency or abuse.
> • As a medical assistant, you may be responsible for maintaining or reminding the physician about professional records and licensure, including registration with the DEA.
> • Drug dependence, sometimes referred to as addiction, can be either psychological, physical, or both.

Inventory, Storage, Dispensation, and Disposal of Medications _____

_____

☐ **LEARNING OBJECTIVE 4:** Name the legal regulations and branches of government that impact prescription medications and controlled substances.

Sources of Drugs _____

_____

_____

Drug Actions and Interactions _____

_____

_____

Pharmacodynamics _____

Key Term: pharmacodynamics
Key Point:
• All drugs cause cellular change (drug action) and some degree of physiological change (drug effect).

Pharmacokinetics _____

Key Term: pharmacokinetics
Key Point:
• Specifically, the processes included in **pharmacokinetics** include absorption (getting the drug into the bloodstream); distribution (movement of the drug from the bloodstream into the cells and tissues); metabolism (the physical and chemical breakdown of drugs by the body, including the liver); and excretion (byproducts sent to the kidneys to be removed from the body).

Drug Interactions _____

Key Terms: interactions; synergism; antagonism; potentiation
Key Point:
• When two or more drugs are taken simultaneously, one drug may increase, decrease, or cancel the effects of the other.

☐ **LEARNING OBJECTIVE 5:** Explain the various drug actions and interactions including pharmacodynamics and pharmacokinetics.

Side Effects and Allergies _____

Key Terms: allergy; anaphylaxis; side effects
Key Points:
• Allergic reactions can be immediate or delayed 2 hours or longer, depending on the route of administration; however, many allergic reactions occur within minutes if the medication is administered by injection.
• Because of the possibility of an anaphylactic reaction, patients should never be given medications that they have had an allergic reaction to in the past.
• Side effects are reactions to medications that are predictable (as noted by the manufacturer of the medication) and that occur in some patients who take the medication.
• Some offices require all patients receiving injections to wait for a specific amount of time (15 to 20 minutes) before leaving the office.

☐ **LEARNING OBJECTIVE 6:** Describe the difference between medication side effects and allergies.

Sources of Information _____

Key Points:
- The *Physician's Desk Reference* (PDR) is widely used as a reference for drugs in current use.
- All prescribed medications must be documented in full in the patient's record.

☐ **LEARNING OBJECTIVE 7:** Name the sources for locating information on pharmacology.

Prescriptions _____

Key Point:
- Medications may be administered (given in the office), dispensed (a supply given for later use), or prescribed (a written order to be filled by a pharmacist).

Refilling Prescriptions _____

Content Review

FOUNDATIONAL KNOWLEDGE

1. Chemical, Generic, and Trade Names

Every medication has three names: its chemical, generic, and trade name. Mark in the table below which drug characteristic corresponds with what name.

	Chemical Name	Generic Name	Trade Name
a. The name of a drug that begins with a lowercase letter			
b. The name assigned to a drug during research and development			
c. The name given to a drug when it is available for commercial use			
d. The first name given to any medication			
e. The name that is registered by the U.S. patent office			
f. The name that identifies the chemical components of the drug			

2. Review the following statements. Circle the correct answer to indicate if they are true or false.

    a. The DEA is concerned with controlled substances only.   True   False

    b. Drugs are derived from natural and synthetic sources.   True   False

    c. Children have a slower response to drug intakes.   True   False

    d. Allergic reactions are always immediate.   True   False

    e. Side effects from drugs are often life threatening.   True   False

Pharmacodynamics and Pharmacokinetics

3. What are pharmacodynamics and pharmacokinetics? Explain the relationship between these two processes.

_____

_____

4. What four processes are connected to pharmacokinetics?

    a. _____

    b. _____

    c. _____

    d. _____

Drug Interactions

5. Fill in the chart below to describe the different types of drug interactions.

Type of Drug Interaction	Effects
a. Synergism	
b. Antagonism	
c. Potentiation	

6. Why is it important for patients to know about food-drug interactions?

_____

_____

7. Side Effects and Allergies

Louise asks Mr. Fujiwara about his medical history and if he has any allergies to any medications. Mr. Fujiwara says that he has an allergy to aspirin. Louise marks Mr. Fujiwara's drug allergy prominently on the front of his medication record before giving the record to the physician. What else should the medical assistant do?

_____

_____

8. Explain the difference between drug side effects and allergic reactions.

_____

_____

9. List three common and predictable drug side effects.

a. _____

b. _____

c. _____

10. Sources of Information

Determine if the information below can be found in the *Physician's Desk Reference* (*PDR*) or the *United States Pharmacopeia Dispensing Information* (*USPDI*). Place a check mark in the appropriate box below.

	Physician's Desk Reference (PDR)	United States Pharmacopeia Dispensing Information (USPDI)
a. Drug sources		
b. Indications		
c. Dosages		
d. Pictures		
e. Chemistry		
f. Physical properties		
g. Side effects		
h. Tests for identity		
i. Storage		
j. Contraindications		

11. Prescriptions

Place the following elements of prescription protocol into sequential order.

Patient's name and address	Line 1.
Date	Line 2.
Inscription	Line 3.
Superscription	Line 4.
Subscription	Line 5.
Physician's signature	Line 6.
Signature	Line 7.
Generic	Line 8.
Refills	Line 9.

12. Read the following scenario.

Ms. Schemer calls in for a refill of digoxin. You should:

a. consult with the physician before refilling Ms. Schemer's prescription.

b. consult with the physician and then ask Ms. Schemer to come in for blood monitoring before refilling her prescription.

c. check with the physician before calling any prescriptions in to the pharmacy.

d. authorize a refill of the medication.

13. Complete the following sentence:

You must understand the _____, _____, and _____ of drugs to carry out a physician's order.

14. List the effect or action of the following therapeutic classifications.

a. Stimulants _____

b. Diuretics _____

c. Emetics _____

d. Immunologic agents _____

Controlled Substances

15. Place a check mark in the box below to indicate each drug's controlled substance category.

	I	II	III	IV	V
a. morphine					
b. Tylenol with codeine					
c. cocaine					
d. codeine in cough medications					
e. marijuana					
f. Valium					
g. LSD					
h. Ritalin					
i. Librium					

16. Match the following terms with their meanings.

a. Therapeutic classification	**1.** Relates the level of risk to fetal or maternal health. These rank from Category A through D, with increasing danger at each level. Category X indicates that the particular drug should never be given during pregnancy.
b. Idiosyncratic Reaction	**2.** Refers to an excessive reaction to a particular drug; also known as a drug allergy. The body must build this response; the first exposures may or may not indicate that a problem is developing.
c. Indications	**3.** Indicates conditions or instances for which the particular drug should not be used.
d. Teratogenic Category	**4.** States the purpose for the drug's use (e.g., cardiotonic, anti-infective, antiarrhythmic).
e. Hypersensitivity	**5.** Refers to an abnormal or unexpected reaction to a drug peculiar to the individual patient; not technically an allergy.
f. Contraindications	**6.** Gives diseases for which the particular drug would be prescribed.
g. Adverse reactions	**7.** Refers to undesirable side effects of a particular drug.

17. Each of the following statements about inventory of controlled substances is false or incomplete. Rewrite each statement to make it true and complete.

a. List only category III controlled substances on the appropriate inventory form.

_____

_____

b. When you receive controlled substances, make sure that only the physician signs the receipt.

_____

_____

c. Keep all controlled substance inventory forms for ten years.

_____

_____

d. When a controlled substance leaves the medical office inventory, record the following information: drug name and patient.

_____

_____

e. Notify the office manager immediately if these drugs are lost or stolen.

_____

_____

f. Store controlled substances in the same cabinet as other medications and supplies.

_____

_____

18. Responsibilities

Check all the duties below that you are responsible for as a medical assistant.

Medical Assistant Responsibilities	Yes	No
a. Maintaining and reminding physician about medical licensure		
b. Keeping medication area clean, neat, and organized		
c. Administering medications to patients on your own		
d. Making sure the physician's office is on the DEA mailing list		
e. Gathering information about "lost" or "stolen" medications and reporting illegal activities to authorities		
f. Advising patients on the therapeutic effects of over-the-counter medications		
g. Gathering information about the patient's medical history and inquiring about allergies		
h. Notifying the AMA if you suspect a patient of diverting illegal substances		
i. Taking primary responsibility for disposing of controlled substances		
j. Always checking with the physician before authorizing the refill of any medication		

19. Match the following key terms to their definitions.

Key Terms

a. allergy _____
b. anaphylaxis _____
c. antagonism _____
d. chemical name _____
e. contraindication _____
f. drug _____
g. generic name _____

Definitions

1. effects, positive and negative, of two or more drugs taken by a patient
2. situation or condition that prohibits the prescribing or administering of a drug or medication
3. any substance that may modify one or more of the functions of an organism
4. study of drugs and their origin, nature, properties, and effects upon living organisms
5. exact chemical descriptor of a drug
6. official name given to a drug whose patent has expired

h. interaction _____

i. pharmacodynamics _____

j. pharmacokinetics _____

k. pharmacology _____

l. potentiation _____

m. synergism _____

n. trade name _____

7. name given to a medication by the company that owns the patent

8. study of the effects and reactions of drugs within the body

9. study of the action of drugs within the body from administration to excretion

10. harmonious action of two agents, such as drugs or organs, producing an effect that neither could produce alone or that is greater than the total effects of each agent operating by itself

11. mutual opposition or contrary action with something else; opposite of synergism

12. describes the action of two drugs taken together in which the combined effects are greater than the sum of the independent effects

13. acquired abnormal response to a substance (allergen) that does not ordinarily cause a reaction

14. severe allergic reaction that may result in death

20. True or False. Determine whether the following statements are true or false. If false, explain why.

a. A drug is a chemical substance that affects body function or functions.

_____

_____

b. A drug administered for a systemic effect is applied topically.

_____

_____

c. Women may react differently to certain drugs than men.

_____

_____

d. Medications should always be taken on a full stomach.

_____

_____

APPLICATION

Critical Thinking Practice

1. You are doing an inventory of the controlled substances in your office and notice that the office's supply of morphine is off count. You double-check all written records of medications given for administration and still cannot account for the missing morphine. After realizing this, you immediately tell the physician. The physician tells you not to worry about it. Three weeks later you notice that more morphine is missing. What do you do?

_____

_____

2. A patient just received a shot of penicillin. Before the shot was administered, you advised the patient that she needs to remain in the physician's office for 30 minutes before leaving. However, the patient just remembers that she must pick her mother up for an appointment that her mother needs to attend. The patient is adamant that she must leave right away so as not to be late. What do you do?

_____

_____

Patient Education

1. You have an elderly patient who is taking lasix for his high blood pressure. This patient has recently called in to the office complaining of muscle weakness. What is the first thing that you must advise this patient about?

_____

_____

Documentation

1. The physician has prescribed a patient 250 milligrams of amoxicillin for an ear infection. The patient should take this medication 3 times a day by mouth for 9 days. Write a note to document this in the patient's chart.

_____

_____

Active Learning

1. You have just begun working in a medical office and are getting yourself acquainted with the types of medications that the physician frequently prescribes. You know that many medications interact with food; however, you don't know a lot about specific food–drug interactions. Choose 10 common drugs from different therapeutic classifications in Table 23-1. Then research any possible food interactions. Make a chart for patients showing how common drugs and foods interact with one another.

2. Familiarize yourself with the *Physician's Desk Reference, United States Pharmacopeia Dispensing Information*, and *Compendium of Drug Therapy*. Look up five specific drugs in all three sources and create a chart to compare information that is found in each reference guide.

Professional Journal

REFLECT

(Prompts and Ideas: Have you ever experienced any side effects from a prescription medication? Did you know there might be side effects in advance? Did you have to switch medications or were you able to find a way to reduce the side effects, for example by taking the medicine with food? Do you or a loved one have any drug allergies?)

_____

_____

_____

_____

_____

_____

PONDER AND SOLVE

1. You have a patient with hepatic disease. After she consults with the physician, she asks you some general questions to clarify how her body processes medication. Think about the pharmacokinetic effects of drugs on her body. What processes would you discuss with her?

_____

_____

_____

_____

_____

_____

2. You feel like you're coming down with a cold and have had a sore throat since yesterday. You mention this to a friend, and she tells you that she still has antibiotics that she was prescribed when she had strep throat last month. She offers the medicine to you and suggests that you can finish the rest of it. What would you say to her?

_____

_____

_____

_____

_____

_____

Work Product 1

Apply pharmacology principles to prepare and administer oral and parenteral (excluding IV) medications.

Tavon Lake came to the office with an infection. Dr. Foley prescribed 250 mg tablets of erythromycin to be taken 4 times a day for 10 days. The first tablet was to be taken at the office. You watched as Mr. Lake took the first tablet, which you provided, and you gave him oral and written directions for taking the rest of the medicine. The prescription was called into his pharmacy for him to pick up.

If you are currently working in a medical office, use a blank paper patient chart from the office. If this is not available to you, use the space below to record the information above in the chart.

_____

_____

_____

_____

_____

_____

_____

Chapter Self-Assessment Quiz

1. A physician needs to register with the U.S. Attorney General:
   a. every 3 years.
   b. every 2 years.
   c. every 4 years.
   d. only once; registration is for life.
   e. every year.

2. When a drug is contraindicated, it:
   a. is not properly eliminated.
   b. is distributed throughout the bloodstream.
   c. should not be used.
   d. is detected in urine excretion.
   e. should be retested for accuracy.

3. Emetics are used to:
   a. dilate bronchi.
   b. prevent symptoms of menopause.
   c. control diabetes.
   d. dissolve blood clots.
   e. promote vomiting.

4. Which substance is an example of a Schedule I controlled substance?
   a. Morphine
   b. Ritalin
   c. Amphetamines
   d. Opium
   e. Tylenol with codeine

5. Which drug below is an example of an antipyretic?
   a. Aspirin
   b. Dramamine
   c. Lanoxin
   d. Zantac
   e. Benylin

6. A symptom of an allergic reaction is:
   a. nausea.
   b. drowsiness.
   c. dryness of mouth.
   d. hives.
   e. fever.

7. Two drugs when taken together that can create synergism are:
   a. sedatives and barbiturates.
   b. antacids and antibiotics.
   c. diuretics and decongestants.
   d. antibiotics and antifungals.
   e. antihypertensives and expectorants.

8. The DEA is a branch of the:
   a. BNDD.
   b. DOJ.
   c. FDA.
   d. AMA.
   e. AHFS.

9. All drugs cause:
   a. cellular and physiological change.
   b. cellular and psychological change.
   c. physiological and psychological change.
   d. physiological changes.
   e. cellular, physiological, and psychological change.

10. Green leafy vegetables can sometimes interact with:
    a. coumadin.
    b. verapamil.
    c. ibuprofen.
    d. amoxicillin.
    e. phenobarbital.

11. Drugs with a potential for abuse and currently accepted medicinal use are:
    a. Schedule I drugs.
    b. Schedule II drugs.
    c. Schedule III drugs.
    d. Schedule IV drugs.
    e. Schedule I and IV drugs.

12. A drug is given a brand name when it:
    a. is first developed in laboratories.
    b. is used in field testing and studies.
    c. is assigned a sponsor for the research.
    d. is approved by the FDA.
    e. is available for commercial use.

Scenario: A teenaged patient has called in saying that the pharmacy will not refill her painkiller prescription. It has been just over a month since she last refilled her prescription.

13. What is the first step you should take?

a. Check her records to see how many more refills she has left.

b. Inform the physician about the situation for directions.

c. Call the pharmacy to find out how many refills she has gotten.

d. Write out another prescription and fax it to the pharmacy.

e. Inform the patient that she has no more refills remaining.

14. The patient still has three remaining refills on her prescription. After you call the pharmacy, however, you are informed that the patient has been purchasing over-the-counter painkillers along with her prescription. There is suspicion that the patient might be selling her medication and taking over-the-counter drugs. What do you do?

a. Call the patient and confront her about the purchases.

b. Discuss the possibility of drug abuse with the physician.

c. Call the police immediately and report the patient.

d. Tell the pharmacy to give her the prescriptions anyway.

e. Gather information and report your findings.

End Scenario

15. The study of how drugs act on the body, including cells, tissues, and organs, is:

a. pharmacokinetics.

b. pharmacodynamics.

c. synergism.

d. antagonism.

e. potentiation.

16. What kind of drug is used to increase the size of arterial blood vessels?

a. Anticonvulsants

b. Emetics

c. Cholinergics

d. Antihypertensives

e. Immunologic agents

17. Which of the following is a trait of a Schedule I drug?

a. No accepted safety standards

b. Cannot be prescribed by a physician

c. Lowest potential for abuse

d. May be filled up to five times in six months

e. Requires a handwritten prescription

18. When you are administering a controlled substance in a medical office, you must include:

a. drug schedule.

b. time of administration.

c. patient allergies.

d. your name.

e. location.

19. If a patient is receiving a medication that has a high incidence of allergic reactions, how long should the patient wait before leaving the office?

a. No wait time necessary

b. 5 to 10 minutes

c. 10 to 20 minutes

d. 30 minutes to an hour

e. Overnight observation

20. The chemical name of a drug is the:

a. last name a drug is given before it is put on the market.

b. description of the chemical compounds found in the drug.

c. name given to the drug during research and development.

d. name given to the drug by the FDA and AMA.

e. name of the chemical the drug supplements in the body.

Preparing and Administering Medications

Chapter Checklist

☐ Read textbook chapter and take notes within the Chapter Notes outline. Answer the Learning Objectives as you reach them in the content, and then check them off.

☐ Work the Content Review questions—both Foundational Knowledge and Application.

☐ Perform the Active Learning exercise(s).

☐ Complete Professional Journal entries.

☐ Complete Skill Practice Activity(s) using Competency Evaluation Forms and Work Products, when appropriate.

☐ Take the Chapter Self-Assessment Quiz.

☐ Insert all appropriate pages into your portfolio.

Learning Objectives

1. Spell and define the key terms.
2. List the safety guidelines for medication administration.
3. Explain and demonstrate how to correctly calculate an adult medication dosage.
4. Explain the differences between various parenteral and non-parenteral routes of medication administration.
5. Describe the parts of a syringe and needle and name those parts that must be kept sterile.
6. List the various needle lengths, gauges, and preferred site for each type of injection.
7. Compare the types of injections and locate the sites where each may be administered safely.
8. Describe principles of intravenous (IV) therapy.

Chapter Notes

Note: Bold-faced headings are the major headings in the text chapter; headings in regular font are lower-level headings (i.e., the content is subordinate to, or falls "under," the major headings). Make sure you understand the key terms used in the chapter, as well as the concepts presented as Key Points.

TEXT SUBHEADINGS   **NOTES**

Introduction _____

_____

_____

☐ **LEARNING OBJECTIVE 1:** Spell and define the key terms.

_____

Medication Administration Basics

Key Point:
- As a clinical medical assistant, you must look up any drugs you are not familiar with to determine the drug classification, the usual dosage, and the route of administration.

Safety Guidelines

Key Point:
- To ensure safety when administering medications, follow these guidelines.

☐ **LEARNING OBJECTIVE 2:** List the safety guidelines for medication administration.

Seven Rights for Correct Medication Administration

Key Terms: parenteral; otic; ophthalmic; topical
Key Point:
- By observing the seven rights during medication administration, you will eliminate the potential for many errors.

Systems of Measurement

Key Terms: metric system; apothecary system of measurement
Key Point:
- Both the **apothecary** and the household systems of measurement should be avoided in the medical setting, since the measurements are not as accurate as in the **metric system**.

Metric, Household, and Apothecary

Key Points:
- Because the metric system is based on multiples of 10, decimals, not fractions, are used in calculating and recording dosages.
- The apothecary system is used less frequently now than in the past and is gradually being replaced by the metric system.
- While this system is not used in the medical office for calculating doses, patients may need to be instructed on the proper household measurement for taking medications ordered in the metric system.

Converting between Systems of Measurement _____

_____

_____

Apothecary or Household to Metric _____

_____

_____

Metric to Metric _____

_____

_____

Calculating Adult Dosages _____

_____

Key Point:
- Although the physician will order the amount of medication to be administered to the patient, you may have to calculate the amount of medication to withdraw into a syringe or pour into a medicine cup.

Ratio and Proportion _____

_____

_____

The Formula Method _____

_____

_____

☐ **LEARNING OBJECTIVE 3:** Explain and demonstrate how to correctly calculate an adult medication dosage.

_____

Calculating Pediatric Dosages _____

_____

Key Point:
- Although several formulas may be used to calculate children's doses, one method uses the body surface area (BSA) and is considered to be the most accurate method for children up to 12 years of age or adults who are below normal percentiles for body weight.

Routes of Medication Administration _____

_____

Key Point:
- Medication can be administered in many ways and is chosen by the physician after considering many factors.

_____

Oral, Sublingual, and Buccal Routes

Key Terms: sublingual; buccal
Key Points:
- Of all of the medication routes, the oral route is most preferred by patients and is the easiest to administer.
- Medication taken sublingually is placed under the patient's tongue; it must not be swallowed.
- Medication given by the **buccal** route is placed in the pouch between the cheek and gum at the side of the mouth.

Parenteral Administration

Key Point:
- Administration by injection is the most efficient method of parenteral drug administration, but it can also be the most hazardous.

☐ **LEARNING OBJECTIVE 4:** Explain the differences between various parenteral and non-parenteral routes of medication administration.

Equipment for Injections

Ampules, Vials, and Cartridges

Key Terms: ampules; vials; diluent
Key Points:
- **Ampules** are small glass containers that must be broken at the neck so that the solution can be aspirated into the syringe.
- **Vials** are glass or plastic containers sealed at the top by a rubber stopper.
- Prefilled syringes contain a premeasured amount of medication in a disposable cartridge with a needle attached.

Needles and Syringes

Key Term: gauge
Key Points:
- All syringes consist of a plunger, body or barrel, flange, and tip.
- Needle lengths vary from 3/8 inch to 1 1/2 inch for standard injections.
- Needle **gauge** varies from 18 (large) to 30 (small); the higher the number, the smaller the gauge.
- Choose the package with a needle length and gauge appropriate for the route of the injection.
- The insulin syringe is used strictly for administering insulin subcutaneously to diabetic patients.

☐ **LEARNING OBJECTIVE 5:** Describe the parts of a syringe and needle and name those parts that must be kept sterile.

☐ **LEARNING OBJECTIVE 6:** List the various needle lengths, gauges, and preferred site for each type of injection.

Types of Injections

Intradermal Injections

Key Terms: Mantoux; induration
Key Points:
- Intradermal medications are administered into the dermal layer of the skin by inserting the needle at a 10 to 15 degree angle, almost parallel to the skin.
- A positive **Mantoux** reaction has **induration**, a hard raised area over the injection site, larger than 10 mm. This positive reaction indicates the possibility of exposure to tuberculosis; however, it does not indicate that the patient has active tuberculosis.

Subcutaneous Injections

Key Point:
- The subcutaneous route is chosen for drugs that should not be absorbed as rapidly as through the intramuscular or intravenous (IV) route.

Intramuscular Injections

Key Points:
• Absorption of IM medications is fairly rapid because of the rich vascularity of muscle.
• The muscle chosen for the injection depends on the preference of the medical assistant, the patient, and the amount of medication to be administered.

Z-Track Method of Intramuscular Injections

Key Point:
• This method is used for IM administration of medications that may irritate or damage the tissues if allowed to leak back along the line of injection.

☐ **LEARNING OBJECTIVE 7:** Compare the types of injections and locate the sites where each may be administered safely.

Other Medication Routes

Rectal Administration

Key Point:
• Rectal medications may be used for patients who are NPO (allowed nothing by mouth) or who have nausea and vomiting, but they are never used for patients who have diarrhea.

Vaginal Administration

Key Point:
• Very few medications other than those for local effects are prescribed for vaginal administration.

Transdermal Administration

Key Term: topical medications
Key Point:
• **Topical medications** (creams, ointments, sprays, and lotions) produce local effects, while transdermal medications produce systemic effects.

Inhalation _____

_____

Key Term: nebulizer
Key Point:
- Medication administered by inhalation is absorbed quickly through the alveolar walls into the capillaries, but a disease condition may make absorption difficult to predict.

Principles of Intravenous (IV) Therapy _____

_____

Key Point:
- IV medication has the quickest action because it enters the bloodstream immediately.

Intravenous Equipment _____

_____

Key Point:
- Examples of fluids that come prepackaged for use in IV therapy are Ringer's lactate (RL), dextrose 5% and water (D_5W), 0.9% normal saline, 0.45% normal saline, or a combination (D_5NS, D_5RL).

Troubleshooting Problems _____

_____

Key Term: infiltration
Key Points:
- The medical assistant must be vigilant about watching the IV fluids and the site of venipuncture.
- In case of **infiltration**, stop the flow of fluids, remove the catheter, and notify the physician.
- Phlebitis may occur when the intravenous catheter has caused inflammation in the vein or when there is an infection present.

☐ **LEARNING OBJECTIVE 8:** Describe principles of intravenous (IV) therapy.

Content Review

FOUNDATIONAL KNOWLEDGE

Measurements

1. Physician's Orders

As a medical assistant, you may be called on to prepare medications. The patient's safety relies on good communication between the physician and yourself. Identify the safety rules you should use to prevent communication errors.

Rule	Yes	No
a. Confirm all medications verbally. Do not try to interpret the physician's handwriting.		
b. Use previous medications and dosages listed on the patient's chart as a safety check.		
b. Check with the physician if you have any doubt about a medication or an order.		

The Right Stuff

2. Once you have correctly interpreted the medications ordered by the physician, you must locate the correct drugs to dispense. Identify which rules prevent errors with dispensing incorrect drugs.

	Yes	No
a. Check the label when taking the medication from the shelf, when preparing it, and again when replacing it on the shelf or disposing of the empty container.		
b. Peel off the label from the medication and place it in the patient's record.		
c. Place the order and the medication side by side to compare for accuracy.		
d. Only fill prescriptions written using brand names.		
e. Read labels carefully. Do not scan labels or medication orders.		
f. Use a resource like the Internet to cross-reference generic and brand names for medications.		
g. It is always safer to give a medication poured or drawn up by someone more experienced.		

3. Once you have correctly interpreted and identified the medications ordered by the physician, you must safely dispense and administer these drugs. Identify which rules prevent mistakes in dispensing and administering medications.

	Yes	No
a. Know the policies of your office regarding the administration of medications.		
b. Never question the physician's written orders.		
c. Prepare medications in the presence of the patient so you can discuss what you are doing and answer the patient's questions.		
d. Check the strength of the medication (e.g., 250 versus 500 mg) and the route of administration.		
e. If you are interrupted, return the medicine to its original container so you can correctly identify it when you come back and finish.		
f. Work in a quiet, well-lit area.		
g. Check the patient's medical record for allergies to the actual medication or its components before administering.		

h. Measure exactly. Always read a meniscus where it touches the glass.		
i. Shake liquid medications vigorously before measuring to ensure they are well mixed.		
j. Never give a medication poured or drawn up by someone else.		
k. Stay with the patient while he or she takes oral medication. Watch for any reaction and record the patient's response.		

4. It's All About Me

Self-protection has many aspects. Review these steps and correctly identify those that protect you.

	Yes	No
a. Have sharps containers as close to the area of use as possible.		
b. Put on gloves for all procedures that might result in contact with blood or bodily fluids.		
c. Recap used needles to protect against accidental jabs.		
d. Bend or break used needles to prevent accidental reuse.		
e. Never document medication given by someone else, and do not ask someone else to document medication that you have administered.		

5. Protecting the Drugs

The medications themselves have to be protected for the patient's health. Identify which rules protect your office's medications.

	Yes	No
a. Check the medication's expiration date. Outdated medications should be used quickly.		
b. Be alert for color changes, precipitation, odor, or any indication that the medication's properties have changed. If the medication has changed in consistency, color, or odor, discard it appropriately.		
c. Keep narcotics on your person so others do not have access to them.		
d. Never leave the medication cabinet unlocked when it is not in use.		
e. Never give keys for the medication cabinet to an unauthorized person. Limit access to the medication cabinet by limiting access to the cabinet keys.		

6. How Much?

The physician orders enoxaparin 75 mg SC. The label on the package reads 150 mg/mL. Find the correct dosage for this patient. Show your work.

7. Where Did It Go?

What are the primary differences between enteral, parenteral, and topical medications? Give your answer in terms of where the medication is supposed to have an effect and how it is meant to get there.

8. The Syringe

List the four parts of a syringe that must be kept sterile.

a. _____

b. _____

c. _____

d. _____

Administration Routes

9. What size needle would you use for the following administration routes?

Route	Gauge	Length
IM		
SC		

10. Match the injection to the proper locations.

a. intradermal (ID)	**1.** abdomen
b. adult intramuscular (IM)	**2.** anterior forearm
c. juvenile (<2 years old) intramuscular (IM)	**3.** back
d. Z-track intramuscular (IM)	**4.** deltoid
e. subcutaneous (SC)	**5.** dorsalgluteal
	6. rectus femoris
	7. thigh
	8. upper arm
	9. vastus lateralis
	10. ventrogluteal

11. What is a major advantage of starting an IV line on a patient?

_____

_____

12. What are the components of an IV setup?

a. _____

b. _____

c. _____

d. _____

13. You are directed to give a heroin addict 30 mg of methadone. Convert this dosage to micrograms and grams.

_____

_____

14. Name two routes that are enteral, or passing through the GI tract.

a. _____

b. _____

15. Identify the route indicated below.

    a. ear drops _____

    b. eye drops _____

    c. fentanyl patch _____

    d. lotion _____

    e. Mantoux test _____

    f. nebulizer _____

    g. suppositories _____

    h. syrup taken by mouth _____

16. Identify whether the following administration routes are normally local, systemic, or both.

Route	Local	Systemic
a. buccal		
b. dermal		
c. inhalation		
d. intradermal		
e. intramuscular		
f. intravenous		
g. ophthalmic		
h. oral		
i. otic		
j. rectal		
k. subcutaneous		
l. sublingual		
m. transdermal		
n. vaginal		

17. Identify the following as parenteral or enteral.

Route	Parenteral	Enteral
a. buccal		
b. inhalation		
c. intramuscular		
d. intravenous		
e. oral		
f. rectal		
g. subcutaneous		
h. sublingual		
i. transdermal		

18. Circle the preferred sites for applying a transdermal patch.

abdomen	axilla	back	chest
behind the ear	forehead	groin	neck
scalp	thigh	upper arm	

19. Match the following key terms to their definitions.

Key Terms

a. ampule _____

b. apothecary system of measurement _____

c. buccal _____

d. diluent _____

e. gauge _____

f. induration _____

g. infiltration _____

h. Mantoux _____

i. metric system _____

j. nebulizer _____

k. ophthalmic _____

l. otic _____

m. parenteral _____

n. sublingual _____

o. topical _____

p. vial _____

Definitions

1. leakage of intravenous fluids into surrounding tissues

2. administration of medication between the cheek and gum of the mouth

3. all systemic administration routes excluding the gastrointestinal tract

4. a system of measurement that uses grams, liters, and meters

5. diameter of a needle lumen

6. device for administering respiratory medications as a fine inhaled spray

7. a tuberculosis screening test

8. small glass container that must be broken at the neck so that the solution can be aspirated into the syringe

9. administration route to a local spot on the outside of the body

10. administration route to the eyes

11. a system of measures based on drops, minims, grains, drams, and ounces

12. administration route to or by way of the ears

13. hardened area at the injection site after an intradermal screening test for tuberculosis

14. administration beneath the tongue

15. glass or plastic container sealed at the top by a rubber stopper

16. specified liquid used to reconstitute powder medications for injection

20. True or False? Determine whether the following statements are true or false. If false, explain why.

a. It is normal for frightened patients to have trouble breathing after taking a medication.

_____

_____

b. A sip of water will help a patient take nitroglycerine sublingually.

_____

_____

c. During SC and IM injections, a small amount of blood appears in the syringe when there is good penetration.

_____

_____

d. Redness, swelling, pain, and discomfort are normal complications of IV therapy.

_____

_____

APPLICATION

Critical Thinking Practice

1. Why shouldn't children under 2 years of age be given IM injections through the gluteal muscles?

_____

_____

2. Where would you insert a new IV when a patient has developed complications?

_____

_____

Patient Education

1. Your patient is a type I diabetic who is beginning to take insulin. She will have to begin calculating dosages and injecting herself. Assume a one-unit dose and write a sheet of instructions that clearly explains to the patient how to properly draw and inject this drug.

Documentation

1. The physician has asked you to prepare an administration of gr iii Haldol IM for a patient. The dispenser is labeled in milligrams. How do you convert this dosage to the metric system, and how many milligrams of Haldol should you dispense? Write the preparation as a chart note.

_____

_____

Active Learning

1. Accidental needlesticks are one of the most frightening occupational hazards you will encounter as a medical assistant. The greatest fear is centered on human immunodeficiency virus (HIV) and hepatitis B (HBV). Research the incubation, signs and symptoms, treatment, and prognosis associated with these two diseases. Prepare a one-page handout on each.

2. You may encounter abbreviations in the medical office where you work. Table 24-1 in the chapter lists the abbreviations that are safe to use in patients' charts as identified by the Joint Commission on the Accreditation of Health Organizations. Create flash cards for all abbreviations that are acceptable for use in the medical office. Then work with a partner to commit these abbreviations to memory.

Professional Journal

REFLECT

(Prompts and Ideas: What would you do if you received a needlestick injury? Have you considered the hazards of this profession? What are your feelings about working with potentially infectious patients?)

_____

_____

_____

_____

PONDER AND SOLVE

1. One of the physicians in your medical office would like to change office policy so that no abbreviations are used in the patients' medical charts for fear of potentially harmful errors. The office is divided on the issue. What's your opinion?

_____

_____

_____

_____

2. You are directed to give a Z-track IM injection to a patient. The patient's spouse observes you deliberately draw a bubble into the syringe and panics because you are about to inject air into the patient. How do you address the spouse's concerns?

_____

_____

_____

_____

EXPERIENCE

Skills related to this chapter include:

1. Administering Oral Medications (Procedure 24-1).
2. Preparing Injections (Procedure 24-2).
3. Administering an Intradermal Injection (Procedure 24-3).
4. Administering a Subcutaneous Injection (Procedure 24-4).
5. Administering an Intramuscular Injection (Procedure 24-5).
6. Administering an Intramuscular Injection Using the Z-track Method (Procedure 24-6).
7. Applying Transdermal Medications (Procedure 24-7).
8. Obtaining and Preparing an Intravenous Site (Procedure 24-8).

Record any common mistakes, lessons learned, and/or tips you discovered during your experience of practicing and demonstrating these skills:

_____

_____

_____

_____

Skill Practice

PERFORMANCE OBJECTIVES:

1. Administering oral medications (Procedure 24-1).
2. Preparing injections (Procedure 24-2).
3. Administering an intradermal injection (Procedure 24-3).
4. Administering a subcutaneous injection (Procedure 24-4).
5. Administering an intramuscular injection (Procedure 24-5).
6. Administering an intramuscular injection using the Z-track method (Procedure 24-6).
7. Applying transdermal medications (Procedure 24-7).
8. Obtaining and preparing an intravenous site (Procedure 24-8).

Name_____   Date _____   Time _____

Procedure 24-1:	ADMINISTERING ORAL MEDICATIONS

EQUIPMENT/SUPPLIES: Physician's order, oral medication, disposable calibrated cup, glass of water, patient's medical record

STANDARDS: Given the needed equipment and a place to work, the student will perform this skill with _____% accuracy in a total of _____ minutes. *(Your instructor will tell you what the percentage and time limits will be before you begin practicing.)*

KEY: 4 = Satisfactory   0 = Unsatisfactory   NA = This step is not counted

PROCEDURE STEPS	SELF	PARTNER	INSTRUCTOR
1. Wash your hands.	☐	☐	☐
2. Review the physician's medication order and select the correct oral medication. **a.** Compare the label with the physician's instructions. **b.** Note the expiration date. **c.** Check the label three times: when taking it from the shelf, while pouring, and when returning to the shelf.	☐	☐	☐
3. Calculate the correct dosage to be given if necessary.	☐	☐	☐
4. If using a multidose container, remove cap from container. For single-dose medications, obtain the correct amount of medication.	☐	☐	☐
5. Remove the correct dose of medication. **a.** For solid medications: (1) Pour the capsule/tablet into the bottle cap, (2) Transfer the medication to a disposable cup. **b.** For liquid medications: (1) Open the bottle lid: place it on a flat surface with open end up. (2) Palm the label to prevent liquids from dripping onto the label. (3) With opposite hand, place the thumbnail at the correct calibration. (4) Pour the medication until the proper amount is in the cup.	☐	☐	☐
6. Greet and identify the patient. Explain the procedure.	☐	☐	☐
7. Ask the patient about medication allergies that might not be noted on the chart.	☐	☐	☐
8. Give the patient a glass of water, unless contraindicated. Hand the patient the disposable cup containing the medication or pour the tablets or capsules into the patient's hand.	☐	☐	☐
9. Remain with the patient to be sure that all of the medication is swallowed. **a.** Observe any unusual reactions and report them to the physician. **b.** Record in the medical record.	☐	☐	☐
10. Thank the patient and give any appropriate instructions.	☐	☐	☐
11. Wash your hands.	☐	☐	☐
12. Record the procedure in the patient's medical record. Note the date, time, name of medication, dose administered, route of administration, and your name.	☐	☐	☐

CALCULATION

Total Possible Points: _____
Total Points Earned: _____ Multiplied by 100 = _____ Divided by Total Possible Points = _____%

Pass　**Fail**
☐　　☐　　Comments:

Student's signature _____ Date _____
Partner's signature _____ Date _____
Instructor's signature _____ Date _____

Name _____   Date _____   Time _____

Procedure 24-2:	**PREPARING INJECTIONS**

EQUIPMENT/SUPPLIES: Physician's order, medication for injection in ampule or vial, antiseptic wipes, appropriate-size needle and syringe, small gauze pad, biohazard sharps container, patient's medical record

STANDARDS: Given the needed equipment and a place to work, the student will perform this skill with _____% accuracy in a total of _____ minutes. *(Your instructor will tell you what the percentage and time limits will be before you begin practicing.)*

KEY: 4 = Satisfactory   0 = Unsatisfactory   NA = This step is not counted

PROCEDURE STEPS	SELF	PARTNER	INSTRUCTOR
1. Wash your hands.	☐	☐	☐
2. Review the physician's medication order and select the correct medication.	☐	☐	☐
a. Compare the label with the physician's instructions. Note the expiration date.			
b. Check the label three times: when taking it from the shelf, while drawing it up into the syringe, and when returning to the shelf.			
3. Calculate the correct dosage to be given, if necessary.	☐	☐	☐
4. Choose the needle and syringe according to the route of administration, type of medication, and size of the patient.	☐	☐	☐
5. Open the needle and syringe package. Assemble if necessary. Secure the needle to the syringe.	☐	☐	☐
6. Withdraw the correct amount of medication:	☐	☐	☐
a. From an ampule:			
(1) Tap the stem of the ampule lightly.			
(2) Place a piece of gauze around the ampule neck.			
(3) Grasp the gauze and ampule firmly. Snap the stem off the ampule.			
(4) Dispose of the ampule top in a biohazard sharps container.			
(5) Insert the needle lumen below the level of the medication.			
(6) Withdraw the medication.			
(7) Dispose of the ampule in a biohazard sharps container.			
(8) Remove any air bubbles in the syringe.			
(9) Draw back on the plunger to add a small amount of air; then gently push the plunger forward to eject the air out of the syringe.			
b. From a vial:			
(1) Using the antiseptic wipe, cleanse the rubber stopper of the vial.			
(2) Pull air into the syringe with the amount equivalent to the amount of medication to be removed from the vial.			
(3) Insert the needle into the vial top. Inject the air from the syringe.			
(4) With the needle inside the vial, invert the vial.			
(5) Hold the syringe at eye level.			

PROCEDURE STEPS	SELF	PARTNER	INSTRUCTOR
(6) Aspirate the desired amount of medication into the syringe. **(7)** Displace any air bubbles in the syringe by gently tapping the barrel. **(8)** Remove the air by pushing the plunger slowly and forcing the air into the vial.			
7. Carefully recap the needle using one-hand technique.	☐	☐	☐

CALCULATION

Total Possible Points: _____
Total Points Earned: _____ Multiplied by 100 = _____ Divided by Total Possible Points = _____%

Pass **Fail**
☐   ☐   Comments:

Student's signature _____ Date _____
Partner's signature _____ Date _____
Instructor's signature _____ Date _____

Name _____ Date _____ Time _____

Procedure 24-3:	ADMINISTERING AN INTRADERMAL INJECTION

EQUIPMENT/SUPPLIES: Physician's order, medication for injection in ampule or vial, antiseptic wipes, appropriate-size needle and syringe, small gauze pad, biohazard sharps container, clean examination gloves, patient's medical record

STANDARDS: Given the needed equipment and a place to work, the student will perform this skill with _____% accuracy in a total of _____ minutes. *(Your instructor will tell you what the percentage and time limits will be before you begin practicing.)*

KEY: 4 = Satisfactory   0 = Unsatisfactory   NA = This step is not counted

PROCEDURE STEPS	SELF	PARTNER	INSTRUCTOR
1. Wash your hands.	☐	☐	☐
a. Review the physician's medication order and select the correct medication.			
b. Compare the label with the physician's instructions. Note the expiration date.			
c. Check the label three times: when taking it from the shelf, while drawing it up into the syringe, and when returning it to the shelf.			
2. Prepare the injection according to the steps in Procedure 24-2.	☐	☐	☐
3. Greet and identify the patient. Explain the procedure.	☐	☐	☐
4. Ask patient about medication allergies.	☐	☐	☐
5. Select the appropriate site for the injection.	☐	☐	☐
6. Prepare the site by cleansing with an antiseptic wipe.	☐	☐	☐
7. Put on gloves. Remove the needle guard.	☐	☐	☐
8. Using your nondominant hand, pull the patient's skin taut.	☐	☐	☐
9. With the bevel of the needle facing upward, insert needle at a 10- to 15-degree angle into the upper layer of the skin.	☐	☐	☐
a. When the bevel of the needle is under the skin, stop inserting the needle.			
b. The needle will be slightly visible below the surface of the skin.			
c. It is not necessary to aspirate when performing an intradermal injection.			
10. Inject the medication slowly by depressing the plunger.	☐	☐	☐
a. A wheal will form as the medication enters the dermal layer of the skin.			
b. Hold the syringe steady for proper administration.			
11. Remove the needle from the skin at the same angle at which it was inserted.	☐	☐	☐
a. Do not use an antiseptic wipe or gauze pad over the site.			
b. Do not press or massage the site. Do not apply an adhesive bandage.			
12. Do not recap the needle.	☐	☐	☐

PROCEDURE STEPS	SELF	PARTNER	INSTRUCTOR
13. Dispose of the needle and syringe in an approved biohazard sharps container.	☐	☐	☐
14. Remove your gloves, and wash your hands.	☐	☐	☐
15. Depending upon the type of skin test administered, the length of time required for the body tissues to react, and the policies of the medical office, perform one of the following: **a.** Read the test results. Inspect and palpate the site for the presence and amount of induration. **b.** Tell the patient when to return (date and time) to the office to have the results read. **c.** Instruct the patient to read the results at home. **d.** Make sure the patient understands the instructions.	☐	☐	☐
16. Document the procedure, the site, and the results. If instructions were given to the patient, document these also.	☐	☐	☐

CALCULATION

Total Possible Points: _____
Total Points Earned: _____ Multiplied by 100 = _____ Divided by Total Possible Points = _____%

Pass   **Fail**
☐   ☐   Comments:

Student's signature _____ Date _____
Partner's signature _____ Date _____
Instructor's signature _____ Date _____

Name_____ Date _____ Time _____

Procedure 24-4:	ADMINISTERING A SUBCUTANEOUS INJECTION

EQUIPMENT/SUPPLIES: Physician's order, medication for injection in ampule or vial, antiseptic wipes, appropriate size needle and syringe, small gauze pad, biohazard sharps container, clean examination gloves, adhesive bandage, patient's medical record

STANDARDS: Given the needed equipment and a place to work, the student will perform this skill with _____% accuracy in a total of _____ minutes. *(Your instructor will tell you what the percentage and time limits will be before you begin practicing.)*

KEY: 4 = Satisfactory   0 = Unsatisfactory   NA = This step is not counted

PROCEDURE STEPS	SELF	PARTNER	INSTRUCTOR

1. Wash your hands.
  a. Review the physician's medication order and select the correct medication.
  b. Compare the label with the physician's instructions. Note the expiration date.
  c. Check the label three times: when taking it from the shelf, while drawing it up into the syringe, and when returning it to the shelf.
	☐	☐	☐

2. Prepare the injection according to the steps in Procedure 24-2.	☐	☐	☐
3. Greet and identify the patient. Explain the procedure.	☐	☐	☐
4. Ask the patient about medication allergies.	☐	☐	☐
5. Select the appropriate site for the injection.	☐	☐	☐
6. Prepare the site by cleansing with an antiseptic.	☐	☐	☐
7. Put on gloves.	☐	☐	☐
8. Using your nondominant hand, hold the skin surrounding the injection site.	☐	☐	☐
9. With a firm motion, insert the needle into the tissue at a 45-degree angle to the skin surface.	☐	☐	☐
10. Hold the barrel between the thumb and the index finger of your dominant hand.	☐	☐	☐
11. Insert the needle completely to the hub.	☐	☐	☐
12. Remove your nondominant hand from the skin.	☐	☐	☐
13. Holding the syringe steady, pull back on the syringe gently. If blood appears in the hub or the syringe, do not inject the medication; remove the needle and prepare a new injection.	☐	☐	☐
14. Inject the medication slowly by depressing the plunger.	☐	☐	☐

15. Place a gauze pad over the injection site and remove the needle.
  a. Gently massage the injection site with the gauze pad.
  b. Do not recap the used needle; place it in the biohazard sharps container.
  c. Apply an adhesive bandage if needed.
	☐	☐	☐

16. Remove your gloves and wash your hands.	☐	☐	☐

PROCEDURE STEPS	SELF	PARTNER	INSTRUCTOR

17. An injection given for allergy desensitization requires:
    a. Keeping the patient in the office for at least 30 minutes for observation.
    b. Notifying the doctor of any reaction. (Be alert, anaphylaxis is possible.)
	☐	☐	☐

18. Document the procedure, the site, and the results. If instructions were given to the patient, document these also.	☐	☐	☐

CALCULATION

Total Possible Points: _____
Total Points Earned: _____ Multiplied by 100 = _____ Divided by Total Possible Points = _____%

Pass   **Fail**
☐   ☐

Comments:

Student's signature _____ Date _____
Partner's signature _____ Date _____
Instructor's signature _____ Date _____

Name_____ Date _____ Time _____

Procedure 24-7:	**APPLYING TRANSDERMAL MEDICATIONS**

EQUIPMENT/SUPPLIES: Physician's order, medication, clean examination gloves, patient's medical record

STANDARDS: Given the needed equipment and a place to work, the student will perform this skill with _____% accuracy in a total of _____ minutes. *(Your instructor will tell you what the percentage and time limits will be before you begin practicing.)*

KEY: 4 = Satisfactory   0 = Unsatisfactory   NA = This step is not counted

PROCEDURE STEPS	SELF	PARTNER	INSTRUCTOR
1. Wash your hands.	☐	☐	☐

2. Review the physician's medication order and select the correct medication.
  a. Compare the label with the physician's instructions. Note the expiration date.
  b. Check the label three times: when taking it from the shelf, while drawing it up into the syringe, and when returning to the shelf.
	☐	☐	☐

3. Greet and identify the patient. Explain the procedure.	☐	☐	☐
4. Ask the patient about medication allergies that might not be noted on the medical record.	☐	☐	☐

5. Select the appropriate site and perform any necessary skin preparation. The sites are usually the upper arm, the chest or back surface, or behind the ear.
  a. Ensure that the skin is clean, dry, and free from any irritation.
  b. Do not shave areas with excessive hair; trim the hair closely with scissors.
	☐	☐	☐

6. If there is a transdermal patch already in place, remove it carefully while wearing gloves. Discard the patch in the trash container. Inspect the site for irritation.	☐	☐	☐
7. Open the medication package by pulling the two sides apart. Do not touch the area of medication.	☐	☐	☐

8. Apply the medicated patch to the patient's skin, following the manufacturer's directions.
  a. Press the adhesive edges down firmly all around, starting at the center and pressing outward.
  b. If the edges do not stick, fasten with tape.
	☐	☐	☐

9. Wash your hands.	☐	☐	☐
10. Document the procedure and the site of the new patch in the medical record.	☐	☐	☐

CALCULATION

Total Possible Points: _____
Total Points Earned: _____ Multiplied by 100 = _____ Divided by Total Possible Points = _____%

Pass   **Fail**
☐   ☐   Comments:

Student's signature _____ Date _____
Partner's signature _____ Date _____
Instructor's signature _____ Date _____

Name_____ Date _____ Time _____

Procedure 24-8:	OBTAINING AND PREPARING AN INTRAVENOUS SITE

EQUIPMENT/SUPPLIES: Physician's order including the type of fluid to be used and the rate, intravenous solution, infusion administration set, IV pole, blank labels, appropriate size intravenous catheter, antiseptic wipes, tourniquet, small gauze pad, biohazard sharps container, clean examination gloves, bandage tape, adhesive bandage, patient's medical record, intravenous catheter (angiocath)

STANDARDS: Given the needed equipment and a place to work, the student will perform this skill with _____% accuracy in a total of _____ minutes. *(Your instructor will tell you what the percentage and time limits will be before you begin practicing.)*

KEY: 4 = Satisfactory   0 = Unsatisfactory   NA = This step is not counted

PROCEDURE STEPS	SELF	PARTNER	INSTRUCTOR
1. Wash your hands.	☐	☐	☐
2. Review the physician's order and select the correct IV catheter, solution, and administration set. **a.** Compare the label on the infusate solution and administration set with the physician's order. **b.** Note the expiration dates on the infusion solution and the administration set.	☐	☐	☐
3. Prepare the infusion solution by attaching a label to the solution indicating the date, time and name of the patient who will be receiving the IV. **a.** Hang the solution on an IV pole. **b.** Remove the administration set from the package and close the roller clamp.	☐	☐	☐
4. Remove the end of the administration set by removing the cover on the spike (located above the drip chamber). **a.** Remove the cover from the solution infusion port (located on the bottom of the bag). **b.** Insert the spike end of the administration set into the IV fluid.	☐	☐	☐
5. Fill the drip chamber on the administration set by squeezing the drip chamber until about half full.	☐	☐	☐
6. Open the roller clamp and allow fluid to flow from the drip chamber through the length of the tubing, displacing any air. Do not remove the cover protecting the end of the tubing. **a.** Close the roller clamp when the fluid has filled the tubing and no air is noted. **b.** Drape the filled tubing over the IV pole and proceed to perform a venipuncture.	☐	☐	☐
7. Greet and identify the patient. Explain the procedure.	☐	☐	☐
8. Ask the patient about medication allergies that might not be noted on the medical record.	☐	☐	☐
9. Prepare the IV start equipment by tearing or cutting 2 to 3 strips of tape that will be used to secure the IV catheter after insertion; also, inspect each arm for the best available vein.	☐	☐	☐
10. Wearing gloves, apply the tourniquet 1 to 2 inches above the intended venipuncture site. **a.** The tourniquet should be snug, but not too tight. **b.** Ask the patient to open and close the fist of the selected arm to distend the veins.	☐	☐	☐

PROCEDURE STEPS	SELF	PARTNER	INSTRUCTOR
11. Secure the tourniquet by using the half-bow.	☐	☐	☐
12. Make sure the ends of the tourniquet extend upward to avoid contaminating the venipuncture site.	☐	☐	☐
13. Select a vein by palpating with your gloved index finger to trace the path of the vein and judge its depth.	☐	☐	☐
14. Release the tourniquet after palpating the vein if it has been left on for more than 1 minute.	☐	☐	☐
15. Prepare the site by cleansing with an antiseptic wipe using a circular motion.	☐	☐	☐
16. Place the end of the administration set tubing on the examination table for easy access after the venipuncture.	☐	☐	☐
17. Anchor the vein to be punctured by placing the thumb of your nondominant hand below the intended site and holding the skin taut.	☐	☐	☐
18. Remove the needle cover from the IV catheter. **a.** While holding the catheter by the flash chamber, not the hub of the needle, use the dominant hand to insert the needle and catheter unit directly into the top of the vein, with the bevel of the needle up at a 15- to 20-degree angle for superficial veins. **b.** Observe for a blood flashback into the flash chamber.	☐	☐	☐
19. When the blood flashback is observed, lower the angle of the needle until it is flush with the skin and slowly advance the needle and catheter unit about 1\4 inch.	☐	☐	☐
20. Once the needle and catheter unit has been inserted slightly into the lumen of the vein hold the flash chamber of the needle steady with the nondominant hand **a.** Slide the catheter (using the catheter hub) off the needle and into the vein with the dominant hand. **b.** Advance the catheter into the vein up to the hub.	☐	☐	☐
21. With the needle partly occluding the catheter, release the tourniquet.	☐	☐	☐
22. Remove the needle and discard into a biohazard sharps container. **a.** Connect the end of the administration tubing to the end of the IV catheter that has been inserted into the vein. **b.** Open the roller clamp and adjust the flow according the physician's order.	☐	☐	☐
23. Secure the hub of the IV catheter with tape. **a.** Place one small strip, sticky side up, under the catheter. **b.** Cross one end over the hub and adhere onto the skin on the opposite side of the catheter. **c.** Cross the other end of the tape in the same fashion and adhere to the skin on the opposite side of the hub. **d.** A transparent membrane adhesive dressing can then be applied over the entire hub and insertion site.	☐	☐	☐
24. Make a small loop with the administration set tubing near the IV insertion site and secure with tape.	☐	☐	☐
25. Remove your gloves, wash your hands, and document the procedure in the medical record indicating the size of the IV catheter inserted, the location, the type of infusion, and the rate.	☐	☐	☐

CALCULATION

Total Possible Points: _____
Total Points Earned: _____ Multiplied by 100 = _____ Divided by Total Possible Points = _____%

Pass   **Fail**
☐   ☐   Comments:

Student's signature _____ Date _____
Partner's signature _____ Date _____
Instructor's signature _____ Date _____

Work Product 1

Apply pharmacology principles to prepare and administer oral and parenteral (excluding IV) medications.

Dr. Fosworth asked you to administer 125 milligrams of ampicillin in tablet form, along with a cup of water, to Stephanie Ciazzo at 9:15 in the morning. You observed the patient swallow the pill and gave her instructions on how to take the rest of the prescription.

If you are currently working in a medical office, use a blank paper patient chart from the office. If this is not available to you, use the space below to record the medication in the chart.

_____

_____

_____

_____

Work Product 2

Maintain medication and immunization records.

Janice Jones brought her 6-month-old daughter Akeelah to the office for her well-child visit. During this visit, Akeelah received all of the necessary immunizations suggested by the recommended schedule for immunization. First, research which immunizations should be administered at 6 months of age. Then document the administration of these immunizations below as if all recommended shots were given in the right and left thighs.

During the visit, Mrs. Jones asked if it was okay to give her daughter any medication to reduce swelling. The physician recommends 0.8 mL of infant acetaminophen to reduce discomfort.

If you are currently working in a medical office, use a blank paper patient chart from the office. If this is not available to you, use the space below to record the immunizations in the chart.

_____

_____

_____

_____

Work Product 3

Document appropriately.

Rita Morris is required to have a TB test to participate in her university volunteer corps. She comes to the office and you administer the Mantoux test for tuberculosis. After administering the shot in her right forearm, you give her instructions for when to return to the office. Document this in the patient's chart or the lines below.

When Ms. Morris returns to the office 3 days later, there is a hard, raised area over the spot where you administered her injection. Now make a new note in the patient's chart documenting the results of her test and any further actions that are necessary.

_____

_____

_____

_____

1. When administering an unfamiliar drug, you should look up information on:
   a. alternate formulations.
   b. the chemical name.
   c. generic alternatives.
   d. side effects.
   e. the route of administration.

2. When preparing medications you should:
   a. use previous medications and dosages listed on the patient's chart as a safety check.
   b. use a resource like the Internet to cross-reference generic and brand names for medications.
   c. work in a quiet, well-lighted area.
   d. shake liquid medications vigorously before measuring to ensure they are well mixed.
   e. recap used needles to protect against accidental jabs.

3. Patient safety is protected by ensuring:
   a. the patient answers when you address him or her by name.
   b. you are administering the right drug.
   c. medications are delivered to the right room.
   d. you are using the right type of syringe.
   e. you write down and document medications before you give them.

4. When dispensing drugs be sure to convert units to:
   a. apothecary units.
   b. units used by the doctor.
   c. imperial units.
   d. units used on the labeling.
   e. metric units.

5. The basic unit of weight in the metric system is the:
   a. grain.
   b. gram.
   c. liter.
   d. newton.
   e. pound.

6. By what do you multiply the base metric unit if the prefix is "milli"?
   a. 0.000001
   b. 0.001
   c. 0.01
   d. 1000
   e. 1,000,000

7. What does 2 cc equal?
   a. 2 mg
   b. 2 mL
   c. 30 gr
   d. 120 mg
   e. 200 grains

8. What does 45 mL equal?
   a. 0.75 fl oz
   b. 1.5 fl oz
   c. 3.0 fl oz
   d. 4.5 fl oz
   e. 20.5 fl oz

9. The physician orders chloroquine syrup 100 mg oral for a 20-kg child. The concentration of the syrup is 50 mg/mL. How much medication do you give the child?
   a. 0.5 mL
   b. 2 mL
   c. 10 mL
   d. 40 mL
   e. 250 mL

10. Which method is the most accurate means of calculating pediatric dosages?
    a. Body weight method
    b. BSA method
    c. Clarke's rule
    d. Fried's rule
    e. Young's rule

11. Medicine administered under the tongue follows the:
    a. buccal route.
    b. dental route.
    c. dermal route.
    d. oral route.
    e. sublingual route.

12. Which item below is a multiple-dose dispenser?

   a. Ampule

   b. Cartridge

   c. Carpuject

   d. Tubex

   e. Vial

13. How large is a tuberculin syringe?

   a. 0.1 mL

   b. 1 mL

   c. 3 mL

   d. 5 mL

   e. 10 U

14. A possible site for an intradermal injection is the:

   a. antecubital fossa.

   b. anterior forearm.

   c. upper arm.

   d. deltoid.

   e. vastus lateralis.

Scenario: You are directed to set up an IV line delivering RL 30 mL/hr TKO with a 10 gtt/mL system.

15. How many drips per minute should the IV deliver?

   a. 1 gtt/min

   b. 3 gtt/min

   c. 5 gtt/min

   d. 10 gtt/min

   e. 20 gtt/min

16. A good site for the angiocatheter would be the:

   a. antecubital fossa.

   b. anterior forearm.

   c. upper arm.

   d. deltoid.

   e. vastus lateralis.

End Scenario

17. A good place to administer a 0.25 mL IM injection on a child is the:

   a. antecubital fossa.

   b. anterior forearm.

   c. upper arm.

   d. deltoid.

   e. vastus lateralis.

18. The physician orders Demerol 150 mg SC for a patient. The dispenser contains 20 mL at 100 mg/ml. Find the dosage.

   a. 0.67 mL

   b. 1.5 mL

   c. 2.5 mL

   d. 7.5 mL

   e. 30 mL

19. A good site to inject Demerol SC would be the:

   a. antecubital fossa.

   b. anterior forearm.

   c. upper arm.

   d. deltoid.

   e. vastus lateralis.

20. You are told to administer a medicine by the otic route. This medicine should be given by:

   a. the ears.

   b. inhaler.

   c. injection into the bone.

   d. the mouth.

   e. the nose.

Diagnostic Imaging

Chapter Checklist

- ☐ Read textbook chapter and take notes within the Chapter Notes outline. Answer the Learning Objectives as you reach them in the content, and then check them off.
- ☐ Work the Content Review questions—both Foundational Knowledge and Application.
- ☐ Perform the Active Learning exercise(s).
- ☐ Complete Professional Journal entries.
- ☐ Complete Skill Practice Activity(s) using Competency Evaluation Forms and Work Products, when appropriate.
- ☐ Take the Chapter Self-Assessment Quiz.
- ☐ Insert all appropriate pages into your Portfolio.

Learning Objectives

1. Spell and define the key terms.
2. Explain the theory and function of x-rays and x-ray machines.
3. State the principles of radiology.
4. Describe routine and contrast media, fluoroscopy, computed tomography, sonography, magnetic resonance imaging, nuclear medicine, and mammographic examinations.
5. Explain the role of the medical assistant in radiological procedures.

Chapter Notes

Note: Bold-faced headings are the major headings in the text chapter; headings in regular font are lower-level headings (i.e., the content is subordinate to, or falls "under," the major headings). Make sure you understand the key terms used in the chapter, as well as the concepts presented as Key Points.

TEXT SUBHEADINGS   **NOTES**

Introduction _____

_____

_____

☐ **LEARNING OBJECTIVE 1:** Spell and define the key terms.

_____

Principles of Radiology _____

_____

Key Terms: x-rays; magnetic resonance imaging; nuclear medicine; radiology

X-rays and X-ray Machines _____

_____

Key Terms: film; cassette; radiograph; radiography; radiolucent; radiopaque; radiologists
Key Points:
- X-rays are high-energy waves that cannot be seen, heard, felt, tasted, or smelled, and that can penetrate fairly dense objects, such as the human body.
- Images are formed on the x-ray film as the rays either pass through or are absorbed by the tissues of the body.

☐ **LEARNING OBJECTIVE 2:** Explain the theory and function of x-rays and x-ray machines.

☐ **LEARNING OBJECTIVE 3:** State the principles of radiology.

Outpatient X-rays _____

_____

Key Point:
- In some states, you may be permitted to take and process simple images such as bone or chest radiographs.

Patient Positioning _____

_____

Key Point:
- Because the human body is a three-dimensional structure, x-ray examinations usually require a minimum of two exposures taken at 90 degrees to each other.

Examination Sequencing _____

_____

Key Term: contrast medium
Key Point:
- Most radiographic procedures can be performed in any order of convenience, but certain procedures must follow certain sequences in specific situations.

Radiation Safety

Key Points:
- X-rays have the potential to cause cellular or genetic damage to the body, and the results of this damage may not manifest for several years after exposure.
- For both patients and medical assistants working around radiation, these concerns can be summed up in what is called the ALARA concept: doing whatever is necessary to keep radiation exposure *as low as reasonably achievable*.

Diagnostic Procedures

Mammography

Key Point:
- Mammography, x-ray examination of the breast, is used as a screening tool for breast cancer.

Contrast Medium Examinations

Key Points:
- The use of a radiopaque contrast medium helps differentiate between body structures by artificially changing the absorption rate of a particular structure.
- Contrast media may be introduced into the body in several ways, including by mouth, intravenously, or through a catheter, depending on the material and area of the body being examined.
- Although this type of radiographic procedure is not performed in the medical office, you must ensure that the patient has proper instructions for preparing for the procedure and is notified of the scheduled time and facility.

Fluoroscopy

Key Term: fluoroscopy
Key Point:
- **Fluoroscopy**, or fluoro studies, use x-rays to observe movement within the body.

Computed Tomography

Key Term: tomography
Key Point:
- CT uses a combination of x-rays from a tube circling the patient and analyzed by computers to create cross-sectional images of the body.

Sonography

Key Term: ultrasound
Key Point:
- **Ultrasound**, or sonography, uses high-frequency sound waves, not x-rays, to create cross-sectional still or real-time (motion) images of the body, usually with the help of a computer.

Magnetic Resonance Imaging

Key Point:
- Magnetic resonance imaging (MRI) uses a combination of high-intensity magnetic fields, radio waves, and computer analysis to create cross-sectional images of the body. MRI does not use x-rays.

Nuclear Medicine

Key Term: radionuclides

Interventional Radiological Procedures

Key Point:
- Interventional radiological techniques are designed to treat specific disease conditions.

Radiation Therapy

Key Points:
- Used in conjunction with surgery, chemotherapy, or both, radiation is possibly the best-known treatment for cancer.
- Treatment consists of a precise, carefully planned regimen of therapy, including the frequency and amount of radiation to be used and the number of exposures during a given period.

☐ **LEARNING OBJECTIVE 4:** Describe routine and contrast media, fluoroscopy, computed tomography, sonography, magnetic resonance imaging, nuclear medicine, and mammographic examinations.

The Medical Assistant's Role in Radiological Procedures

Calming the Patient's Fears

Key Points:
- Being sensitive to patients' feelings is one of the greatest talents anyone in medicine can possess and should be an important part of your training and personality.
- The key to success in explaining radiology procedures to patients is simplicity, leaving the details to the physician.

Assisting with Examinations

Handling and Storing Radiographic Films

Key Point:
- Unexposed film must be protected from moisture, heat, and light by storage in a cool, dry place, preferably in a lead-lined box.

Transfer of Radiographic Information

Key Point:
- X-ray films belong to the site where the study was performed.

Teleradiology _____

_____

Key Term: teleradiology

☐ **LEARNING OBJECTIVE 5:** Explain the role of the medical assistant in radiological procedures.

Content Review

FOUNDATIONAL KNOWLEDGE

Radiography

1. List the four processes by which radiographic film is produced.

   a. _____

   b. _____

   c. _____

   d. _____

2. What is the difference between radiolucent and radiopaque tissues? Give an example of each. How do these tissues appear differently on a radiograph?

	Radiolucent Tissues	**Radiopaque Tissues**
Explanation:		
Example:		
How they appear on a radiograph:		

3. Why do x-ray examinations require a minimum of two exposures?

   _____

   _____

4. **Radiation Safety**

   List five radiation safety procedures for patients.

   a. _____

   b. _____

   c. _____

   d. _____

   e. _____

Radiographic Procedures

5. Fill in the full names for the abbreviations below.

   a. PET _____

   b. SPECT _____

   c. ALARA _____

6. Routine radiographic examinations are used primarily for viewing _____ or _____.

7. Match the different types of radiography techniques with their individual characteristics.

a. Fluoroscopy	**1.** the image depends on the chemical makeup of the body, commonly used in prenatal testing
b. Tomography	**2.** can create three-dimensional images, so that organs can be viewed from all angles
c. Mammography	**3.** the area of the body exposed must be defined exactly so that each treatment is identical
d. Ultrasound	**4.** used as an aid to other types of treatment, such as reducing fractures and implanting devices such as pacemakers
e. Magnetic resonance imaging	**5.** a vital adjunct to biopsy
f. Nuclear medicine	**6.** designed to concentrate on specific areas of the body
g. Radiation therapy	

Contrast Mediums

8. Name two contrast mediums.

   a. _____

   b. _____

9. Give an example of one invasive and one noninvasive contrast medium procedure, and explain each one.

Invasive Contrast Medium Procedure	**Noninvasive Contrast Medium Procedure**

10. Why is it imperative to have an esophagogastroduodenoscopy done before other barium studies?

_____

_____

11. Compare and contrast fluoroscopy with tomography. How do these procedures use movement? How do they use contrast media?

_____

_____

12. Name four types of interventional radiological procedures.

a. _____

b. _____

c. _____

d. _____

All About Radiology

13. X-rays have the potential to cause _____ or _____ to the body.

14. List five side effects of radiation therapy.

a. _____

b. _____

c. _____

d. _____

e. _____

15. Name three tasks that the medical assistant performs in the field of radiology.

a. _____

b. _____

c. _____

16. What are some of the advancements that have been made in the medical field of radiology? How has radiology changed the need for certain surgical procedures?

_____

_____

17. What are the three ways contrast media may be introduced into the body?

a. _____

b. _____

c. _____

18. List and briefly describe the four lying-down positions used for radiography.

a. _____

b. _____

c. _____

d. _____

19. Match the following key terms to their definitions.

Key Terms

a. cassette _____

b. contrast medium _____

c. film _____

Definitions

1. invisible electromagnetic radiation waves used in diagnosis and treatment of various disorders

2. a lightproof holder in which film is exposed

3. imaging technique that uses a strong magnetic field

d. fluoroscopy _____

e. magnetic resonance imaging _____

f. nuclear medicine _____

g. radiograph _____

h. radiography _____

i. radiologist _____

j. radiology _____

k. radiolucent _____

l. radionuclide _____

m. radiopaque _____

n. teleradiology _____

o. tomography _____

p. ultrasound _____

q. x-rays _____

4. a radioactive material with a short life that is used in small amounts in nuclear medicine studies

5. physician who interprets images to provide diagnostic information

6. imaging technique that uses sound waves to diagnose or monitor various body structures

7. not permeable to passage of x-rays

8. processed film that contains a visible image

9. a substance ingested or injected into the body to facilitate imaging of internal structures

10. the use of computed imaging and information systems to transmit diagnostic images to distant locations

11. a procedure in which the x-ray tube and film move in relation to each other during exposure, blurring out all structures except those in the focal plane

12. a raw material on which x-rays are projected through the body; prior to processing, this does not contain a visible image

13. permitting the passage of x-rays

14. a special x-ray technique for examining a body part by immediate projection onto a fluorescent screen

15. the branch of medicine involving diagnostic and therapeutic applications of x-rays

16. a branch of medicine that uses radioactive isotopes to diagnose and treat disease

17. the art and science of producing diagnostic images with x-rays

20. True or False. Determine whether the following statements are true or false. If false, explain why.

a. A patient may hear noises during an x-ray procedure.

_____

_____

b. A mammogram is a minimally invasive procedure.

_____

_____

c. You need to be proficient in the operation of your facility's equipment.

_____

_____

d. The best way to explain procedures to a patient is with lots of detail.

_____

_____

APPLICATION

Critical Thinking Practice

1. You have a patient who will have a radiographic exam using contrast media next week. You find out this patient has an allergy to shellfish. What should you do?

_____

_____

2. Mrs. Kay has had several radiographic and contrast media studies over the past 5 years. She is now moving to another state and wants to know how to get copies of the films and reports to her new physician. What will you tell her about transferring these records?

_____

_____

Patient Education

1. You have a patient with a fear of enclosed spaces who is not able to have an open MRI at your outpatient radiographic center. How would you console this patient and explain x-ray procedures?

_____

_____

Documentation

1. You have just taken a chest x-ray to rule out pneumonia. Write a narrative note detailing this procedure to be included in the patient's chart.

_____

_____

Active Learning

1. Research the current recommendations by the American Cancer Society for mammography. At what age does the ACS recommend that women get their first mammogram? How can women perform a self-examination at home? What other important information do women need to know about breast cancer? Create a poster to hang up in your office outlining this information and addressing women of all ages and stages of life.

2. Pair up with another student and take turns practicing to prepare a patient for an x-ray. Practice procedures before, during, and after an x-ray is taken. What information or instructions will the patient need to know? Make notes about how to best convey necessary information. If you are playing the role of the patient, what questions might you have? If you are the medical assistant, how would you answer these questions? After you have taken several turns as both patient and medical assistant, discuss your scenarios with the class. What did it feel like to be a patient on the other end of the procedure? What did you find most challenging as the medical assistant? Being sensitive to patients' feelings is one of the greatest talents anyone in medicine can possess and should be an important part of your training.

3. The x-ray has come a long way since Wilhelm Roentgen published his discoveries in 1895. New technologies, new procedures, and new applications have made the x-ray an integral part of medicinal practices around the world. It is an ever-evolving, ever-improving field of study. Research some of the new studies, procedures, applications, and equipment that are currently being developed. Who is working on it? Where is their study being conducted? What problems have they encountered? What improvements are they hoping to achieve? You need to stay current with new procedures and surgical techniques so that you can be informed and reassure patients and their families, who may not be aware of the advances made in health care.

Professional Journal

REFLECT

(Prompts and Ideas: Have you ever had an x-ray? What were your concerns and fears before the examination? What did the medical assistant, radiologist, or physician tell you that assuaged your fears?)

_____

_____

_____

_____

_____

_____

_____

PONDER AND SOLVE

1. You have a patient coming in for radiation therapy, who has been experiencing side effects such as weight loss, loss of appetite, and hair loss. She has concerns about the radiation therapy that she has been receiving and feels that it may be too much for her body. What would you say to her to help her better understand the situation?

_____

_____

_____

_____

_____

_____

2. You have a patient who has had radiographs taken with a referring physician. This patient has already spoken to his referral physician about the finding in his x-rays and would now like to consult with his primary care physician. However, the referring physician has not yet sent a summary of findings. Your patient is very anxious. What should you say?

_____

_____

_____

_____

_____

_____

EXPERIENCE

Skills related to this chapter include:

1. Assist with an X-ray Procedure (Procedure 25-1).

Record any common mistakes, lessons learned, and/or tips you discovered during your experience of practicing and demonstrating these skills:

_____

_____

_____

_____

_____

_____

_____

Skill Practice

PERFORMANCE OBJECTIVES:

1. Assist with x-ray procedures (Procedure 25-1).

Name_____ Date _____ Time _____

Procedure 25-1:	**ASSIST WITH AN X-RAY PROCEDURE**

PURPOSE: Prepare the patient for a general x-ray procedure.

EQUIPMENT: Patient gown and drape

STANDARDS: Given the needed equipment and a place to work, the student will perform this skill with _____% accuracy in a total of _____ minutes. *(Your instructor will tell you what the percentage and time limits will be before you begin practicing.)*

KEY: 4 = Satisfactory   0 = Unsatisfactory   NA = This step is not counted

PROCEDURE STEPS	SELF	PARTNER	INSTRUCTOR
1. Wash your hands.	☐	☐	☐
2. Greet the patient by name, introduce yourself, and escort him or her to the room where the x-ray equipment is maintained.	☐	☐	☐
3. Ask female patients about the possibility of pregnancy. If the patient is unsure or indicates pregnancy in any trimester, consult with the physician before proceeding with the x-ray procedure.	☐	☐	☐
4. After explaining what clothing should be removed, if any, give the patient a gown and privacy.	☐	☐	☐
5. Notify the x-ray technician or physician that the patient is ready for the x-ray procedure. Stay behind the lead-lined wall during the x-ray procedure to avoid exposure to x-rays during the procedure.	☐	☐	☐
6. After the x-ray, ask the patient to remain in the room until the film has been developed and checked for accuracy and readability.	☐	☐	☐
7. Once you have determined that the exposed film is adequate for the physician to view for diagnosis, have the patient get dressed and escort him or her to the front desk.	☐	☐	☐
8. Document the procedure in the medical record.	☐	☐	☐

CALCULATION

Total Possible Points: _____
Total Points Earned: _____ Multiplied by 100 = _____ Divided by Total Possible Points = _____%

Pass   **Fail**
☐   ☐   Comments:

Student's signature _____ Date _____
Partner's signature _____ Date _____
Instructor's signature _____ Date _____

Work Product 1

Document appropriately.

Ms. Molly Espinoza is a 43-year-old female patient. Dr. Cord ordered a routine screening mammogram for this patient. You confirm with her that she is not pregnant and explain the procedure. Then you prepare the patient, and two radiographs are taken of each breast, repositioning the patient between each image. All four radiographs are developed and are readable and accurate.

If you are currently working in a medical office, use a blank paper patient chart from the office. If this is not available to you, use the space below to record the incident in the chart.

_____

_____

_____

_____

_____

_____

_____

_____

_____

Chapter Self-Assessment Quiz

1. Which term below means lying face downward?
  a. Supine
  b. Prone
  c. Decubitus
  d. Recumbent
  e. Relaxed

2. Which of the following is a form of nuclear medicine?
  a. Radiopaque
  b. Barium
  c. Iodine
  d. Radionuclides
  e. Radiolucent

3. Noises heard during an x-ray exposure may come from:
  a. the x-ray tube.
  b. x-rays.
  c. the positioning aid.
  d. high voltage.
  e. the sheet of film.

4. Which of the following is an example of a radiopaque tissue?
  a. Lungs
  b. Bone
  c. Muscle
  d. Fat
  e. Veins

5. A minimum of two x-rays should be taken at:
  a. 180 degrees of each other.
  b. 30 degrees of each other.
  c. 70 degrees of each other.
  d. 90 degrees of each other.
  e. 50 degrees of each other.

6. A type of radiography that creates cross-sectional images of the body is:
  a. fluoroscopy.
  b. MRI.
  c. tomography.
  d. ultrasound.
  e. mammography.

7. Which of the following form of radiography does <u>not</u> use x-rays?

   a. MRI

   b. Nuclear medicine

   c. Fluoroscopy

   d. Teleradiology

   e. Tomography

8. Which procedure creates an image that depends on the chemical makeup of the body?

   a. Tomography

   b. Fluoroscopy

   c. MRI

   d. Mammography

   e. Nuclear medicine

9. Sonograms create images using:

   a. radioactive material.

   b. contrast media.

   c. magnetic resonance.

   d. chemotherapy.

   e. ultrasound.

10. X-rays can be harmful to infants and young children because:

    a. their immune systems are not fully developed.

    b. their cells divide at a rapid pace.

    c. they have less muscle mass than adults.

    d. they are more sensitive to the rays than adults.

    e. they have less body fat than adults.

11. Which of the following procedures is done in a confined space?

    a. MRI

    b. Nuclear medicine

    c. Fluoroscopy

    d. Teleradiology

    e. Tomography

12. A physician who specializes in interpreting the images on the processed film is a(n):

    a. pulmonologist.

    b. internist.

    c. immunologist.

    d. ophthalmologist.

    e. radiologist.

Scenario: A patient has come in for an x-ray. The physician wants you to get a clear image of the patient's liver.

13. What is another possible way to view the patient's liver without injections?

    a. Mammalogy

    b. Sonography

    c. Fluoroscopy

    d. Teleradiology

    e. Tomography

14. Which position would allow you to take the best images of the liver?

    a. Supine

    b. Decubitus

    c. Posterior

    d. Left anterior oblique

    e. Right anterior oblique

End Scenario

15. Who has the rights for x-ray film after it has been developed?

    a. The patient

    b. The physician who ordered the x-rays

    c. The physician who will use the x-rays

    d. The lab that developed the film

    e. The site where the study was performed

16. You should wear a dosimeter to

    a. lower the level of radiation.

    b. protect against radiation effects.

    c. monitor personal radiation exposure.

    d. enhance radiography images.

    e. collect data on different procedures.

17. Why do some tests require patients to be NPO before an administration of barium?

    a. Gastric juices may interfere with the readings.

    b. A full stomach may distort or alter an image.

    c. Patients are not allowed to relieve themselves.

    d. Undigested food might counteract contrast media.

    e. Instruments might become soiled during the procedure.

18. Images that partially block x-rays are called:

   a. radiographs.

   b. radiolucent.

   c. radiopaque.

   d. radionuclides.

   e. radiograms.

19. Why is radiology used as a form of cancer treatment?

   a. X-rays show the exact location of cancer.

   b. Radioactive cells produce more white blood cells.

   c. Radiation can destroy or weaken cancer cells.

   d. Radiation makes cancerous tumors benign.

   e. Chemotherapy is not as effective as radiation.

20. When explaining procedures to patients:

   a. let the physician go into detail.

   b. answer all the questions they ask.

   c. do not worry them with potential risk.

   d. soothe their fears without telling them anything.

   e. allow only the nurse to explain the procedure.

26 Medical Office Emergencies

Chapter Checklist

- ☐ Read textbook chapter and take notes within the Chapter Notes outline. Answer the Learning Objectives as you reach them in the content, and then check them off.
- ☐ Work the Content Review questions—both Foundational Knowledge and Application.
- ☐ Perform the Active Learning exercise(s).

- ☐ Complete Professional Journal entries.
- ☐ Complete Skill Practice Activity(s) using Competency Evaluation Forms and Work Products, when appropriate.
- ☐ Take the Chapter Self-Assessment Quiz.
- ☐ Insert all appropriate pages into your portfolio.

Learning Objectives

1. Spell and define the key terms.
2. Describe the role of the medical assistant in an emergency.
3. Identify the five types of shock and the management of each.
4. Describe how burns are classified and managed.
5. Explain the management of allergic reactions.

6. Describe the management of poisoning and the role of the poison control center.
7. List the three types of hyperthermic emergencies and the treatment for each type.
8. Discuss the treatment of hypothermia.
9. Describe the role of the medical assistant in managing psychiatric emergencies.

Chapter Notes

Note: Bold-faced headings are the major headings in the text chapter; headings in regular font are lower-level headings (i.e., the content is subordinate to, or falls "under," the major headings). Make sure you understand the key terms used in the chapter, as well as the concepts presented as Key Points.

TEXT SUBHEADINGS   **NOTES**

Introduction _____

_____

_____

☐ **LEARNING OBJECTIVE 1:** Spell and define the key terms.

_____

Medical Office Emergency Procedures _____

Key Point:
• In a life-threatening situation, the well-prepared medical assistant can obtain important information and perform life-saving procedures before the ambulance or rescue squad arrives, increasing the patient's chance for survival.

☐ **LEARNING OBJECTIVE 2:** Describe the role of the medical assistant in an emergency.

Emergency Action Plan _____

Key Point:
• Whether confronted with a cardiac emergency or psychiatric crisis, medical assistants must be able to coordinate multiple ongoing events while rendering patient care.

Emergency Medical Kit _____

Key Point:
• Although the office's equipment and supplies vary with the medical specialty, emergency equipment and supplies are fairly standard.

The Emergency Medical Services System _____

Key Term: shock
Key Points:
• Most communities have a 911 system to report emergencies and summon help by telephone.
• You should know the emergency system used in your community.
• In the medical office, an emergency requiring notification of the EMS includes situations that are life threatening or have the potential to become life threatening, such as the symptoms of a heart attack, **shock**, or severe breathing difficulties.

Patient Assessment _____

Key Point:
• The two primary objectives in assessment of the patient are to identify and correct any life-threatening problems and provide necessary care

Recognizing the Emergency _____

The Primary Assessment _____

Key Points:
- Once you are at the victim's side, an initial survey of the patient is the first step in emergency care.
- Checking for responsiveness means noting whether the patient is conscious or unconscious.
- If the patient is not breathing, artificial respiration must be started immediately.
- Evaluate circulation in adults and children by checking the carotid pulse.

The Secondary Assessment _____

Key Term: seizures
Key Point:
- The secondary assessment includes asking the patient questions to obtain additional information and performing a more thorough physical evaluation to find less obvious problems than those noted in the primary assessment.

The Physical Examination _____

Key Point:
- A head-to-toe survey that includes examination of the head and neck, chest and back, abdomen, and extremities, in this sequence, should be done only after completing the primary and secondary surveys.

Head and Neck _____

Key Point:
- If a cervical spine injury is suspected, immediately immobilize the spine and avoid manipulating the neck during examination of the head.

Chest and Back _____

Key Point:
- The anterior chest is evaluated to some degree when the patient's respiratory status is evaluated.

Abdomen _____

_____

Key Term: melena
Key Points:
- The abdomen of all patients is evaluated, but it is particularly important for those with GI symptoms or suspicion of blood or fluid loss as seen in vaginal bleeding, vomiting, or **melena** (blood in the stool).
- Inspect the arms and legs for swelling, deformity, and tenderness. Also note any tremors in the hands.

Types of Emergencies _____

_____

Shock _____

_____

Key Points:
- Shock is lack of oxygen to the individual cells of the body, including the brain, as a result of a decrease in blood pressure.
- As shock progresses, the body has more difficulty trying to adjust, and eventually tissues and body organs have such severe damage that the shock becomes irreversible and death ensues.

Types of Shock _____

_____

Key Terms: hypovolemic shock; cardiogenic shock; neurogenic shock; anaphylactic shock; septic shock

☐ **LEARNING OBJECTIVE 3:** Identify the five types of shock and the management of each.

Management of the Patient in Shock _____

_____

Key Point:
- Because shock can result from many types of medical situations or trauma, you should always be prepared to treat the patient for shock in any emergency situation that occurs in the medical office.

Bleeding

Key Terms: contusions; hematomas; ecchymosis
Key Points:
• Soft tissue injuries involve damage to the skin and/or underlying musculature.
• A blood clot that forms at the injury site, generally when large areas of tissue are damaged, is a **hematoma**.

Management of Bleeding and Soft Tissue Injuries

Key Points:
• Management of open soft tissue injuries includes controlling bleeding by applying direct pressure.
• An impaled object should not be removed but requires careful immobilization of the patient and the injured area of the body.

Burns

Key Point:
• The four major sources of burn injury are thermal, electrical, chemical, and radiation.

Classification of Burn Injuries

Key Point:
• Classification of burn injuries depends on the depth, or tissue layers involved.

Calculation of Body Surface Area Burned

Key Point:
• The extent of body surface area (BSA) injured by the burn is most commonly estimated by a method called the *rule of nines*.

Management of the Burn Victim

☐ **LEARNING OBJECTIVE 4:** Describe how burns are classified and managed.

Musculoskeletal Injuries _____

Key Point:
- Injuries to muscles, bones, and joints are some of the most common problems encountered in providing emergency care.

Management of Musculoskeletal Injuries _____

Key Point:
- Splinting helps prevent further injury to soft tissues, blood vessels, and nerves from sharp bone fragments and relieves pain by stopping motion at the fracture site.

Types of Splints _____

Key Terms: splint; ischemia; infarction
Key Point:
- Splinting material may be soft or rigid and can be improvised from almost any object that can provide stability.

Cardiovascular Emergencies _____

Key Point:
- Approximately two-thirds of sudden deaths from coronary artery disease occur out of the hospital, and most occur within 2 hours of the onset of symptoms.

Neurological Emergencies _____

Key Points:
- A seizure is caused by an abnormal discharge of electrical activity in the brain.
- In managing a patient having a seizure, you must give priority to assessing the patient's responsiveness, airway, breathing, and circulation.

Allergic and Anaphylactic Reactions

Key Point:
- An allergic reaction is a generalized reaction that can occur within minutes to hours after the body has been exposed to a substance recognized by the immune system as foreign and to which it is oversensitive.

Common Allergens

Key Term: allergen
Key Point:
- A person may have symptoms within seconds after exposure to an **allergen**, or the reaction may be delayed for several hours.

Signs and Symptoms

Key Points:
- The initial signs and symptoms of an allergic reaction may include severe itching, a feeling of warmth, tightness in the throat or chest, or a rash.
- Since the primary cause of death in an anaphylactic reaction is swelling of the tissues in the airway, leading to airway obstruction, observe the patient closely for signs of airway involvement, including wheezing, shortness of breath, and coughing.

Management of Allergic and Anaphylactic Reactions

Key Point:
- The primary goal when treating a patient having an anaphylactic reaction is restoring respiratory and circulatory function.

☐ **LEARNING OBJECTIVE 5:** Explain the management of allergic reactions.

Poisoning

Key Point:
- Most toxic exposures occur in the home, and almost 50% occur in children aged 1 to 3 years

Poison Control Center _____

_____

Key Point:
- When information about a poisoning or drug overdose is not readily available, the poison control center is a valuable resource, and the phone number should be posted near all phones in the medical office.

Management of Poisoning Emergencies _____

_____

Key Points:
- The patient may go to the medical office after the poisoning, or more commonly, the patient or caregiver telephones the office requesting information.
- Never give a patient syrup of ipecac or otherwise induce vomiting unless directed to do so by the professionals at the poison control center.

☐ **LEARNING OBJECTIVE 6:** Describe the management of poisoning and the role of the poison control center.

Heat and Cold Related Emergencies _____

_____

Key Terms: hyperthermia; hypothermia

Hyperthermia _____

_____

Key Terms: heat cramps; heat exhaustion; heat stroke
Key Point:
- Hyperthermia is the general condition of excessive body heat.

☐ **LEARNING OBJECTIVE 7:** List the three types of hyperthermic emergencies and the treatment for each type.

Hypothermia _____

_____

Key Point:
- Basic management of hypothermia includes handling the patient gently, removing wet clothing, and covering the patient to prevent further cooling.

☐ **LEARNING OBJECTIVE 8:** Discuss the treatment of hypothermia.

Frostbite

Key Term: frostbite
Key Points:
- The type and duration of contact are the two most important factors in determining the extent of frostbite injury.
- The combination of wind and cold is dangerous.

Behavioral and Psychiatric Emergencies

Key Point:
- A psychiatric emergency is any situation in which the patient's moods, thoughts, or actions are so disordered or disturbed that harm or death may result for the patient or others if no intervention occurs.

☐ **LEARNING OBJECTIVE 9:** Describe the role of the medical assistant in managing psychiatric emergencies.

Content Review

FOUNDATIONAL KNOWLEDGE

1. In Case of Emergency . . .

As a medical assistant, you may be called on to assist during an emergency. Review the list of tasks below and determine which tasks you may be responsible for as a medical assistant. Place a check mark in the "Yes" column for those duties you might assist with as a medical assistant and place a check mark in the "No" column for those tasks that fall to another member of the team.

Task	Yes	No
a. Obtain important patient information.		
b. Perform CPR.		
c. Set and splint bone fractures.		
d. Remove foreign body airway obstructions.		
e. Remain calm and react competently and professionally during a psychiatric crisis.		
f. Coordinate multiple ongoing events while rendering patient care in a cardiac emergency.		
g. Negotiate with or attempt to calm a violent patient during a psychiatric crisis.		
h. Know what emergency system is used in the community.		
i. Provide immediate care to the patient while the physician is notified.		

Task	Yes	No
j. Perform rapid sequence intubation (RSI) on a patient who is suffering respiratory failure.		
k. Administer first aid.		
l. Document all actions taken.		
m. Complete routine scheduled tasks.		
n. Assist EMS personnel as necessary.		
o. Allow EMS personnel to examine the patient.		
p. Direct care of the patient by EMS personnel.		
q. Remove any obstacles that prevent speedy evacuation of the patient by stretcher.		
r. Direct family members to the reception area or a private room.		

Shocking

2. Identify the type of shock described in the following scenarios. How should you position the patient for each of these? What special intervention or management is required for each form of shock?

   a. A very ill patient has been complaining of increasing pain in the pelvis and legs. Blood is present in the urine. The patient's temperature was elevated but is dropping.

   _____

   _____

   b. An elderly patient falls on her back while attempting to get out of bed. Her heart rate becomes rapid and thready, and her blood pressure drops quickly.

   _____

   _____

   c. A patient presents with fluid in the lungs, difficulty breathing, and chest pain.

   _____

   _____

   d. A patient presents with labored breathing, grunting, wheezing, and swelling followed by fainting.

   _____

   _____

   e. A child is brought in for diarrhea. She has poor skin turgor and capillary refill. Her mental status appears to be deteriorating.

   _____

   _____

3. Put a check mark next to the proper signs and symptoms for shock.

low blood pressure	high blood pressure
calm or lethargic	restlessness or signs of fear
thirst	polyuria
hunger	nausea
hot, sweaty skin	cool, clammy skin
pale skin with cyanosis (bluish color) at the lips and earlobes	flushed skin
rapid and weak pulse	bounding pulse

Burn Control

4. Classify the type, severity, and coverage of the burns in each of these scenarios.

   a. A contractor installing medical equipment accidentally touches exposed wires. He has burns on his right arm, but no sensation of pain.

   _____

   _____

   b. A child spills bleach on one leg. The leg is blistering and causing severe pain.

   _____

   _____

   c. A man watches a welder install handrails on your office's handicapped ramp. Now his face is red and painful, and his eyes have a painful itching sensation.

   _____

   _____

   d. A patient spills hot coffee while driving to your office, painfully blistering his genital area.

   _____

   _____

5. List nine interventions or steps to manage burns.

   a. _____

   b. _____

   c. _____

   d. _____

   e. _____

   f. _____

   g. _____

   h. _____

   i. _____

6. **Wheal of Fortune**

   What are your responsibilities for managing an allergic reaction? Circle all that apply.

   a. Leave the patient to bring the emergency kit or cart, oxygen, and to get a physician to evaluate the patient.

   b. Assist the patient to a supine position.

   c. Scrub patient's skin to remove allergens and urticaria.

   d. Assess the patient's respiratory and circulatory status by obtaining the blood pressure, pulse, and respiratory rates.

   e. Observe skin color and warmth.

   f. If the patient complains of being cold or is shivering, cover with a blanket.

   g. Intubate the patient.

   h. Upon the direction of the physician, start an intravenous line and administer oxygen.

   i. Administer medications as ordered by the physician.

   j. Document vital signs and any medications and treatments given, noting the time each set of vital signs is taken or medications are administered.

   k. Communicate relevant information to the EMS personnel, including copies of the progress notes or medication record as needed.

7. I Drank What?

A teenage patient is given an instant coldpack for an injury to the mouth. A few minutes later you discover the teenager misunderstood, and drank the contents of the cold pack. What information do you need to collect to prepare for a call to the poison control center?

_____

_____

Hot or Cold?

8. Identify the hyperthermic and hypothermic emergencies from the list below and match them with the proper treatment.

a. heat cramps	**1.** Remove wet clothing. Cover the patient. Give warm fluids by mouth if patient is alert and oriented.
b. frostbite	**2.** Move the patient to a cool area. Remove clothing that may be keeping in the heat. Place cool, wet cloths or a wet sheet on the scalp, neck, axilla, and groin. Administer oxygen as directed by the physician and apply a cardiac monitor. Notify the EMS for transportation to the hospital as directed by the physician.
c. heat stroke	**3.** Immerse the affected tissue in lukewarm water (41°C, 105°F) until the area becomes pliable and the color and sensation return. Do not apply dry heat. Do not massage the area; massage may cause further tissue damage. Avoid breaking any blisters that may form. Notify the EMS for transportation to a hospital.
d. hypothermia	**4.** Move the patient to a cool area. Give fluids (commercial electrolyte solution) by mouth if uncomplicated. Give IV fluids if patient presents with nausea.

9. Dante commutes to your office by public transportation. On a particularly cold day, Dante arrives late with cool, pale skin. He is lethargic and confused, with slow and shallow respirations and a slow and faint pulse. Describe what actions are appropriate.

_____

_____

It's an Emergency!

10. A sullen and moody patient suddenly becomes threatening. Name three things the medical assistant should do.

a. _____

b. _____

c. _____

11. What six pieces of information should be included in your office's emergency plan?

a. _____

b. _____

c. _____

d. _____

e. _____

f. _____

12. What are the elements of the AVPU scale for assessing a patient's level of consciousness?

A	
V	
P	
U	

13. List the first three steps you should use to control bleeding from an open wound.

a. _____

b. _____

c. _____

14. You enter an exam room and unexpectedly find someone sprawled on the floor. What four things do you check on your primary assessment?

a. _____

b. _____

c. _____

d. _____

15. At what point do you assess the general appearance of the patient?

_____

_____

16. A patient is found unconscious. You do not suspect trauma. In what order would you perform the physical examination?

_____

_____

17. An examination of the eyes can be done according to the acronym "PEARL," meaning *P*upils *E*qual *A*nd *R*eactive to *L*ight. What does this examination reveal?

_____

_____

18. A 55-year-old male begins complaining about nausea. He is clearly anxious or agitated. What could this be an early symptom of?

_____

_____

19. Match the following key terms to their definitions.

Key Terms

a. allergen _____

b. anaphylactic shock _____

c. cardiogenic shock _____

d. contusion _____

e. ecchymosis _____

Definitions

1. an abnormal discharge of electrical activity in the brain, resulting in erratic muscle movements, strange sensations, or a complete loss of consciousness

2. black, tarry stools caused by digested blood from the gastrointestinal tract

3. severe allergic reaction within minutes to hours after exposure to a foreign substance

4. an emergency where the body cannot compensate for elevated temperatures

f. full-thickness burn _____

g. heat cramps _____

h. heat stroke _____

i. hematoma _____

j. hyperthermia _____

k. hypothermia _____

l. hypovolemic shock _____

m. infarction _____

n. ischemia _____

o. melena _____

p. neurogenic shock _____

q. partial-thickness burn _____

r. seizure _____

s. septic shock _____

t. shock _____

u. splint _____

v. superficial burn _____

5. a bruise or collection of blood under the skin or in damaged tissue

6. a burn limited to the epidermis

7. any device used to immobilize a sprain, strain, fracture, or dislocated limb

8. shock that results from dysfunction of the nervous system following a spinal cord injury

9. muscle cramping that follows a period of physical exertion and profuse sweating in a hot environment

10. a penetrating burn that has destroyed all skin layers

11. a characteristic black and blue mark from blood accumulation

12. below-normal body temperature

13. the general condition of excessive body heat

14. a blood clot that forms at an injury site

15. a burn that involves epidermis and varying levels of the dermis

16. a decrease in oxygen to tissue

17. a substance that causes manifestations of an allergy

18. shock that results from general infection in the bloodstream

19. shock caused by loss of blood or other body fluids

20. death of tissue due to lack of oxygen

21. condition resulting from the lack of oxygen to individual cells of the body

22. type of shock in which the left ventricle fails to pump enough blood for the body to function

20. True or False? Determine whether the following statements are true or false. If false, explain why.

a. During a primary assessment, you find a patient has inadequate respirations. You should proceed to the secondary assessment and physical examination to find out why.

_____

_____

b. An impaled object should not be removed but requires careful immobilization of the patient and the injured area of the body.

_____

_____

c. An allergic reaction will be evident immediately after exposure to an allergen.

_____

_____

d. Closed wounds are not life threatening.

_____

_____

APPLICATION

Critical Thinking Practice

1. An elderly man falls in an exam room. He is conscious, but agitated and anxious. You are the first to discover him struggling on the floor. What is the only duty you will perform until others arrive, and why?

_____

_____

2. A patient in your office is in respiratory arrest. The physician is attending this patient. You have collected notes on the patient's vitals and SAMPLE history (signs and symptoms, allergies, medications, past pertinent history, last oral intake, and the events that led to the problem). A family member of the patient is present and is growing upset and intrusive. The EMTs arrive on the scene. What is your immediate responsibility? Explain.

_____

_____

Patient Education

1. You have just had a patient suffer anaphylactic shock and respiratory arrest due to an unsuspected penicillin allergy. EMS has transported the patient to a local hospital. The following week, the patient calls to ask what she can do to prevent this from happening in the future. Write a sheet of instructions that clearly explains the nature of the emergency and recommends future precautions this patient should take.

_____

_____

Documentation

1. A patient received penicillin for a sexually transmitted infection, and this was the last event documented in the patient's chart. Fifteen minutes later the patient began wheezing and gasping, and within five minutes was clearly suffering anaphylactic shock. A first injection of epinephrine administered SC at that time was ineffective, and the patient was in respiratory arrest when EMS arrived. Mask-to-mouth respirations were given with supplemental oxygen at 15 liters per minute for 2 minutes before EMS assumed care of the patient. How would you document this interaction in the patient's chart?

_____

_____

Active Learning

1. Some medical professionals live on the front line of emergency medical care. Locate an EMT-Basic (EMT-B) textbook at a library, bookstore, or other source.
   • Research the different procedures EMT-Bs use to assess trauma and medical emergencies.

   • Compare the EMT's perspective with your own professional approach to a medical emergency.

   • Outline how someone in your specialty can be better prepared to communicate with EMTs during a crisis.

   • Create an emergency checklist for turning a patient's care over to the EMS system.

2. Develop a set of scenarios for different emergencies you might find in your office, including:
   • Shock

   • Bleeding

   • Burns

   • Musculoskeletal injuries

   • Cardiovascular emergencies

   • Neurological emergencies

   • Allergic and anaphylactic reactions

   • Poisoning

   • Heat- and cold-related emergencies

   • Behavioral and psychiatric emergencies

These scenarios should include a patient history and the signs and symptoms a first responder would encounter. Then practice three different emergency scenarios developed above with two other students. For each scenario, one student will take the role of evaluator, a second student will act as patient or victim, and a third student will take the role of medical assistant. The evaluator will give the medical assistant verbal cues when asked, such as skin appearance, heart rate, and breathing, and the medical assistant should attempt to evaluate the patient's condition and take appropriate actions. The goal is for students to practice the steps of patient assessment and management through delivery to the EMS providers.

3. Prepare a list of emergency contacts in the area, including the contact information of local hospitals, poison control centers, and emergency medical services.

Professional Journal

REFLECT

(Prompts and Ideas: How do you think you would handle an emergency in the office? What can you do to be better prepared and level headed in such a situation?)

_____

_____

_____

_____

_____

PONDER AND SOLVE

1. You have a 35-year-old patient who has religious reservations about some medical procedures. Normally, you and the physician carefully explain procedures to this patient so she has the opportunity to make informed consent decisions. Now she is lying unconscious in front of you with a medical emergency. How do you handle informed consent with an unconscious patient?

_____

_____

_____

_____

_____

2. You have an elderly patient with a "do not resuscitate" order, because he does not want to receive CPR in the event of a heart attack. During treatment for another condition, he collapses in apparent anaphylactic shock. Do you provide emergency medical assistance?

_____

_____

_____

_____

_____

EXPERIENCE

Skills related to this chapter include:

1. Administer Oxygen (Procedure 26-1).
2. Perform Cardiopulmonary Resuscitation (Adult) (Procedure 26-2).
3. Use an Automatic External Defibrillator (AED) (Procedure 26-3).
4. Manage a Foreign Body Airway Obstruction (Adult) (Procedure 26-4).
5. Control External Bleeding (Procedure 26-5).

Record any common mistakes, lessons learned, and/or tips you discovered during your experience of practicing and demonstrating these skills:

_____

_____

_____

_____

_____

_____

_____

Skill Practice

PERFORMANCE OBJECTIVES:

1. Administer oxygen (Procedure 26-1)
2. Perform CPR (adult) (Procedure 26-2)
3. Use an AED (Procedure 26-3)
4. Manage a foreign body airway obstruction (adult) (Procedure 26-4)
5. Control external bleeding (Procedure 26-5)

Name _____ Date _____ Time _____

PROCEDURE 26-1:   ADMINISTER OXYGEN

EQUIPMENT/SUPPLIES: Oxygen tank with a regulator and flowmeter, an oxygen delivery system (nasal cannula or mask)

STANDARDS: Given the needed equipment and a place to work, the student will perform this skill with _____ % accuracy in a total of _____ minutes. (*Your instructor will tell you what the percentage and time limits will be before you begin.*)

KEY: 4 = Satisfactory   0 = Unsatisfactory   NA = This step is not counted

PROCEDURE STEPS	SELF	PARTNER	INSTRUCTOR
1. Wash your hands.	☐	☐	☐
2. Check the physician order.	☐	☐	☐
3. Obtain the oxygen tank and nasal cannula or mask.	☐	☐	☐
4. Greet and identify the patient.	☐	☐	☐
5. Connect the distal end of the nasal cannula or mask tubing to the adapter on the oxygen tank regulator, which is attached to the oxygen tank.	☐	☐	☐
6. Place the oxygen delivery device into the patient's nares (nasal cannula) or over the patient's nose and mouth (mask).	☐	☐	☐
7. Turn the regulator dial to the liters per minute ordered by the physician.	☐	☐	☐
8. Record the procedure in the patient's medical record.	☐	☐	☐

CALCULATION

Total Possible Points: _____
Total Points Earned: _____ Multiplied by 100 = _____ Divided by Total Possible Points = _____%

Pass   **Fail**
☐   ☐   Comments:

Chart Documentation

_____
_____

Student's signature _____ Date _____
Partner's signature _____ Date _____
Instructor's signature _____ Date _____

Name_____ Date _____ Time _____

| Procedure 26-2: | PERFORM CARDIOPULMONARY RESUSCITATION (ADULT) |

EQUIPMENT/SUPPLIES: CPR mannequin, mouth-to-mouth barrier device, gloves

STANDARDS: Given the needed equipment and a place to work, the student will perform this skill with _____ % accuracy in a total of _____ minutes. (*Your instructor will tell you what the percentage and time limits will be before you begin.*)

KEY:　　4 = Satisfactory　　　0 = Unsatisfactory　　　NA = This step is not counted

NOTE: All health care professionals should receive training for proficiency in CPR in an approved program. This skill sheet is not intended to substitute for proficiency training with a mannequin and structured protocol.

PROCEDURE STEPS	SELF	PARTNER	INSTRUCTOR
1. Determine unresponsiveness by shaking the patient and shouting "Are you okay?"	☐	☐	☐
2. Assess for airway patency and respiratory effort with the patient in the supine position.	☐	☐	☐
3. Instruct another staff member to get the physician.	☐	☐	☐
4. Apply gloves if readily available.	☐	☐	☐
5. If respiratory effort adequate, but patient is unresponsive, place the patient in the recovery position until the patient regains consciousness or the physician instructs you to call the EMS.	☐	☐	☐
6. For minimal or absent respiratory effort, give 2 rescue breaths according to the national standard protocol.	☐	☐	☐
7. Check for cardiac function by checking for the presence of a pulse using the carotid artery on the side of the neck.	☐	☐	☐
8. If cardiac function is adequate, continue rescue breathing according to standard protocol.	☐	☐	☐
9. If cardiac function is minimal or absent, begin chest compressions and rescue breathing for an adult using either one-rescuer or two-rescuer protocol according to the standards of the training provided by an approved provider of CPR training.	☐	☐	☐
10. Continue CPR until the patient has adequate cardiac function and respiratory effort or you are relieved by another health care provider.	☐	☐	☐
11. Document the procedure and copy any records necessary for transport with EMS.	☐	☐	☐

CALCULATION

Total Possible Points: _____
Total Points Earned: _____ Multiplied by 100 = _____ Divided by Total Possible Points = _____%

Pass   **Fail**
☐   ☐   Comments:

Chart Documentation

_____

_____

Student's signature _____ Date _____
Partner's signature _____ Date _____
Instructor's signature _____ Date _____

Name _____ Date _____ Time _____

Procedure 26-3:	USE AN AUTOMATIC EXTERNAL DEFIBRILLATOR

EQUIPMENT/SUPPLIES: Practice mannequin, training automatic external defibrillator with chest pads and connection cables, scissors, gauze, gloves

STANDARDS: Given the needed equipment, and a place to work, the student will perform this skill with _____ % accuracy in a total of _____ minutes. (*Your instructor will tell you what the percentage and time limits will be before you begin.*)

KEY: 4 = Satisfactory   0 = Unsatisfactory   NA = This step is not counted

NOTE: All health care professionals should receive training for proficiency in CPR and using an AED in an approved program. This skill sheet is not intended to substitute for proficiency training with a mannequin and structured protocol.

PROCEDURE STEPS	SELF	PARTNER	INSTRUCTOR
1. Determine unresponsiveness by shaking the patient and shouting "Are you okay?"	☐	☐	☐
2. Follow the procedure for assessing airway patency, respiratory effort, and cardiac function using standard protocol.	☐	☐	☐
3. Instruct another health care worker to notify the physician and get the AED.	☐	☐	☐
4. Begin CPR and rescue breathing for inadequate cardiac function and respiratory effort.	☐	☐	☐
5. Continue CPR and rescue breathing while a second rescuer with the AED removes the patient's shirt and prepares the chest for the electrodes.	☐	☐	☐
6. After opening the AED, the second rescuer removes the sticky backing on the chest electrodes and applies one to the upper right chest area and the other on the lower chest area.	☐	☐	☐
7. Explain what should be done in the event the patient has an implantable device or medication patch in the area where the chest electrodes should be applied.	☐	☐	☐
8. With the electrodes securely on the chest, connect the wire from the electrodes to the AED unit and turn the AED on.	☐	☐	☐
9. Do not touch the patient while the AED is analyzing the heart rhythm.	☐	☐	☐
10. If no shock is advised by the AED, check for adequate breathing and cardiac function and resume CPR if necessary.	☐	☐	☐
11. If a shock is advised by the AED, the second rescuer will make sure no one is touching the patient before pressing the appropriate button on the AED.	☐	☐	☐
12. After a shock is delivered by the AED, follow the instructions for additional shocks or resuming CPR, always reassessing the patient's respirations and cardiac function before resuming CPR.	☐	☐	☐
13. Do not touch the patient while the heart rhythm is be reanalyzed at any point during the procedure.	☐	☐	☐
14. Continue to follow the instructions given by the AED and the physician until EMS has been notified and has arrived.	☐	☐	☐

CALCULATION

Total Possible Points: _____

Total Points Earned: _____ Multiplied by 100 = _____ Divided by Total Possible Points = _____%

Pass **Fail**

☐ ☐ Comments:

Chart Documentation

_____

_____

Student's signature _____ Date _____

Partner's signature _____ Date _____

Instructor's signature _____ Date _____

Name _____ Date _____ Time _____

Procedure 26-4:	**MANAGE A FOREIGN BODY AIRWAY OBSTRUCTION (ADULT)**

EQUIPMENT/SUPPLIES: Mouth-to-mouth barrier device, gloves, mannequin

STANDARDS: Given the needed equipment and a place to work the student will perform this skill with _____ % accuracy in a total of _____ minutes. (*Your instructor will tell you what the percentage and time limits will be before you begin.*)

KEY: 4 = Satisfactory   0 = Unsatisfactory   NA = This step is not counted

NOTE: All health care professionals should receive training for proficiency in managing a foreign body airway obstruction in an approved program. This skill sheet is not intended to substitute for proficiency training with a mannequin and structured protocol.

PROCEDURE STEPS	SELF	PARTNER	INSTRUCTOR
1. If the patient is conscious and appears to be choking, ask the patient "Are you choking?"	☐	☐	☐
2. Do not perform abdominal thrusts if the patient can speak or cough since these are signs that the obstruction is not complete.	☐	☐	☐
3. If the patient cannot speak or cough but has indicated the he/she is choking, move behind the patient, wrapping your arms around his/her abdomen.	☐	☐	☐
4. Place the fist of your dominant hand with the thumb against the patient's abdomen, between the navel and xiphoid process.	☐	☐	☐
5. Put your other hand against your dominant hand and give quick, upward thrusts, forceful enough to dislodge the obstruction in the airway.	☐	☐	☐
6. If the patient is obese or pregnant, place your hands against the middle of the sternum, above the xiphoid process and proceed with quick thrusts inward.	☐	☐	☐
7. Continue with the abdominal thrusts until the object is expelled and the patient can breathe or the patient becomes unconscious.	☐	☐	☐
8. If the patient becomes unconscious or is found unconscious, open the airway and give 2 rescue breaths.	☐	☐	☐
9. If rescue breaths are obstructed, reposition the head and try again.	☐	☐	☐
10. If rescue breaths continue to be obstructed after repositioning, begin abdominal thrusts by placing your palm against the patients abdomen with your fingers facing his/her head (you may need to straddle the patients hips). The palm of the hand should be located between the navel and the xiphoid process.	☐	☐	☐
11. Lace the fingers of the other hand into the fingers of the hand on the abdomen and give 5 abdominal thrusts.	☐	☐	☐
12. After 5 abdominal thrusts, open the mouth using a tongue-jaw lift maneuver and do a finger-sweep of the mouth, removing any objects that may have been dislodged.	☐	☐	☐
13. If an item has been dislodged and can be removed easily, remove the object and attempt rescue breaths. Continue rescue breaths and chest compressions as necessary and appropriate.	☐	☐	☐

PROCEDURE STEPS	SELF	PARTNER	INSTRUCTOR
14. If the item has not been dislodged, attempt rescue breaths. If rescue breaths are successful, continue rescue breathing and chest compressions as necessary and appropriate.	☐	☐	☐
15. If the item has not been dislodged and rescue breaths are not successful, continue with abdominal thrusts.	☐	☐	☐
16. Repeat the pattern of abdominal thrusts, finger-sweep, and rescue breaths and follow the physician orders until EMS is notified and arrives.	☐	☐	☐

CALCULATION

Total Possible Points: _____
Total Points Earned: _____ Multiplied by 100 = _____ Divided by Total Possible Points = _____%

Pass   **Fail**
☐   ☐   Comments:

Chart Documentation

_____

_____

Student's signature _____ Date _____
Partner's signature _____ Date _____
Instructor's signature _____ Date _____

Name _____   Date _____   Time _____

Procedure 26-5:	CONTROL EXTERNAL BLEEDING

EQUIPMENT/SUPPLIES: Gloves, sterile gauze pads

STANDARDS: Given the needed equipment and a place to work the student will perform this skill with _____ % accuracy in a total of _____ minutes. (*Your instructor will tell you what the percentage and time limits will be before you begin.*)

KEY: 4 = Satisfactory   0 = Unsatisfactory   NA = This step is not counted

PROCEDURE STEPS	SELF	PARTNER	INSTRUCTOR
1. Identify the patient and assess the extent of the bleeding and type of accident.	☐	☐	☐
2. Take the patient to an examination room and notify the physician if appropriate.	☐	☐	☐
3. Give the patient some gauze pads and have him/her apply pressure to the area while you put on a pair of clean examination gloves and open additional sterile gauze pads.	☐	☐	☐
4. Observe the patient for signs of dizziness or lightheadedness. Have the patient lie down if needed.	☐	☐	☐
5. Using several sterile gauze pads, apply direct pressure to the wound.	☐	☐	☐
6. Maintain pressure until the bleeding stops.	☐	☐	☐
7. If the bleeding continues or seeps through the gauze, apply additional gauze on top of the saturated gauze while continuing to apply direct pressure.	☐	☐	☐
8. If directed by the physician to do so, apply pressure to the artery delivering blood to this area while continuing to apply direct pressure to the wound to control bleeding.	☐	☐	☐
9. Once the bleeding is controlled, prepare to assist the physician with a minor office surgical procedure to close the wound.	☐	☐	☐
10. Continue to monitor the patient for signs of shock and be prepared to treat the patient appropriately.	☐	☐	☐
11. Document the treatment in the patient's medical record.	☐	☐	☐

CALCULATION

Total Possible Points: _____
Total Points Earned: _____ Multiplied by 100 = _____ Divided by Total Possible Points = _____%

Pass   **Fail**

☐   ☐   Comments:

Chart Documentation

_____

_____

Student's signature _____ Date _____
Partner's signature _____ Date _____
Instructor's signature _____ Date _____

Work Product 1

Document appropriately.

During a routine visit, Carlos Delgado, a 55-year-old male, complains of tightness in his chest and nausea. He is short of breath and appears hypoxic. You notify the physician, and when you return Mr. Delgado is in respiratory arrest. EMS is called. The physician orders bag-to-mouth respirations with 6 L supplemental oxygen, which you provide. An AED is not available. After 5 minutes of artificial respirations, the patient enters full cardiac arrest, and the physician begins chest compressions. Five minutes later EMS arrives to take the patient.

If you are currently working in a medical office, use a blank paper patient chart from the office. If this is not available to you, use the space below to record the incident in the chart.

_____

_____

_____

_____

_____

_____

_____

_____

Chapter Self-Assessment Quiz

1. During a primary assessment, you should check:

   a. AVPU.

   b. pupils.

   c. responsiveness.

   d. vital signs.

   e. patient identification.

2. What signs and symptoms are consistent with heat stroke?

   a. Cyanotic skin

   b. Pale wet skin

   c. Ecchymosis

   d. Dry, flushed skin

   e. Waxy, gray skin

3. Superficial burns are categorized as:

   a. first degree.

   b. second degree.

   c. third degree.

   d. partial thickness.

   e. full thickness.

4. Which is an example of a closed wound?

   a. Abrasion

   b. Avulsion

   c. Contusion

   d. Laceration

   e. Ecchymosis

5. What is the BSA of the anterior portion of an adult's trunk?

   a. 1%

   b. 9%

   c. 13.5%

   d. 18%

   e. 36%

6. A patient with pneumonia is at risk for:

   a. hypothermia.

   b. hypovolemic shock.

   c. septic shock.

   d. seizures.

   e. hyperthermia.

7. The first step to take when discovering an unresponsive patient is to:

   a. begin CPR.

   b. check circulation.

   c. establish an airway.

   d. go find help.

   e. identify the patient.

8. During a physical examination of an emergency patient's abdomen, check for:

   a. cerebral fluid.

   b. distal pulses.

   c. paradoxical movement.

   d. tenderness, rigidity, and distension.

   e. lethargy and slow movements.

9. A potential complication from a splint could be:

   a. compartment syndrome.

   b. dislocation.

   c. hematoma.

   d. injury from sharp bone fragments.

   e. tissue ischemia and infarction.

10. Circulation after splinting can be tested using:

   a. blood pressure.

   b. brachial pulse.

   c. carotid pulse.

   d. distal pulse.

   e. femoral pulse.

Scenario: A patient complains about tightness in the chest, a feeling of warmth, and itching. After a minute the patient's breathing is labored.

11. You are most likely watching the early warning signs of:

   a. an allergic reaction.

   b. cardiogenic shock.

   c. a myocardial infarction.

   d. poisoning.

   e. ecchymosis.

12. What action is contraindicated should this patient go into shock?

   a. Cardiac monitoring

   b. Epinephrine (1:1000)

   c. Establishing an IV line

   d. Intubation

   e. Providing high-flow oxygen

End Scenario

13. If a patient is having a seizure, you should:

   a. force something into the patient's mouth to protect the tongue.

   b. maintain spine immobilization.

   c. protect the patient from injury.

   d. restrain the patient.

   e. assist patient to supine position.

14. What is the difference between an emotional crisis and a psychiatric emergency?

   a. A psychiatric emergency results from substance abuse.

   b. A patient in a psychiatric emergency poses a physical threat to himself or others.

   c. An emotional crisis is a case of bipolar disorder.

   d. A psychiatric emergency involves a patient diagnosed with a psychiatric disorder.

   e. An emotional crisis does not include delusions.

15. A patient suffering hypothermia should be given:

   a. alcohol to promote circulation.

   b. hot chocolate to provide sugar.

   c. IV fluids for rehydration.

   d. warm coffee to raise his or her level of consciousness.

   e. dry heat to warm the surface.

16. What agency should be contacted first when a patient is exposed to a toxic substance?

   a. AMAA

   b. EMS

   c. MSDS

   d. the National Centers for Disease Control

   e. the Poison Control Center

17. Which form of shock is an acute allergic reaction?

   a. Neurogenic shock

   b. Anaphylactic shock

   c. Cardiogenic shock

   d. Septic shock

   e. Hypovolemic shock

18. What does the "V" in AVPU stand for?

   a. Vocalization

   b. Vital signs

   c. Viscosity

   d. Voice recognition

   e. Verbal response

19. To manage open soft tissue injuries, you should:

  a. leave them open to the air.

  b. wrap loosely in bandages.

  c. immediately stitch closed.

  d. elevate the wound.

  e. apply direct pressure.

20. Which of the following items should be included in an emergency kit?

  a. Alcohol wipes

  b. Syringe

  c. Penicillin

  d. Oscilloscope

  e. Sample containers

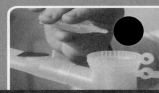

Chapter Checklist

☐ Read textbook chapter and take notes within the Chapter Notes outline. Answer the Learning Objectives as you reach them in the content, and then check them off.

☐ Work the Content Review questions—both Foundational Knowledge and Application.

☐ Perform the Active Learning exercise(s).

☐ Complete Professional Journal entries.

☐ Complete Skill Practice Activity(s) using Competency Evaluation Forms and Work Products, when appropriate.

☐ Take the Chapter Self-Assessment Quiz.

☐ Insert all appropriate pages into your Portfolio.

Learning Objectives

1. Spell and define the key terms.
2. Describe common skin disorders.
3. Explain common diagnostic procedures.
4. Prepare the patient for examination of the integument.
5. Assist the physician with examination of the integument.
6. Explain the difference between bandages and dressings and give the purpose of each.
7. Identify the guidelines for applying bandages.

Chapter Notes

Note: Bold-faced headings are the major headings in the text chapter; headings in regular font are lower-level headings (i.e., the content is subordinate to, or falls "under," the major headings). Make sure you understand the key terms used in the chapter, as well as the concepts presented as Key Points.

TEXT SUBHEADINGS   **Notes**

Introduction _____

_____

_____

☐ **LEARNING OBJECTIVE 1:** Spell and define the key terms.

Common Disorders of the Integumentary System

Key Point:
• Although it has many functions, including maintaining homeostasis, one of the most important functions of the integumentary system is to protect the underlying tissues and organs from the external environment.

Skin Infections

Key Point:
• When working with a patient who may have a skin infection, you should always wear protective equipment, such as examination gloves, since the drainage from any lesions may be infective.

Bacterial Infections

Key Terms: impetigo; macule; vesicle; bulla; pustule; erythema; folliculitis; furuncle; carbuncle; cellulitis
Key Points:
• Scratching must be discouraged to prevent the spread of the infection, and patients must be instructed to wash towels, washcloths, and bed linens daily.
• An abscess is formed when a small sac of pus, or purulent material, accumulates at the site of inflammation.
• Treatment of a **furuncle** includes application of moist heat to assist in ripening it, or bringing it to a head, and antibiotic therapy.
• **Carbuncles** are hard, round, extremely painful swellings that enlarge over several days to a week.
• When an existing wound is infected and the infection spreads to the surrounding connective tissue, **cellulitis** results.

Viral Infections

Key Terms: herpes zoster; verruca
Key Points:
• Herpes simplex infections produce lesions commonly known as cold sores or fever blisters.
• **Herpes zoster**, or shingles, is caused by the same virus that causes chickenpox.
• **Verruca** may occur singly or in groups and may be found anywhere on the skin or mucous membranes.

Fungal Infections

Key Terms: dermatophytosis; alopecia
Key Points:
- Fungal infection of the skin (**dermatophytosis**) is caused by a group of molds called dermatophytes.
- Tinea capitis affects the scalp.
- Tinea corporis (also known as tinea circinata) manifests on hairless portions of the body.
- Tinea cruris, known in lay terms as jock itch, is found on the skin in the groin area and the gluteal folds.
- Tinea pedis, or athlete's foot, is characterized by itching, burning, and stinging between the toes and on the soles of the feet.
- Also known as onychomycosis, tinea unguium causes thickening, discoloration, and crumbling of the nails, most often the toenails.
- Diagnosis of tinea versicolor is determined with a Wood's light, an ultraviolet light used in a darkened room to show abnormalities in the skin as fluorescent.

Parasitic Infections

Key Term: pediculosis
Key Points:
- Scabies is a contagious skin disorder caused by the itch mite *Sarcoptes scabiei*.
- **Pediculosis** is an infestation of the skin with a parasite known commonly as lice.
- The infestation is transmitted through physical contact with an infested person, by sitting on an infested toilet seat, or by sharing a comb, brush, clothing, or bedding that is infested.

Inflammatory Reactions

Eczema

Key Terms: eczema; pruritus
Key Point:
- **Eczema** is an inflammatory skin disorder usually involving only the epidermal layer of the skin.

Seborrheic Dermatitis _____

_____

Key Terms: seborrhea
Key Point:
• It is a chronic disorder resulting in greasy yellow scales primarily on the scalp, where it is called seborrheic dandruff.

Urticaria _____

_____

Key Term: urticaria
Key Point:
• **Urticaria**, or hives, is an acute inflammatory reaction of the dermis.

Acne Vulgaris _____

_____

Key Point:
• Acne vulgaris is an inflammatory disease of the sebaceous glands.

Psoriasis _____

_____

Key Point:
• Psoriasis is a chronic inflammatory skin disorder characterized by bright red plaques covered with dry, silvery scales.

Disorders of Wound Healing _____

_____

_____

Keloids _____

_____

Key Point:
• Keloids, an overproduction of scar tissue, occur as a complication of wound healing.

Disorders Caused by Pressure _____

_____

_____

Callus and Corn

Key Point:
• A callus, sometimes called a callosity, is a raised painless thickening of the epidermis.

Decubitus Ulcers

Key Point:
• Decubitus ulcers are also called pressure sores and are caused by prolonged pressure to an area of the body, usually over a bony prominence.

Intertrigo

Key Point:
• Intertrigo is a disorder of skin breakdown that occurs in the body folds of obese persons.

Alopecia

Key Term: alopecia
Key Point:
• **Alopecia**, or baldness, may be the result of physical trauma, systemic disease, bacteria or fungal infection, chemotherapy, excessive radiation, hormonal imbalance, or genetic predisposition.

Disorders of Pigmentation

Albinism

Key Point:
• Albinism is a genetically determined condition of partial or total absence of the pigment melanin in the skin, hair, and eyes.

Vitiligo _____

_____

Key Point:
- Vitiligo is a progressive, chronic destruction of melano-cytes, cells in the epidermis that produce melanin, a skin pigment.

Leukoderma _____

_____

Key Point:
- Leukoderma is a permanent local loss of skin pigment that results from damage caused by skin trauma.

Nevus _____

_____

Key Point:
- A nevus, also known as a birthmark or mole, is a congeni-tal pigmented skin blemish. It is usually circumscribed and may involve the epidermis, connective tissue, nerves, or blood vessels.

Skin Cancers _____

_____

_____

Basal Cell Carcinoma _____

_____

Key Point:
- Basal cell carcinoma is a slow-growing cancer that appears most commonly on exposed areas of the body, usually the face, but may also occur on the shoulders or chest.

Squamous Cell Carcinoma _____

_____

Key Term: neoplasm
Key Point:
- Squamous cell carcinoma is slightly less common than basal cell carcinoma and occurs in any squamous (scaly) epithelial area of the body, such as the lungs, cervix, or anus, but is most frequently found on the skin.

Malignant Melanoma _____

Key Points:
• Malignant melanoma is a cancer of the skin that forms from melanocytes.
• Malignant melanoma, which is thought to be caused by excessive exposure to sunlight, is the leading cause of death due to skin disease.

☐ **LEARNING OBJECTIVE 2:** Describe common skin disorders.

Diagnostic Procedures _____

Physical Examination of the Skin _____

Key Point:
• Examination of the skin is performed primarily by inspection.

Wound Cultures _____

Key Point:
• Obtain a wound culture by getting a sample of wound exudate (drainage) using a sterile swab, applying the specimen to a growth medium, and allowing the microorganisms to grow.

Skin Biopsy _____

Key Point:
• The purpose of a skin biopsy is to remove a small piece of tissue from a lesion so that it may be examined under a microscope to determine whether it is a benign or malignant growth.

Urine Melanin _____

Key Point:
• Melanin is not normally present in the urine unless the patient has malignant melanoma.

Wood's Light Analysis _____

_____

Key Point:
- Wood's light is an ultraviolet light that is used to detect fungal and bacterial infections, scabies, and alterations in pigment.

☐ **LEARNING OBJECTIVE 3:** Explain common diagnostic procedures.

☐ **LEARNING OBJECTIVE 4:** Prepare the patient for examination of the integument.

☐ **LEARNING OBJECTIVE 5:** Assist the physician with examination of the integument.

Bandaging _____

_____

Types of Bandages _____

_____

☐ **LEARNING OBJECTIVE 6:** Explain the difference between bandages and dressings and give the purpose of each.

Bandage Application Guidelines _____

_____

Key Points:
- When properly applied, bandages should feel comfortably snug and should be fastened securely enough to remain in place until removed.
- Never place a bandage directly over an open wound.

☐ **LEARNING OBJECTIVE 7:** Identify the guidelines for applying bandages.

Content Review

FOUNDATIONAL KNOWLEDGE

Common Skin Disorders

1. Take a look at the following information. The list on the left describes some common skin disorders. The list on the right contains the names of the disorders. Draw lines to match the descriptions with the correct disorder.

a. A skin disease characterized by pimples, comedones, and cysts

b. A pigmentation disorder thought to be an autoimmune disorder in patients with an inherited predisposition

c. An infection in an interconnected group of hair follicles

d. A skin inflammation caused by an overproduction of sebum that affects the scalp, eyelids, face, back, umbilicus, and body folds

e. A hard, raised thickening of the stratum corneum on the toes

f. An ulcerative lesion caused by impaired blood supply and insufficient oxygen to an area

g. A type of skin cancer that is a slow-growing, malignant tumor

1. Vitiligo
2. Decubitus ulcer
3. Corn
4. Acne vulgaris
5. Carbuncle
6. Squamous cell carcinoma
7. Seborrheic dermatitis

2. Which of the following skin disorders cannot be treated? Circle the correct answer.

a. Impetigo

b. Folliculitis

c. Albinism

d. Malignant melanoma

e. Decubitus ulcers

3. What are the symptoms of psoriasis?

_____

_____

4. A man brings his 85-year-old mother to the physician's office. He tells you that his mother lives in a local care home. When the physician examines the patient, you notice multiple decubitus ulcers on her body. Explain why this would be a particular cause of concern.

_____

_____

5. How would a physician be able to confirm a suspected case of malignant melanoma? Circle the correct answer.

a. Wood's light analysis

b. inspection

c. urine test

6. List the three types of skin biopsy performed by a physician.

a. _____

b. _____

c. _____

The Medical Assistant's Role

7. As a medical assistant, you'll be responsible for helping the physician perform physical examinations of the skin. Review the list of tasks below and determine which tasks you may be responsible for as a medical assistant. Place a check mark in the "Yes" column for duties that you might assist with and a check mark in the "No" column for tasks that would be completed by someone else.

Task	Yes	No
a. Assemble the equipment required by the physician.		
b. Perform a skin biopsy.		
c. Inject local anesthetic when needed.		

Task	Yes	No
d. Direct specimens to the appropriate laboratories.		
e. Clean and disinfect the examination room.		
f. Diagnose and treat common skin inflammations.		
g. Reinforce the physician's instructions about caring for a skin condition at home.		

8. You are applying a bandage to a patient. Read the statements below and check the appropriate box to show whether the bandage has been applied correctly or incorrectly.

	Applied Correctly	Applied Incorrectly
a. You have fastened the bandage with adhesive tape.		
b. The area that you are about to bandage is clean and damp.		
c. You have dressed two burned fingers separately and then bandaged them together.		
d. The skin around the bandaged arm is pale and cool.		
e. You have bandaged a wounded foot by covering the toes to make it neater.		
f. You have bandaged an elbow with extra padding.		

9. Match the following types of bandages with the correct statement below them.

Bandage

a. Roller bandages _____

b. Elastic bandages _____

c. Tubular gauze bandages _____

Description

1. These bandages can be given to the patient to take home to wash and reuse. You should be careful when applying them so as not to compromise circulation.

2. These bandages are made of soft, woven materials and are available in various lengths and widths. They can be either sterile or clean.

3. These bandages are very stretchy and are used to enclose fingers, toes, arms, legs, head, and trunk.

More Skin Disorders

10. List the three bacterial skin infections that develop in the hair follicles.

a. _____

b. _____

c. _____

11. A patient has a band of lesions on his back made up of small red papules. What skin disorder does this person most likely have? Explain what causes the condition.

_____

_____

12. A father brings his 8-year-old son to the physician, who diagnoses the child with pediculosis. What advice could you give the father to ensure that no other members of the family become infected? List three things that the father could do to contain the problem.

a. _____

b. _____

c. _____

13. What is the full version of the cancer prevention message "Slip! Slop! Slap! Wrap!"?

_____

_____

14. Take a look at the case studies in the chart below. Place a check mark in the appropriate box to show whether the person is at a high risk or a low risk of developing impetigo.

Case Study	High Risk	Low Risk
a. A slightly overweight 34-year-old woman who showers twice a day		
b. A 55-year-old man who works at a hospital laundry room and does not wash his hands		
c. A 22-year-old woman with severe anorexia		
d. An 18-year-old drug addict who lives in an abandoned warehouse		
e. A 40-year-old mother of three who enjoys reading in the tub		

15. Match the following skin disorders with the appropriate treatment.

Disorder

a. Decubitus ulcers _____
b. Basal cell carcinoma _____
c. Cellulitis _____
d. Folliculitis _____
e. Verruca _____
f. Urticaria _____

Treatment

1. Saline soaks or compresses
2. Antihistamines
3. Antibiotic powder
4. Surgical removal
5. Keratolytic agents
6. Antibiotics

16. The physician suspects that a patient has ringworm. Explain what method you would use to confirm the physician's suspicion and describe the procedure.

_____

_____

17. A clinically obese patient comes into the office in the middle of summer, complaining of itching and stinging sensations all over the body. Name the skin disorder that the patient is probably suffering from and describe how it should be treated.

_____

_____

18. Read these descriptions of five of Dr. Marsh's patients. Then decide which of his patients is at the highest risk of developing malignant melanoma. Circle the correct answer.

a. Mrs. Pearson, 42-year-old mother of two. Light brown hair, brown eyes, enjoys reading and watching movies.
b. Mr. Stevens, 50-year-old widower. Gray hair, brown eyes, enjoys walking and playing golf.
c. Jessica Phillips, 24-year-old college student. Red hair, blue eyes, enjoys playing volleyball and surfing.
d. Todd Andrews, 18-year-old student. Black hair, green eyes, enjoys running and swimming.
e. Mr. Archer, 39-year-old father of three. Blond hair, blue eyes, lives in Minnesota and enjoys skiing.

19. Match the following key terms to their definitions.

Key Terms

a. alopecia _____
b. bulla _____
c. carbuncle _____
d. cellulitis _____
e. dermatophytosis _____
f. eczema _____
g. erythema _____
h. folliculitis _____
i. furuncle _____
j. herpes simplex _____
k. herpes zoster _____
l. impetigo _____
m. macule _____
n. neoplasm _____
o. pediculosis _____
p. pruritus _____
q. psoriasis _____
r. seborrhea _____
s. urticaria _____
t. verruca _____
u. vesicle _____
v. pustule _____

Definitions

1. a highly infectious skin infection causing erythema and progressing to honey-colored crusts
2. redness of the skin
3. an inflammation of hair follicles
4. a small, flat discoloration of the skin
5. an abnormal growth of new tissue; tumor
6. an infection of an interconnected group of hair follicles or several furuncles forming a mass
7. an inflammation or infection of the skin and deeper tissues that may result in tissue destruction if not treated properly
8. an infection caused by the herpes simplex virus
9. hives
10. an infection caused by reactivation of varicella zoster virus, which causes chickenpox
11. a wart
12. a large blister or vesicle
13. an infestation with parasitic lice
14. baldness
15. superficial dermatitis
16. itching
17. an overproduction of sebum by the sebaceous glands
18. an infection in a hair follicle or gland; characterized by pain, redness, and swelling with necrosis of tissue in the center
19. a skin lesion that appears as a small sac containing fluid; a blister
20. a fungal infection of the skin
21. a vesicle filled with pus
22. a chronic skin disorder that appears as red patches covered with thick, dry, silvery scales

20. True or False? Determine whether the following statements are true or false. If false, explain why.

a. Before applying a bandage, you should perform surgical asepsis.

_____

_____

b. Young women are more likely to develop keloids than young men.

_____

_____

c. A wound culture is obtained by excising the wound.

_____

_____

d. Erythema is best treated with antihistamines.

_____

_____

APPLICATION

Critical Thinking Practice

1. A patient has come into the physician's office for a skin biopsy on his thigh. After the physician has removed the tissue, she asks you to bandage the area. List three things you should do while you are bandaging the patient's thigh to ensure that it is both sterile and secure. Explain why they are important.

_____

_____

2. There are three patients waiting to be seen by a physician, and all of the appointments are slightly behind schedule. One of the patients is a young man who has clusters of wheals on his left arm. The second patient is a 7-year-old girl who has dry scaly crusts on her face and neck. The third patient is a 5-year-old boy with dried skin flakes and bald patches on his scalp. All three patients are itching, and the receptionist is concerned that they might be contagious. You have only one spare examination room. Which patient would you isolate in the examination room? Explain your answer.

_____

_____

Patient Education

1. Your patient is a 25-year-old female who has been to see the physician several times for severe sunburn. You know that her lifestyle can lead to long-term skin problems and that she is in a high-risk category for developing malignant melanoma. Write a list of useful guidelines for the patient to educate her about staying safe in the sun. Include some of the early warning signs of skin cancer that she should keep an eye out for.

_____

_____

Documentation

1. Your patient is a 9-year-old girl who suffers from severe eczema. The physician has recommended that she wear bandages at night to protect against scratching. You demonstrate to the patient's mother how to apply the bandages. The patient's mother asks how often she should apply ointment to her daughter's skin, and you repeat the physician's instructions to use it twice a day. How would you document this interaction in the patient's chart?

_____

_____

Active Learning

1. Use the Internet to research the major causes of fungal infections and find out how they can be prevented. Produce a poster to display in the office, educating patients about the main types of fungal infection, how they are spread, and how patients can protect their families from outbreaks.
2. Work with a partner to practice applying bandages and dressings. Ask your partner to tell you what type of injury needs dressing and make sure that you select the correct type of bandage for the task. Make sure you apply the bandage snugly but not too tightly in each case.

3. Use the Internet to research the differences between eczema and psoriasis. Produce a one-page leaflet to help patients understand the disorders. Include causes, symptoms, and treatments for each.

Professional Journal

REFLECT

(Prompts and Ideas: Have you or a loved one ever had a skin cancer scare? Did you have to undergo a skin biopsy? How were you or your loved one treated by medical staff throughout the procedure? Do you think there is enough awareness about the dangers of skin cancer? What steps do you take to prevent it?)

_____

_____

_____

_____

_____

_____

_____

PONDER AND SOLVE

1. A mother brings her 8-year-old son to the physician's office and the child is diagnosed with pediculosis. She insists that her child cannot possibly have lice because they live in a very clean home. The mother demands that the physician examine the child again. What do you say to the mother to calm her down? How do you reassure her?

_____

_____

_____

_____

_____

_____

2. A 14-year-old boy comes into the physician's office with severe acne vulgaris on his face and neck. He is embarrassed and depressed about his condition and is worried that it will never get better. He says that he has tried every over-the-counter medication and that this is his last hope. What can you say to the patient to ease his mind?

_____

_____

_____

_____

_____

_____

EXPERIENCE

Skills related to this chapter include:

1. Apply a Warm or Cold Compress (Procedure 27-1).
2. Assist with Therapeutic Soaks (Procedure 27-2).
3. Apply a Tubular Gauze Bandage (Procedure 27-3).

Record any common mistakes, lessons learned, and/or tips you discovered during your experience of practicing and demonstrating these skills:

_____

_____

_____

_____

_____

_____

_____

Skill Practice

PERFORMANCE OBJECTIVES:

1. Apply a warm or cold compress (Procedure 27-1).
2. Assist with therapeutic soaks (Procedure 27-2).
3. Apply a tubular gauze bandage (Procedure 27-3).

Name_____ Date _____ Time _____

Procedure 27-1:	**APPLY A WARM OR COLD COMPRESS**

EQUIPMENT/SUPPLIES: Warm compresses—appropriate solution (water with possible antiseptic if ordered), warmed to 110°F or recommended temperature; bath thermometer; absorbent material (cloths, gauze); waterproof barriers; hot water bottle (optional); clean or sterile basin; gloves. Cold compresses—appropriate solution; ice bag or cold pack; absorbent material (cloths, gauze); waterproof barriers; gloves

STANDARDS: Given the needed equipment and a place to work, the student will perform this skill with _____% accuracy in a total of _____ minutes. *(Your instructor will tell you what the percentage and time limits will be before you begin practicing.)*

KEY: 4 = Satisfactory   0 = Unsatisfactory   NA = This step is not counted

PROCEDURE STEPS	SELF	PARTNER	INSTRUCTOR
1. Wash your hands and put on gloves.	☐	☐	☐
2. Check the physician's order and assemble the equipment and supplies.	☐	☐	☐
3. Pour the appropriate solution into the basin. For hot compresses, check the temperature of the warmed solution.	☐	☐	☐
4. Greet and identify the patient. Explain the procedure.	☐	☐	☐
5. Ask patient to remove appropriate clothing.	☐	☐	☐
6. Gown and drape accordingly.	☐	☐	☐
7. Protect the examination table with a waterproof barrier.	☐	☐	☐
8. Place absorbent material or gauze into the prepared solution. Wring out excess moisture.	☐	☐	☐
9. Place the compress on the patient's skin and ask about comfort of temperature.	☐	☐	☐
10. Observe the skin for changes in color.	☐	☐	☐
11. Arrange the wet compress over the area.	☐	☐	☐
12. Insulate the compress with plastic or another waterproof barrier.	☐	☐	☐
13. Check the compress frequently for moisture and temperature. **a.** Hot water bottles or ice packs may be used to maintain the temperature. **b.** Rewet absorbent material as needed.	☐	☐	☐
14. After the prescribed amount of time, usually 20–30 minutes. Remove the compress. **a.** Discard disposable materials. **b.** Disinfect reusable equipment.	☐	☐	☐
15. Remove your gloves and wash your hands.	☐	☐	☐
16. Document the procedure including: **a.** Length of treatment, type of solution, temperature of solution **b.** Skin color after treatment, assessment of the area, and patient's reactions	☐	☐	☐

CALCULATION

Total Possible Points: _____
Total Points Earned: _____ Multiplied by 100 = _____ Divided by Total Possible Points = _____%

Pass **Fail**
☐   ☐   Comments:

Student's signature _____ Date _____
Partner's signature _____ Date _____
Instructor's signature _____ Date _____

Name_____   Date _____   Time _____

Procedure 27-2:	ASSIST WITH THERAPEUTIC SOAKS

EQUIPMENT/SUPPLIES: Clean or sterile basin or container to comfortably contain the body part to be soaked; solution and/or medication; dry towels; bath thermometer; gloves

STANDARDS: Given the needed equipment and a place to work, the student will perform this skill with _____ % accuracy in a total of _____ minutes. *(Your instructor will tell you what the percentage and time limits will be before you begin practicing.)*

KEY: 4 = Satisfactory   0 = Unsatisfactory   NA = This step is not counted

PROCEDURE STEPS	SELF	PARTNER	INSTRUCTOR
1. Wash your hands and apply your gloves.	☐	☐	☐
2. Assemble the equipment and supplies, including the appropriately sized basin or container. Pad surfaces of container for comfort.	☐	☐	☐
3. Fill the container with solution and check the temperature with a bath thermometer. The temperature should be below 110°F.	☐	☐	☐
4. Greet and identify the patient. Explain the procedure.	☐	☐	☐
5. Slowly lower the patient's extremity or body part into the container.	☐	☐	☐
6. Arrange the part comfortably and in easy alignment.	☐	☐	☐
7. Check for pressure areas and pad the edges as needed for comfort.	☐	☐	☐
8. Check the solution every 5–10 minutes for proper temperature.	☐	☐	☐
9. Soak for the prescribed amount of time, usually 15–20 minutes.	☐	☐	☐
10. Remove the body part from the solution and carefully dry the area with a towel.	☐	☐	☐
11. Properly care for the equipment and appropriately dispose of single-use supplies.	☐	☐	☐
12. Document the procedure including: a. Length of treatment, type of solution, temperature of solution b. Skin color after treatment, assessment of the area, and patient's reactions	☐	☐	☐

CALCULATION

Total Possible Points: _____
Total Points Earned: _____ Multiplied by 100 = _____ Divided by Total Possible Points = _____%

Pass   **Fail**
☐   ☐   Comments:

Student's signature _____ Date _____
Partner's signature _____ Date _____
Instructor's signature _____ Date _____

Name _____ Date _____ Time _____

Procedure 27-3:　APPLY A TUBULAR GAUZE BANDAGE

EQUIPMENT/SUPPLIES: Tubular gauze, applicator, tape, scissors

STANDARDS: Given the needed equipment and a place to work, the student will perform this skill with _____% accuracy in a total of _____ minutes. *(Your instructor will tell you what the percentage and time limits will be before you begin practicing.)*

KEY:　　4 = Satisfactory　　　0 = Unsatisfactory　　　NA = This step is not counted

PROCEDURE STEPS	SELF	PARTNER	INSTRUCTOR
1. Wash your hands and assemble the equipment.	☐	☐	☐
2. Greet and identify the patient. Explain the procedure.	☐	☐	☐
3. Choose the appropriate-size tubular gauze applicator and gauze width.	☐	☐	☐
4. Select and cut or tear adhesive tape in lengths to secure the gauze ends.	☐	☐	☐
5. Place the gauze bandage on the applicator in the following manner: 　**a.** Be sure that the applicator is upright (open end up) and placed on a flat surface. 　**b.** Pull a sufficient length of gauze from the stock box, ready to cut. 　**c.** Open the end of the length of gauze and slide it over the upper end of the applicator. 　**d.** Push estimated amount of gauze needed for this procedure onto the applicator. 　**e.** Cut the gauze when the required amount of gauze has been transferred to the applicator.	☐	☐	☐
6. Place applicator over the distal end of the affected part. Hold it in place as you move to step 7.	☐	☐	☐
7. Slide applicator containing the gauze up to the proximal end of the affected part.	☐	☐	☐
8. Pull the applicator 1–2 inches past the end of the affected part if the part is to be completely covered.	☐	☐	☐
9. Turn the applicator one full turn to anchor the bandage.	☐	☐	☐
10. Move the applicator toward the proximal part as before.	☐	☐	☐
11. Move the applicator forward about 1 inch beyond the original starting point.	☐	☐	☐
12. Repeat the procedure until the desired coverage is obtained.	☐	☐	☐
13. The final layer should end at the proximal part of the affected area. Remove the applicator.	☐	☐	☐
14. Secure the bandage in place with adhesive tape or cut the gauze into two tails and tie them at the base of the tear.	☐	☐	☐
15. Tie the two tails around the closest proximal joint.	☐	☐	☐

PROCEDURE STEPS	SELF	PARTNER	INSTRUCTOR
16. Use the adhesive tape sparingly to secure the end if not using a tie.	☐	☐	☐
17. Properly care for or dispose of equipment and supplies.	☐	☐	☐
18. Clean the work area. Wash your hands.	☐	☐	☐
19. Record the procedure.	☐	☐	☐

CALCULATION

Total Possible Points: _____
Total Points Earned: _____ Multiplied by 100 = _____ Divided by Total Possible Points = _____%

Pass   **Fail**
  ☐   ☐

Comments:

Student's signature _____ Date _____
Partner's signature _____ Date _____
Instructor's signature _____ Date _____

Work Product 1

Document appropriately.

Anne Thomas is a 34-year-old inpatient recovering from a surgical procedure. Two days after the procedure, she presents with a stage III decubitus ulcer measuring 10 cm across, centered in the thoracic region of her lower back. The physician orders a punch biopsy, and you are instructed to bandage the area after the procedure.

If you are currently working in a medical office, use a blank paper patient chart from the office. If this is not available to you, use the space below to record the incident in the chart.

_____

_____

_____

_____

_____

_____

_____

Chapter Self-Assessment Quiz

1. Which of the following groups of people are most likely to develop impetigo?

   a. The elderly

   b. Women

   c. Young children

   d. Men

   e. Teenagers

2. What type of infection is herpes simplex?

   a. Bacterial

   b. Fungal

   c. Parasitic

   d. Viral

   e. Genetic

3. Public showers and swimming pools are common places to pick up fungal infections because:

   a. fungi thrive in moist conditions.

   b. areas that are highly populated increase the risk factor.

   c. sharing towels passes fungal infections from one person to another.

   d. fungi grow quickly on tile surfaces.

   e. antifungal medications do not work once they come into contact with water.

4. Which of these skin disorders may be caused by food allergies?

   a. Keloids

   b. Intertrigo

   c. Alopecia

   d. Eczema

   e. Seborrheic dermatitis

5. Which of the following statements is true about albinism?

   a. Respiratory problems are common among sufferers of albinism.

   b. Albinism is treated with benzoyl peroxide.

   c. Albinism usually occurs in exposed areas of the skin.

   d. People who suffer from albinism should have regular checkups.

   e. People who suffer from albinism should take particular care of their eyes in the sun.

6. Which statements are true about decubitus ulcers?

   a. They are frequently diagnosed in school-aged children.

   b. They are most common in aged, debilitated, and immobilized patients.

   c. They are highly contagious.

   d. They generally occur on the chin and forehead.

   e. They are effectively treated with antifungal creams.

7. When bandaging a patient, you should:

   a. fasten bandages only with safety pins.

   b. complete surgical asepsis before you begin.

   c. keep the area to be bandaged warm.

   d. leave fingers and toes exposed when possible.

   e. wrap the bandage as tightly as possible to prevent it from coming loose.

8. A person suffering from high stress levels is most likely to develop:

   a. urticaria.

   b. acne vulgaris.

   c. impetigo.

   d. leukoderma.

   e. herpes zoster.

9. How many people in the United States will typically develop malignant melanoma?

   a. 1 in 5

   b. 1 in 500

   c. 1 in 105

   d. 1 in 1005

   e. 1 in 5000

10. Which of the following conditions would be treated with topical antifungal cream?

    a. Folliculitis

    b. Vitiligo

    c. Tinea versicolor

    d. Urticaria

    e. Decubitus ulcers

11. What should patients do if they have an absence of melanin in their skin?

    a. Avoid coming into contact with other people.

    b. Protect their skin from the sun.

    c. Seek immediate medical assistance.

    d. Take supplementary vitamin pills.

    e. Stop sharing towels and bedding.

Scenario: A male patient comes into the physician's office to have a wart removed from his finger. While you are preparing him for the procedure, he tells you that he regularly gets verrucas on his feet.

12. How would you advise the patient to avoid further viral infections?

    a. Wash all bedding and clothing at high temperatures.

    b. Avoid sharing combs and toiletries with anyone.

    c. Avoid coming into direct contact with skin lesions.

    d. Wear comfortable footwear and avoid walking long distances.

    e. Frequently wash hands with antibacterial soap.

13. The patient should look for over-the-counter wart medication that contains:

    a. podophyllum resin.

    b. acyclovir.

    c. selenium sulfide.

    d. permethrin.

    e. prednisone.

End Scenario

14. Before you apply a bandage to an open wound, you should:

    a. moisten the bandage.

    b. keep the bandage at room temperature.

    c. apply pressure to the wound.

    d. apply a sterile dressing to the wound.

    e. check to see how the patient would like the bandage fastened.

15. How can you tell that a patient is suffering from Stage I decubitus ulcers?

    a. The skin is blistered, peeling, or cracked.

    b. Red skin does not return to normal when massaged.

    c. The skin is scaly, dry, and flaky.

    d. The skin is extremely itchy.

    e. The patient is unable to feel pressure on the area.

16. When a physician performs a shave biopsy, he:

    a. cuts the lesion off just above the skin line.

    b. removes a small section from the center of the lesion.

    c. removes the entire lesion for evaluation.

    d. cuts the lesion off just below the skin line.

    e. removes a small section from the edge of the lesion.

17. Which of these is thought to be a cause of skin cancer in areas not exposed to the sun?

    a. Chemicals in toiletries

    b. Pet allergies

    c. Frequent irritation

    d. Second-hand smoke

    e. Excessive scratching

18. Treatment of impetigo involves:

    a. washing the area two to three times a day followed by application of topical antibiotics.

    b. cleaning with alcohol sponges twice a day.

    c. washing towels, washcloths, and bed linens daily.

    d. oral antibiotics for severe cases.

    e. the physician removing the infected area.

19. Which of the following statements is true about nevi?

    a. Nevi are usually malignant.

    b. Nevi are usually found on the back or legs.

    c. It is common for nevi to bleed occasionally.

    d. Nevi are congenital pigmented skin blemishes.

    e. Nevi are extremely rare in young patients.

20. Which part of the body is affected by tinea capitis?

    a. Hands

    b. Feet

    c. Hair follicles

    d. Groin

    e. Scalp

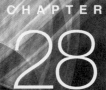

CHAPTER 28

Orthopedics

Chapter Checklist

☐ Read textbook chapter and take notes within the Chapter Notes outline. Answer the Learning Objectives as you reach them in the content, and then check them off.

☐ Work the Content Review questions—both Foundational Knowledge and Application.

☐ Perform the Active Learning exercise(s).

☐ Complete Professional Journal entries.

☐ Complete Skill Practice Activity(s) using Competency Evaluation Forms and Work Products, when appropriate.

☐ Take the Chapter Self-Assessment Quiz.

☐ Insert all appropriate pages into your Portfolio.

Learning Objectives

1. Spell and define the key terms.
2. List and describe disorders of the musculoskeletal system.
3. Compare the different types of fractures.
4. Identify and explain diagnostic procedures of the musculoskeletal system.
5. Discuss the role of the medical assistant in caring for the patient with a musculoskeletal system disorder.
6. Describe the various types of ambulatory aids.

Chapter Notes

Note: Bold-faced headings are the major headings in the text chapter; headings in regular font are lower-level headings (i.e., the content is subordinate to, or falls "under," the major headings). Make sure you understand the key terms used in the chapter, as well as the concepts presented as Key Points.

TEXT SUBHEADINGS   **NOTES**

Introduction _____

_____

_____

☐ **LEARNING OBJECTIVE 1:** Spell and define key terms.

_____

The Musculoskeletal System and Common Disorders _____

_____

Key Points:
- Muscles allow movement of the body through contraction and relaxation.
- The most common disorders of the musculoskeletal system are sprains, dislocations, fractures, joint disruptions, and degeneration.

Sprains and Strains _____

_____

Key Point:
- Injury to a joint capsule and its supporting ligaments is called a sprain, and injury to a muscle and its supporting tendons is called a strain.

Dislocations _____

_____

Key Point:
- Dislocation of a joint, also called a luxation, occurs when the end of the bone is displaced from its articular surface.

Fractures _____

_____

Key Terms: contusion; reduction
Key Point:
- A fracture is a break or disruption in a bone caused by falls, other trauma, disease, tumors, and unusual stress.

Casts _____

_____

Key Point:
- Fractures must be immobilized to facilitate healing of the bone in the proper alignment.

Assisting With Plaster or Fiberglass Cast Application _____

_____

_____

Plaster or Fiberglass Cast Removal _____

_____

_____

Healing of Fractures

Key Terms: callus; prosthesis; embolus
Key Point:
- The most important criterion for successful healing of a fracture is an adequate blood supply.

Bursitis

Key Term: bursae
Key Point:
- The subdeltoid bursa in the shoulder between the deltoid muscle and the joint capsule is the most common site of bursitis, an inflammation of the bursa.

Arthritis

Key Term: ankylosing spondylitis
Key Points:
- Osteoarthritis, or degenerative joint disease, is caused by wear and tear on the weight-bearing joints.
- Rheumatoid arthritis is a systemic autoimmune disease that attacks the synovial membrane lining of the joint.

Tendonitis

Key Term: iontophoresis
Key Point:
- The most common site of tendonitis is at the supraspinatus tendon in the shoulder, one of the rotator cuff muscles.

Fibromyalgia

Key Point:
- Fibromyalgia causes multiple often nonspecific symptoms including widespread pain in specific body areas, muscular stiffness, fatigue, and difficulty sleeping.

Gout

Key Point:
- Gout, a metabolic disease of overproduction of uric acid, is a form of arthritis caused by the deposit of uric acid crystals into a joint, usually in the great toe.

Muscular Dystrophy

Key Term: electromyography
Key Point:
- The congenital disorders collectively known as muscular dystrophy are characterized by varying degrees of progressive wasting of skeletal muscles.

Osteoporosis

Key Point:
- Porous bones, or osteoporosis, is a condition in which the bones are deficient in calcium and phosphorus, making them brittle and vulnerable to fractures.

Bone Tumors

Key Point:
- Bone tissue is rarely the primary site for malignancies but is frequently a site of metastasis.

Spine Disorders

Key Point:
- However, back injuries are common and are a leading cause of work-related injury among health care professionals.

Abnormal Spine Curvatures

Key Terms: lordosis; kyphosis; scoliosis
Key Point:
- Exaggerated or abnormal curvatures of the spine affect the posture and the alignment of the shoulders and hips.

Herniated Intervertebral Disc _____

_____

Key Point:
• A disc herniates when its soft center, known as the nucleus, ruptures through its tough outer layer to protrude into the spinal canal, sometimes pressing on the spinal cord.

Disorders of the Upper Extremities _____

_____

_____

Rotator Cuff Injury _____

_____

Key Point:
• Injury to the rotator cuff muscles in the shoulder can cause severe pain, weakness, and loss of function.

Adhesive Capsulitis, or Frozen Shoulder _____

_____

Key Term: contracture
Key Point:
• **Contractures** develop when the joint is immobilized, allowing the collagen fibers to stick to each other and thereby limiting the movement in the joint.

Lateral Epicondylitis, or Tennis Elbow _____

_____

Key Term: phonophoresis
Key Point:
• Lateral epicondylitis, often called tennis elbow, is a common elbow injury, a sprain or strain of the tendons of origin of the wrist and finger extensor muscles.

Carpal Tunnel Syndrome _____

_____

Key Point:
• A repetitive motion injury, carpal tunnel syndrome occurs when the carpal bones and transverse carpal ligaments compress the median nerve at the wrist.

Dupuytren Contracture _____

_____

Key Point:
- Dupuytren contracture results in flexion deformities of the fingers, most often the ring and little fingers.

Disorders of the Lower Extremities _____

_____

_____

Chondromalacia Patellae _____

_____

Key Terms: arthroscopy; arthroplasty
Key Point:
- Chondromalacia patellae is a degenerative disorder affecting the cartilage that covers the back of the patella, or kneecap.

Plantar Fasciitis _____

_____

Key Point:
- Plantar fasciitis, inflammation of the plantar fascia ligament that stretches across the bottom of the foot, is the most frequent cause of pain in the bottom of the foot.

☐ **LEARNING OBJECTIVE 2:** List and describe disorders of the musculoskeletal system.

☐ **LEARNING OBJECTIVE 3:** Compare the different types of fractures.

Common Diagnostic Procedures _____

_____

_____

Physical Examination _____

_____

Key Point:
- The physician's evaluation of the musculoskeletal system usually includes an assessment of structure and function, movement, and pain.

Diagnostic Studies _____

Key Terms: arthrogram; goniometer
Key Point:
• The most frequently used tools for detecting disorders of the musculoskeletal system are radiology and diagnostic imaging, which are used to diagnose fractures, dislocations, and degeneration or diseases of the bones and joints.

☐ **LEARNING OBJECTIVE 4:** Identify and explain diagnostic procedures of the musculoskeletal system.

The Role of the Medical Assistant _____

Warm and Cold Applications _____

Precautions _____

Key Point:
• The body responds to extremes of temperature for extended periods by exerting an opposite effect called the rebound phenomenon.

Ambulatory Assist Devices _____

Crutches _____

Key Point:
• Axillary crutches, which are the most common form, extend from just under the patient's axillae to the floor with hand grips to distribute weight to the palms.

Canes _____

Key Point:
• A cane is used when the patient needs extra support and stability but requires only a small measure of assistance with weight bearing.

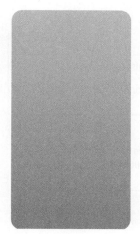

Walkers _____

_____

Key Point:
• A walker is a comfortable aid for the elderly and others with conditions that cause weakness or poor coordination.

☐ **LEARNING OBJECTIVE 5:** Discuss the role of the medical assistant in caring for the patient with a musculoskeletal system disorder.

☐ **LEARNING OBJECTIVE 6:** Describe the various types of ambulatory aids.

Content Review

FOUNDATIONAL KNOWLEDGE

Sprains, Strains, and Fractures

1. What is the difference between a sprain and a strain? How are they similar?

_____

_____

2. Name four common sites of dislocations.

  a. _____

  b. _____

  c. _____

  d. _____

3. Complete this chart to show the different types of fractures.

Type of Fracture	Description
Avulsion	Tearing away of bone fragments caused by sharp twisting force applied to ligaments or tendons attached to bone
Comminuted	**a.**
Compound or open	Broken end of bone punctures and protrudes through skin
b.	Damage to bone caused by strong force on both ends of the bone, such as through a fall
Depressed	Fracture of flat bones (typically the skull) which causes bone fragment to be driven below the surface of the bone
Greenstick	**c.**
Impacted	One bone segment driven into another
d.	Break is slanted across the axis of the bone
Pathological	Related to a disease such as osteoporosis, Paget disease, bone cysts, tumors, or cancers

Type of Fracture	Description
Simple or closed	**e.**
Spiral	Appears as an S-shaped fracture on radiographs and occurs with torsion or twisting injuries
f.	A fracture at right angles to axis of bone that is usually caused by excessive bending force or direct pressure on bone

4. Your patient is complaining of pain in his wrist. You learn that the pain began after he fell from a ladder and used his hand to break his fall. You suspect a fracture. What signs of a fracture could you look for to confirm your suspicions?

_____

_____

5. Draw a bone with a simple or closed fracture. Then, use your illustration to show where callus is applied.

6. What is the difference between a spiral fracture and an avulsion fracture?

_____

_____

Musculoskeletal Disorders

7. Complete this chart, which shows the variations of arthritis, the affected site, and the characteristics of the variation.

Disease	Affected Site	Characteristics
Osteoarthritis	Weight-bearing joints	**a.**
b.	Synovial membrane lining of the joint	Usually begins in nonweight-bearing joints, but can spread to many other joints; results in inflammation, pain, stiffness, and crippling deformities
Ankylosing spondylitis (or Marie-Strumpell disease)	**c.**	Rheumatoid arthritis of the spine; results in extreme forward flexion of the spine and tightness in the hip flexors
d.	Joint, usually the great toe	An overproduction of uric acid leads to a deposit of uric acid crystals in the joint; results in a painful, hot, inflamed joint; can become chronic

8. A patient has come to your medical office complaining of pain in her shoulder. She tells you that she recently strained her rotator cuff. Now, she experiences pain when she uses her shoulder. The pain is greater when she resists movement. There is no pain when she does not use her shoulder. The site of the pain is tender. What musculoskeletal disorder does this patient likely have, and what are some options for treatment?

_____

_____

9. What is Duchenne and how is it treated?

_____

_____

10. Complete this chart to describe three abnormal spine curvatures.

Abnormal Spine Curvature	Description
Lordosis	**a.**
Kyphosis	**b.**
Scoliolis	**c.**

11. What test is performed that determines whether back pain results from a herniated intervertebral disc? How is the test done, and what is a positive indicator?

_____

_____

Diagnosis and Treatment

12. Radiology and diagnostic imaging are the most frequently used tools for detecting musculoskeletal disorders. Name two methods of radiology and two methods of diagnostic imaging.

Radiology	Diagnostic Imaging
a. _____	**a.** _____
b. _____	**b.** _____

13. As a medical assistant, you will need to assist the physician with orthopedic diagnosis and treatment. Review the list of tasks below and determine which tasks you may be responsible for as a medical assistant. Place a check in the "Yes" column for those duties you might assist with as a medical assistant and place a check in the "No" column for those tasks that fall to another member of the team.

Task	Yes	No
a. Instruct patients on how to use crutches, a cane, a walker, or a wheelchair.		
b. Inform patients of the potential injury associated with heating-pad use.		
c. Perform arthroplasty to repair or remove cartilage damaged by chondromalacia patellae.		
d. Assemble the supplies needed to cast a fractured bone.		
e. Treat tendonitis with a transverse friction massage.		
f. Help elderly patients avoid hip fractures by reviewing fall-prevention techniques.		
g. Observe and report signs of a musculoskeletal disorder, such as skin color, temperature, tone, and tenderness.		
h. Give patients specific and detailed instructions for applying heat or cold at home.		
i. Identify the type of fracture and decide the method of treatment.		

14. Match the following patient descriptions with the ambulatory assist device most suited to the patient's condition.

Patient

a. Patient A is a 53-year-old female who has recently undergone hip replacement surgery. She is able to walk and needs only slight assistance until she has fully healed from her surgery. _____

b. Patient B is a 17-year-old male with a sprained ankle. His condition is temporary, but he needs assistance walking with one affected leg. _____

c. Patient C is a 79-year-old female with osteoarthritis. She has trouble maintaining her balance when walking. _____

Ambulatory Assist Device

1. crutches
2. cane
3. walker

15. Both heat and cold treatments are used to relieve pain, but how do their uses differ?

_____

_____

16. List the five gaits utilized by patients who use crutches to assist them with walking.

a. _____

b. _____

c. _____

d. _____

e. _____

17. Use the word bank to fill in the blanks in this paragraph about bone tumors.

The cause of malignant skeletal tumors is unknown but may be linked to rapid development of _____ during youth. An early sign of bone tumors is bone pain, which is most intense at night. Some bone tumors have the potential to spread to the skin and muscles. Bone tumors are identified by _____ after a bone scan reveals the need for further diagnosis. Treatments include surgery, amputation, and _____.

Word Bank:

biopsy	bone tissue	chemotherapy
CT scan	osteosarcomas	

18. Deirdre is a 52-year-old patient. She visits the office with a complaint of joint pain. After taking Deirdre's height and weight measurements, you notice that she is 1½ inches shorter than she was just 2 years ago. After speaking with the patient, you learn that she does not exercise. What do you suspect may be Deirdre's condition? If it turns out that Deirdre is not afflicted with a musculoskeletal disorder, what preventative medicine information might be useful for Deirdre?

_____

_____

19. Match the following key terms to their definitions.

Key Terms

a. ankylosing spondylitis _____
b. arthrogram _____
c. arthroscopy _____
d. arthroplasty _____
e. bursae _____
f. callus _____
g. contracture _____
h. contusion _____
i. electromyography _____
j. embolus _____
k. goniometer _____
l. iontophoresis _____
m. kyphosis _____
n. lordosis _____
o. Paget disease _____
p. phonophoresis _____
q. prosthesis _____
r. reduction _____
s. scoliosis _____

Definitions

1. introduction of various chemical ions into the skin by means of electrical current

2. a deposit of new bone tissue that forms between the healing ends of broken bones

3. any artificial replacement for a missing body part, such as false teeth or an artificial limb

4. a mass of matter (thrombus, air, fat globule) freely floating in the circulatory system

5. small sacs filled with clear synovial fluid that surround some joints

6. a lateral curve of the spine, usually in the thoracic area, with a corresponding curve in the lumbar region, causing uneven shoulders and hips

7. an abnormal shortening of muscles around a joint caused by atrophy of the muscles and resulting in flexion and fixation

8. an abnormally deep ventral curve at the lumbar flexure of the spine; also known as swayback

9. ultrasound treatment used to force medications into tissues

10. surgical repair of a joint

11. an abnormally deep dorsal curvature of the thoracic spine; also known as humpback or hunchback

12. an examination of the inside of a joint through an arthroscope

13. x-ray of a joint

14. an instrument used to measure the angle of joints for range of motion

15. a collection of blood in tissues after an injury; a bruise

16. correcting a fracture by realigning the bones; may be closed (corrected by manipulation) or open (requires surgery)

17. a stiffening of the spine with inflammation

18. a recording of electrical nerve transmission in skeletal muscles

19. a degenerative bone disease usually in older persons with bone destruction and poor repair

20. True or False? Determine whether the following statements are true or false. If false, explain why.

a. Heat, such as heat from a heating pad or hot water bottle, should not be applied to the uterus of a pregnant woman.

_____

_____

b. A greenstick fracture is a partial or incomplete fracture in which only one side of the bone is broken.

_____

_____

c. The swing-through gait is the gait most commonly used to train patients to use crutches.

_____

_____

d. Fibromyalgia is easy to diagnose because the symptoms are constant and centrally located in one joint socket.

_____

_____

APPLICATION

Critical Thinking Practice

1. Maddy, a 9-year-old patient, needs to have her arm cast after it is discovered that she has a greenstick fracture. The physician informs Maddy's mother that he will be using a fiberglass cast to immobilize Maddy's arm. Maddy's mother grows concerned after speaking with the physician. She has heard that fiberglass can be dangerous, and she wonders why the physician cannot use a plaster cast, like the one she received when she was a child with a fractured arm. Explain to Maddy's mother the benefits of a fiberglass cast over a plaster cast, especially when the patient is a young, active child.

_____

_____

2. Mr. Hoover is a 37-year-old patient. He is visiting the office because he has been awakened every night for a week by pain in his right wrist and hand. During the day, Mr. Hoover experiences pain and weakness in his wrist and hand. Mr. Hoover also tells you that he is a receptionist and spends many hours a day typing reports and e-mails for his business. What do you suspect to be Mr. Hoover's ailment? What tests can the physician request to confirm your suspicion? What instructions can you give to Mr. Hoover to prevent another onset of this ailment in the future?

_____

_____

Patient Education

1. The physician has just applied a plaster cast to a patient. What instructions and information should you give to the patient regarding her plaster cast?

_____

_____

Documentation

1. Your patient is an elderly man. The physician has determined that the patient requires an ambulatory assist device to assist with mobility. You first attempt to teach the patient to use a cane. The patient is unsteady while using the cane, so you instead teach the patient to use a walker. The patient successfully learns how to use the walker and demonstrates stability and control. You explain to the patient how to use the aid safely, including how to maintain the aid and what changes the patient should make at home to operate the aid safely. The patient verbalizes that he is comfortable using the walker and that he understands his maintenance responsibilities. How would you document this interaction on the patient's chart?

_____

_____

Active Learning

1. School children, especially girls, are commonly screened for scoliosis. Research the methods used for this screening using the Internet or the library. Then, prepare a patient education pamphlet for school children who are about to undergo the screening. Explain the procedure in a way that will calm any anxieties. Include information about scoliosis, as well as preventative measures the children can take and warning signs they should look for in the years following their school screening.

2. The Muscular Dystrophy Association is a voluntary health agency that sponsors research on neuromuscular diseases. Visit the MDA's website and research clinical trials. Choose three clinical trials and write a short report outlining the disease the trial is seeking to cure and the eligibility requirements for participants.

3. Practice teaching patients how to use an ambulatory assist device. Work with a fellow student or a friend or relative. Obtain a pair of crutches, a cane, and a walker. Show the "patient" all five of the crutch gaits and how to use the cane and the walker. Be sure to have the "patient" demonstrate each gait before moving on to ensure that he or she has retained your instructions. Ask for feedback on your instruction technique. Were you clear in your instruction? Was the "patient" ever confused? Did the "patient" feel comfortable? Use this feedback to adjust your instruction technique for future patient interactions.

Professional Journal

REFLECT

(Prompts and Ideas: Have you or a loved one ever had to wear a cast after fracturing a bone? What do you wish you had known once the cast was applied? What minor obstacles did you or your loved one encounter while wearing the cast, and how did you overcome them? What did you or your loved one experience once the cast was removed? What information from your personal experience could you pass on to patients about to receive a cast or about to have a cast removed?)

_____

_____

_____

_____

_____

PONDER AND SOLVE

1. Your coworker Ben is moving some boxes from the reception area to a closet in the office. As you walk by, you observe him bending his back and lifting a box with extended arms. You know that this method of lifting could lead to serious back problems, so you decide to speak to Ben about avoiding back strain. When you approach Ben, he waves you away, insisting that he does not have the time to hear your advice. What should you say to Ben? What will you do next?

_____

_____

_____

_____

2. A 46-year-old patient has been advised by the physician to avoid using his strained knee. After you secure an ice pack to the patient's knee, you begin to instruct the patient in how to care for his knee at home. While you are speaking, the patient interrupts you saying that he has had this injury before and will "just throw a heating pad on there" like he has done in the past. What should you say to the patient? What will you do next?

_____

_____

_____

_____

_____

_____

_____

EXPERIENCE

Skills related to this chapter include:

1. Apply an Arm Sling (Procedure 28-1).
2. Apply Cold Packs (Procedure 28-2).
3. Use a Hot Water Bottle or Commercial Hot Pack (Procedure 28-3).
4. Measure a Patient for Axillary Crutches (Procedure 28-4).
5. Instruct a Patient in Various Crutch Gaits (Procedure 28-5).

Record any common mistakes, lessons learned, and/or tips you discovered during your experience of practicing and demonstrating these skills:

_____

_____

_____

_____

_____

_____

_____

Skill Practice

PERFORMANCE OBJECTIVES:

1. Apply an arm sling (Procedure 28-1).
2. Apply cold packs (Procedure 28-2).
3. Use a hot water bottle or commercial hot pack (Procedure 28-3).
4. Measure a patient for axillary crutches (Procedure 28-4).
5. Instruct a patient in various crutch gaits (Procedure 28-5).

Name_____ Date _____ Time _____

Procedure 28-1:   APPLY AN ARM SLING

EQUIPMENT/SUPPLIES: A canvas triangular arm sling, 2 safety pins

STANDARDS: Given the needed equipment and a place to work, the student will perform this skill with _____% accuracy in a total of _____ minutes. *(Your instructor will tell you what the percentage and time limits will be before you begin practicing.)*

KEY: 4 = Satisfactory   0 = Unsatisfactory   NA = This step is not counted

PROCEDURE STEPS	SELF	PARTNER	INSTRUCTOR
1. Wash your hands.	☐	☐	☐
2. Assemble the equipment and supplies.	☐	☐	☐
3. Greet and identify the patient; explain the procedure.	☐	☐	☐
4. Position the affected limb with the hand at slightly less than a 90° angle.	☐	☐	☐
5. Place the affected arm into the sling with the elbow snugly against the back of the sling, and the arm extended through the sling with the hand and/or fingers protruding out of the oppsite end of the sling.	☐	☐	☐
6. Position the strap from the back of the sling around the patient's back, over the opposite shoulder.	☐	☐	☐
7. Secure the strap by inserting the end through the two metal rings on the top of the sling and further bringing the end of the strap back, looping it through the top metal ring only.	☐	☐	☐
8. Tighten the strap so that the patient's arm in the sling is slightly elevated. Make sure the strap coming around the patient's shoulder and neck is comfortable, padding if necessary to prevent friction and pressure areas.	☐	☐	☐
9. Check the patient's level of comfort and distal extremity circulation.	☐	☐	☐
10. Document the appliance in the patient's chart.	☐	☐	☐

CALCULATION

Total Possible Points: _____
Total Points Earned: _____ Multiplied by 100 = _____ Divided by Total Possible Points = _____%

Pass   **Fail**
☐   ☐   Comments:

Student's signature _____ Date _____
Partner's signature _____ Date _____
Instructor's signature _____ Date _____

Name_____ Date _____ Time _____

Procedure 28-2:	**APPLY COLD PACKS**

EQUIPMENT/SUPPLIES: Ice bag and ice chips or small cubes, or disposable cold pack; small towel or cover for ice pack; gauze or tape

STANDARDS: Given the needed equipment and a place to work, the student will perform this skill with _____% accuracy in a total of _____ minutes. *(Your instructor will tell you what the percentage and time limits will be before you begin practicing.)*

KEY: 4 = Satisfactory   0 = Unsatisfactory   NA = This step is not counted

PROCEDURE STEPS	SELF	PARTNER	INSTRUCTOR
1. Wash your hands.	☐	☐	☐
2. Assemble the equipment and supplies, checking the ice bag, if used, for leaks. If using a commercial cold pack, read the manufacturer's directions.	☐	☐	☐
3. Fill a nondisposable ice bag about two-thirds full. 　**a.** Press it flat on a surface to express air from the bag. 　**b.** Seal the container.	☐	☐	☐
4. If using a commercial chemical ice pack, activate it now.	☐	☐	☐
5. Cover the bag in a towel or other suitable cover.	☐	☐	☐
6. Greet and identify the patient. Explain the procedure.	☐	☐	☐
7. After assessing skin for color and warmth, place the covered ice pack on the area.	☐	☐	☐
8. Secure the ice pack with gauze or tape.	☐	☐	☐
9. Apply the treatment for the prescribed amount of time, but no longer than 30 minutes.	☐	☐	☐
10. During the treatment, assess the skin under the pack frequently for mottling, pallor, or redness.	☐	☐	☐
11. Properly care for or dispose of equipment and supplies. Wash your hands.	☐	☐	☐
12. Document the procedure, the site of the application, the results including the condition of the skin after the treatment, and the patient's reactions.	☐	☐	☐

CALCULATION

Total Possible Points: _____
Total Points Earned: _____ Multiplied by 100 = _____ Divided by Total Possible Points = _____%

Pass   **Fail**
☐   ☐   Comments:

Student's signature _____ Date _____
Partner's signature _____ Date _____
Instructor's signature _____ Date _____

Name_____ Date_____ Time_____

Procedure 28-3:	USE A HOT WATER BOTTLE OR COMMERCIAL HOT PACK

EQUIPMENT/SUPPLIES: A hot water bottle or commercial hot pack, towel or other suitable covering for the hot pack

STANDARDS: Given the needed equipment and a place to work, the student will perform this skill with _____% accuracy in a total of _____ minutes. *(Your instructor will tell you what the percentage and time limits will be before you begin practicing.)*

KEY: 4 = Satisfactory   0 = Unsatisfactory   NA = This step is not counted

PROCEDURE STEPS	SELF	PARTNER	INSTRUCTOR
1. Wash your hands.	☐	☐	☐
2. Assemble equipment and supplies, checking the hot water bottle for leaks.	☐	☐	☐
3. Fill the hot water bottle about two-thirds full with warm (110°F) water. **a.** Place the bottle on a flat surface and the opening up; "burp" it by pressing out the air. **b.** If using a commercial hot pack, follow the manufacturer's directions for activating it.	☐	☐	☐
4. Wrap and secure the pack or bottle before placing it on the patient's skin.	☐	☐	☐
5. Greet and identify the patient. Explain the procedure.	☐	☐	☐
6. After assessing the color of the skin where the treatment is to be applied, place the covered hot pack on the area.	☐	☐	☐
7. Secure the hot pack with gauze or tape.	☐	☐	☐
8. Apply the treatment for the prescribed length of time, but no longer than 30 minutes.	☐	☐	☐
9. During treatment, assess the skin every 10 minutes for pallor (an indication of rebound), excessive redness (indicates temperature may be too high), and swelling (indicates possible tissue damage).	☐	☐	☐
10. Properly care for or dispose of equipment and supplies. Wash your hands.	☐	☐	☐
11. Document the procedure, the site of the application, the results including the condition of the skin after the treatment, and the patient's reactions.	☐	☐	☐

CALCULATION

Total Possible Points: _____
Total Points Earned: _____ Multiplied by 100 = _____ Divided by Total Possible Points = _____%

Pass   **Fail**
☐   ☐

Comments:

Student's signature _____ Date _____
Partner's signature _____ Date _____
Instructor's signature _____ Date _____

Name _____ Date _____ Time _____

| Procedure 28-4: | **MEASURE A PATIENT FOR AXILLARY CRUTCHES** |

EQUIPMENT/SUPPLIES: Axillary crutches with tips, pads for the axillae, and hand rests, as needed; tools to tighten bolts

STANDARDS: Given the needed equipment and a place to work, the student will perform this skill with _____% accuracy in a total of _____ minutes. *(Your instructor will tell you what the percentage and time limits will be before you begin practicing.)*

KEY: 4 = Satisfactory   0 = Unsatisfactory   NA = This step is not counted

PROCEDURE STEPS	SELF	PARTNER	INSTRUCTOR
1. Wash your hands.	☐	☐	☐
2. Assemble the equipment including the correct-size crutches.	☐	☐	☐
3. Greet and identify the patient.	☐	☐	☐
4. Ensure that the patient is wearing low-heeled shoes with safety soles.	☐	☐	☐
5. Have the patient stand erect. Support the patient as needed.	☐	☐	☐
6. While standing erect, have the patient hold the crutches in the tripod position.	☐	☐	☐

7. Using the tools as needed, adjust the central support in the base.
   a. Tighten the bolts for safety when the proper height is reached.
   b. Adjust the handgrips. Tighten bolts for safety.
   c. If needed, pad axillary bars and handgrips.
	☐	☐	☐

8. Wash your hands and record the procedure.	☐	☐	☐

CALCULATION

Total Possible Points: _____
Total Points Earned: _____ Multiplied by 100 = _____ Divided by Total Possible Points = _____%

Pass   **Fail**
☐   ☐ | Comments: |

Student's signature _____ Date _____
Partner's signature _____ Date _____
Instructor's signature _____ Date _____

Name_____ Date _____ Time _____

Procedure 28-5:	INSTRUCT A PATIENT IN VARIOUS CRUTCH GAITS

EQUIPMENT/SUPPLIES: Axillary crutches measured appropriately for a patient

STANDARDS: Given the needed equipment and a place to work, the student will perform this skill with _____% accuracy in a total of _____ minutes. *(Your instructor will tell you what the percentage and time limits will be before you begin practicing.)*

KEY: 4 = Satisfactory   0 = Unsatisfactory   NA = This step is not counted

PROCEDURE STEPS	SELF	PARTNER	INSTRUCTOR
1. Wash your hands.	☐	☐	☐
2. Have the patient stand up from a chair: **a.** The patient holds both crutches on the affected side. **b.** Then the patient slides to the edge of the chair. **c.** The patient pushes down on the chair arm on the unaffected side. **d.** Then the patient pushes to stand.	☐	☐	☐
3. With one crutch in each hand, rest on the crutches until balance is restored.	☐	☐	☐
4. Assist the patient to the tripod position.	☐	☐	☐
5. Depending upon the patient's weight-bearing ability, coordination, and general state of health, instruct the patient in one or more of the following gaits: **a.** *Three-point gait:* (1) Both crutches are moved forward with the unaffected leg bearing the weight. (2) With the weight supported by the crutches on the handgrips, the unaffected leg is brought past the level of the crutches. (3) The steps are repeated. **b.** *Two-point gait:* (1) The right crutch and left foot are moved forward. (2) As these points rest, the right foot and left crutch are moved forward. (3) The steps are repeated. **c.** *Four-point gait:* (1) The right crutch moves forward. (2) The left foot is moved to a position just ahead of the left crutch. (3) The left crutch is moved forward (4) The right foot moves to a position just ahead of the right crutch. (5) The steps are repeated.	☐	☐	☐

PROCEDURE STEPS	SELF	PARTNER	INSTRUCTOR
d. *Swing-through gait:*			
(1) Both crutches are moved forward.			
(2) With the weight on the hands, the body swings through to a position ahead of the crutches with both legs leaving the floor together.			
(3) The crutches are moved ahead.			
(4) The steps are repeated.			
e. *Swing-to gait:*			
(1) Both crutches are moved forward.			
(2) With the weight on the hands, the body swings to the level of the crutches with both legs leaving the floor.			
(3) The crutches are moved ahead.			
(4) The steps are repeated.			
6. Wash your hands and record the procedure.	☐	☐	☐

CALCULATION

Total Possible Points: _____

Total Points Earned: _____ Multiplied by 100 = _____ Divided by Total Possible Points = _____%

Pass   **Fail**
☐   ☐   Comments:

Student's signature _____ Date _____

Partner's signature _____ Date _____

Instructor's signature _____ Date _____

Work Product 1

Document appropriately.

John Beck is a 17-year-old male with a sports injury. The physician diagnoses the injury as a moderately sprained ankle and orders cold packs applied to the ankle for 30 minutes. Following the cold pack application, she directs you to wrap the injury to stabilize his ankle and check distal circulation when complete. Finally, you measure axillary crutches and instruct the patient in their use.
If you are currently working in a medical office, use a blank paper patient chart from the office. If this is not available to you, use the space below to record the incident in the chart.

_____

_____

_____

_____

_____

_____

_____

Chapter Self-Assessment Quiz

1. The rebound phenomenon is:
   a. when the body secretes callus, which fills in fractures and mends damaged bone.
   b. when the body experiences bulging discs or biomechanical stress as a result of poor posture.
   c. when the body overcompensates for a muscle sprain by increasing use of unaffected muscles.
   d. when the body responds to extremes of temperature for long periods of time by exerting an opposite effect.
   e. when the body releases fat droplets from the yellow marrow of the long bones.

2. In which crutch gait do both legs leave the floor together?
   a. One-arm gait
   b. Two-point gait
   c. Three-point gait
   d. Four-point gait
   e. Swing-through gait

3. A fracture that occurs in flat bones (like those of the skull) and results in fragment to be driven below the surface of the bone is called a(n):
   a. depressed fracture.
   b. impacted fracture.
   c. pathological fracture.
   d. compression fracture.
   e. spiral fracture.

4. A possible cause of gout is:
   a. a liver disorder.
   b. a degenerative strain.
   c. a diet high in purines.
   d. the wear and tear on weight-bearing joints.
   e. the release of fat droplets from the marrow of long bones.

Scenario: The physician has determined that a male patient will need to wear a short arm cast on his left arm as part of the treatment for his fracture. The physician asks you to help her apply the cast to the patient. You assemble the items needed to apply the cast. As the physician prepares the limb for casting, you soak the casting material and press it until it is no longer dripping. Then, the physician wraps the affected limb with the material. After the cast has dried, the physician asks you to apply an arm sling to the patient's left arm.

5. How should the physician wrap the patient's affected arm with the soaked casting material?

 a. From the axilla to mid palm

 b. From mid palm to the axilla

 c. From the elbow to mid palm

 d. From mid palm to the elbow

 e. From the axilla to the elbow

6. Which of these steps will you follow when applying the arm sling?

 a. Cover the left arm with soft knitted tubular material.

 b. Position the hand of the left arm at a 90-degree angle.

 c. Instruct the patient in various gaits using auxiliary crutches.

 d. Check the patient's circulation by pinching each of his fingers.

 e. Insert the elbow of the right arm into the pouch end of the sling.

End Scenario

7. Rheumatoid arthritis is a(n):

 a. joint failure.

 b. bone fracture.

 c. skeletal tumor.

 d. autoimmune disease.

 e. spine disorder.

8. Tendonitis that is caused by calcium deposits is called:

 a. fibromyalgia.

 b. iontophoresis.

 c. hardened tendons.

 d. calcific tendonitis.

 e. depository tendonitis.

Scenario: A 20-year-old female patient is visiting your office because of pain in her knee. During the patient interview, the patient tells you that she experiences pain when walking down stairs and getting out of bed. You learn that she is very active and is a member of her university's track and field team.

9. What musculoskeletal disorder does this patient have?

 a. Plantar fasciitis

 b. Lateral humeral epicondylitis

 c. Dupuytren contracture

 d. Chondromalacia patellae

 e. Ankylosing spondylitis

10. What surgical procedure may need to be performed to repair or remove damaged cartilage if the patient's case is severe?

 a. Arthrogram

 b. Arthroplasty

 c. Arthroscopy

 d. Phonophoresis

 e. Electromyography

End Scenario

11. You should *not* apply cold to:

 a. open wounds.

 b. the pregnant uterus.

 c. acute inflammation.

 d. the very young and the elderly.

 e. a contusion.

12. Proper cane length calls for the cane to be level with the user's greater trochanter and for the user's elbow to be bent at a:

 a. 30-degree angle.

 b. 50-degree angle.

 c. 60-degree angle.

 d. 80-degree angle.

 e. 90-degree angle.

13. A subluxation is a(n):

 a. dislocation of a facet joint.

 b. partial dislocation of a joint.

 c. complete dislocation of a joint.

 d. dislocation that damages the tendons.

 e. injury to a joint capsule.

14. How is immobilization during closed reduction achieved?

  a. Casting

  b. Surgery

  c. Exercise

  d. Splinting

  e. Ultrasound

15. You and the physician must wear goggles during a cast removal to protect against:

  a. flying particles.

  b. dangerous waves.

  c. unsanitary material.

  d. blood-borne pathogens.

  e. disease and infection.

16. If a fat embolus becomes lodged in a patient's pulmonary or coronary vessels, the patient may experience:

  a. limited mobility.

  b. pain and swelling.

  c. a warm sensation.

  d. an infarction and death.

  e. swelling and numbness.

17. The most common site of bursitis is the:

  a. foot.

  b. wrist.

  c. elbow.

  d. shoulder.

  e. ankle.

18. Your patient has just received a fiberglass leg cast. Which of the following is a sign that proper circulation is present?

  a. Red, hot toes

  b. Swollen toes

  c. Clammy toes

  d. Cold, blue toes

  e. Warm, pink toes

19. Osteoporosis is a condition in which the bones lack:

  a. bursae.

  b. calcium.

  c. vitamin D.

  d. malignancies.

  e. marrow.

20. Your patient is recovering from a strain in his Achilles' tendon. He is unable to use one leg, but he has coordination and upper body strength. Which of the following ambulatory assist devices should this patient use to gain mobility?

  a. Cast

  b. Cane

  c. Sling

  d. Walker

  e. Crutches

Ophthalmology and Otolaryngology

Chapter Checklist

☐ Read textbook chapter and take notes within the Chapter Notes outline. Answer the Learning Objectives as you reach them in the content, and then check them off.

☐ Work the Content Review questions—both Foundational Knowledge and Application.

☐ Perform the Active Learning exercise(s).

☐ Complete Professional Journal entries.

☐ Complete Skill Practice Activity(s) using Competency Evaluation Forms and Work Products, when appropriate.

☐ Take the Chapter Self-Assessment Quiz.

☐ Insert all appropriate pages into your Portfolio.

Learning Objectives

1. Spell and define the key terms.
2. List and define disorders associated with the eye and identify commonly performed diagnostic procedures.
3. List and define disorders associated with the ear and identify commonly performed diagnostic procedures.

4. List and define disorders associated with the nose and throat and identify commonly performed diagnostic procedures.
5. Describe patient education procedures associated with the eye, ear, nose, and throat.

Chapter Notes

Note: Bold-faced headings are the major headings in the text chapter; headings in regular font are lower-level headings (i.e., the content is subordinate to, or falls "under," the major headings). Make sure you understand the key terms used in the chapter, as well as the concepts presented as Key Points.

TEXT SUBHEADINGS

NOTES

Introduction _____

_____

Key Terms: ophthalmologist; otolaryngologist

☐ **LEARNING OBJECTIVE 1:** Spell and define the key terms.

Common Disorders of the Eye

Key Point:
- Light waves are reflected off of all objects and are transmitted through various structures of the eye including the cornea, lens, and retina.

Cataract

Key Term: ophthalmoscope
Key Point:
- A cataract is an opacity, or clouding, of the lens that leads to decreased visual acuity.

Sty or Hordeolum

Key Point:
- A sty, or hordeolum, is an infection of any of the lacrimal glands of the eyelids, causing redness, swelling, and pain.

Conjunctivitis

Key Points:
- Conjunctivitis, an infection of the mucous membrane covering the sclera and cornea (conjunctiva) of the eye, is caused by several species of bacteria or viruses.
- Bacterial and viral conjunctivitis, or pink eye, is highly contagious and can rapidly spread through schools and day care centers.

Corneal Ulcer

Key Point:
- A corneal ulcer is erosion of the surface of the cornea, leaving scar tissue that may lead to visual disturbances or blindness.

Retinopathy

Key Terms: retinal degeneration; fluorescein angiography
Key Point:
- Retinopathy is a general term for disease or disorder affecting the retina.

Glaucoma _____

Key Term: tonometry
Key Point:
• Glaucoma describes a group of disorders that result in increased intraocular pressure, or pressure within the eye.

Refractive Errors _____

Key Terms: refraction; hyperopia; myopia; astigmatism; presbyopia; optometrist; optician
Key Points:
• **Hyperopia**, also known as farsightedness, occurs in an eyeball that is too short from front to back to allow the lines of vision to reflect distinctly on the fovea centralis.
• **Myopia**, also known as nearsightedness, results when the eyeball is too long.
• **Astigmatism** is unfocused refraction of light rays on the retina resulting from lens or corneal irregularities.
• **Presbyopia** is vision change resulting from loss of lens elasticity with age.

Strabismus _____

Key Point:
• Strabismus is a misalignment of eye movements, usually caused by muscle incoordination.

Color Deficit _____

Key Point:
• Color deficit is an absence of or a defect in color perception.

Diagnostic Studies of the Eye _____

Key Term: ophthalmoscope

Visual Acuity Testing _____

Key Point:
• Visual acuity, or clearness, is commonly assessed in the medical office using the Snellen eye chart.

Color Deficit Testing _____

_____

Key Point:
• The Ishihara method is used to test for color deficits.

Tonometry and Gonioscopy _____

_____

Key Points:
• Using a tonometer, the physician measures the intraocular pressure or tension in the eye.
• Gonioscopy, also performed at the ophthalmologist's or optometrist's office, is use of a special instrument (gonioscope) to measure the angle of the anterior chamber between the iris and the cornea.

☐ **LEARNING OBJECTIVE 2:** List and define disorders associated with the eye and identify commonly performed diagnostic procedures.

Therapeutic Procedures for the Eye _____

_____

_____

Instilling Eye Medications _____

_____

Key Point:
• Instillations are used to treat infection or irritation, to dilate the pupil for retinal examination, and to apply anesthetic for treatment or testing.

Common Disorders of the Ear _____

_____

Key Point:
• Patients who have problems with the ear or hearing are often referred to an otolaryngologist.

Ceruminosis _____

_____

Key Terms: cerumen; tinnitus; otoscope
Key Point:
• Ceruminosis, or impacted earwax, is a frequent reason for diminished hearing.

Conductive and Perceptual Hearing Loss _____

_____

Key Term: presbycusis
Key Points:
- Conductive and perceptual hearing loss are the two categories of hearing impairment.
- Treatment is aimed at addressing the underlying cause of the hearing loss if possible.

Ménière Disease _____

_____

Key Point:
- Ménière disease, a degenerative condition of unknown cause, affects the inner ear and upsets the body's ability to maintain equilibrium in addition to causing loss of hearing.

Otitis Externa _____

_____

Key Point:
- Also known as swimmer's ear, otitis externa is an inflammation or infection of the external ear.

Otitis Media _____

_____

Key Term: myringotomy
Key Point:
- Otitis media, an inflammation or infection of the middle ear, is frequently caused by an upper respiratory infection.

Otosclerosis _____

_____

Key Point:
- Otosclerosis is a disorder of the ossicles of the inner ear, especially the stapes bone.

Diagnostic Studies of the Ear _____

_____

_____

Visual Examination _____

_____

_____

Audiometry and Tympanometry _____

_____

Key Point:
• An audiometer can be used to detect hearing loss.

Tuning Fork Tests _____

_____

Key Point:
• Two tests that may be performed using the tuning fork are the Rinne test and the Weber test.

☐ **LEARNING OBJECTIVE 3:** List and define disorders associated with the ear and identify commonly performed diagnostic procedures.

Therapeutic Procedures for the Ear _____

_____

_____

Irrigations and Instillations _____

_____

Key Point:
• Ear irrigations are performed to relieve pain, to remove debris or foreign objects, or to apply medication solutions.

Common Disorders of the Nose and Throat _____

_____

_____

Allergic Rhinitis _____

_____

Key Point:
• Allergic rhinitis is inflammation of the mucous membranes of the nasal passages usually resulting from exposure to an allergen.

Epistaxis _____

_____

Key Point:
• Commonly known as nosebleed, epistaxis generally occurs from trauma to the nasal membranes, but it may be secondary to another disorder, such as hypertension, malignancy, polyps, or the fragile capillaries associated with pregnancy.

Nasal Polyps _____

_____

Key Point:
• Nasal polyps are small pendulous tissues that obstruct breathing.

Sinusitis _____

_____

Key Point:
• Sinusitis, or inflammation of one or more of the sinus cavities, can be either acute or chronic.

Pharyngitis and Tonsillitis _____

_____

Key Point:
• Inflammation of the epithelial tissues of the throat and of the tonsils produces similar symptoms of sore throat and difficulty swallowing.

Laryngitis _____

_____

Key Point:
• Inflammation of the larynx can result from an infection, irritation, or overuse of the voice.

Diagnostic Studies of the Nose and Throat _____

_____

Visual Inspection _____

_____

Key Point:
• Examination of the nose and throat entails visually inspecting the nose using a nasal speculum or viewing the throat using a penlight and tongue depressor.

☐ **LEARNING OBJECTIVE 4:** List and define disorders associated with the nose and throat and identify commonly performed diagnostic procedures.

Therapeutic Procedures for the Nose and Throat _____

_____

Throat Culture _____

_____

Key Point:
• A throat culture in cases of suspected pharyngitis or tonsillitis can help determine what microorganism is causing the problem.

☐ **LEARNING OBJECTIVE 5:** Describe patient education procedures associated with the eye, ear, nose, and throat.

Content Review

FOUNDATIONAL KNOWLEDGE

All About Eyes

1. Fill in the chart below with three types of vision testing charts, and when you should use each.

Type of Vision Testing Chart	When You Would Use It
a.	
b.	
c.	

2. A patient calls in to the physician's office saying that pink eye is going around her son's school. He has not been complaining of pain in either eye, but she has noticed that his eyes are red and that he has been sniffing and coughing lately. She wants to know if she should bring him in for a checkup. What should you tell her?

_____

_____

3. List five preventive eye care tips that you can tell patients to follow.

a. _____

b. _____

c. _____

d. _____

e. _____

4. A patient complains of loss of vision and blurring, and cataracts are found in both eyes. How would surgery correct these symptoms?

_____

_____

5. What is the difference between an optometrist and an optician? Fill in the chart below to explain.

Optometrist	Optician
.	

6. What is astigmatism?

_____

_____

7. An examination of a patient's eye reveals an irregular corneal surface. What is the method used to diagnose a corneal ulcer?

_____

_____

8. If the lines of vision converge after they reach the fovea centralis, what kind of eye is this?
   a. normal
   b. myopic
   c. hyperopic
   d. astigmatic
   e. presbyopic

I'm All Ears

9. A patient comes in complaining of vertigo, nausea, and slight hearing loss. What might the patient be suffering from?

_____

_____

10. What are seven causes of hearing loss?
   a. _____
   b. _____
   c. _____
   d. _____
   e. _____
   f. _____
   g. _____

11. Why is otitis media so common in infants and young children?

_____

_____

12. What is the difference between audiometry and tympanometry?

Audiometry	Tympanometry

Nose and Throat Conditions

13. List the initial therapy for common epistaxis.

_____

_____

14. Why is it so important to treat upper respiratory infections?

_____

_____

15. When is the physician likely to suggest that a patient receive a tonsillectomy?

_____

_____

16. Draw a picture in the space below to show the proper initial method of treatment for epistaxis.

_____

17. What is a way to isolate the protein causing allergic reactions in a patient directly?

_____

_____

18. Where do nasal polyps usually occur?

_____

_____

19. Match the following key terms to their definitions.

Key Terms

a. astigmatism _____

b. cerumen _____

c. decibel _____

Definitions

1. physician who specializes in treatment of diseases and disorders of the ears, nose, and throat

2. an extraneous noise heard in one or both ears, described as whirring, ringing, whistling, roaring, etc.; may be continuous or intermittent

d. fluorescein angiography _____

e. hyperopia _____

f. intraocular pressure _____

g. myopia _____

h. myringotomy _____

i. ophthalmologist _____

j. ophthalmoscope _____

k. optician _____

l. optometrist _____

m. otolaryngologist _____

n. otoscope _____

o. presbycusis _____

p. presbyopia _____

q. refraction _____

r. retinal degeneration _____

s. tinnitus _____

t. tonometry _____

u. upper respiratory infection (URI) _____

3. specialist who can measure for errors of refraction and prescribe lenses but who cannot treat diseases of the eye or perform surgery

4. an instrument used for visual examination of the ear canal and tympanic membrane

5. an incision into the tympanic membrane to relieve pressure

6. unit of intensity of sound

7. an unfocused refraction of light rays on the retina

8. nearsightedness

9. loss of hearing associated with aging

10. specialist who grinds lenses to correct errors of refraction according to prescriptions

11. yellowish or brownish waxlike secretion in the external ear canal; earwax

12. physician who specializes in treatment of disorders of the eyes

13. farsightedness

14. pathological changes in the cell structure of the retina that impair or destroy its function, resulting in blindness

15. infection of the nasopharynx, throat, and bronchi

16. intravenous injection of fluorescent dye; photographing blood vessels of the eye as dye moves through the vessels

17. measurement of intraocular pressure using a tonometer

18. lighted instrument used to examine the inner surfaces of the eye

19. bending of light rays that enter the pupil to reflect exactly on the fovea centralis, the area of greatest visual acuity

20. pressure within the eyeball

21. vision change (farsightedness) associated with aging

20. True or False? Determine whether the following statements are true or false. If false, explain why.

a. Diagnosis of vision loss of any type is done by testing the hearing using an audiometer.

_____

_____

b. Swimmer's ear goes away on its own and does not need to be treated.

_____

_____

c. Allergic rhinitis is another name for hay fever.

_____

_____

d. A patient with tonsillitis should be told to rest his voice and speak as little as possible.

_____

_____

APPLICATION

Critical Thinking Practice

1. A patient is interested in getting LASIK surgery to correct her nearsightedness. She is 24 years old, and both of her parents have strong prescriptions for nearsightedness as well. She asks you what the surgery will be like, and if there is any chance that her

eyes might revert back to their previous state. Discuss some of the advantages and disadvantages to LASIK surgery. Be sure to mention possible side effects.

_____

_____

2. A middle-aged patient comes in for a routine checkup, and mentions a slight loss of hearing since the last exam. What tests can you give to the patient to check his hearing? What suggestions can you give him about dealing with gradual hearing loss?

_____

_____

Patient Education

1. A swimmer comes into the office complaining of swimmer's ear. She says she has used cotton swabs in the past to clear her ear canals, and asks if there is any particular solvent she can apply to the tip to help keep her canal clear. Write down advice for the patient on how to care for her ears and prevent otitis externa from developing in the future.

_____

_____

Documentation

1. A patient has come in for ceruminosis treatment. Document the steps that were taken to complete this procedure, as well as any complications that might have arisen during the procedure. Be sure to include any instructions that were given to the patient after the procedure.

_____

_____

Active Learning

1. The composer Beethoven was afflicted with hearing loss that left him completely deaf. Many music lovers today suffer from hearing loss as well, and they rely on the technology available to help them enjoy the subtle tones that are written into compositions. Research the new programs and software that are being installed in hearing aids that are specifically aimed toward listening to music. List differences between listening to music and listening to speech, and make a note of tips for listening to music that physicians can give to patients with hearing aids.

2. Refraction is the bending of light. Lenses are used to correct eyes that do not focus the refracted light properly. Different-shaped lenses are used to correct myopia, hyperopia, and astigmatism. Find information on convex, concave, bioconvex, plano-convex, convex-concave, meniscus, plano-concave, and bioconcave lenses. Create a chart that describes what each type of lens does to correct eyesight.

3. Work with a partner and obtain three types of lenses. Place a sheet of paper on a table, and place the edge of the lens in the middle of the paper. Next, use three laser pointers to shine through the lens on one side of the paper. Use a pencil to sketch the path of the light to the lens and to show where the lens refracts the light. Shift the light source left, then right, marking each path as you go. Determine the focal point for each lens.

Professional Journal

REFLECT

(Prompts and Ideas: Have you ever thought about what it would be like to have hearing loss? What sounds would you miss the most? How do people treat deaf individuals?)

_____

_____

_____

_____

_____

_____

PONDER AND SOLVE

1. A young man comes in for a routine checkup, and mentions that he will soon be learning to drive. However, the physician gives him the Ishihara test, and the teen fails to differentiate between colors. What would be the best way to break the news to him? What information can you give him about color blindness, and what encouragement can you give him in regard to his upcoming driving test?

_____

_____

_____

_____

_____

_____

_____

2. A young boy is brought in because he is complaining of headaches in school. The physician determines that the boy needs glasses and that the headaches are from eye strain. The boy does not want glasses, however, because he is afraid his classmates will make fun of him. What can you say to the boy to help soothe his concerns?

_____

_____

_____

_____

_____

_____

EXPERIENCE

Skills related to this chapter include:

1. Measure Distance Visual Acuity with a Snellen Chart (Procedure 29-1).
2. Measure Color Perception with an Ishihara Color Plate Book (Procedure 29-2).

3. Instill Eye Medication (Procedure 29-3).

4. Irrigate the Eye (Procedure 29-4).

5. Administer an Audiometric Hearing Test (Procedure 29-5).

6. Irrigate the Ear (Procedure 29-6).

7. Instill Ear Medication (Procedure 29-7).

8. Instill Nasal Medication (Procedure 29-8).

Record any common mistakes, lessons learned, and/or tips you discovered during your experience of practicing and demonstrating these skills:

_____

_____

_____

_____

_____

_____

_____

Skill Practice

PERFORMANCE OBJECTIVES:

1. Measure distance visual acuity with a Snellen chart (Procedure 29-1).

2. Measure color perception with an Ishihara color plate book (Procedure 29-2).

3. Instill eye medication (Procedure 29-3).

4. Irrigate the eye (Procedure 29-4).

5. Administer an audiometric hearing test (Procedure 29-5).

6. Irrigate the ear (Procedure 29-6).

7. Instill ear medication (Procedure 29-7).

8. Instill nasal medication (Procedure 29-8).

Name_____   Date_____   Time_____

Procedure 29-1:   MEASURE DISTANCE VISUAL ACUITY WITH A SNELLEN CHART

EQUIPMENT/SUPPLIES: Snellen eye chart, paper cup or eye paddle

STANDARDS: Given the needed equipment and a place to work, the student will perform this skill with _____% accuracy in a total of _____ minutes. *(Your instructor will tell you what the percentage and time limits will be before you begin practicing.)*

KEY: 4 = Satisfactory   0 = Unsatisfactory   NA = This step is not counted

PROCEDURE STEPS	SELF	PARTNER	INSTRUCTOR
1. Wash your hands.	☐	☐	☐
2. Prepare the examination area (well lit, distance marker 20 feet from the chart).	☐	☐	☐
3. Make sure the chart is at eye level.	☐	☐	☐
4. Greet and identify the patient. Explain the procedure.	☐	☐	☐
5. Position the patient in a standing or sitting position at the 20-foot marker.	☐	☐	☐
6. If not wearing glasses, ask patient about contact lenses. Mark results accordingly.	☐	☐	☐
7. Have patient cover left eye with eye paddle.	☐	☐	☐
8. Instruct patient not to close the left eye, but to keep both eyes open during the test.	☐	☐	☐
9. Stand beside the chart and point to each row as the patient reads aloud. **a.** Point to the lines, starting with the 20/200 line. **b.** Record the smallest line that the patient can read with no errors.	☐	☐	☐
10. Repeat the procedure with the right eye covered and record.	☐	☐	☐
11. Wash your hands and document the procedure.	☐	☐	☐

CALCULATION

Total Possible Points: _____
Total Points Earned: _____ Multiplied by 100 = _____ Divided by Total Possible Points = _____%

Pass   **Fail**
☐   ☐   Comments:

Student's signature _____ Date _____
Partner's signature _____ Date _____
Instructor's signature _____ Date _____

Name_____   Date _____   Time _____

Procedure 29-2:	MEASURE COLOR PERCEPTION WITH AN ISHIHARA COLOR PLATE BOOK

EQUIPMENT/SUPPLIES: Ishihara color plates, gloves

STANDARDS: Given the needed equipment and a place to work, the student will perform this skill with _____% accuracy in a total of _____ minutes. *(Your instructor will tell you what the percentage and time limits will be before you begin practicing.)*

KEY: 4 = Satisfactory   0 = Unsatisfactory   NA = This step is not counted

PROCEDURE STEPS	SELF	PARTNER	INSTRUCTOR
1. Wash your hands, put on gloves, and obtain the Ishihara color plate book.	☐	☐	☐
2. Prepare the examination area (adequate lighting).	☐	☐	☐
3. Hold the first bookplate about 30 inches from the patient.	☐	☐	☐
4. Ask if the patient can see the "number" within the series of dots. **a.** Record results of test by noting the number or figure the patient reports. **b.** If patient cannot distinguish a pattern, record plate number–x (e.g., 4–x).	☐	☐	☐
5. The patient should not take more than 3 seconds when reading the plates. **a.** The patient should not squint nor guess. These indicate patient is unsure. **b.** Record as plate number–x.	☐	☐	☐
6. Record the results for plates 1 through 10. **a.** Plate number 11 requires patient to trace a winding line between x's. **b.** Patients with a color deficit will not be able to trace the line.	☐	☐	☐
7. Store the book in a closed, protected area to protect the integrity of the colors.	☐	☐	☐
8. Remove your gloves and wash your hands.	☐	☐	☐

CALCULATION

Total Possible Points: _____
Total Points Earned: _____ Multiplied by 100 = _____ Divided by Total Possible Points = _____%

Pass   **Fail**
☐   ☐   Comments:

Student's signature _____ Date _____
Partner's signature _____ Date _____
Instructor's signature _____ Date _____

Name _____   Date _____   Time _____

Procedure 29-3:   INSTILL EYE MEDICATION

EQUIPMENT/SUPPLIES: Physician's order and patient record, ophthalmic medications, sterile gauze, tissues, gloves

STANDARDS: Given the needed equipment and a place to work, the student will perform this skill with _____% accuracy in a total of _____ minutes. *(Your instructor will tell you what the percentage and time limits will be before you begin practicing.)*

KEY: 4 = Satisfactory   0 = Unsatisfactory   NA = This step is not counted

PROCEDURE STEPS	SELF	PARTNER	INSTRUCTOR
1. Wash your hands.	☐	☐	☐
2. Obtain the physician order, the correct medication, sterile gauze, and tissues.	☐	☐	☐
3. Greet and identify the patient. Explain the procedure.	☐	☐	☐
4. Ask the patient about any allergies not recorded in the chart.	☐	☐	☐
5. Position the patient comfortably.	☐	☐	☐
6. Put on gloves. Ask the patient to look upward.	☐	☐	☐

7. Use sterile gauze to gently pull lower lid down. Instill the medication.
 a. *Ointment:* Discard first bead of ointment without touching the end of the tube.
    (1) Place a thin line of ointment across inside of lower eyelid.
    (2) Move from the inner canthus outward.
    (3) Release ointment by twisting the tube slightly.
    (4) Do not touch the tube to the eye.
 b. *Drops:* Hold dropper close to conjunctival sac, but do not touch the patient.
    (1) Release the proper number of drops into the sac.
    (2) Discard any medication left in the dropper.
	☐	☐	☐

8. Release the lower lid. Have patient gently close the eyelid and roll the eye.	☐	☐	☐
9. Wipe off any excess medication with tissue.	☐	☐	☐
10. Instruct patient to apply light pressure on puncta lacrimale for several minutes.	☐	☐	☐
11. Properly care for or dispose of equipment and supplies. Clean the work area.	☐	☐	☐
12. Wash your hands.	☐	☐	☐
13. Record the procedure.	☐	☐	☐

CALCULATION

Total Possible Points: _____

Total Points Earned: _____ Multiplied by 100 = _____ Divided by Total Possible Points = _____%

Pass **Fail**

☐ ☐ Comments:

Student's signature _____ Date _____

Partner's signature _____ Date _____

Instructor's signature _____ Date _____

Name_____ Date _____ Time _____

Procedure 29-4:	**IRRIGATE THE EYE**

EQUIPMENT/SUPPLIES: Physician's order and patient record, small sterile basin, irrigating solution and medication if ordered, protective barrier or towels, emesis basin, sterile bulb syringe, tissues, gloves

STANDARDS: Given the needed equipment and a place to work, the student will perform this skill with _____% accuracy in a total of _____ minutes. *(Your instructor will tell you what the percentage and time limits will be before you begin practicing.)*

KEY: 4 = Satisfactory   0 = Unsatisfactory   NA = This step is not counted

PROCEDURE STEPS	SELF	PARTNER	INSTRUCTOR
1. Wash your hands and put on your gloves.	☐	☐	☐

2. Assemble the equipment, supplies, and medication if ordered by the physician.
  a. Check solution label three times.
  b. Make sure that the label indicates for ophthalmic use.
	☐	☐	☐

3. Greet and identify the patient. Explain the procedure.	☐	☐	☐

4. Position the patient comfortably.
  a. Sitting with head tilted with the affected eye lower.
  b. Lying with the affected eye downward.
	☐	☐	☐

5. Drape patient with the protective barrier or towel to avoid wetting the clothing.	☐	☐	☐

6. Place emesis basin against upper cheek near eye with the towel under the basin.
  a. Wipe the eye from the inner canthus outward with gauze to remove debris.
  b. Separate the eyelids with your thumb and forefinger.
  c. Lightly support your hand, holding the syringe, on bridge of patient's nose.
	☐	☐	☐

7. Holding syringe 1 inch above the eye, gently irrigate from inner to outer canthus.
  a. Use gentle pressure and do not touch the eye.
  b. Physician will order the period of time or amount of solution required.
	☐	☐	☐

8. Use tissues to wipe any excess solution from the patient's face.	☐	☐	☐
9. Properly dispose of equipment or sanitize as recommended.	☐	☐	☐
10. Remove your gloves. Wash your hands.	☐	☐	☐
11. Record procedure, including amount, type, and strength of solution; which eye was irrigated; and any observations.	☐	☐	☐

CALCULATION

Total Possible Points: _____

Total Points Earned: _____ Multiplied by 100 = _____ Divided by Total Possible Points = _____%

Pass   **Fail**

☐   ☐   Comments:

Student's signature _____ Date _____
Partner's signature _____ Date _____
Instructor's signature _____ Date _____

Name _____ Date _____ Time _____

Procedure 29-5:	ADMINISTER AN AUDIOMETRIC HEARING TEST

EQUIPMENT/SUPPLIES: Audiometer, otoscope

STANDARDS: Given the needed equipment and a place to work, the student will perform this skill with _____% accuracy in a total of _____ minutes. *(Your instructor will tell you what the percentage and time limits will be before you begin practicing.)*

KEY: 4 = Satisfactory 0 = Unsatisfactory NA = This step is not counted

PROCEDURE STEPS	SELF	PARTNER	INSTRUCTOR
1. Wash your hands.	☐	☐	☐
2. Greet and identify patient. Explain the procedure.	☐	☐	☐
3. Take patient to a quiet area or room for testing.	☐	☐	☐
4. Visually inspect the ear canal and tympanic membrane before the examination.	☐	☐	☐
5. Choose the correct-size tip for the end of the audiometer.	☐	☐	☐
6. Attach a speculum to fit the patient's external auditory meatus.	☐	☐	☐
7. With the speculum in the ear canal, retract the pinna: 　**a.** *Adults:* Gently pull up and back to straighten the auditory canal. 　**b.** *Children:* Gently pull slightly down and back to straighten the auditory canal.	☐	☐	☐
8. Follow audiometer instrument directions for use: 　**a.** Screen right ear. 　**b.** Screen left ear.	☐	☐	☐
9. If the patient fails to respond at any frequency, rescreening is required.	☐	☐	☐
10. If the patient fails rescreening, notify the physician.	☐	☐	☐
11. Record the results in the medical record.	☐	☐	☐

CALCULATION

Total Possible Points: _____
Total Points Earned: _____ Multiplied by 100 = _____ Divided by Total Possible Points = _____%

Pass **Fail**
☐　　☐ | Comments:

Student's signature _____ Date _____
Partner's signature _____ Date _____
Instructor's signature _____ Date _____

Name _____ Date _____ Time _____

Procedure 29-6:	IRRIGATE THE EAR

EQUIPMENT/SUPPLIES: Physician's order and patient record, emesis basin or ear basin, waterproof barrier or towels, otoscope, irrigation solution, bowl for solution, gauze

STANDARDS: Given the needed equipment and a place to work, the student will perform this skill with _____% accuracy in a total of _____ minutes. *(Your instructor will tell you what the percentage and time limits will be before you begin practicing.)*

KEY: 4 = Satisfactory   0 = Unsatisfactory   NA = This step is not counted

PROCEDURE STEPS	SELF	PARTNER	INSTRUCTOR
1. Wash your hands.	☐	☐	☐
2. Assemble the equipment and supplies.	☐	☐	☐
3. Greet and identify the patient. Explain the procedure.	☐	☐	☐
4. Position the patient comfortably in an erect position.	☐	☐	☐
5. View the affected ear with an otoscope to locate the foreign matter or cerumen. **a.** *Adults:* Gently pull up and back to straighten the auditory canal. **b.** *Children:* Gently pull slightly down and back to straighten the auditory canal.	☐	☐	☐
6. Drape the patient with a waterproof barrier or towel.	☐	☐	☐
7. Tilt the patient's head toward the affected side.	☐	☐	☐
8. Place the drainage basin under the affected ear.	☐	☐	☐
9. Fill the irrigating syringe or turn on the irrigating device.	☐	☐	☐
10. Gently position the auricle as described above using your nondominant hand.	☐	☐	☐
11. With dominant hand, place the tip of the syringe into the auditory meatus.	☐	☐	☐
12. Direct the flow of the solution gently upward toward the roof of the canal.	☐	☐	☐
13. Irrigate for the prescribed period of time or until the desired results are obtained.	☐	☐	☐
14. Dry the patient's external ear with gauze.	☐	☐	☐
15. Have patient sit for a while with the affected ear downward to drain the solution.	☐	☐	☐
16. Inspect the ear with the otoscope to determine the results.	☐	☐	☐
17. Properly care for or dispose of equipment and supplies. Clean the work area.	☐	☐	☐
18. Wash your hands.	☐	☐	☐
19. Record the procedure in the patient's chart.	☐	☐	☐

CALCULATION

Total Possible Points: _____
Total Points Earned: _____ Multiplied by 100 = _____ Divided by Total Possible Points = _____%

Pass **Fail**
□ □ Comments:

Student's signature _____ Date _____
Partner's signature _____ Date _____
Instructor's signature _____ Date _____

Name_____ Date _____ Time _____

Procedure 29-7:   INSTILL EAR MEDICATION

EQUIPMENT/SUPPLIES: Physician's order and patient record, otic medication with dropper, cotton balls

STANDARDS: Given the needed equipment and a place to work, the student will perform this skill with _____% accuracy in a total of _____ minutes. *(Your instructor will tell you what the percentage and time limits will be before you begin practicing.)*

KEY: 4 = Satisfactory   0 = Unsatisfactory   NA = This step is not counted

PROCEDURE STEPS	SELF	PARTNER	INSTRUCTOR
1. Wash your hands.	☐	☐	☐
2. Assemble the equipment, supplies, and medication if ordered by the physician. **a.** Check solution label three times. **b.** Make sure that the label indicates for otic use.	☐	☐	☐
3. Greet and identify the patient. Explain the procedure.	☐	☐	☐
4. Ask patient about any allergies not documented.	☐	☐	☐
5. Have the patient seated with the affected ear tilted upward.	☐	☐	☐
6. Draw up the ordered amount of medication. **a.** *Adults:* Pull the auricle slightly up and back to straighten S-shaped canal. **b.** *Children:* Pull the auricle slightly down and back to straighten S-shaped canal.	☐	☐	☐
7. Insert the tip of dropper without touching the patient's skin. **a.** Let the medication flow along the side of the canal. **b.** Have patient sit or lie with affected ear upward for about 5 minutes.	☐	☐	☐
8. To keep medication in the canal, gently insert a moist cotton ball into the external auditory meatus.	☐	☐	☐
9. Properly care for or dispose of equipment and supplies. Clean the work area.	☐	☐	☐
10. Wash your hands.	☐	☐	☐
11. Record the procedure in the patient record.	☐	☐	☐

CALCULATION

Total Possible Points: _____
Total Points Earned: _____ Multiplied by 100 = _____ Divided by Total Possible Points = _____%

Pass   **Fail**

☐   ☐   Comments:

Student's signature _____ Date _____
Partner's signature _____ Date _____
Instructor's signature _____ Date _____

Name_____   Date _____   Time _____

Procedure 29-8:	**INSTILL NASAL MEDICATION**

EQUIPMENT/SUPPLIES: Physician's order and patient record; nasal medication, drops, or spray; tissues; gloves

STANDARDS: Given the needed equipment and a place to work, the student will perform this skill with _____% accuracy in a total of _____ minutes. *(Your instructor will tell you what the percentage and time limits will be before you begin practicing.)*

KEY: 4 = Satisfactory   0 = Unsatisfactory   NA = This step is not counted

PROCEDURE STEPS	SELF	PARTNER	INSTRUCTOR
1. Wash your hands and put on gloves.	☐	☐	☐
2. Assemble the equipment and supplies. Check the medication label three times.	☐	☐	☐
3. Greet and identify the patient. Explain the procedure.	☐	☐	☐
4. Ask patient about any allergies not documented.	☐	☐	☐

5. Position the patient in a comfortable recumbent position.
  a. Extend patient's head beyond edge of examination table.
  b. Or place a pillow under the patient's shoulders.
  c. Support the patient's neck to avoid strain as the head is tilted back.
	☐	☐	☐

6. Administering nasal medication:
  a. Nasal drops
    (1) Hold the dropper upright just above each nostril.
    (2) Drop the medication one drop at a time without touching the nares.
    (3) Keep the patient in a recumbent position for 5 minutes.
  b. Nasal spray
    (1) Place tip of the bottle at the naris opening without touching the patient.
    (2) Spray as the patient takes a deep breath.
	☐	☐	☐

7. Wipe any excess medication from the patient's skin with tissues.	☐	☐	☐
8. Properly care for or dispose of equipment and supplies. Clean the work area.	☐	☐	☐
9. Remove your gloves and wash your hands.	☐	☐	☐
10. Record the procedure in the patient's chart.	☐	☐	☐

CALCULATION

Total Possible Points: _____
Total Points Earned: _____ Multiplied by 100 = _____ Divided by Total Possible Points = _____%

Pass **Fail**
☐   ☐   Comments:

Student's signature _____ Date _____
Partner's signature _____ Date _____
Instructor's signature _____ Date _____

16. What important advice can you give children when dealing with contagious diseases like pink eye?

    a. Keep your hands washed and clean.

    b. Do not play with children who are sick.

    c. If you sneeze, immediately cover your face with your hand.

    d. Do not go to school if you are sick.

    e. Try to keep from touching anything others have already touched.

17. You test for pharyngitis or tonsillitis by:

    a. blood sample.

    b. urine sample.

    c. reflex test.

    d. throat culture.

    e. radiology.

18. Which form of strabismus is known as convergent eyes, when the eyes are crossed?

    a. Esotropic

    b. Exotropic

    c. Hypotropic

    d. Hypertropic

    e. Nonconcomitant

19. The purpose of a hearing aid is to:

    a. fully restore the ability to hear.

    b. assist patients with permanent nerve damage.

    c. amplify sound waves.

    d. differentiate between tones.

    e. correct hearing disabilities.

20. The best treatment for allergic rhinitis is:

    a. sleep.

    b. antihistamine medication.

    c. surgery.

    d. antibiotics.

    e. ear irrigation.

Chapter Checklist

☐ Read textbook chapter and take notes within the Chapter Notes outline. Answer the Learning Objectives as you reach them in the content, and then check them off.

☐ Work the Content Review questions—both Foundational Knowledge and Application.

☐ Perform the Active Learning exercise(s).

☐ Complete Professional Journal entries.

☐ Complete Skill Practice Activity(s) using Competency Evaluation Forms and Work Products, when appropriate.

☐ Take the Chapter Self-Assessment Quiz.

☐ Insert all appropriate pages into your Portfolio.

Learning Objectives

1. Spell and define the key terms.
2. Identify the primary defense mechanisms of the respiratory system.
3. List and describe disorders of the respiratory system.
4. Explain various diagnostic procedures of the respiratory system.
5. Describe the physician's examination of the respiratory system.
6. Discuss the role of the medical assistant with regard to various diagnostic and therapeutic procedures.

Chapter Notes

Note: Bold-faced headings are the major headings in the text chapter; headings in regular font are lower-level headings (i.e., the content is subordinate to, or falls "under," the major headings). Make sure you understand the key terms used in the chapter, as well as the concepts presented as Key Points.

TEXT SUBHEADINGS   **NOTES**

Introduction _____

_____

_____

☐ **LEARNING OBJECTIVE 1:** Spell and define the key terms.

_____

☐ **LEARNING OBJECTIVE 2:** Identify the primary defense mechanisms of the respiratory system.

_____

Common Respiratory Disorders _____

_____

_____

Upper Respiratory Disorders _____

_____

Key Point:
• The most common problems of the upper respiratory tract are caused by infectious microorganisms and by allergic reactions that produce inflammation.

Lower Respiratory Disorders _____

_____

_____

Bronchitis _____

_____

Key Point:
• Bronchitis is an inflammation of the mucous membranes of the bronchi caused by infection or irritation that induces increased production of mucus in the trachea, bronchi, and bronchioles.

Pneumonia _____

_____

Key Term: dyspnea
Key Points:
• Pneumonia is a bacterial or viral infection in the alveoli, or tiny air sacs, that are the site of gas exchange in the lungs.
• Viral pneumonia is usually more gradual in onset but can be just as serious as bacterial pneumonia.

Asthma _____

_____

Key Term: status asthmaticus
Key Point:
• Asthma is a reversible inflammatory process involving primarily the small airways such as the bronchi and bronchioles

Chronic Obstructive Pulmonary Disease _____

Key Term: chronic obstructive pulmonary disease
Key Points:
• Chronic bronchitis is a chronic inflammation and swelling of the airways with excessive mucus production, obstruction of the bronchi, and trapping of air behind mucus plugs.
• Emphysema is a disease process in which the walls of the damaged alveoli stretch and break down after repeated exposure to irritants such as cigarette smoke and air pollution.

Tuberculosis _____

Key Point:
• Tuberculosis is an infectious disease spread by respiratory droplets from a person infected with *Mycobacterium tuberculosis.*

☐ **LEARNING OBJECTIVE 3:** List and describe disorders of the respiratory system.

Common Cancers of the Respiratory System _____

Laryngeal Cancer _____

Key Terms: laryngectomy; tracheostomy
Key Point:
• Cancer of the larynx is seen most commonly in heavy smokers and alcoholics.

Lung Cancer _____

Key Term: hemoptysis; thoracentesis; palliative
Key Point:
• Lung cancer is one of the most common causes of death in both men and women.

Common Diagnostic and Therapeutic Procedures _____

Physical Examination of the Respiratory System

Key Point:
• The traditional examination of the chest consists of four parts: inspection, palpation, percussion, and auscultation.

Inspection

Key Point:
• Inspection consists of a visual examination of the chest and the patient's respiratory pattern.

Palpation

Key Point:
• In palpation, the physician uses his or her hands to feel the patient's throat for lumps, areas of tenderness, and location of the trachea, which may be displaced by a tumor.

Percussion

Key Term: atelectasis
Key Point:
• Percussion is placing a finger or fingers on the chest and striking it with the fingers of the other hand.

Auscultation

Key Point:
• Auscultation is listening to the patient's lungs and airway passages with a stethoscope.

Sputum Culture and Cytology

Key Point:
• Sputum cultures are obtained to aid with diagnosis and treatment decisions in patients with suspected pneumonia, tuberculosis, or other infectious diseases of the lower airway.

Chest Radiography _____

_____

Key Point:
• Chest radiography can help in the diagnosis of a large variety of pulmonary problems, including pneumonia, lung cancer, emphysema, tuberculosis, and pulmonary edema.

Bronchoscopy _____

_____

Key Point:
• Bronchoscopy is an endoscopic procedure in which a lighted scope is inserted into the trachea and bronchi for direct visualization.

Pulmonary Function Tests _____

_____

Key Terms: tidal volume; forced expiratory volume
Key Point:
• Pulmonary function tests are performed with a spirometer that measures the amount of air a patient can move in and out of the lungs.

Arterial Blood Gasses _____

_____

Key Point:
• Arterial blood gas (ABG) determinations measure the pH and pressures of oxygen and carbon dioxide in arterial blood.

Pulse Oximetry _____

_____

Key Point:
• Many medical offices have a pulse oximeter, which quickly and painlessly determines the percentage of oxygen saturation on a patient's capillary blood cells.

☐ **LEARNING OBJECTIVE 4:** Explain various diagnostic procedures of the respiratory system.

☐ **LEARNING OBJECTIVE 5:** Describe the physician's examination of the respiratory system.

☐ **LEARNING OBJECTIVE 6:** Discuss the role of the medical assistant with regard to various diagnostic and therapeutic procedures.

Content Review

FOUNDATIONAL KNOWLEDGE

Understanding Respiratory Disorders

1. Read the following chart listing practices that might promote good pulmonary health. Mark whether the remedy is appropriate for promoting good pulmonary health. Assume the patient is generally healthy.

Practice	Appropriate	Inappropriate
a. Avoid exercise.		
b. Take rapid, deep breaths.		
c. Avoid smoking cigarettes.		
d. Use oxygen treatment.		
e. Avoid excessive pollution.		
f. Have a physician check pulmonary function regularly.		
g. Avoid allergens such as dust and mold.		

2. What is the most common cause of chronic obstructive pulmonary disease?

_____

_____

3. Why is the term *chronic obstructive pulmonary disease* used to characterize a patient suffering from emphysema and chronic bronchitis?

_____

_____

4. What are two of the most common causes of upper respiratory problems?

a. _____

b. _____

5. In the case of a pneumonia patient, what prevents effective gas exchange?

_____

_____

6. Place a check mark in the appropriate box to indicate if each symptom is considered a presenting symptom of laryngeal cancer.

Symptom	
a. hoarseness lasting longer than three weeks	
b. pain in the throat when drinking hot liquids	
c. wheezing	
d. a feeling of a lump in the throat	
e. chest pain	

Symptom

f. burning in the throat when drinking citrus juice	
g. dyspnea	
h. night sweats	
i. general malaise	

7. What is usually the etiology of chronic bronchitis?

_____

_____

Diagnosing Respiratory Disorders

8. What is a symptomatic difference between viral and bacterial pneumonia?

_____

_____

9. What is the role of the medical assistant in the collection and analysis of a sputum specimen?

_____

_____

10. What is the purpose of a peak flow meter?

_____

_____

11. Which of the following is/are an element/elements of the traditional examination of the chest? Circle all that apply.
   a. Palpation
   b. Auscultation
   c. Sputum culture
   d. Chest radiography
   e. Inspection

12. Which of the following pulmonary diagnostic methods is considered invasive?
   a. Percussion
   b. Bronchoscopy
   c. Auscultation
   d. Sputum Culture
   e. Posteroanterior x-ray

13. Under what circumstance would a physician perform a laryngectomy?

_____

_____

Treating Respiratory Disorders

14. Describe the difference between palliative care and a cure.

Palliative Care	Cure

15. What measures ought to be taken in the case of an asthmatic patient who does not respond to medication?

_____

_____

16. If a patient is prescribed two inhaled bronchodilators, what is the most likely explanation? Why would two be prescribed?

_____

_____

17. Describe the typical prognosis of a lung cancer patient.

_____

_____

18. Why would a medical assistant not perform an arterial blood gas test?

_____

_____

19. Match the following key terms to their definitions.

Key Terms

a. atelectasis _____
b. chronic obstructive pulmonary disease (COPD) _____
c. dyspnea _____
d. forced expiratory volume (FEV) _____
e. hemoptysis _____
f. laryngectomy _____
g. palliative _____
h. status asthmaticus _____
i. thoracentesis _____
j. tidal volume _____
k. tracheostomy _____

Definitions

1. coughing up blood from the respiratory tract
2. easing symptoms without curing
3. a permanent surgical stoma in the neck with an indwelling tube
4. a surgical puncture into the pleural cavity for aspiration of serous fluid or for injection of medication
5. a progressive, irreversible condition with diminished respiratory capacity
6. the volume of air forced out of the lungs
7. difficulty breathing
8. the amount of air inhaled and exhaled during normal respiration
9. an asthma attack that is not responsive to treatment
10. collapsed lung fields; incomplete expansion of the lungs, either partial or complete
11. the surgical removal of the larynx

20. True or False? Determine whether the following statements are true or false. If false, explain why.

a. An asthma patient will, upon contracting the disease, suffer from it for her entire life.

_____

_____

b. Emphysema entails chronic inflammation of the airways.

_____

_____

c. A patient who tests positive for tuberculosis is contagious.

_____

_____

d. Lung cancer, one of the most common causes of death in men and women, is believed to result usually from cigarette smoking.

_____

_____

APPLICATION

Critical Thinking Practice

1. A patient with a severe lung disease explains that she has been smoking for decades. You explain that she ought to quit, but she contends that it does not matter. She says she has already damaged her lungs enough that continuing to smoke will do no further harm. How do you respond to this patient?

_____

_____

2. A patient receiving oxygen therapy calls to complain that his machine is not working. He does not know what to do. What will you say to the patient? What will you do to assist him?

_____

_____

Patient Education

1. Your patient has just been diagnosed with tuberculosis. Explain to him ways in which he should act to protect others while he undergoes treatment.

_____

_____

Documentation

1. Write a patient care note for a patient recovering from bacterial pneumonia. Explain what her symptoms are as well as what remedies the physician recommends/prescribes. Also, indicate how these remedies are intended to combat specific elements of the disease. You do not need to explain the details of how a remedy works, only what it is intended to do (i.e., a glucocorticoid is prescribed to reduce inflammation).

_____

_____

Active Learning

1. Most people are aware of the dangers of smoking. However, it is still important to educate children about the long-term dangers of smoking. Working with a group, create a role-playing skit that could be presented to a middle school classroom to show the dangers of smoking. Then create a pamphlet outlining the dangers of smoking to be presented to the same class. Be prepared to perform your skit in front of your classmates.

2. Find ICD-9 codes for emphysema, bronchitis, allergic rhinitis, asthma, pneumonia, and sinusitis.

3. There is a wide variety of medication used in the treatment of asthma and allergic rhinitis. Some medications are corticosteroids. Some common ones are budesonide, ciclesonide, and fluticasone. Select one of these compounds, research its intended effects and side effects, and formulate an explanation that you might give to a patient who was recently prescribed your drug of choice.

Professional Journal

REFLECT

(Prompts and Ideas: Patients afflicted by severe pulmonary ailments are sometimes despondent. Their conditions are probably worsening and it may not be long before they succumb to disease. Reflect on how such a patient ought to be treated. As a medical assistant, what can you do to ease their pain?)

_____

_____

_____

_____

_____

_____

PONDER AND SOLVE

1. A healthy patient worries that his exposure to secondhand smoke might cause his health to deteriorate. You are aware of research suggesting that this is so; however, much of the research is controversial. How would you advise the patient?

_____

_____

_____

_____

_____

2. A patient has just been diagnosed with lung cancer that the physician described as "not terribly aggressive and potentially curable." The patient asks you if this means that he will be okay. How do you respond?

_____

_____

_____

_____

_____

_____

EXPERIENCE

Skills related to this chapter include:

1. Instructing a Patient on Using the Peak Flowmeter (Procedure 30-1).
2. Performing a Nebulized Breathing Treatment (Procedure 30-2).
3. Perform a Pulmonary Function Test (Procedure 30-3).

Record any common mistakes, lessons learned, and/or tips you discovered during your experience of practicing and demonstrating these skills:

_____

_____

_____

_____

_____

_____

_____

Skill Practice

PERFORMANCE OBJECTIVES:

1. Instruct a patient in the use of the peak flowmeter (Procedure 30-1).
2. Administer a nebulized breathing treatment (Procedure 30-2).
3. Perform a pulmonary function test (Procedure 30-3).

Name _____ Date _____ Time _____

Procedure 30-1: INSTRUCTING A PATIENT ON USING THE PEAK FLOW METER

EQUIPMENT/SUPPLIES: Peak flow meter, recording documentation form

STANDARDS: Given the needed equipment and a place to work, the student will perform this skill with _____% accuracy in a total of _____ minutes. *(Your instructor will tell you what the percentage and time limits will be before you begin practicing.)*

KEY: 4 = Satisfactory 0 = Unsatisfactory NA = This step is not counted

PROCEDURE STEPS	SELF	PARTNER	INSTRUCTOR
1. Wash your hands.	☐	☐	☐
2. Assemble the peak flow meter, disposable mouthpiece, and patient documentation form.	☐	☐	☐
3. Greet and identify the patient and explain the procedure.	☐	☐	☐
4. Holding the peak flow meter upright, explain how to read and reset the gauge after each reading.	☐	☐	☐
5. Instruct the patient to place the peak flow meter mouthpiece into the mouth, forming a tight seal with the lips. After taking a deep breath, the patient should blow hard into the mouthpiece without blocking the back of the flowmeter.	☐	☐	☐
6. Note the number on the flowmeter denoting the level at which the sliding gauge stopped after the hard blowing into the mouthpiece. Reset the gauge to zero.	☐	☐	☐
7. Instruct the patient to perform this procedure a total of three times consecutively, in both the morning and at night, and to record the highest reading on the form.	☐	☐	☐
8. Explain to the patient the procedure for cleaning the mouthpiece of the flowmeter by washing with soapy water and rinsing without immersing the flowmeter in water.	☐	☐	☐
9. Document the procedure.	☐	☐	☐

CALCULATION

Total Possible Points: _____
Total Points Earned: _____ Multiplied by 100 = _____ Divided by Total Possible Points = _____%

Pass **Fail**
☐   ☐   Comments:

Student's signature _____ Date _____
Partner's signature _____ Date _____
Instructor's signature _____ Date _____

Name_____ Date _____ Time _____

Procedure 30-2:	PERFORMING A NEBULIZED BREATHING TREATMENT

EQUIPMENT/SUPPLIES: Physician's order and patient's medical record, inhalation medication, saline for inhalation, nebulizer disposable setup, nebulizer machine

STANDARDS: Given the needed equipment and a place to work, the student will perform this skill with _____% accuracy in a total of _____ minutes. *(Your instructor will tell you what the percentage and time limits will be before you begin practicing.)*

KEY: 4 = Satisfactory   0 = Unsatisfactory   NA = This step is not counted

PROCEDURE STEPS	SELF	PARTNER	INSTRUCTOR
1. Wash your hands.	☐	☐	☐
2. Assemble the equipment and medication, checking the medication label three times as indicated when administering any medications.	☐	☐	☐
3. Greet and identify the patient and explain the procedure.	☐	☐	☐
4. Remove the nebulizer treatment cup from the setup and add the exact amount of medication ordered by the physician.	☐	☐	☐
5. Add 2–3 mL of saline for inhalation therapy to the cup that contains the medication.	☐	☐	☐
6. Place the top on the cup securely, attach the "T" piece to the top of the cup, and position the mouthpiece firmly on one end of the "T" piece.	☐	☐	☐
7. Attach one end of the tubing securely to the connector on the cup and the other end to the connector on the nebulizer machine.	☐	☐	☐
8. Ask the patient to place the mouthpiece into the mouth and make a seal with the lips, without biting the mouthpiece. Instruct the patient to breathe normally during the treatment, occasionally taking a deep breath.	☐	☐	☐
9. Turn the machine on using the on/off switch. The medication in the reservoir cup will become a fine mist that is inhaled by the patient breathing through the mouthpiece.	☐	☐	☐
10. Before, during, and after the breathing treatment, take and record the patient's pulse.	☐	☐	☐
11. When the treatment is over and the medication/saline is gone from the cup, turn the machine off and have the patient remove the mouthpiece.	☐	☐	☐
12. Disconnect the disposable treatment setup and dispose of all parts into a biohazard container. Properly put away the machine.	☐	☐	☐
13. Wash your hands and document the procedure, including the patient's pulse before, during, and after the treatment.	☐	☐	☐

CALCULATION

Total Possible Points: _____

Total Points Earned: _____ Multiplied by 100 = _____ Divided by Total Possible Points = _____%

Pass   **Fail**

☐   ☐   Comments:

Student's signature _____ Date _____

Partner's signature _____ Date _____

Instructor's signature _____ Date _____

Name _____ Date _____ Time _____

Procedure 30-3:	PERFORM A PULMONARY FUNCTION TEST (PFT)

EQUIPMENT/SUPPLIES: Physician's order and patient's medical record, spirometer and appropriate cables, calibration syringe and log book, disposable mouthpiece, printer, nose clip

STANDARDS: Given the needed equipment and a place to work, the student will perform this skill with _____% accuracy in a total of _____ minutes. *(Your instructor will tell you what the percentage and time limits will be before you begin practicing.)*

KEY: 4 = Satisfactory   0 = Unsatisfactory   NA = This step is not counted

PROCEDURE STEPS	SELF	PARTNER	INSTRUCTOR
1. Wash your hands.	☐	☐	☐
2. Assemble the equipment, greet and identify the patient, and explain the procedure.	☐	☐	☐
3. Turn the PFT machine on and if the spirometer has not been calibrated according to the office policy, calibrate the machine using the calibration syringe according to the manufacturer's instructions, and record the calibration in the appropriate log book.	☐	☐	☐
4. With the machine on and calibrated, attach the appropriate cable, tubing, and mouthpiece for the type of machine being used.	☐	☐	☐
5. Using the keyboard on the machine, input patient data into the machine including the patient's name or identification number, age, weight, height, sex, race, and smoking history.	☐	☐	☐
6. Ask the patient to remove any restrictive clothing such as a necktie and instruct the patient in applying the nose clip.	☐	☐	☐
7. Ask the patient to stand, breathe in deeply, and blow into the mouthpiece as hard as possible. He or she should continue to blow into the mouthpiece until the machine indicates that it is appropriate to stop blowing. A chair should be available in case the patient becomes dizzy or lightheaded.	☐	☐	☐
8. During the procedure, coach the patient as needed to obtain an adequate reading.	☐	☐	☐
9. Continue the procedure until three adequate readings or maneuvers are performed.	☐	☐	☐
10. After printing the results, properly care for the equipment and dispose of the mouthpiece into the biohazard container. Wash your hands.	☐	☐	☐
11. Document the procedure and place the printed results in the patient's medical record.	☐	☐	☐

CALCULATION

Total Possible Points: _____
Total Points Earned: _____ Multiplied by 100 = _____ Divided by Total Possible Points = _____%

Pass   **Fail**

☐   ☐   Comments:

Student's signature _____ Date _____
Partner's signature _____ Date _____
Instructor's signature _____ Date _____

Work Product 1

Perform Respiratory Testing.

Use the equipment available to you at a medical office or at school to perform the following tests on at least one patient or volunteer. Take three consecutive measurements using the peak flow meter. Record the results in the chart below and attach any additional test results to this sheet.

Peak Flow Meter Daily Record

Name: _____

Date	3/05	3/06	3/07							
Time	8AM	8:30	8:15							
750										
650										
550										
450										
350										
250										
150										

Work Product 2

Document appropriately.

Perform a pulmonary function test on a patient or volunteer. Perform three consecutive tests using a calibrated spirometer. Print the results and attach to this sheet. Then record the procedure in the patient's chart.

If you are currently working in a medical office, use a blank paper patient chart from the office. If this is not available to you, use the space below to record the incident in the chart.

_____

_____

_____

_____

_____

_____

_____

Chapter Self-Assessment Quiz

1. A pulmonary function test measures:

   a. arterial blood gases.

   b. oxygen saturation.

   c. sputum cells.

   d. tidal volume.

   e. fluid in lungs.

2. A patient in need of an artificial airway will likely undergo:

   a. laryngectomy.

   b. tracheostomy.

   c. chemotherapy.

   d. bronchoscopy.

   e. pneumonectomy.

3. Which procedure necessitates a stethoscope?

   a. Percussion

   b. Palpation

   c. Inspection

   d. Radiation

   e. Auscultation

4. Which of the following is a normal pulse oximetry result?

   a. 96%

   b. 94%

   c. 92%

   d. 90%

   e. 88%

5. One lower respiratory disorder is:

   a. laryngitis.

   b. bronchitis.

   c. sinusitis.

   d. pharyngitis.

   e. tonsillitis.

6. Which of the following is anesthetized by cigarette smoke?

   a. Alveoli

   b. Bronchioles

   c. Mucus

   d. Cilia

   e. Trachea

7. The most prominent symptom of bronchitis is:

   a. severe wheezing.

   b. repeated sneezing.

   c. productive cough.

   d. shortness of breath.

   e. coughing blood.

8. Viral pneumonia differs from bacterial pneumonia in that:

   a. it can be treated by antibiotics.

   b. it might result in hospitalization.

   c. it affects gas exchange in the lungs.

   d. it may lead to a fever and cough.

   e. it spreads throughout the lungs.

9. People with asthma have difficulty breathing because their:

   a. airways are narrow.

   b. cilia are inoperative.

   c. alveoli are collapsed.

   d. bronchioles are too wide.

   e. lungs are underdeveloped.

10. A productive cough refers to a cough that produces:

    a. blood.

    b. nasal mucus.

    c. respiratory mucus.

    d. oxygen.

    e. antibodies.

11. A type of medication that opens the bronchioles and controls bronchospasms is a(n):

    a. corticosteroid.

    b. bronchodilator.

    c. antibiotic.

    d. antihistamine.

    e. decongestant.

12. The public health department should be alerted about a diagnosis of:

    a. tuberculosis.

    b. pneumonia.

    c. bronchitis.

    d. asthma.

    e. COPD.

13. Which of the following is true of emphysema?

    a. It is not associated with bronchitis.

    b. It causes inflammation of the airways.

    c. It can be treated with steroids.

    d. It is usually reversible.

    e. It usually takes many years to develop.

14. The purpose of a nebulizer is to:

    a. turn a vaporous medicine into a liquid.

    b. administer an asthma treatment.

    c. turn a liquid medicine into a vapor.

    d. cure COPD.

    e. pump oxygen.

15. Of the following diseases affecting the respiratory system, which, in most cases, is linked to cigarette smoking?

    a. Bronchitis

    b. Cystic fibrosis

    c. Laryngitis

    d. Lung cancer

    e. Allergic rhinitis

16. In the case of a patient receiving oxygen treatment, a cannula:

    a. stores the oxygen.

    b. separates oxygen from the air in a room.

    c. delivers oxygen to the airways.

    d. ensures proper flow of oxygen.

    e. prevents accidents caused by oxygen's flammability.

17. COPD patients may take medications for which disease, even if they have not been diagnosed with it?

    a. Influenza

    b. Pneumonia

    c. Emphysema

    d. Lung cancer

    e. Asthma

18. One acute disease of the lower respiratory tract is:

    a. asthma.

    b. pneumonia.

    c. emphysema.

    d. bronchitis.

    e. COPD.

19. The best way to keep mucus in the airways thin is:

    a. oxygen therapy.

    b. steroid medication.

    c. good fluid intake.

    d. a balanced diet.

    e. frequent exercise.

20. A physician may perform an arterial blood gas test to:

    a. determine how much gas is in a patient's lungs.

    b. determine whether a patient is breathing normally.

    c. determine when a patient will be ready for respiratory surgery.

    d. determine whether a patient will be receptive to oxygen therapy.

    e. determine whether the patient's lungs are adequately exchanging gases.

Cardiology

Chapter Checklist

☐ Read textbook chapter and take notes within the Chapter Notes outline. Answer the Learning Objectives as you reach them in the content, and then check them off.

☐ Work the Content Review questions—both Foundational Knowledge and Application.

☐ Perform the Active Learning exercise(s).

☐ Complete Professional Journal entries.

☐ Complete Skill Practice Activity(s) using Competency Evaluation Forms and Work Products, when appropriate.

☐ Take the Chapter Self-Assessment Quiz.

☐ Insert all appropriate pages into your Portfolio.

Learning Objectives

1. Spell and define the key terms.

2. List and describe common cardiovascular disorders.

3. Identify and explain common cardiovascular procedures and tests.

4. Describe the role and responsibilities of the medical assistant during cardiovascular examinations and procedures.

5. Discuss the information recorded on a basic 12-lead electrocardiogram.

6. Explain the purpose of a Holter monitor.

Chapter Notes

Note: Bold-faced headings are the major headings in the text chapter; headings in regular font are lower-level headings (i.e., the content is subordinate to, or falls "under," the major headings). Make sure you understand the key terms used in the chapter, as well as the concepts presented as Key Points.

TEXT SUBHEADINGS

NOTES

Introduction _____

_____

Key Point:
• The cardiologist is a physician who specializes in disorders of the heart, and many patients with chronic cardiac conditions are referred to the cardiology office for treatment and follow-up.

☐ **LEARNING OBJECTIVE 1:** Spell and define the key terms.

Common Disorders of the Cardiovascular System _____

_____

_____

Disorders of the Heart _____

_____

_____

Carditis _____

_____

Key Terms: pericarditis; myocardial infarction; myocarditis; cardiomegaly; endocarditis

Key Point:
• Cardiac inflammation, or carditis, may affect any of the layers of the heart muscle, and although other factors may be involved, it is usually the result of a systemic infection.

Congestive Heart Failure _____

_____

Key Point:
• Congestive heart failure (CHF) is a condition in which the heart cannot pump effectively.

Myocardial Infarction _____

_____

Key Terms: angina pectoris; electrocardiography; percutaneous transluminal coronary angioplasty; coronary artery bypass graft

Key point:
• Death of any part of the heart muscle, called myocardial infarction (MI), occurs when one or more of the coronary arteries becomes totally occluded, usually by atherosclerotic plaques or by an embolism.

Cardiac Arrhythmia _____

_____

Key Terms: bradycardia; tachycardia

Key Point:
• Cardiac arrhythmia or dysrhythmia is an abnormal heart rhythm that may occur as a primary disorder or as a response to a systemic problem.

Artificial Pacemakers _____

_____

_____

Congenital and Valvular Heart Disease

Key Points:
- Valvular disease is an acquired or congenital abnormality of any of the four cardiac valves.
- Rheumatic heart disease, an acquired valvular disease, presents clinically as a generalized inflammatory disease occurring 10 to 21 days after an upper respiratory infection caused by group A beta-hemolytic streptococci.

Disorders of the Blood Vessels

Atherosclerosis

Key Term: atherosclerosis
Key Point:
- Diseases of blood vessels—arteries or veins—often begin with collection of fatty plaques made of calcium and cholesterol inside the walls of the vessels. These plaques narrow the lumen, or opening, of the blood vessels and impede blood flow.

Hypertension

Key Point:
- Hypertension cannot be diagnosed on the basis of one blood pressure measurement, since other factors, such as emotional upset or anxiety may cause a temporary increase in blood pressure.

Varicose Veins

Key Point:
- Varicosities, the most common circulatory disease of the lower extremities, occur when the superficial veins of the legs swell and distend.

Venous Thrombosis and Pulmonary Embolism _____

_____

Key Term: cerebrovascular accident
Key Point:
• Thrombi, or blood clots, in the peripheral or pulmonary veins commonly affect patients with underlying cardiovascular disease.

Cerebrovascular Accident _____

_____

Key Term: transient ischemic attack
Key Point:
• Cerebrovascular accident (CVA), sometimes called stroke, results suddenly when damage to the blood vessels in the brain occurs.

Aneurysm _____

_____

Key Term: aneurysm
Key Point:
• Weakened blood vessel walls are predisposed to abnormal dilation. Dilation in the form of an **aneurysm** may occur in any vessel, but arteries are most often affected.

Anemia _____

_____

Key Term:
• Deficiencies in hemoglobin or in the numbers of red blood cells result in anemia.

☐ **LEARNING OBJECTIVE 2:** List and describe common cardiovascular disorders.

Common Diagnostic and Therapeutic Procedures _____

_____

_____

Physical Examination of the Cardiovascular System _____

_____

Key Point:
• The cardiovascular examination is the most basic noninvasive procedure used to assess the heart and blood vessels.

Electrocardiogram

Key Term: leads
Key Point:
• One of the most valuable diagnostic tools for evaluating the electrical pathway through the heart is the electrocardiogram, known by the acronym ECG or EKG.

ECG Leads

Key Points:
• Each lead records the electrical impulse through the heart from a different angle. Viewing the conduction of the electrical impulses in these various angles gives the physician a fairly complete view of the entire heart.
• The first three combinations, standard bipolar leads also known as Einthoven leads, allow frontal visualization of the heart's electrical activity from side to side.
• These second three combinations, the augmented unipolar limb leads, allow visualization from a frontal view top to bottom.

ECG Interpretation

Key Term: artifacts
Key Point:
• The physician's interpretation of the standard 12-lead ECG includes an examination of various wave forms associated with the cardiac cycle.

☐ **LEARNING OBJECTIVE 3:** Identify and explain common cardiovascular procedures and tests.

☐ **LEARNING OBJECTIVE 4:** Describe the roles and responsibilities of the medical assistant during cardiovascular examinations and procedures.

☐ **LEARNING OBJECTIVE 5:** Discuss the information recorded on a basic 12-lead electrocardiogram.

Holter Monitor

Key Point:
• The Holter monitor is small and portable and can be worn comfortably for long periods without interfering with daily activities.

☐ **LEARNING OBJECTIVE 6:** Explain the purpose of a Holter monitor.

Chest Radiography _____

_____

Key Point:
- Chest radiography provides valuable basic information about the anatomical location and gross structures of the heart, great vessels, and lungs.

Cardiac Stress Test _____

_____

Key Term: palpitations
Key Point:
- To measure the response of the cardiac muscle to increased demands for oxygen, the physician may request a cardiac stress test. The heart is usually tested with the patient walking on a treadmill.

Echocardiography _____

_____

Key Term: cardiomyopathy
Key Point:
- An echocardiogram, or echo, uses sound waves generated by a small device called a transducer. These waves travel through the cardiac chambers, walls, and valves and are transmitted back to a screen, where they can be viewed and interpreted.

Cardiac Catheterization and Coronary Arteriography _____

_____

Key Point:
- Cardiac catheterization is a common invasive procedure used to help diagnose or treat conditions affecting the coronary arterial circulation.

Content Review

FOUNDATIONAL KNOWLEDGE

Heart Disorders

1. List five symptoms of the various heart disorders.

   a. _____

   b. _____

c. _____

d. _____

e. _____

2. Cardiac inflammation, or carditis, is a disorder of the heart that is usually the result of infection. In the table below are descriptions of the three types of carditis. Read the descriptions and fill in the missing boxes with the correct type of carditis.

Disorder	Causes	Signs and Symptoms	Treatment
a. _____	a pathogen, neoplasm, or autoimmune disorder, such as lupus erythematosus or rheumatoid arthritis	sharp pain in the same locations as myocardial infarction	relieving the symptoms and, if possible, correcting the underlying cause, including administering an antibiotic for bacterial infection
b. _____	radiation, chemicals, and bacterial, viral, or parasitic infection	early signs: fever, fatigue, and mild chest pain chronic: cardiomegaly, arrhythmias, valvulitis	supportive care and medication as ordered by the physician to kill the responsible pathogen
c. _____	infection or inflammation of the inner lining of the heart, the endocardium	reflux, or backflow, of the valves or blood	directed at eliminating the infecting organism

3. List the four causes of congestive heart failure.

a. _____

b. _____

c. _____

d. _____

4. Match the condition with its description.

a. congestive heart failure	**1.** occurs when some of the electrical signals originate in the ventricles rather than in the SA node
b. myocardial infarction	**2.** a shock administered to restore normal cardiac electrical activity
c. ventricular tachycardia	**3.** symptoms may be similar to those felt during angina pectoris
d. ventricular fibrillation	**4.** may occur if the SA node initiates electrical impulses too fast or too slowly
e. arrhythmia	**5.** failure of the left ventricle leads to pulmonary congestion

5. Explain how a pacemaker helps the heart maintain normal sinus rhythm.

_____

_____

6. Valvular disease is:

a. inflammatory lesions of the connective tissues, particularly in the heart joints, and subcutaneous tissues.

b. an acquired or congenital abnormality of any of the four cardiac valves.

c. a collection of fatty plaques made of calcium and cholesterol inside the walls of blood vessels.

d. a disordered blood flow within the valvular walls of the heart.

7. Atherosclerosis can sometimes result in:

    a. rheumatic heart disease.

    b. valvular disease.

    c. coronary artery disease.

    d. congestive heart failure.

8. Cerebrovascular accident (CVA) is sometimes called:

    a. heart attack.

    b. paralysis.

    c. blood clot.

    d. stroke.

9. List six potential causes of anemia.

    a. _____

    b. _____

    c. _____

    d. _____

    e. _____

    f. _____

Diagnosing Cardiovascular Conditions

10. Explain angiography, one of the procedures used to diagnose atherosclerosis.

_____

_____

11. Explain why a physician often requires several blood pressure readings before making the diagnosis of hypertension.

_____

_____

12. Which of the following is a question you should ask the patient before a cardiovascular examination?

    a. Are you currently pregnant?

    b. How long have you had the pain/discomfort?

    c. How often do you exercise?

    d. What do you like to do in your free time?

13. Risky Business

Risk factors for developing thrombi may either be primary (inherited) or secondary (acquired). Read the risk factors below and place a check mark in the appropriate column.

Risk Factor for Developing Thrombi	Primary	Secondary
a. hemolytic anemia		
b. long-term immobility		
c. chronic pulmonary disease		
d. thrombophlebitis		

e. sickle cell disease		
f. varicosities		
g. defibrillation after cardiac arrest		

The ABCs of EKGs

14. Explain the role of the medical assistant during an electrocardiogram (ECG).

_____

_____

15. Match the lead with its measurements.

a. Lead I	**1.** measures the difference in electrical potential between the right arm (RA) and the left leg (LL).
b. Lead II	**2.** measures the difference in electrical potential between the right arm (RA) and the left arm (LA).
c. Lead III	**3.** measures the difference in electrical potential between the left arm (LA) and the left leg (LL).

16. List the six elements that are taken into consideration during the ECG.

a. _____

b. _____

c. _____

d. _____

e. _____

f. _____

17. A Holter monitor is used for:

a. the diagnosis of intermittent cardiac arrhythmias and dysfunctions.

b. obtaining a good-quality ECG without avoidable artifacts.

c. obtaining basic information about the anatomical location and gross structures of the heart, great vessels, and lungs.

d. measuring the response of the cardiac muscle to increased demands for oxygen.

18. Match the procedure with the correct description.

Procedure	**Description**
a. electrocardiogram	**1.** provides valuable information about the anatomical location and gross structures of the heart, great vessels, and lungs
b. chest radiography	**2.** uses sounds waves generated by a small device called a transducer
c. cardiac stress test	**3.** a graphic record of the electrical current as it progresses through the heart
d. echocardiography	**4.** common invasive procedure used to help diagnose or treat conditions affecting coronary arterial circulation
e. cardiac catheterization	**5.** measures the response of the cardiac muscle to increased demands for oxygen

19. Match the following key terms to their definitions.

Key Terms

a. aneurysm _____

b. angina pectoris _____

c. artifact _____

d. atherosclerosis _____

e. bradycardia _____

f. cardiomegaly _____

g. cardiomyopathy _____

h. cerebrovascular accident (CVA) _____

i. congestive heart failure _____

j. electrocardiography _____

k. coronary artery bypass graft _____

l. endocarditis _____

m. leads _____

n. myocardial infarction (MI) _____

o. myocarditis _____

p. palpitations _____

q. percutaneous transluminal coronary angioplasty (PTCA) _____

r. pericarditis _____

s. tachycardia _____

t. transient ischemic attack (TIA) _____

Definitions

1. a heart rate of less than 60 beats per minute

2. any disease affecting the myocardium

3. a surgical procedure that increases the blood flow to the heart by bypassing the occluded or blocked vessel with a graft

4. any activity recorded in an electrocardiogram caused by extraneous activity such as patient movement, loose lead, or electrical interference

5. a procedure that improves blood flow through a coronary artery by pressing the plaque against the wall of an artery with a balloon on a catheter, allowing for more blood flow

6. an inflammation of the inner lining of the heart

7. a death of cardiac muscle due to lack of blood flow to the muscle; also known as heart attack

8. a local dilation in a blood vessel wall

9. a heart rate of more than 100 beats per minute

10. an acute episode of cerebrovascular insuffiency, usually a result of narrowing of an artery by atherosclerotic plaques, emboli, or vasospasm; usually passes quickly, but should be considered a warning for predisposition to cerebrovascular accidents

11. electrodes or electrical connections attached to the body to record electrical impulses in the body, especially the heart or brain

12. paroxysmal chest pain usually caused by a decrease in blood flow to the heart muscle due to coronary occlusion

13. ischemia of the brain due to an occlusion of the blood vessels supplying blood to the brain, resulting in varying degrees of debilitation

14. a buildup of fatty plaque on the interior lining of arteries

15. the feeling of an increased heart rate or pounding heart that may be felt during an emotional response or a cardiac disorder

16. a condition in which the heart cannot pump effectively

17. an inflammation of the sac that covers the heart

18. a procedure that produces a record of the electrical activity of the heart

19. an enlarged heart muscle

20. an inflammation of the myocardial layer of the heart

20. True or False? Determine whether the following statements are true or false. If false, explain why.

a. Congestive heart failure (CHF) is a condition in which the heart cannot pump effectively.

_____

_____

b. Ventricular fibrillation is a medical emergency that occurs when the heart is contracting rather than quivering in an organized fashion.

_____

_____

c. Diagnosis of atherosclerosis is often made by electrocardiography.

_____

_____

d. Patients who have cerebrovascular accidents usually have varying degrees of weakness or paralysis of one side of the body.

_____

_____

APPLICATION

Critical Thinking Practice

1. You are interviewing a patient prior to a physical examination of the cardiovascular system. This is his first time in a medical office after many years' absence, and he is considerably anxious. What do you say to him to calm him down? How would you explain the procedure?

_____

_____

2. A patient comes into the office complaining of chest pain, nausea, and vomiting. Will he likely be admitted to the hospital right away? Why or why not?

_____

_____

Patient Education

1. A patient is given an artificial pacemaker. She would like to know how the device works and what changes she can expect from it. What do you tell her?

_____

_____

Documentation

1. When interviewing a patient prior to a physical examination of the cardiovascular system, what should you ask the patient and document in his chart?

_____

_____

Active Learning

1. Pretend you are a patient who is keeping a Holter monitor diary. Create a diary based on experiences a patient is likely to have. What kinds of activities do you participate in during the day? How are these activities influencing your symptoms?

2. Research your family's health history by conducting interviews with family members. Document your findings in a chart or other graphic organizer. Are there any cardiac conditions that run in your family? If so, are there ways to prevent the onset of these medical conditions? Think about the ways in which you take care of your heart. What would you like to modify or improve?

3. Make a KWL chart about a topic of your choice from the chapter. After reading and reviewing this chapter, fill in the "What I Know" section. Are there any gaps in information? Are you still unclear about something? Fill in the "What I Would Like to Know" section with this information. Then research your topic at the library or using the Internet. If you search for information online, make sure the website is legitimate. Then fill out the last section of your chart, "What I Learned."

Professional Journal

REFLECT

(Prompts and Ideas: Are you concerned about assisting the physician during procedures? Are you more concerned about your technical skills or soft skills? In what ways? How will you ensure that you do a good job?)

_____

_____

_____

_____

_____

_____

PONDER AND SOLVE

1. Why is it important that a patient continue taking her prescribed antihypertensive medication, even if her blood pressure has reached a manageable level?

_____

_____

_____

_____

_____

_____

2. Many cardiac conditions are preventable with proper diet and exercise. It's important to stress prevention over cure, because in most instances, there is no quick "cure." How will you send this message to patients? What kinds of tools will you use?

_____

_____

_____

_____

_____

_____

EXPERIENCE

Skills related to this chapter include:

1. Perform a Basic 12-lead Electrocardiogram (Procedure 31-1).
2. Apply a Holter Monitor for a 24-hour Test (Procedure 31-2).

Record any common mistakes, lessons learned, and/or tips you discovered during your experience of practicing and demonstrating these skills:

_____

_____

_____

_____

_____

_____

_____

Skill Practice

PERFORMANCE OBJECTIVES:

1. Perform a basic 12-lead electrocardiogram (Procedure 31-1).

2. Apply a Holter monitor for a 24-hour test (Procedure 31-2).

Name _____   Date _____   Time _____

Procedure 31-1:	PERFORM A BASIC 12-LEAD ELECTROCARDIOGRAM

EQUIPMENT/SUPPLIES: Physician order, ECG machine with cable and lead wires, ECG paper, disposable electrodes that contain coupling gel, patient gown and drape, skin preparation materials including a razor and antiseptic wipes

STANDARDS: Given the needed equipment and a place to work, the student will perform this skill with _____% accuracy in a total of _____ minutes. *(Your instructor will tell you what the percentage and time limits will be before you begin practicing.)*

KEY: 4 = Satisfactory   0 = Unsatisfactory   NA = This step is not counted

PROCEDURE STEPS	SELF	PARTNER	INSTRUCTOR
1. Wash your hands.	☐	☐	☐
2. Assemble the equipment.	☐	☐	☐
3. Greet and identify the patient. Explain the procedure.	☐	☐	☐
4. Turn the ECG machine on and enter appropriate data into it. Include the patient's name and/or identification number, age, sex, height, weight, blood pressure, and medications.	☐	☐	☐
5. Instruct the patient to disrobe above the waist. **a.** Provide a gown for privacy. **b.** Female patients should also be instructed to remove any nylons or tights.	☐	☐	☐
6. Position patient comfortably in a supine position. **a.** Provide pillows as needed for comfort. **b.** Drape the patient for warmth and privacy.	☐	☐	☐
7. Prepare the skin as needed. **a.** Wipe away skin oil and lotions with the antiseptic wipes. **b.** Shave hair that will interfere with good contact between skin and electrodes.	☐	☐	☐
8. Apply the electrodes snugly against the fleshy, muscular parts of upper arms and lower legs according to the manufacturer's directions. Apply the chest electrodes, V_1 through V_6.	☐	☐	☐
9. Connect the lead wires securely according to the color codes. **a.** Untangle the wires before applying them to prevent electrical artifacts. **b.** Each lead must lie unencumbered along the contours of the patient's body to decrease the incidence of artifacts. **c.** Double-check the placement.	☐	☐	☐
10. Determine the sensitivity and paper speed settings on the ECG machine.	☐	☐	☐
11. Depress the automatic button on the ECG machine to obtain the 12-lead ECG.	☐	☐	☐
12. When tracing is printed, check the ECG for artifacts and standardization mark.	☐	☐	☐

PROCEDURE STEPS	SELF	PARTNER	INSTRUCTOR

13. If the tracing is adequate, turn off the machine.
   a. Remove the electrodes from the patient's skin.
   b. Assist the patient to a sitting position and help with dressing if needed.
	☐	☐	☐

14. For a single-channel machine, roll the ECG strip.
   a. Do not secure the roll with clips.
   b. This ECG will need to be mounted on an 8 × 11-inch paper or form.
	☐	☐	☐

15. Record the procedure in the patient's medical record.	☐	☐	☐
16. Place the ECG tracing and the patient's medical record on the physician's desk or give it directly to the physician as instructed.	☐	☐	☐

CALCULATION

Total Possible Points: _____

Total Points Earned: _____ Multiplied by 100 = _____ Divided by Total Possible Points = _____%

Pass **Fail**
☐   ☐

Comments:

Student's signature _____ Date _____

Partner's signature _____ Date _____

Instructor's signature _____ Date _____

Name _____ Date _____ Time _____

Procedure 31-2:	APPLY A HOLTER MONITOR FOR A 24-HOUR TEST

EQUIPMENT/SUPPLIES: Physician's order, Holter monitor with appropriate lead wires, fresh batteries, carrying case with strap, disposable electrodes that contain coupling gel, adhesive tape, patient gown and drape, skin preparation materials including a razor and antiseptic wipes, patient diary

STANDARDS: Given the needed equipment and a place to work, the student will perform this skill with _____% accuracy in a total of _____ minutes. *(Your instructor will tell you what the percentage and time limits will be before you begin practicing.)*

KEY: 4 = Satisfactory   0 = Unsatisfactory   NA = This step is not counted

PROCEDURE STEPS	SELF	PARTNER	INSTRUCTOR
1. Wash your hands.	☐	☐	☐
2. Assemble the equipment.	☐	☐	☐
3. Greet and identify the patient.	☐	☐	☐
4. Explain the procedure and importance of carrying out all normal activities.	☐	☐	☐
5. Explain the reason for the incident diary, emphasizing the need for the patient to carry it at all times during the test.	☐	☐	☐
6. Ask the patient to remove all clothing from the waist up; gown and drape appropriately for privacy.	☐	☐	☐
7. Prepare the patient's skin for electrode attachment. **a.** Provide privacy and have the patient in a sitting position. **b.** Shave the skin if necessary and cleanse with antiseptic wipes.	☐	☐	☐
8. Apply the Holter electrodes at the specified sites: **a.** The right manubrium border **b.** The left manubrium border **c.** The right sternal border at the fifth rib level **d.** The fifth rib at the anterior axillary line **e.** The right lower rib cage over the cartilage as a ground lead	☐	☐	☐
9. To do this, expose the adhesive backing of the electrodes and follow the manufacturer's instructions to attach each firmly. Check the security of the attachments.	☐	☐	☐
10. Position electrode connectors downward toward the patient's feet.	☐	☐	☐
11. Attach the lead wires and secure with adhesive tape.	☐	☐	☐
12. Connect the cable and run a baseline ECG by hooking the Holter monitor to the ECG machine with the cable hookup.	☐	☐	☐
13. Assist the patient to carefully redress with the cable extending through the garment opening. Clothing that buttons down the front is more convenient.	☐	☐	☐

PROCEDURE STEPS	SELF	PARTNER	INSTRUCTOR
14. Plug the cable into the recorder and mark the diary.	☐	☐	☐
a. If needed, explain the purpose of the diary to the patient again.			
b. Give instructions for a return appointment to evaluate the recording and the diary.			
15. Record the procedure in the patient's medical record.	☐	☐	☐

CALCULATION

Total Possible Points: _____

Total Points Earned: _____ Multiplied by 100 = _____ Divided by Total Possible Points = _____%

Pass   **Fail**

☐   ☐

Comments:

Student's signature _____ Date _____

Partner's signature _____ Date _____

Instructor's signature _____ Date _____

Work Product 1

Perform electrocardiography.

Use the equipment available to you at a medical office or at school to perform a 12-lead electrocardiogram on at least one patient or volunteer. Print the ECG tracing and attach it to this sheet.

Work Product 2

Document appropriately.

Perform a 12-lead electrocardiogram on a patient or volunteer. If you are currently working in a medical office, use a blank paper patient chart from the office. If this is not available to you, use the space below to record the procedure in the chart.

_____

_____

_____

_____

_____

_____

_____

Chapter Self-Assessment Quiz

1. Chronic cases of myocarditis may lead to heart failure with:
   a. endocarditis.
   b. cardiomegaly.
   c. asthma.
   d. bronchitis.
   e. congestive heart failure.

2. To identify the causative agent, proper diagnosis of endocarditis requires a(n):
   a. chest radiograph.
   b. blood culture.
   c. electrocardiogram.
   d. x-ray.
   e. stool sample.

3. Arrhythmia may occur if the SA node initiates electrical impulses:
   a. too quietly or too loudly.
   b. too roughly or too smoothly.
   c. too fast or too slowly.
   d. always.
   e. never.

4. When a patient's heart conduction system cannot maintain normal sinus rhythm without assistance, an electrical source can be implanted to assist or replace the sinoatrial node. This device is called a(n):
   a. pacemaker.
   b. artifact.
   c. Holter monitor.
   d. aneurysm.
   e. lead.

5. Which condition may result from rheumatic heart disease?

   a. Valvular disease

   b. Cardiac arrhythmia

   c. Angina pectoris

   d. Mitral valve stenosis

   e. Endocarditis

6. One symptom of coronary artery disease is:

   a. bleeding around the heart.

   b. chronic head cold.

   c. swollen tongue.

   d. pressure or fullness in the chest.

   e. back pain.

7. Patients who are considered hypertensive have a resting systolic blood pressure above _____ and a diastolic pressure above _____.

   a. 120 mm Hg; 70 mm Hg

   b. 130 mm Hg; 80 mm Hg

   c. 140 mm Hg; 90 mm Hg

   d. 150 mm Hg; 100 mm Hg

   e. 160 mm Hg; 110 mm Hg

8. Who is predisposed to varicose veins?

   a. People who use their brains more than their bodies

   b. People who run or jog excessively

   c. People who sit or stand for long periods of time without moving

   d. People who are obese over many years

   e. People who play a musical instrument

9. Another term for *thrombi* is:

   a. heart attack.

   b. blood clots.

   c. fever.

   d. racing heart.

   e. stroke.

10. Another term for *anticoagulant medications* is:

   a. coumadin.

   b. deep-vein thrombosis.

   c. peripheral vascular occlusion.

   d. thickening agents.

   e. blood thinners.

11. A common cause of cerebrovascular accident is:

   a. damage to the blood vessels in the brain.

   b. blockage of the cerebral artery by a thrombus.

   c. weakness or paralysis.

   d. pulmonary embolism.

   e. pleuritic chest pain.

12. Another term for *transient ischemic attack* is:

   a. peripheral vascular occlusion.

   b. mini-stroke.

   c. heart attack.

   d. brain damage.

   e. slurred speech.

13. Deficiencies in hemoglobin or in the numbers of red blood cells result in:

   a. tachycardia.

   b. thrombus.

   c. stroke.

   d. anemia.

   e. aneurysm.

14. During the physician's examination, what is used to evaluate the efficiency of the circulatory pathways and peripheral pulses?

   a. Palpitation

   b. Blood pressure

   c. Weight

   d. Height

   e. Sign of fever

15. Electrocardiograms are not used to detect:

   a. ischemia.

   b. delays in impulse conduction.

   c. hypertrophy of the cardiac chambers.

   d. arrhythmias.

   e. heart murmurs.

16. How many leads does the standard ECG have?

   a. 2

   b. 10

   c. 12

   d. 18

   e. 20

17. A patient must keep a daily diary of activities when:

   a. wearing a Holter monitor.

   b. preparing for a cardiac examination.

   c. having an ECG.

   d. taking blood thinners.

   e. completing a cardiac stress test.

18. Many patients with CHF have an enlarged:

   a. chest.

   b. throat.

   c. lung.

   d. heart.

   e. brain.

19. A person who can read and perform echocardiograms is called a(n):

    a. medical assistant.

    b. cardiologist.

    c. ultrasonographer.

    d. sound technician.

    e. neurologist.

20. If atherosclerotic plaques are found during a catheterization, which procedure may be performed?

    a. Bypass graft

    b. Angioplasty

    c. Echocardiogram

    d. ECG

    e. Ultrasonograph

CHAPTER

32 Gastroenterology

Chapter Checklist

- [ ] Read textbook chapter and take notes within the Chapter Notes outline. Answer the Learning Objectives as you reach them in the content, and then check them off.
- [ ] Work the Content Review questions—both Foundational Knowledge and Application.
- [ ] Perform the Active Learning exercise(s).
- [ ] Complete Professional Journal entries.
- [ ] Complete Skill Practice Activity(s) using Competency Evaluation Forms and Work Products, when appropriate.
- [ ] Take the Chapter Self-Assessment Quiz.
- [ ] Insert all appropriate pages into your Portfolio.

Learning Objectives

1. Spell and define the key terms.
2. Describe common disorders of the alimentary canal and accessory organs.
3. Explain the purpose of various diagnostic procedures associated with the GI system.
4. Discuss the role of the medical assistant in diagnosing and treating disorders of the GI system.

Chapter Notes

Note: Bold-faced headings are the major headings in the text chapter; headings in regular font are lower-level headings (i.e., the content is subordinate to, or falls "under," the major headings). Make sure you understand the key terms used in the chapter, as well as the concepts presented as Key Points.

TEXT SUBHEADINGS   **NOTES**

Introduction _____

_____

Key Terms: peristalsis; metabolism

_____

- [ ] **LEARNING OBJECTIVE 1:** Spell and define the key terms.

_____

Common Gastrointestinal Disorders _____

_____

_____

Mouth Disorders _____

_____

Key Point:
• While disorders of the teeth, gums, and oral cavity are typically diagnosed and treated by the dentist, patients requiring a referral to a dentist or oral surgeon may be seen first in the medical office.

Caries _____

_____

Key Term: malocclusion
Key Point:
• Dental caries (tooth decay) is the most widespread disease of the oral cavity.

Stomatitis _____

_____

Key Point:
• Stomatitis, an inflammation of the oral mucosa, may be caused by a virus, bacteria, or fungus.

Gingivitis _____

_____

Key Point:
• Gingivitis is an inflammation of the gingiva, or gums. It may lead to periodontitis, or inflammation and possible destruction of the supporting structures of the teeth, including the gingiva, periodontal ligament, and mandibular or maxillary bone.

Oral Cancers _____

_____

Key Term: leukoplakia
Key Point:
• Cancers of the oral cavity are common, especially among individuals who use tobacco products.

Esophageal Disorders _____

_____

_____

Hiatal Hernia _____

_____

_____

Gastroesophageal Reflux Disease (GERD) _____

_____

_____

Esophageal Varices _____

_____

Key Term: sclerotherapy
Key Point:
• The most common and dangerous problem that results from esophageal varices is hemorrhaging if the distended veins rupture.

Esophageal Cancer _____

_____

Key Term: dysphagia
Key Point:
• Predisposing factors for this type of cancer include chronic gastroesophageal reflux, smoking, and drinking alcohol.

Stomach Disorders _____

_____

_____

Gastritis _____

_____

Key Point:
• Gastritis, an inflammation of the lining of the stomach, can be acute or chronic. The most common causes include irritants such as alcohol and certain drugs, including aspirin and nonsteroidal anti-inflammatory medications (NSAIDs).

Peptic Ulcers _____

_____

Key Terms: melena; hematemesis
Key Point:
• Peptic ulcers occur from the exposure of the lining of the stomach and first part of the small intestine (duodenum) to hydrochloric acid (HCl), a caustic chemical produced and secreted by the lining of the stomach that may cause erosion if too much is excreted.

Gastric Cancer _____

_____

Key Point:
- Gastric cancer has no known cause, although smoking, excessive alcohol intake, ingesting foods high in preservatives, and genetic predisposition may contribute.

Intestinal Disorders _____

_____

_____

Gastroenteritis _____

_____

Key Point:
- Gastroenteritis is general inflammation of the stomach, small intestine, and/or colon. This condition is caused by ingesting food or water that contains bacteria, viruses, parasites, or irritating agents such as spices.

Duodenal Ulcers _____

_____

Key Point:
- Ulcerative lesions in the duodenum are often caused by exposure to highly corrosive gastric acid that is secreted by the stomach or other irritants that pass through the pylorus to the small intestine.

Malabsorption Syndromes _____

_____

Key Point:
- Malabsorption syndromes prevent the normal absorption of certain nutrients through the walls of the small intestines.

Crohn Disease _____

_____

Key Term: anorexia
Key Point:
- Crohn disease, also known as regional enteritis, is an inflammation of deep lining of the bowel ranging from very mild to severe and debilitating. The cause of Crohn disease is unclear, but it is thought to be an autoimmune disorder with a possible genetic link.

Ulcerative Colitis _____

_____

Key Point:
• Like Crohn disease, ulcerative colitis is an inflammatory bowel disease affecting the lining of the colon. It occurs most often in young women but may occur at any age and may affect men also.

Irritable Bowel Syndrome _____

_____

Key Point:
• Although the patient may have signs and symptoms resembling those of Crohn disease or ulcerative colitis, irritable bowel syndrome usually does not result in weight loss, and the prognosis is good.

Diverticulosis _____

_____

Key Point:
• Diverticulosis is a chronic condition of thinning of the bowel wall, causing small out-pouches in the lining of the intestinal wall.

Polyps _____

_____

Key Point:
• Colon polyps are masses of benign mucous membrane lining the large intestine that are usually slow growing but may become cancerous.

Hernias _____

_____

Key Point:
• The anterior abdominal wall is covered with various muscles that assist with movement and support and protect the internal structures of the abdomen. When these muscles weaken, the underlying organs or intestines may protrude through the weakened muscle wall, resulting in a hernia.

Appendicitis _____

_____

Key Point:
• Appendicitis occurs when the vermiform appendix becomes infected and fills with bacteria, pus, and blood.

Hemorrhoids _____

_____

Key Point:
• Hemorrhoids are external or internal dilated veins (varicosities) in the rectum.

Colorectal Cancers _____

_____

Key Term: guaiac
Key Point:
• Although the cause of colorectal cancer is unknown, it has been linked to diets high in animal fats and low in fiber.

Functional Disorders _____

_____

Key Points:
• Functional disorders of the GI tract include the common disorders constipation, diarrhea, and intestinal gas.
• Most constipation is caused by poor bowel habits (avoiding defecation and overusing laxatives), low-fiber diet, and inadequate fluid intake.

Liver Disorders _____

_____

Key Terms: ascites; hepatomegaly; hepatotoxins

Hepatitis _____

_____

Key Points:
• Hepatitis is an inflammation or infection of the liver that may lead to liver destruction and necrosis of hepatic cells.
• While the viruses responsible for the individual types of viral hepatitis are physically different, the symptoms of all types are similar. They may include fatigue, joint pain, flu-like symptoms with fever, jaundice, dark urine, and light stools.

Cirrhosis or Fibrosis _____

_____

Key Point:
• Cirrhosis is a chronic disease characterized by destruction of liver cells and the formation of scar tissue or fibers throughout the liver, altering its function and efficiency.

_____

Liver Cancer _____

_____

Key Point:
• There is no known cause, but primary liver cancers are thought to be due to exposure to carcinogenic chemicals, including hepatotoxins. Patients who have cirrhosis or hepatitis B are more likely than the general population to develop liver cancer.

_____

Gallbladder Disorders _____

_____

_____

Cholelithiasis and Cholecystitis _____

_____

Key Points:
• Cholelithiasis is the formation of gallstones made of cholesterol and bilirubin.
• Signs and symptoms of any gallbladder disorder include acute right upper abdominal quadrant pain that may radiate to the shoulders, back, or chest; indigestion; nausea; and intolerance of fatty foods.

_____

Gallbladder Cancer _____

_____

Key Point:
• Cancer of the gallbladder is rare and difficult to diagnose. Since the symptoms are similar to those of cholecystitis, this cancer is usually discovered during routine gallbladder tests performed to diagnose general gallbladder disease.

_____

Pancreatic Disorders _____

_____

_____

Pancreatitis _____

_____

Key Point:
- Pancreatitis is an inflammation of the pancreas that may be related to alcoholism, trauma, gastric ulcer, or biliary tract disease.

Pancreatic Cancer _____

_____

Key Point:
- There is no definitive cause of pancreatic cancer, but it occurs most often in middle-aged African American men who smoke, who have a diet high in fats and proteins, or who are exposed to industrial chemicals for long periods.

☐ **LEARNING OBJECTIVE 2:** Describe common disorders of the alimentary canal and accessory organs.

Common Diagnostic and Therapeutic Procedures _____

_____

_____

History and Physical Examination of the GI System _____

_____

Key Term: turgor
Key Point:
- Before beginning any patient's care, an adequate history must be obtained. The patient presenting with GI concerns will be assessed for signs (e.g., vomiting) and symptoms (e.g., nausea).

Blood Tests _____

_____

Key Points:
- Blood work ordered by the physician may include white and red blood cell counts.
- Blood may also be drawn and sent to the laboratory to determine liver function. Specifically, alkaline phosphatase, serum bilirubin, prothrombin time, and SGPT (serum glutamic pyruvic transaminase) levels are determined in a test collectively known as a liver panel.

Radiology Studies

Key Points:
- Radiology studies of the stomach and intestines consist of instilling barium, a radiopaque liquid, into the GI tract orally or rectally to outline the organs and identify abnormalities.
- Since the lower GI study requires that the colon be empty of stool, the patient must be given specific instructions to follow before the examination.
- The role of the medical assistant in radiographic procedures includes determining third-party payer (insurance) requirements for referrals or preauthorization, scheduling the procedure in an outpatient facility, and explaining to the patient the preparations for the examination as necessary.

Nuclear Imaging

Key Point:
- Radionuclides, or radioactive elements, are often used in the diagnosis of disorders of the liver. After the elements are injected into the body, images are taken using a nuclear scanning device, and abnormalities can be detected and evaluated by the radiologist.

Ultrasonography

Key Point:
- Abnormalities in the structure of various digestive accessory organs, such as the liver and gallbladder, can be easily viewed using ultrasonography, which requires very little if any preparation by the patient.

Endoscopic Studies

Key Terms: obturator; insufflator
Key Point:
- Fiberoptic technology has enabled physicians to pass soft, flexible tubes down the esophagus into the stomach and small intestine or up into the colon for direct visualization of these organs.

Fecal Tests

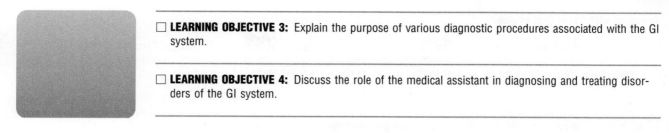

☐ **LEARNING OBJECTIVE 3:** Explain the purpose of various diagnostic procedures associated with the GI system.

☐ **LEARNING OBJECTIVE 4:** Discuss the role of the medical assistant in diagnosing and treating disorders of the GI system.

Content Review

FOUNDATIONAL KNOWLEDGE

Common Gastrointestinal Disorders

1. Review the following list of common gastrointestinal disorders and their descriptions. Draw lines to match the name of the gastrointestinal disorder with the correct description.

Description

a. a chronic disorder characterized by discomfort in the chest due to the backflow of gastric contents into the esophagus

b. a condition that occurs when part of the stomach protrudes up through the diaphragm

c. varicose veins of the esophagus resulting from pressure within the esophageal veins

d. an acute or chronic inflammation of the gall bladder

e. erosions or sores in the GI tract left by sloughed tissue

f. a disorder that usually occurs in the sigmoid colon, attributed to a diet deficient in roughage

g. an inflammation of the oral mucosa, caused by a virus, bacteria, or fungus

Gastrointestinal Disorder

1. esophageal varices
2. cholecystitis
3. peptic ulcers
4. stomatitis
5. gastroesophageal reflux disease (GERD)
6. diverticulosis
7. hiatal hernia

2. A patient comes into the office with abdominal pain and indigestion. The physician diagnoses the patient with a hiatal hernia. Which of the following diet modifications and treatments would the physician most likely suggest to the patient? Circle the correct answers.

a. Eat small, frequent meals.

b. Exercise vigorously three times a week.

c. Elevate the head of the bed when sleeping.

d. Do not eat for two hours before bedtime.

e. Drink less water.

f. Lose weight.

Assisting with Colon Procedures

3. As a medical assistant, you may be called on to assist with colon procedures in the medical office. Take a look at the chart below and review the list of tasks. Place a check mark in the "Yes" column for duties you might assist with, and place a check mark in the "No" column for duties that someone else would be responsible for.

Task	Yes	No
a. Instruct the patient in the procedure of stool sample collection.		
b. Help to educate the patient about diet and the prevention of gastric disorders.		
c. Prescribe pain medication and antibiotics.		
d. Schedule radiographic and ultrasound procedures in an outpatient facility.		
e. Test the stool specimen when it is returned to the office.		
f. Compile detailed dietary regimens for obese patients.		
g. Assist the physician in performing colon examinations.		
h. Diagnose minor gastrointestinal disorders.		

4. Identify the part of the digestive system where the following gastrointestinal disorders occur.

a. appendicitis _____

b. hepatitis _____

c. cholelithiasis _____

d. Crohn disease _____

e. peptic ulcers _____

f. ulcerative colitis _____

g. diverticulosis _____

5. List three symptoms that could indicate a patient is suffering from gastric cancer.

a. _____

b. _____

c. _____

Examining the GI System

6. As a medical assistant, you need to be aware of the different ways that a physician can examine a patient's GI system. Match the following ways of examining the GI system with the correct description.

Description

a. instilling barium into the GI tract orally or rectally to outline the organs and identify abnormalities _____

b. injecting radionuclides into the body and taking images using a nuclear scanning device to detect abnormalities _____

c. using high-frequency sound waves to diagnose disorders of internal structures _____

d. passing soft, flexible tubes into the stomach, small intestine, or colon for direct visualization of the organs _____

GI System Examination Techniques

1. endoscopic studies
2. nuclear imaging
3. ultrasonography
4. radiology studies

7. A 40-year-old woman comes to the physician's office complaining of severe stomach cramps and vomiting. To help assess her condition, the physician obtains some personal information. List four things that the physician will ask the patient before continuing with the exam.

a. _____

b. _____

c. _____

d. _____

8. A 55-year-old woman comes to the physician's office and asks about gastric bypass surgery. She says that she has tried every diet available and is unable to lose weight. She suffers from shortness of breath and an inability to walk for long distances. You take the woman's vital signs and measure her height and weight. She appears to be in good health, but is at least 60 pounds over the ideal weight for her height. The physician later confirms these facts. Is the patient likely to be a candidate for gastric bypass surgery? Explain your answer.

_____

_____

9. Which of these groups of people are at the highest risk of developing esophageal cancer? Circle the correct answer.

a. Teenagers

b. Pregnant women

c. Young children

d. Elderly women

e. Elderly men

10. A male patient comes to the physician's office complaining of an acute pain in his upper abdomen and back. He also suffers from indigestion and nausea, particularly when he tries to eat foods that have a high fat content. Which of the following gastrointestinal disorders does the patient probably have? Circle the correct answer.

a. Cholelithiasis

b. Peptic ulcers

c. Gastritis

d. Leukoplakia

e. Caries

Endoscopic Studies

11. As a medical assistant, it is important that you are able to identify key procedures that might be used during an endoscopic study. Match the procedures with the correct description.

Description

a. a method of injecting dye into the ducts of the gallbladder and pancreas; used to visualize the esophagus, stomach, proximal duodenum, and pancreas with a flexible endoscope _____

b. the insertion of a metal or plastic anoscope into the rectal canal to inspect the anus and rectum and swab for cultures _____

c. a visual examination of the sigmoid colon _____

Procedure

1. sigmoidoscopy examination
2. endoscopic retrograde cholangiopancreatography (ERCP)
3. anoscopy

12. Which is the more widely accepted instrument to use during an endoscopic study: a rigid sigmoidoscope or a flexible fiberoptic sigmoidoscope? Explain your answer.

_____

_____

13. **Risk Factors**

Which of the following factors increase a person's risk of developing pancreatic cancer? Circle all that apply.

a. being female

b. drinking alcohol

c. smoking

d. being of African American descent

e. being male

f. being of Caucasian descent

g. eating high-fat foods

h. a history of working with industrial chemicals

Office Procedures

14. A patient is advised to undergo a radiographic procedure. List the tasks that you would perform, both before and after the procedure.

Before Procedure

a. _____

b. _____

c. _____

After Procedure

a. _____

b. _____

15. A 25-year-old woman comes to the physician's office complaining of fatigue and joint pain. She looks jaundiced, and when the physician asks her for her medical history, she says that she recently returned from a 3-month trip to Ghana. Which two tests will the physician most likely recommend?

a. _____

b. _____

16. As a medical assistant, part of your job may be to educate patients about the care of teeth and gums. List three things that you could tell a patient to do that might help to prevent dental caries.

a. _____

b. _____

c. _____

17. Some gastrointestinal disorders require specialist knowledge and equipment outside of the physician's office. Take a look at the table below. Place a check mark in the appropriate box to state whether a procedure could be carried out in the physician's office or would likely require an outpatient facility.

Procedure	Physician's office	Outpatient facility
a. Ultrasonography		
b. Anoscopy		
c. Endoscopic retrograde cholangiopancreatography		
d. Nuclear imaging		
e. Sigmoidoscopy examination		

18. If certain gastrointestinal disorders are not treated promptly, they can develop into more serious conditions. Match the original disorders below with the conditions they can turn into when left untreated.

Original Disorders	Future Conditions If Left Untreated
a. appendicitis _____	**1.** colon cancer
b. gingivitis _____	**2.** peritonitis
c. gastroesophageal reflux disease _____	**3.** esophageal cancer
d. polyps _____	**4.** periodontitis

19. Match the following key terms to their definitions.

Key Terms

a. anorexia _____

b. ascites _____

c. dysphagia _____

d. guaiac _____

e. hematemesis _____

f. heptomegaly _____

g. hepatotoxin _____

h. insufflator _____

i. leukoplakia _____

j. malocclusion _____

k. melena _____

l. metabolism _____

m. obturator _____

n. peristalsis _____

o. sclerotherapy _____

p. stomatitis _____

q. turgor _____

Definitions

1. an enlarged liver

2. a substance used in a laboratory test for occult blood in the stool

3. a device for blowing air, gas, or powder into a body cavity

4. the sum of chemical processes that result in growth, energy production, elimination of waste, and body functions performed as digested nutrients are distributed

5. black, tarry stools caused by digested blood from the gastrointestinal tract

6. the contraction and relaxation of involuntary muscles of the alimentary canal, producing wavelike movements of products through the digestive system

7. difficulty speaking

8. loss of appetite

9. a substance that can damage the liver

10. an accumulation of serous fluid in the peritoneal cavity

11. the use of chemical agents to treat esophageal varices to produce fibrosis and hardening of the tissue

12. an inflammation of the mucous membranes of the mouth

13. an abnormal contact between the teeth in the upper and lower jaw

14. the normal tension in a cell or the skin

15. vomiting blood or bloody vomitus

16. the smooth, rounded, removable inner portion of a hollow tube, such as an anoscope, that allows for easier insertion

17. white, thickened patches on the oral mucosa or tongue that are often precancerous

20. True or False? Determine whether the following statements are true or false. If false, explain why.

a. Oral cancers are more common among people who smoke.

_____

_____

b. Cancer of the esophagus is common and can easily be treated.

_____

_____

c. A sign that a patient has a problem with malabsorption of fats includes stools that are loose.

_____

_____

d. Irritable bowel syndrome usually results in chronic weight loss.

_____

_____

APPLICATION

Critical Thinking Practice

1. The physician tells a patient that he would like to schedule an endoscopic retrograde cholangiopancreatography in a local outpatient facility. After the physician leaves the room, you notice that the patient looks confused and worried. How would you explain the procedure to the patient to reassure him?

_____

_____

2. Mr. Thompson, a 50-year-old patient, is scheduled to have an endoscopic examination on Wednesday morning. You have given him all the necessary information to prepare for the examination, including taking a laxative the night before and eating only a light meal on Tuesday evening, with no breakfast Wednesday morning. Mr. Thompson calls you an hour before his appointment to tell you that he forgot to take the laxative the previous evening and has eaten breakfast. Explain what you would do.

_____

_____

Patient Education

1. Your patient is a clinically obese 45-year-old male, who comes to the physician's office for advice about gastric bypass surgery. You know that the patient would be a candidate for the surgery because his health is starting to suffer due to his obesity. Write the patient a brief information sheet, explaining what the procedure involves. Include a list of positive and negative effects that he should consider before going ahead with the surgery.

_____

_____

Documentation

1. You need to schedule a patient for an ultrasonography in an outpatient clinic. The patient is a 65-year-old woman named Mary Harp, with suspected gallbladder disease. Explain the documentation process both before and after Mrs. Harp's appointment.

_____

_____

Active Learning

1. One of the deadliest types of cancer is pancreatic cancer, which kills most patients within a year of diagnosis. Research the latest information about the suspected causes of pancreatic cancer on the Internet. Try to find out which treatments are proving the most effective and whether there have been any recent developments.
   - Use the information you find to create an informational poster about pancreatic cancer, educating high-risk patients on how they can lower their chances of developing pancreatic cancer.
   - Write a one-page leaflet for physicians, informing them of the latest treatments for pancreatic cancer.

2. Assess your oral hygiene. Keep a food diary for a week and note which foods could be harmful to your teeth. Check the date of your last dental appointment and schedule a new one if necessary.

3. Trace a rough outline of the digestive system from a medical textbook onto a large sheet of paper. On another piece of paper, write down a list of body parts that make up the digestive system and a list of disorders that affect them. Cut the words out and stick a piece of double-sided tape onto the back of each word. Working with a partner, take turns reading out the name of a body part or a disorder. See who can stick the most pieces of card onto the correct place on the outline.

Professional Journal

REFLECT

(Prompts and Ideas: Have you ever suffered from a gastrointestinal disorder? What do you think would help patients overcome fear or embarrassment during an endoscopic examination? What information would you find helpful to prepare for the procedure? How do you feel about gastric bypass surgery?)

_____

_____

_____

_____

_____

_____

_____

PONDER AND SOLVE

1. A 15-year-old female patient comes into the physician's office with severe abdominal pains. She is extremely underweight for her height, and you suspect she might be anorexic. When the physician leaves the room, she confesses that she has been using laxatives every day to keep her weight down. Explain what you would do next.

_____

_____

_____

_____

_____

_____

2. A 50-year-old male patient has been diagnosed with pancreatic cancer. The patient is clearly devastated and tells you he has heard that people who develop pancreatic cancer have little chance of survival. What do you say to the patient?

_____

_____

_____

_____

_____

_____

EXPERIENCE

Skills related to this chapter include:

1. Assisting with Colon Procedures (Procedure 32-1).

Record any common mistakes, lessons learned, and/or tips you discovered during your experience of practicing and demonstrating these skills:

_____

_____

_____

_____

_____

_____

_____

Skill Practice

PERFORMANCE OBJECTIVES:

1. Assisting with colon procedures (Procedure 32-1).

Name_____ Date _____ Time _____

Procedure 32-1:	ASSISTING WITH COLON PROCEDURES

EQUIPMENT/SUPPLIES: Appropriate instrument (flexible or rigid sigmoidoscope, anoscope, or proctoscope); water-soluble lubricant; patient gown and drape; cotton swabs; suction (if not part of the scope); biopsy forceps; specimen container with preservative; completed laboratory requisition form; personal wipes or tissues; equipment for assessing vital signs; examination gloves

STANDARDS: Given the needed equipment and a place to work, the student will perform this skill with _____% accuracy in a total of _____ minutes. *(Your instructor will tell you what the percentage and time limits will be before you begin practicing.)*

KEY: 4 = Satisfactory   0 = Unsatisfactory   NA = This step is not counted

PROCEDURE STEPS	SELF	PARTNER	INSTRUCTOR
1. Wash your hands.	☐	☐	☐

2. Assemble the equipment and supplies.
  a. Place the name of the patient on label on outside of specimen container.
  b. Complete the laboratory requisition.
	☐	☐	☐

3. Check the illumination of the light source if a flexible sigmoidoscope. Turn off the power after checking for working order.	☐	☐	☐

4. Greet and identify the patient and explain the procedure.
  a. Inform patient that a sensation of pressure may be felt.
  b. Tell the patient that the pressure is from the instrument.
  c. Gas pressure may be felt when air is insufflated during the sigmoidoscopy.
	☐	☐	☐

5. Instruct the patient to empty the urinary bladder.	☐	☐	☐
6. Assess the vital signs and record in the medical record.	☐	☐	☐
7. Have the patient undress from the waist down and gown and drape appropriately.	☐	☐	☐

8. Assist the patient onto the examination table.
  a. If the instrument is an anoscope or a fiberoptic device, Sims' position or a side-lying position is most comfortable.
  b. If a rigid instrument is used, position patient when doctor is ready: knee-chest position or on a proctological table. Drape the patient.
	☐	☐	☐

9. Assist the physician with lubricant, instruments, power, swabs, suction, etc.	☐	☐	☐

10. Monitor the patient's response and offer reassurance.
  a. Instruct the patient to breathe slowly through pursed lips.
  b. Encourage relaxing as much as possible.
	☐	☐	☐

PROCEDURE STEPS	SELF	PARTNER	INSTRUCTOR

11. When the physician is finished:
    a. Assist the patient into a comfortable position and allow a rest period.
    b. Offer personal cleaning wipes or tissues.
    c. Take the vital signs before allowing the patient to stand.
    d. Assist the patient from the table and with dressing as needed.
    e. Give the patient any instructions regarding postprocedure care.
	☐	☐	☐

12. Clean the room and route the specimen to the laboratory with the requisition.	☐	☐	☐
13. Disinfect or dispose of the supplies and equipment as appropriate.	☐	☐	☐
14. Wash your hands.	☐	☐	☐
15. Document the procedure.	☐	☐	☐

CALCULATION

Total Possible Points: _____
Total Points Earned: _____ Multiplied by 100 = _____ Divided by Total Possible Points = _____%

Pass **Fail**
☐   ☐   Comments:

Student's signature _____ Date _____
Partner's signature _____ Date _____
Instructor's signature _____ Date _____

Work Product 1

Document appropriately.

Brian Ward is a 45-year-old male complaining of chronic diarrhea, lower intestinal pain, and bloody stool. The physician, Dr. Bo-hache, directs you to prepare this patient for colonic endoscopy. You assist in the procedure, and a specimen is collected.

If you are currently working in a medical office, use a blank paper patient chart from the office. If this is not available to you, use the space below to record the procedure in the chart.

_____

_____

_____

_____

_____

_____

Chapter Self-Assessment Quiz

1. Which of the following can trigger an outbreak of the herpes simplex virus?

   a. Food allergy

   b. Illness

   c. Lack of sleep

   d. Medication

   e. Poor diet

2. What commonly causes leukoplakia to develop?

   a. Hereditary genes

   b. Excessive alcohol intake

   c. Lack of exercise

   d. Tobacco irritation

   e. Obesity

3. Why should a patient complaining of heartburn be assessed immediately?

   a. The symptoms of gastroesophageal reflux disease may be similar to the chest pain of a patient with cardiac problems.

   b. A patient with heartburn is more likely to develop a serious heart condition.

   c. Heartburn is a symptom of a weak lower esophageal sphincter.

   d. It is important to assess any gastrointestinal disorder immediately because they are usually serious.

   e. Heartburn may be symptomatic of Barrett's esophagus, which requires immediate surgery.

4. Abnormal contact between the upper teeth and lower teeth is:

   a. malocclusion.

   b. dental caries.

   c. stomatitis.

   d. candidiasis.

   e. gingivitis.

5. If a patient is suffering from peptic ulcers, the symptoms will be most severe when the patient:

   a. is hungry.

   b. has a bowel movement.

   c. lies on his back.

   d. chews his food.

   e. is digesting a meal.

6. Gastroenteritis could become life threatening if a patient:

   a. is pregnant.

   b. suffers from diabetes mellitus.

   c. needs a heart operation.

   d. consumes excess alcohol.

   e. does not receive treatment immediately.

7. The study of morbid obesity is called:

a. orthodontistry.

b. gerontology.

c. bariatrics.

d. gastroenterology.

e. pediatrics.

8. What is the minimum body mass index that a patient must have to be considered for gastric bypass surgery?

a. 25

b. 30

c. 35

d. 40

e. 45

9. Crohn disease becomes life threatening when:

a. the bowel walls become inflamed and the lymph nodes enlarge.

b. the fluid from the intestinal contents cannot be absorbed.

c. edema of the bowel wall takes place.

d. scarring narrows the colon and obstructs the bowel.

e. patients have periods of constipation, anorexia, and fever.

10. How does irritable bowel syndrome differ from Crohn disease?

a. It does not involve weight loss.

b. It is easily treatable.

c. It is thought to be genetic.

d. It requires a colectomy.

e. It causes scarring.

Scenario: A patient is diagnosed with diverticulitis.

11. Which of the following treatments would the physician most likely recommend?

a. Antibiotics

b. Bed rest

c. Antifungal agent

d. Bland food

e. Drinking less water

12. What advice could you give to the patient to help maintain good bowel habits in future?

a. Never eat spicy foods.

b. Get some form of daily exercise.

c. Try to force a bowel movement at least once a day.

d. Use laxatives when suffering from constipation.

e. Cut out food products that contain wheat.

End Scenario

13. How can a patient decrease her risk of developing a hernia?

a. Avoid lifting heavy objects.

b. Switch from processed to organic foods.

c. Maintain good bowel habits.

d. Have regular medical checkups.

e. Walk at least a mile every day.

14. What is the most effective treatment for appendicitis?

a. Antibiotics

b. Ileostomy

c. Appendectomy

d. Cryosurgery

e. Radiation

15. Which of these factors increases the production of intestinal gas?

a. Excess water

b. Spicy or fatty foods

c. Peristalsis

d. Fast metabolism

e. Lack of exercise

16. The most likely method of contracting hepatitis B is:

a. contaminated food.

b. poor hygiene.

c. contaminated blood.

d. stagnant water.

e. weak immune system.

17. For which of the following procedures would the patient usually be put under anesthesia?

a. Anoscopy

b. Sigmoidoscopy

c. Nuclear imaging

d. Ultrasonography

e. Endoscopic retrograde cholangiopancreatography

18. What is the caustic chemical secreted by the lining of the stomach that may cause erosion if too much of it is secreted?

a. Pepsin

b. Hydrochloric acid

c. Insulin

d. Oral mucosa

e. Melena

19. How does lithotripsy break down gallstones to make them easy to pass?

   a. Lasers

   b. Sound waves

   c. Acidic liquid

   d. Heat

   e. Air pressure

20. Which piece of advice could best be given to a patient with a malabsorption syndrome?

   a. Drink more water.

   b. Eat less processed food.

   c. Take vitamin supplements.

   d. Cut out spicy foods.

   e. Exercise more often.

CHAPTER

Chapter Checklist

- [ ] Read textbook chapter and take notes within the Chapter Notes outline. Answer the Learning Objectives as you reach them in the content, and then check them off.
- [ ] Work the Content Review questions—both Foundational Knowledge and Application.
- [ ] Perform the Active Learning exercise(s).
- [ ] Complete Professional Journal entries.
- [ ] Complete Skill Practice Activity(s) using Competency Evaluation Forms and Work Products, when appropriate.
- [ ] Take the Chapter Self-Assessment Quiz.
- [ ] Insert all appropriate pages into your Portfolio.

Learning Objectives

1. Spell and define the key terms.
2. Identify common disorders of the nervous system.
3. Describe the physical and emotional effects of degenerative nervous system disorders.
4. List potential complications of a spinal cord injury.
5. Name and describe the common procedures for diagnosing nervous system disorders.

Chapter Notes

Note: Bold-faced headings are the major headings in the text chapter; headings in regular font are lower-level headings (i.e., the content is subordinate to, or falls "under," the major headings). Make sure you understand the key terms used in the chapter, as well as the concepts presented as Key Points.

TEXT SUBHEADINGS   **NOTES**

Introduction _____

_____

- [ ] **LEARNING OBJECTIVE 1:** Spell and define the key terms.

Common Nervous System Disorders

Key Point:
- The complexity of the nervous system and its connections with the muscular system make it subject to many disorders that can be difficult to diagnose and treat effectively.

Infectious Disorders

Key Term: seizure

Meningitis

Key Points:
- Viral meningitis is usually not life threatening and is often short lived, but bacterial meningitis is often severe and may be fatal.
- The treatment for viral meningitis includes fluids and bed rest, and bacterial meningitis is treated with antibiotics and generally requires hospitalization.

Encephalitis

Key Point:
- Encephalitis is an inflammation of the brain that frequently results from a viral infection following a varicella (chicken pox), measles, or mumps infection.

Herpes Zoster

Key Term: herpes zoster
Key Point:
- **Herpes zoster**, or shingles, is caused by the virus that causes chicken pox and occurs only in those who have had a varicella infection.

Poliomyelitis

Key Point:
- Commonly called polio, this highly contagious and resistant virus affects the brain and spinal cord.

Tetanus

Key Term: dysphagia
Key Point:
- Tetanus, commonly called lockjaw, is an infection of nervous tissue caused by the tetanus bacillus, *Clostridium tetani*, which lives in the intestinal tract of animals and is excreted in their feces.
- All deep, dirty wounds should be treated as high risk for tetanus.

Rabies

Key Points:
- Rabies is caused by a virus that is commonly transmitted by animal saliva through a bite wound from an infected animal and spreads to the organs of the central nervous system.
- All animal bites must be reported to the city or county animal control center, and you may be responsible for completing and submitting the report.

Reye Syndrome

Key Point:
- Studies have found that the use of aspirin in the presence of a viral illness increases the risk of developing Reye syndrome.

Degenerative Disorders

Multiple Sclerosis

Key Term: dysphasia
Key Point:
- In MS, the myelin sheaths covering many neurons in the body degenerate and are replaced with plaque, which impairs nerve impulse conduction.

Amyotrophic Lateral Sclerosis _____

_____

Key Point:
- Commonly known as Lou Gehrig disease, amyotrophic lateral sclerosis (ALS) causes a progressive loss of motor neurons.

Parkinson Disease _____

_____

_____

Seizure Disorders _____

_____

Key Term: electroencephalogram (EEG)
Key Points:
- Seizures, commonly called convulsions, are involuntary contractions of voluntary muscles caused by a rapid succession of electrical impulses through the brain.
- The primary treatment during the actual seizure is preventing injury to the patient.

Febrile Seizures _____

_____

Key Point:
- Children with febrile seizures must have a complete physical and neurological examination to rule out the possibility of organic origin of the seizures.

Focal, or Jacksonian, Seizures _____

_____

_____

Developmental Disorders _____

_____

_____

Neural Tube Defects _____

_____

Key Terms: spina bifida occulta; meningocele; myelomeningocele
Key Point:
- An abnormality in development in the distal, or caudal, end of the neural tube results in spina bifida.

Hydrocephalus _____

_____

Key Point:
- Hydrocephalus occurs when the arachnoid and ventricular spaces of the brain contain excessive CSF.

Cerebral Palsy _____

_____

Key Point:
- Cerebral palsy describes a group of neuromuscular disorders that result from CNS damage during the prenatal, neonatal, or postnatal period.

Trauma _____

_____

Key Point:
- Traumatic injuries are the most common causes of neurological disorders and the leading killer of individuals aged 1 to 24 years.

Traumatic Brain Injuries _____

_____

Key Terms: concussion; contusion
Key Point:
- Children are at particularly high risk for head trauma.

Spinal Cord Injuries _____

_____

Key Points:
- The higher in the spinal cord the injury, the more serious the complications and paralysis for the patient.
- The goal of long-term care is to prevent complications, which can include skin ulcerations (pressure ulcers), hypostatic pneumonia, bladder infection, muscle contractures, and psychological depression.

Brain Tumors _____

_____

Key Point:
- A brain tumor may be either malignant or benign and may be a secondary or metastatic site.

Headaches

Key Term: cephalalgia
Key Point:
- Headaches have a variety of origins, including stress, trauma, bone pathology, infection (e.g., sinus), or vascular disturbance.

☐ **LEARNING OBJECTIVE 2:** Identify common disorders of the nervous system.

☐ **LEARNING OBJECTIVE 3:** Describe the physical and emotional effects of degenerative nervous system disorders.

☐ **LEARNING OBJECTIVE 4:** List potential complications of a spinal cord injury.

Common Diagnostic Tests for Disorders of the Nervous System

Physical Examination

Key Term: Romberg test
Key Points:
- The patient's mental status is evaluated by routine questioning to establish mental alertness and orientation.
- Cranial nerves are assessed according to the methods described in Table 33-3.
- Patients with weak or slow responses to stimuli applied during reflex testing may require additional testing to determine the source of the problem.

Radiological Tests

Key Point:
- The most common noninvasive radiological tests include computed tomography (CT) and magnetic resonance imaging (MRI).

Electrical Tests

Key Point:
- The EEG is a noninvasive test that records electrical impulses in the brain.

Lumbar Puncture _____

Key Term: Queckenstedt test
Key Point:
• A lumbar puncture is used to diagnose infectious inflammatory or bleeding disorders affecting the brain and spinal cord or as a means of injecting pain control medication into the spinal column near the nerves producing the pain.

☐ **LEARNING OBJECTIVE 5:** Name and describe the common procedures for diagnosing nervous system disorders.

Content Review

FOUNDATIONAL KNOWLEDGE

1. **Understanding the Nervous System**

   Fill in the diagram below to show the two divisions of the nervous system and the components of each.

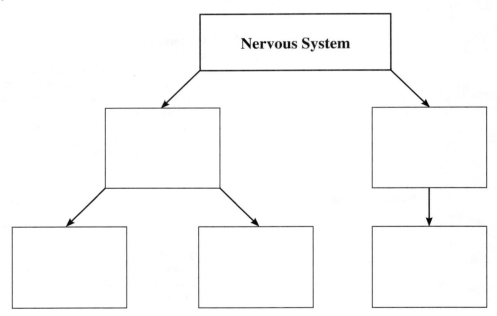

Disorders of the Nervous System

2. Sort the disorders of the nervous system below into their respective groups.

Infectious	Degenerative	Convulsive	Developmental	Traumatic	Neoplastic	Headache

Meningitis	Amyotrophic lateral sclerosis	Encephalitis
Cluster headaches	Brain tumors	Traumatic brain injuries
Spina bifida occulta	Poliomyelitis	Cerebral palsy
Febrile seizures	Febrile seizures	Tetanus
Parkinson disease	Meningocele	Focal or Jacksonian seizures
Tension headaches	Herpes zoster	
Myelomeningocele	Epilepsy	
Multiple sclerosis	Spinal cord injuries	
Reye syndrome	Rabies	
Hydrocephalus	Neural tube defects	

3. Explain the difference between dysphagia and dysphasia.

Dysphagia	Dysphasia

4. Name three viral infections that lead to encephalitis.

   a. _____

   b. _____

   c. _____

5. What kind of outbreak might be caused by a varicella infection? What generally triggers this outbreak?

_____

_____

6. Which age group is most susceptible to traumatic brain injuries? Why? Which age group is most susceptible to spinal cord injuries? Why?

_____

_____

7. Review the list of diseases and then place a check mark in the appropriate column to indicate the age group and or sex that they typically tend to affect.

	Children	Women Aged 20 to 40	Middle-Aged Men	Elderly People
a. Parkinson disease				
b. Amyotrophic lateral sclerosis				
c. Multiple sclerosis				
d. Reye syndrome				
e. Febrile seizures				

8. Divide the following into onset symptoms and symptoms experienced after a migraine begins.

Symptoms	Onset	After Migraine Begins
a. experience of flashing lights		
b. photophobia		
c. nausea		
d. experience of wavy lines		
e. diplopia		

Diagnosing Disorders of the Nervous System

9. Name seven common diagnostic tests.

a. _____

b. _____

c. _____

d. _____

e. _____

f. _____

g. _____

10. Explain the difference between the Romberg test and the Queckenstedt test and how or if you would assist the physician in each procedure.

_____

_____

11. List three responsibilities that you may have when working with patients with neurological disorders.

a. _____

b. _____

c. _____

12. Circle five pieces of equipment you would use to assist the physician with a lumbar puncture.

exam gloves	**lumbar needle**	**local anesthetic**	**x-ray machine**
specimen container	**casting material**	**suturing needles**	**skin staples**
fenestrated drape	**oxygen tank**	**wheelchair**	**IV equipment**

13. Below are the 12 steps you should follow when assisting the patient and physician with a lumbar puncture. Explain the reasons for performing each task.

a. Wash your hands.

_____

_____

b. Assemble the equipment, identify the patient, and explain the procedure.

_____

_____

c. Check that the consent form is signed and in the chart. Warn the patient not to move during the procedure. Tell the patient that the area will be numb but pressure may still be felt after the local anesthetic is administered.

_____

_____

d. Have the patient void. Direct the patient to disrobe and put on a gown with the opening in the back.

_____

_____

e. Prepare the skin unless this is to be done with sterile preparation. If the physician prefers to prepare the skin using sterile forceps after gloving, you may have to add sterile solution to the field. Assist as needed with administration of the anesthetic.

_____

_____

f. When the physician is ready, prepare the sterile field and assist with the initial preparations. Assist the patient into the appropriate position.

_____

_____

g. Throughout the procedure, observe the patient closely for signs such as dyspnea or cyanosis. Monitor the pulse at intervals and record the vital signs after the procedure. Note the patient's mental alertness and any leakage at the site, nausea, or vomiting. Assess lower limb mobility. Assist the physician as necessary.

_____

_____

h. If specimens are to be taken, put on gloves to receive the potentially hazardous bodily fluid. Label the tubes in sequence as you receive them. Label them also with the patient's identification and place them in biohazard bags.

_____

_____

i. If the Queckenstedt test is to be performed, you may be required to press against the patient's jugular veins in the neck (right, left, or both) while the physician monitors the pressure of CSF.

_____

_____

j. At the completion of the procedure, cover the site with an adhesive bandage and assist the patient to a flat position. The physician will determine when the patient is ready to leave the examination room and the office.

_____

_____

k. Route the specimens as required. Clean the examination room and care for or dispose of the equipment as needed. Wash your hands.

_____

_____

l. Chart all observations and record the procedure.

_____

_____

14. Review Table 33-1 in the text. Then, label the disabilities with their corresponding level of injury.

   a. Uses wheelchair with hand controls; eats with hand splints; good elbow flexion _____

   b. Transfers to wheelchair and bed with little or no assistance; good shoulder control _____

   c. Transfers independently to wheelchair and bed; eats with no special devices _____

15. Label the following disabilities as either _C_, Cervical; _L_, Lumbar; or _T_, Thoracic.

   a. Walks with short leg braces with or without crutches _____

   b. Moves from wheelchair to floor with little or no assistance; normal upper extremity function _____

   c. Transfers to wheelchair and bed with little or no assistance; good shoulder control _____

16. Draw lines to match the nerve to its corresponding examination method.

Nerve	**Examination Method**
a. Olfactory (I)	**1.** Ask patient to raise eyebrows, smile, show teeth, puff out cheeks.
b. Trochlear (IV)	**2.** Test for downward, inward eye movement.
c. Facial (VII)	**3.** Test each nostril for smell reception, interpretation.
d. Glossopharyngeal (IX)	**4.** Ask patient to say "ah," yawn to observe upward movement of palate; elicit gag response, note ability to swallow.
e. Vagus (X)	**5.** Ask patient to swallow and speak; note hoarseness.

17. Draw lines to match the following reflexes to their expected responses. Some expected responses may be used more than once.

Reflex	**Expected Response**
a. Brachiordialis	**1.** Closure of eyelid
b. Biceps	**2.** Extension of elbow
c. Triceps	**3.** Flexion of elbow
d. Patellar	**4.** Plantarflexion of foot
e. Achilles	**5.** Extension of leg
f. Corneal	

18. What are the results of the following forms of paralysis?

   a. Hemiplegia _____

   b. Paraplegia _____

   c. Quadriplegia _____

19. Match the following key terms to their definitions.

Key Terms

a. cephalagia _____

b. concussion _____

c. contusion _____

d. convulsion _____

e. dysphagia _____

f. dysphasia _____

g. electroencephalogram (EEG) _____

h. herpes zoster _____

i. meningocele _____

j. migraine _____

k. myelogram _____

l. myelomeningocele _____

m. Queckenstedt test _____

n. Romberg test _____

o. seizure _____

p. spina bifida occulta _____

Definitions

1. tracing of the electrical activity of the brain

2. a headache

3. meninges protruding through the spinal coloumn

4. the protusion of the spinal cord through the spinal defect

5. an invasive radiological test in which dye is injected into the spinal fluid

6. a test to determine presence of obstruction in the CSF flow performed during a lumbar puncture

7. an injury to the brain due to trauma

8. difficulty speaking

9. sudden, involuntary muscle contraction of a voluntary muscle group

10. an infection caused by reactivation of varicella zoster virus, which causes chicken pox

11. a collection of blood tissues after an injury; a bruise

12. a type of severe headache, usually unilateral; may appear in cluster

13. a congenital defect in the spinal column caused by lack of union of the vertebrae

14. an abnormal discharge of electrical activity in the brain, resulting in involuntary contractions of voluntary muscles

15. a test for the inability to maintain body balance when eyes are closed and feet are together; indication of spinal cord disease

16. inability to swallow or difficulty in swallowing

20. True or False? Determine whether the following statements are true or false. If false, explain why.

a. Ice and alcohol and sponge baths are preferable to cool compresses in returning a child's body temperature to normal.

_____

_____

b. If a patient is bitten by an animal, a copy of the animal's rabies tag and certificate should be placed in the patient's chart.

_____

_____

c. Multiple sclerosis is a contagious diease.

_____

_____

d. A lumbar puncture is more commonly performed in outpatient clinics than in the medical office.

_____

_____

APPLICATION

Critical Thinking Practice

1. A patient comes in for treatment because of a severe dog bite. The patient has already cleaned the wound himself and the physician attends to the wound immediately. Your patient then receives antibiotic and vaccine therapy. What is the next course of action and what may you be responsible for?

_____

_____

2. A patient in your clinic has been treated for epilepsy and is now seizure free. This patient has decided that she is going to stop her medication regimen. She has also expressed her excitement about being able to drive again soon. What might you advise this patient before she makes her decisions?

_____

_____

Patient Education

1. There is a patient who has recently started coming to your clinic for treatment for herpes zoster. She doesn't understand why she has shingles. She's a single mom who has been supporting her children and taking care of one child with severe Down syndrome. Her health is suffering because of her stress. What would you explain as the likely cause for the herpes zoster outbreak? What kind of advice might you offer this patient towards improving her health?

_____

_____

Documentation

1. A father brings in his 8-year-old daughter because she fell and hit her head while rollerblading. She was not wearing a helmet and seems to have lost consciousness for just a few seconds. The father is concerned about a possible traumatic brain injury. After a physical examination, the physician finds that the child has suffered a mild concussion. She is sent home, and you give her father instructions regarding her treatment. Write a narrative note documenting this visit for inclusion in the patient's chart.

_____

_____

Active Learning

1. Safe use of car seats can reduce brain and spinal cord injuries in infants and young children. Research the guidelines for car seat use. Then research car seat ratings and find five car seats that receive high safety ratings in each category. Create a handout for parents of young children to promote car seat safety awareness.

2. Many adult brain and spinal cord injuries could be avoided with proper prevention tactics. Working with a group, choose one controllable cause of brain and spinal cord injuries for adults. Create a 90-second public service announcement commercial to increase awareness of safe practices to avoid injury. If possible, videotape your commercial. Present your commercial to the class, either in person or through a video/DVD format.

3. Research various treatments for multiple sclerosis. Choose two specific treatments and create a presentation of your findings using presentation software. Be sure to include a summary of each treatment and any benefits or negative side effects.

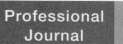

Professional Journal

REFLECT

(Prompts and Ideas: Do you or does anyone you know have a disease or disorder of the nervous system? How did you or your loved one manage to maintain physical and emotional health through this experience? What coping skills have you or your loved one learned from this experience?)

_____

_____

_____

_____

_____

_____

_____

PONDER AND SOLVE

1. A 40-year-old patient has been suffering from severe migraines for the last year. He is concerned about his condition because he is a truck driver. He is worried that it is just a matter time before a migraine sets in while he is driving. Taking rests while he is on the road is a near impossibility. He is usually very tired, and he drinks a lot of coffee to keep himself awake on his long rides. How might you advise and educate this patient?

_____

_____

_____

_____

_____

_____

_____

2. A patient comes in to the office and complains of headaches, blurred vision, and memory loss. What would your immediate concern be? What type of tests may need to be performed to learn more about this patient's symptoms?

_____

_____

_____

_____

_____

_____

_____

EXPERIENCE

Skills related to this chapter include:

1. Assist with a Lumbar Puncture (Procedure 33-1).

Record any common mistakes, lessons learned, and/or tips you discovered during your experience of practicing and demonstrating these skills:

_____

_____

_____

_____

_____

_____

_____

**Skill
Practice**

PERFORMANCE OBJECTIVES:

1. Assist with a lumbar puncture (Procedure 33-1).

Name_____ Date _____ Time _____

Procedure 33-1:   ASSIST WITH A LUMBAR PUNCTURE

EQUIPMENT/SUPPLIES Sterile gloves, examination gloves, 3- to 5-inch lumbar needle with a stylet (physician will specify gauge and length), sterile gauze sponges, specimen containers, local anesthetic and syringe, needle, adhesive bandages, fenestrated drape, sterile drape, antiseptic, skin preparation supplies (razor), biohazard sharps container, biohazard waste container

STANDARDS: Given the needed equipment and a place to work, the student will perform this skill with _____% accuracy in a total of _____ minutes. *(Your instructor will tell you what the percentage and time limits will be before you begin practicing.)*

KEY: 4 = Satisfactory   0 = Unsatisfactory   NA = This step is not counted

PROCEDURE STEPS	SELF	PARTNER	INSTRUCTOR
1. Wash your hands.	☐	☐	☐
2. Assemble the equipment, identify the patient, and explain the procedure.	☐	☐	☐
3. Check that the consent form is signed and available in the chart.	☐	☐	☐
4. Explain the importance of not moving during the procedure and explain that the area will be numbed but pressure may still be felt.	☐	☐	☐
5. Have the patient void.	☐	☐	☐
6. Direct the patient to disrobe and put on a gown with the opening in the back.	☐	☐	☐
7. Prepare the skin unless this is to be done as part of the sterile preparation. **a.** Use a sterile forceps after gloving. **b.** You may be required to add sterile solutions to the field.	☐	☐	☐
8. Assist as needed with administration of the anesthetic.	☐	☐	☐
9. Assist the patient into the appropriate position. **a.** For the side-lying position: (1) Stand in front of the patient and help by holding the patient's knees and top shoulder. (2) Ask the patient to move, so the back is close to the edge of the table. **b.** For the forward-leaning, supported position: (1) Stand in front of the patient and rest your hands on the patient's shoulders. (2) Ask the patient to breathe slowly and deeply.	☐	☐	☐
10. Throughout the procedure, observe the patient closely for signs such as dyspnea or cyanosis. **a.** Monitor the pulse at intervals and record the vital signs after the procedure. **b.** Note the patient's mental alertness. **c.** Watch for any signs of leakage at the site, nausea, or vomiting. **d.** Assess lower limb mobility.	☐	☐	☐

PROCEDURE STEPS	SELF	PARTNER	INSTRUCTOR
11. When the physician has the needle securely in place, if specimens are to be taken: **a.** Put on gloves to receive the potentially hazardous body fluid. **b.** Label the tubes in sequence as you receive them. **c.** Label with the patient's identification and place them in biohazard bags.	☐	☐	☐
12. If the Queckenstedt test is to be performed, you may be required to press against the patient's jugular veins in the neck, either right, left, or both, while the physician monitors the CSF pressure.	☐	☐	☐
13. At the completion of the procedure: **a.** Cover the site with an adhesive bandage and assist the patient to a flat position. **b.** The physician will determine when the patient is ready to leave.	☐	☐	☐
14. Route the specimens as required.	☐	☐	☐
15. Clean the examination room and care for or dispose of the equipment as needed.	☐	☐	☐
16. Wash your hands.	☐	☐	☐
17. Chart all observations and record the procedure.	☐	☐	☐

CALCULATION

Total Possible Points: _____
Total Points Earned: _____ Multiplied by 100 = _____ Divided by Total Possible Points = _____%

Pass   **Fail**
☐   ☐   Comments:

Student's signature _____ Date _____
Partner's signature _____ Date _____
Instructor's signature _____ Date _____

Work Product 1

Document appropriately.

Christopher Guest is a 12-year-old boy brought into your office. He is lethargic and nauseous with a fever and difficulty bending his neck. The physician, Dr. England, orders a lumbar puncture. You assist in the procedure, and CSF is collected and sent to the lab. If you are currently working in a medical office, use a blank paper patient chart from the office. If this is not available to you, use the space below to record the procedure in the chart.

_____

_____

_____

_____

_____

_____

_____

_____

_____

Chapter Self-Assessment Quiz

1. Initial symptoms of tetanus include:
  a. muscle spasms and stiff neck.
  b. paralysis and stiff neck.
  c. drooling and thick saliva.
  d. seizures and dysphagia.
  e. muscle spasms and clenched teeth.

2. What is another name for grand mal seizures?
  a. Absence seizures
  b. Tonic-clonic seizures
  c. Partial seizures
  d. Nervous seizures
  e. Flashing seizures

3. Febrile seizures occur in:
  a. teenagers.
  b. middle-aged men.
  c. young children.
  d. elderly women.
  e. people of all ages.

4. There are no signs of external deformity with:
  a. meningocele.
  b. myelomeningocele.
  c. spina bifida occulta.
  d. amyotrophic lateral sclerosis.
  e. poliomyelitis.

5. To diagnose meningitis, the physician may order a(n):
  a. urine sample.
  b. x-ray.
  c. MRI.
  d. throat culture.
  e. complete blood count.

6. Hydrophobia often occurs after the onset of:
  a. rabies.
  b. tetanus.
  c. encephalitis.
  d. cerebral palsy.
  e. meningitis.

7. A herpes zoster breakout typically develops on:

   a. the legs and arms.

   b. the genitals and mouth.

   c. the stomach and chest.

   d. the face, back, and chest.

   e. the face and neck.

8. A disease closely related to poliomyelitis is:

   a. encephalitis.

   b. meningitis.

   c. Parkinson disease.

   d. PPMA syndrome.

   e. chicken pox.

9. Treatment for brain tumors may include:

   a. chemotherapy and drug therapy.

   b. surgery and radiation therapy.

   c. surgery and drug therapy.

   d. drug therapy and radiation therapy.

   e. physical therapy and drug therapy.

10. CSF removed and sent to the laboratory may be tested for:

   a. glucose and protein.

   b. bacteria and viruses.

   c. cell counts and white blood cells.

   d. red blood cells and white blood cells.

   e. glucose and fatty acids.

11. You should encourage slow, deep breathing for:

   a. electrical tests.

   b. a lumbar puncture.

   c. radiological tests.

   d. physical tests.

   e. the Romberg test.

12. Contrast medium helps distinguish between the soft tissues of the nervous system and:

   a. bones.

   b. tendons.

   c. tumors.

   d. muscles.

   e. arteries.

13. When assisting with a Queckenstedt test, you will be directed to:

   a. assist the patient into a side-curled position.

   b. support a forward-bending sitting position.

   c. maintain sterility of instruments.

   d. press against the patient's jugular vein.

   e. encourage the patient in slow, deep breathing.

14. AFP is generally performed:

   a. during the second trimester.

   b. during the first trimester

   c. during the third trimester.

   d. before a woman gets pregnant.

   e. after a baby is born.

15. Which of the following is true of Lou Gehrig disease?

   a. It is officially known as multiple sclerosis.

   b. It is highly contagious.

   c. It is caused by a spinal cord injury.

   d. It is found most often in children.

   e. It is a terminal disease.

16. During the second phase of a grand mal seizure, the patient experiences:

   a. a tingling in extremities.

   b. a sensitivity to light.

   c. a complete loss of consciousness.

   d. an increased awareness of smell.

   e. a sense of drowsiness.

17. Which of the following is a cause of febrile seizures?

   a. Spinal cord damage

   b. Elevated body temperature

   c. Hypothermia

   d. Reye syndrome

   e. Neural tube defects

18. Paraplegia is:

   a. paralysis of all limbs.

   b. paralysis of the high thoracic vertebrae.

   c. paralysis on one side of the body, opposite the side of involvement.

   d. paralysis from the waist up.

   e. paralysis of any part of the body below the point of involvement.

19. Which of the following is an infectious disorder of the nervous system?

   a. Tumors

   b. ALS

   c. Multiple sclerosis

   d. Encephalitis

   e. Febrile seizures

20. Parkinson disease is a:

   a. convulsive disorder.

   b. degenerative disorder.

   c. developmental disorder.

   d. neoplastic disorder.

   e. traumatic disorder.

Urology

Chapter Checklist

☐ Read textbook chapter and take notes within the Chapter Notes outline. Answer the Learning Objectives as you reach them in the content, and then check them off.

☐ Work the Content Review questions—both Foundational Knowledge and Application.

☐ Perform the Active Learning exercise(s).

☐ Complete Professional Journal entries.

☐ Complete Skill Practice Activity(s) using Competency Evaluation Forms and Work Products, when appropriate.

☐ Take the Chapter Self-Assessment Quiz.

☐ Insert all appropriate pages into your Portfolio.

Learning Objectives

1. Spell and define the key terms.

2. List and describe the disorders of the urinary system and the male reproductive system.

3. Describe and explain the purpose of various diagnostic procedures associated with the urinary system.

4. Discuss the role of the medical assistant in diagnosing and treating disorders of the urinary system and the male reproductive system.

Chapter Notes

Note: Bold-faced headings are the major headings in the text chapter; headings in regular font are lower-level headings (i.e., the content is subordinate to, or falls "under," the major headings). Make sure you understand the key terms used in the chapter, as well as the concepts presented as Key Points.

TEXT SUBHEADINGS

NOTES

Introduction _____

_____

Key Point:
- The urinary system also removes waste from the blood while regulating fluid volume, important electrolytes, blood pressure, and pH (acid-base) balance.

☐ **LEARNING OBJECTIVE 1:** Spell and define the key terms.

Common Urinary Disorders _____

_____

_____

Renal Failure _____

_____

Key Terms: oliguria; dialysis
Key Points:
- Renal failure is an acute or chronic disorder of kidney function manifested by the inability of the kidney to excrete wastes, concentrate urine, and aid in homeostatic electrolyte conservation.
- With hemodialysis, toxins are removed from the blood by routing the patient's blood through a dialysis machine containing synthetic filters and a dialysate, a substance used to balance the electrolyte concentration in the blood.
- Patients receiving peritoneal dialysis often perform the procedure at home. An appropriately balanced dialysate is administered through a catheter into the abdominal cavity, allowed to remain in the abdominal cavity for a specified time, and then drained into a collecting bag.

Calculi _____

_____

Key Term: lithotripsy
Key Point:
- Calculi are stone formations that may be found anywhere in the urinary system and may range from granular particles to staghorn structures that fill the renal pelvis.

Tumors _____

_____

Key Point:
- Tumors are more common in the urinary bladder but may also occur in the kidney.

Hydronephrosis _____

_____

Key Terms: cystoscopy; nephrostomy; ureterostomy
Key Point:
- Hydronephrosis is distention of the renal pelvis and calyces resulting from an obstruction in the kidney or ureter that causes a backup of urine.

Urinary System Infections

Key Terms: proteinuria; hematuria; pyuria; urinary frequency; dysuria; anuria; enuresis; incontinence

Key Points:

• Glomerulonephritis is inflammation of the glomerulus, or filtering unit, of the kidney.
• Pyelonephritis is inflammation of the renal pelvis and the body of the kidney.
• Cystitis is an inflammation of the urinary bladder.
• Urethritis is inflammation of the urethra that may occur before the signs and symptoms of cystitis appear, or it may indicate a sexually transmitted disease, such as gonorrhea or nongonococcal urethritis.

Common Disorders of the Male Reproductive System

Benign Prostatic Hyperplasia

Key Term: nocturia

Key Point:

• As most men reach their middle years, the prostate begins to enlarge, or hypertrophy.

Prostate Cancer

Key Term: prostate-specific antigen

Key Point:

• Prostate cancer, like most cancers, is best treated when detected early.

Testicular Cancer

Key Point:

• Although testicular cancer accounts for only about 1% of all malignancies, the metastatic and mortality rates are high.

Hydrocele _____

_____

Key Point:
• Hydrocele, a collection of fluid in the scrotum and around the testes, may result from trauma or infection or may simply be due to aging.

Cryptorchidism _____

_____

Key Point:
• Cryptorchidism refers to either one or both undescended testes.

Inguinal Hernia _____

_____

Key Point:
• The patient with an inguinal hernia is often asymptomatic unless the intestines protrude through the weakened area, which may result in a noticeable bulge and pain.

Infections _____

_____

Key Point:
• The most common infections of the male reproductive system are epididymitis, orchitis, and prostatitis.

Impotence _____

_____

Key Terms: impotence; psychogenic
Key Point:
• Impotence, also known as erectile dysfunction, is the inability to achieve or maintain an erection; it may be psychological or organic.

☐ **LEARNING OBJECTIVE 2:** List and describe the disorders of the urinary system and the male reproductive system.

Common Diagnostic and Therapeutic Procedures _____

_____

_____

Urinalysis _____

Key Terms: urinalysis; specific gravity; catheterization
Key Point:
- The single most important step in diagnosing urinary diseases is the examination of the patient's urine, or **urinalysis**.

Blood Tests _____

Key Term: blood urea nitrogen (BUN)

Cystoscopy or Cystourethroscopy _____

Key Point:
- Cystoscopy is direct visualization of the bladder and urethra with a lighted instrument called a cystoscope.

Intravenous Pyelogram and Retrograde Pyelogram _____

Key Point:
- An intravenous pyelogram (IVP) is radiographic examination of the kidneys and urinary tract using a radiopaque dye injected into the circulatory system.

Ultrasound _____

Key Point:
- Ultrasound is noninvasive use of sound waves to show stones and obstructions in the urinary system and tissues.

Rectal and Scrotal Examinations _____

Key Point:
- At home, male patients should perform the testicular self-examination, since this is the best method for early detection of testicular cancer.

Vasectomy _____

_____

Key Point:
• A popular form of reproductive control is the vasectomy, or surgical removal of all or a segment of the vas deferens to prevent the passage of sperm from the testes.

☐ **LEARNING OBJECTIVE 3:** Describe and explain the purpose of various diagnostic procedures associated with the urinary system.

☐ **LEARNING OBJECTIVE 4:** Discuss the role of the medical assistant in diagnosing and treating disorders of the urinary system and the male reproductive system.

Content Review

FOUNDATIONAL KNOWLEDGE

Understanding Urinary System Disorders

1. What is the difference between hemodialysis and peritoneal dialysis?

_____

_____

2. What are calculi?

_____

_____

3. List five microorganisms that may cause epididymitis.

a. _____

b. _____

c. _____

d. _____

e. _____

4. What are the symptoms of a possible tumor in the urinary system?

_____

_____

5. Are stones more likely to form when urine is alkaline or acidic?

_____

_____

6. Why is a woman more likely to have cystitis than a man?

_____

_____

7. Why are infections in the male urinary tract likely to spread to the reproductive system?

_____

_____

Diagnostic Procedures

8. What are the three factors a physician is checking when performing a digital rectal examination?

a. _____

b. _____

c. _____

9. A patient comes in complaining of chills, fever, nausea, and some vomiting. She also complains of a pain in her side. When a urinalysis is performed, the urine appears cloudy. The physician prescribes medication to acidify the urine and an antibiotic. What did the patient have?

_____

_____

10. When is a herniorrhaphy performed?

_____

_____

11. An elderly male patient with prostatic hypertrophy must be given a catheter in order to obtain a urine sample. What is the best type of catheter to use, and why?

_____

_____

12. Why is proteinuria a serious occurrence to look for when performing urinalysis?

_____

_____

13. If hydronephrosis occurs, what are the three methods used to restore the flow of urine?

a. _____

b. _____

c. _____

14. What does PSA stand for?

_____

_____

Your Role in the Medical Office

15. List three suggestions to help patients avoid urinary tract infections.

a. _____

b. _____

c. _____

16. What is the difference between an intravenous pyelogram and a retrograde pyelogram, and what might you as a medical assistant be responsible for?

_____

_____

17. When you are giving a woman a catheter, why is it important not to move your nondominant hand, and when can you move your hand out of position?

_____

_____

18. One of the patients has come in because he is thinking about getting a vasectomy, but he wants to know everything that the surgery entails. Indicate where the physician will make the incisions, and write a brief description of what occurs during surgery to give to the patient.

_____

_____

19. Match the following key terms to their definitions.

Key Terms

a. anuria _____
b. blood urea nitrogen _____
c. catheterization _____
d. cystoscopy _____
e. dialysis _____
f. dysuria _____
g. enuresis _____
h. hematuria _____
i. impotence _____
j. incontinence _____
k. intravenous pyelogram (IVP) _____
l. lithotripsy _____
m. nephrostomy _____
n. nocturia _____
o. oliguria _____
p. prostate-specific antigen _____
q. proteinuria _____
r. psychogenic _____
s. pyuria _____
t. retrograde pyelogram _____
u. specific gravity _____

Definitions

1. an inability to achieve or maintain an erection
2. painful or difficult urination
3. crushing a stone with sound waves
4. the removal of waste in blood not filtered by kidneys by passing fluid through a semipermeable barrier that allows normal electrolytes to remain, either with a machine with circulatory access or by passing a balanced fluid through the peritoneal cavity
5. excessive urination at night
6. a blood test to determine the amount of nitrogen in blood or urea, a waste product normally excreted in urine
7. of psychological origin
8. a normal protein produced by the prostate that usually elevates in the presence of prostate cancer
9. the density of a liquid, such as urine, compared with water
10. radiography using contrast medium to evaluate kidney function
11. direct visualization of the urinary bladder through a cystoscope inserted through the urethra
12. an examination of the physical, chemical, and microscopic properties of urine
13. failure of kidneys to produce urine
14. blood in the urine
15. the presence of large quantities of protein in the urine; usually a sign of renal dysfunction
16. scant urine production

v. ureterostomy _____

w. urinalysis _____

x. urinary frequency _____

17. the urge to urinate occurring more often than is required for normal bladder elimination

18. a surgical opening to the outside of the body from the ureter to facilitate drainage of urine from an obstructed kidney

19. pus in the urine

20. bed wetting

21. the placement of a catheter in the kidney pelvis to drain urine from an obstructed kidney

22. the inability to control elimination of urine, feces, or both

23. a procedure for introducing a flexible tube into the body

24. an x-ray of the urinary tract using contrast medium injected through the bladder and ureters; useful in diagnosing obstructions

20. True or False? Determine whether the following statements are true or false. If false, explain why.

a. Orchiopexy refers to either one or both undescended testes.

_____

_____

b. A nephrologist is a physician who specializes in the physical characteristics of the urinary system.

_____

_____

c. No other form of birth control is needed after a man receives a vasectomy.

_____

_____

d. Your office is obligated to notify a patient if a procedure or medication is still in clinical trials, but likely to be approved.

_____

_____

APPLICATION

Critical Thinking Practice

1. A middle-aged patient in good shape comes in complaining of some pain in his groin. The physician suspects he might have an inguinal hernia. What is the procedure to diagnosis this, and how is it corrected?

_____

_____

2. An elderly patient has been diagnosed with renal failure and will need to undergo dialysis. However, he is not sure if hemodialysis or peritoneal dialysis would be better for his lifestyle. What information can you tell him about the two different processes, including the advantages and disadvantages of each?

_____

_____

Patient Education

1. The physician asks you to give information to one of the patients about passing small calculi. What would you tell the patient about calculi, and what suggestions would you give to help the patient pass the stones?

_____

_____

Documentation

1. You have just spoken with a 20-year-old patient about cystitis and have given her tips on how to avoid cystitis in the future. Record what you would write on the woman's chart, and make a note of any handout materials you might give the patient.

_____

_____

Active Learning

1. Prostate cancer is most common in men over the age of 50, and like many other cancers, it is best treated in the early stages. Testicular cancer is another form of cancer, but it occurs most often in younger men, aged 15 to 34. Go online and research more information about these diseases. Then, using your notes, create a presentation to give to the class. Be sure to include information about the causes, the symptoms, the ways to diagnose them, and the treatments available. Design the presentation to be educational for both your classmates and patients alike.

2. Sometimes, it is necessary to use a catheter to obtain a urine sample. Familiarize yourself with the steps, for both men and women. Then, if anatomical models are available, practice administering a catheter to both sexes.

3. Dialysis is a method of filtering the blood of waste products in renal failure. Both hemodialysis and peritoneal dialysis can indefinitely extend a patient's life, but they also significantly affect the patient's lifestyle. Research both hemodialysis and peritoneal dialysis, and write a short paper about your findings. What kinds of waste products do they filter out? What substances might be added? How is this technology improving, and how does it affect the patients who receive the treatment?

Professional Journal

REFLECT

(Prompts and Ideas: For many patients, receiving a catheter can be embarrassing and uncomfortable. What would you say to someone who must get a catheter? To someone you must give a catheter to?)

_____

_____

_____

_____

_____

_____

_____

PONDER AND SOLVE

1. A man in his early 20s has come in for his physical, and the physician has instructed you to teach him about testicular disease. You will also need to teach him how to perform a self-examination. However, the man is shy and embarrassed about the procedure. What can you say to him to help him overcome his discomfort?

_____

_____

_____

_____

2. An elderly woman has chronic renal failure, and the physician decides that she will need a catheter for peritoneal dialysis. The woman is upset that she needs this, because she believes that it will limit her movement and ability to participate in activities she likes. What can you tell her about catheters and how her lifestyle will change that might put her more at ease?

_____

_____

_____

_____

_____

EXPERIENCE

Skills related to this chapter include:

1. Perform a Female Urinary Catheterization (Procedure 34-1).
2. Perform a Male Urinary Catheterization (Procedure 34-2).
3. Instruct a Male Patient on the Self Testicular Examination (Procedure 34-3).

Record any common mistakes, lessons learned, and/or tips you discovered during your experience of practicing and demonstrating these skills:

_____

_____

_____

_____

_____

_____

_____

Skill Practice

PERFORMANCE OBJECTIVES:

1. Perform a female urinary catheterization (Procedure 34-1).
2. Perform a male urinary catheterization (Procedure 34-2).
3. Instruct a male patient on the self testicular examination (Procedure 34-3).

Name_____ Date _____ Time _____

| Procedure 34-1: | PERFORM A FEMALE URINARY CATHETERIZATION |

EQUIPMENT/SUPPLIES: Straight catheterization tray that includes a #14 or #16 French catheter, a sterile tray, sterile gloves, antiseptic, a specimen cup with a lid, lubricant, and a sterile drape; an examination light; an anatomically correct female torso model for performing the catheterization; a biohazard container

STANDARDS: Given the needed equipment and a place to work, the student will perform this skill with _____% accuracy in a total of _____ minutes. *(Your instructor will tell you what the percentage and time limits will be before you begin practicing.)*

KEY: 4 = Satisfactory   0 = Unsatisfactory   NA = This step is not counted

PROCEDURE STEPS	SELF	PARTNER	INSTRUCTOR
1. Wash your hands.	☐	☐	☐
2. Identify the patient. **a.** Explain the procedure and have the patient disrobe from the waist down. **b.** Provide adequate gowning and draping materials.	☐	☐	☐
3. Place the patient in the dorsal recumbent or lithotomy position. **a.** Drape carefully to prevent unnecessary exposure. **b.** Open the tray and place it between the legs of the patient. **c.** Adjust examination light to allow adequate visualization of the perineum.	☐	☐	☐
4. Remove the sterile glove package and put on the sterile gloves.	☐	☐	☐
5. Remove sterile drape and place it under buttocks of the patient.	☐	☐	☐
6. Open the antiseptic swabs and place them upright inside the catheter tray.	☐	☐	☐
7. Open lubricant and squeeze a generous amount onto tip of the catheter.	☐	☐	☐
8. Remove sterile urine specimen cup and lid and place them to the side of the tray.	☐	☐	☐
9. Using your nondominant hand, carefully expose the urinary meatus.	☐	☐	☐
10. Using your sterile dominant hand, use antiseptic swabs to cleanse the urinary meatus by starting at the top and moving the swab down each side of the urinary meatus and down the middle, using a new swab for each side and the middle. Do not contaminate the glove on this hand.	☐	☐	☐
11. Pick up the catheter with the sterile, dominant hand and: **a.** Carefully insert the lubricated tip into the urinary meatus approximately 3 inches. **b.** Leave the other end of the catheter in the tray.	☐	☐	☐
12. Once the urine begins to flow into the catheter tray, hold the catheter in position with your nondominant hand.	☐	☐	☐
13. Use your dominant hand to direct the flow of urine into the specimen cup.	☐	☐	☐

PROCEDURE STEPS	SELF	PARTNER	INSTRUCTOR
14. Remove catheter when urine flow slows or stops or 1000 mL has been obtained.	☐	☐	☐
15. Wipe the perineum carefully with the drape that was placed under the buttocks.	☐	☐	☐
16. Dispose of urine appropriately and discard supplies in a biohazard container. **a.** Label the specimen container and complete the necessary laboratory requisition. **b.** Process the specimen according to the guidelines of the laboratory.	☐	☐	☐
17. Remove your gloves and wash your hands.	☐	☐	☐
18. Instruct patient to dress and give any follow-up information.	☐	☐	☐
19. Document the procedure in the patient's medical record.	☐	☐	☐

CALCULATION

Total Possible Points: _____
Total Points Earned: _____ Multiplied by 100 = _____ Divided by Total Possible Points = _____%

Pass   **Fail**
☐   ☐

Comments:

Student's signature _____ Date _____
Partner's signature _____ Date _____
Instructor's signature _____ Date _____

Name _____ Date _____ Time _____

| Procedure 34-2: | **PERFORM A MALE URINARY CATHETERIZATION** |

EQUIPMENT/SUPPLIES: Straight catheterization tray that includes a #14 or #16 French catheter, a sterile tray, sterile gloves, antiseptic, a specimen cup with a lid, lubricant, a sterile drape, an examination light, an anatomically correct male torso model for performing the catheterization, a biohazard container

STANDARDS: Given the needed equipment and a place to work, the student will perform this skill with _____% accuracy in a total of _____ minutes. *(Your instructor will tell you what the percentage and time limits will be before you begin practicing.)*

KEY: 4 = Satisfactory   0 = Unsatisfactory   NA = This step is not counted

PROCEDURE STEPS	SELF	PARTNER	INSTRUCTOR
1. Wash your hands.	☐	☐	☐

2. Identify the patient.
  a. Explain the procedure and have the patient disrobe from the waist down.
  b. Provide adequate gowning and draping materials.
	☐	☐	☐

3. Place the patient in the supine position.
  a. Drape carefully to prevent unnecessary exposure.
  b. Open the tray and place it to the side or on the patient's thighs.
  c. Adjust examination light to allow adequate visualization of the perineum.
	☐	☐	☐

4. Remove the sterile glove package and put on the sterile gloves.	☐	☐	☐
5. Carefully remove the sterile drape and place it under the glans penis.	☐	☐	☐
6. Open the antiseptic swabs and place them upright inside the catheter tray.	☐	☐	☐
7. Open lubricant and squeeze a generous amount onto the tip of the catheter.	☐	☐	☐
8. Remove sterile urine specimen cup and lid and place them to the side of the tray.	☐	☐	☐
9. Using your nondominant hand, pick up the penis to expose the urinary meatus.	☐	☐	☐
10. Using your sterile dominant hand, use antiseptic swabs to cleanse the urinary meatus by starting at the top and moving the swab around each side of the urinary meatus and down the middle, using a new swab for each side and the middle. Do not contaminate the glove on this hand.	☐	☐	☐

11. Using your sterile dominant hand, pick up the catheter.
  a. Carefully insert the lubricated tip into the meatus approximately 4 to 6 inches.
  b. The other end of the catheter should be left in the tray.
	☐	☐	☐

12. Once the urine begins to flow into the catheter tray, hold the catheter in position.	☐	☐	☐

PROCEDURE STEPS	SELF	PARTNER	INSTRUCTOR
13. Use your dominant hand to direct the flow of urine into the specimen cup.	☐	☐	☐
14. Remove the catheter when urine flow slows or stops or 1000 mL has been obtained.	☐	☐	☐
15. Wipe the glans penis carefully with the drape that was placed under the buttocks.	☐	☐	☐
16. Dispose of urine appropriately and discard supplies in a biohazard container.	☐	☐	☐
17. Label the specimen container and complete the necessary laboratory requisition.	☐	☐	☐
18. Process specimen according to the guidelines of the laboratory.	☐	☐	☐
19. Remove your gloves and wash your hands.	☐	☐	☐
20. Instruct patient to dress and give any follow-up information.	☐	☐	☐
21. Document the procedure in the patient's medical record.	☐	☐	☐

CALCULATION

Total Possible Points: _____
Total Points Earned: _____ Multiplied by 100 = _____ Divided by Total Possible Points = _____%

Pass   **Fail**
☐   ☐

Comments:

Student's signature _____ Date _____
Partner's signature _____ Date _____
Instructor's signature _____ Date _____

Name _____ Date _____ Time _____

Procedure 34-3:	INSTRUCT A MALE PATIENT ON THE SELF TESTICULAR EXAMINATION

EQUIPMENT/SUPPLIES: A patient instruction sheet if available; a testicular examination model or pictures

STANDARDS: Given the needed equipment and a place to work, the student will perform this skill with _____% accuracy in a total of _____ minutes. *(Your instructor will tell you what the percentage and time limits will be before you begin practicing.)*

KEY: 4 = Satisfactory   0 = Unsatisfactory   NA = This step is not counted

PROCEDURE STEPS	SELF	PARTNER	INSTRUCTOR
1. Wash your hands.	☐	☐	☐
2. Identify the patient and explain the procedure.	☐	☐	☐
3. Using the testicular model or pictures, explain the procedure. **a.** Tell the patient to examine each testicle by gently rolling between the fingers and the thumb with both hands. **b.** Check for lumps or thickenings.	☐	☐	☐
4. Explain that the epididymis is located on top of each testicle. **a.** Palpate to avoid incorrectly identifying it as an abnormal growth or lump. **b.** Instruct patient to report abnormal lumps or thickenings to the physician.	☐	☐	☐
5. Allow the patient to ask questions related to the testicular self-examination.	☐	☐	☐
6. Document the procedure in the patient's medical record.	☐	☐	☐

CALCULATION

Total Possible Points: _____
Total Points Earned: _____ Multiplied by 100 = _____ Divided by Total Possible Points = _____%

Pass   **Fail**
☐   ☐   Comments:

Student's signature _____ Date _____
Partner's signature _____ Date _____
Instructor's signature _____ Date _____

Work Product 1

Document appropriately.

Livia Havran is a 42-year-old female with complaints of fever, pain, and difficulty urinating. The physician, Dr. Smith, orders a urinary sample by catheterization. You assist in the procedure, and a sample is collected and sent to the laboratory.

If you are currently working in a medical office, use a blank paper patient chart from the office. If this is not available to you, use the space below to record the procedure in the chart.

_____

_____

_____

_____

_____

_____

_____

_____

Chapter Self-Assessment Quiz

1. Cystoscopy is:

  a. an inflammation of the urinary bladder.

  b. the direct visualization of the bladder and urethra.

  c. a procedure used to help patients pass calculi.

  d. the treatment used for men with an inguinal hernia.

  e. the use of a small camera inserted into the rectum.

2. Which of the following might contribute to psychogenic impotence?

  a. Disease in any other body system

  b. Injury to pelvic organs

  c. Medication

  d. Exhaustion

  e. Cardiovascular problems

3. Before a patient receives an IVP or a retrograde pyelogram, you must check for a(n):

  a. protein allergy.

  b. lubricant allergy.

  c. iodine allergy.

  d. rubber allergy.

  e. latex allergy.

4. A procedure that cleanses the blood of waste products and excess fluid is:

  a. oliguria.

  b. lithotripsy.

  c. proteinuria.

  d. cystoscopy.

  e. dialysis.

5. Young girls are prone to urethritis because they:

  a. forget to practice good hand-washing technique.

  b. have a short urethra.

  c. don't take enough baths.

  d. urinate too frequently.

  e. wipe from front to back.

6. Which of the following instructions would be helpful for a patient trying to pass a stone?

  a. Eat a large amount of fiber.

  b. Get plenty of bed rest and relaxation.

  c. Drink lots of water.

  d. Go to the hospital when the stone passes.

  e. Do not consume anything until the stone has passed.

7. Orchiopexy is surgery to correct:

   a. undescended testes.

   b. enlarged prostate.

   c. inguinal hernia.

   d. impotence.

   e. hydrocele.

8. One common urinary disorder in females is:

   a. benign prostatic hyperplasia.

   b. nocturia.

   c. hydrocele.

   d. cryptorchidism.

   e. urinary tract infection.

Scenario: An elderly patient comes in for a routine checkup, and the physician discovers his prostate gland is very enlarged.

9. What is a blood test you can run to look for prostate cancer?

   a. PSA test

   b. Proteinuria

   c. Snellen test

   d. Digital rectal exam

   e. Dialysis

10. A urinary condition that might indicate an enlarged prostate gland is:

    a. proteinuria.

    b. oliguria.

    c. nocturia.

    d. hematuria.

    e. pyuria.

11. Seventy-five percent of men with prostate cancer are over the age of:

    a. 15.

    b. 30.

    c. 34.

    d. 50.

    e. 75.

End Scenario

12. What kind of juice is recommended to patients to acidify urine?

    a. Tomato juice

    b. Orange juice

    c. Grape juice

    d. Cranberry juice

    e. Grapefruit juice

13. A patient should be given a catheter when:

    a. the patient suffers from nocturia.

    b. the patient has a urinary tract infection.

    c. the patient's urine has high PSA levels.

    d. the patient has calculi.

    e. the patient has dysuria.

14. Which of the following instruments is used to view the bladder and urethra?

    a. Catheter

    b. Cystoscope

    c. Dialysis machine

    d. Ultrasound

    e. Pyelogram

15. Which of the following patients is most likely to develop a urinary tract infection?

    a. A young boy who frequently urinates

    b. A teenaged girl who takes bubble baths

    c. An elderly woman who only wears loose-fitting dresses

    d. An adult woman who showers immediately after sexual intercourse

    e. A middle-aged man who does not wash his hands very often

16. Which of the following is the initial step in catheterization of a patient?

    a. Wash your hands.

    b. Identify the patient.

    c. Put on sterile gloves.

    d. Use antiseptic swabs to clean area.

    e. Assist patient to assume position.

17. What is a symptom of hydronephrosis?

    a. Proteinuria

    b. Chills

    c. Swollen prostate

    d. Back pain

    e. High PSA levels

18. Which of the following is true for catheterizing both men and women?

    a. Tray may be placed on patient's lap for easy access to tools.

    b. Patient's position is on his or her back, legs apart.

    c. Catheter is inserted 5 inches.

    d. Nondominant hand is contaminated.

    e. Coude catheter may be used.

19. Which of the following is a cause of organic impotence?

 a. Exhaustion

 b. Anxiety

 c. Depression

 d. Stress

 e. Endocrine imbalance

20. Ultrasonography can be used to treat which of the following?

 a. Renal failure

 b. Hydronephrosis

 c. Calculi

 d. Urinary tract infection

 e. Inguinal hernia

Chapter
Checklist

☐ Read textbook chapter and take notes within the Chapter Notes outline. Answer the Learning Objectives as you reach them in the content, and then check them off.

☐ Work the Content Review questions—both Foundational Knowledge and Application.

☐ Perform the Active Learning exercise(s).

☐ Complete Professional Journal entries.

☐ Complete Skill Practice Activity(s) using Competency Evaluation Forms and Work Products, when appropriate.

☐ Take the Chapter Self-Assessment Quiz.

☐ Insert all appropriate pages into your Portfolio.

Learning Objectives

1. Spell and define the key terms.
2. List and describe common gynecological disorders.
3. Explain the diagnostic and therapeutic procedures associated with the female reproductive system.
4. Identify your role in the care of gynecological patients.

5. Describe the components of prenatal and postpartum patient care.
6. List and describe common obstetric disorders.
7. Explain common obstetric tests and procedures and identify your role in caring for obstetric patients.
8. Identify the various methods of contraception.
9. Describe menopause.

Chapter Notes

Note: Bold-faced headings are the major headings in the text chapter; headings in regular font are lower-level headings (i.e., the content is subordinate to, or falls "under," the major headings). Make sure you understand the key terms used in the chapter, as well as the concepts presented as Key Points.

TEXT SUBHEADINGS

NOTES

Introduction _____

_____

Key Terms: menses; menarche
Key Point:
• Gynecology is a specialty of medicine that deals with development and disorders of the female reproductive system, including the internal and external organs. Obstetrics is the branch of medicine that cares for female patients through pregnancy, childbirth, and the postpartum period.

☐ **LEARNING OBJECTIVE 1:** Spell and define the key terms.

Gynecological Disorders

Dysfunctional Uterine Bleeding

> **Key Terms:** menorrhagia; metrorrhagia; polymenorrhea; curettage
> **Key Point:**
> • Dysfunctional uterine bleeding is abnormal or irregular uterine bleeding, including heavy, irregular, or light bleeding caused by an endocrine imbalance.

Premenstrual Syndrome

Endometriosis

> **Key Terms:** dysmenorrhea; dyspareunia; laparoscopy; salpingo-oophorectomy
> **Key Point:**
> • Endometriosis is a condition of unknown cause in which endometrial tissue grows outside the uterine cavity.

Uterine Prolapse and Displacement

> **Key Terms:** cystocele; rectocele; colporrhaphy; colpocleisis; pessary
> **Key Points:**
> • Prolapse of the uterus is an abnormal condition in which the uterus droops or protrudes down into the vagina.
> • While many women do not have symptoms, others complain of pelvic pressure, dyspareunia, urinary problems, or constipation.

Leiomyomas

> **Key Point:**
> • Leiomyomas are benign tumors of the uterus, including fibroid tumors, myomas, and fibromyomas.

Ovarian Cysts _____

_____

Key Terms: amenorrhea; hirsutism
Key Point:
• Numerous types of ovarian cysts, including functional cysts and polycystic ovaries, are benign.

Gynecological Cancers _____

_____

Key Term: colposcopy
Key Point:
• Cervical and breast cancers have an excellent prognosis when detected and treated early, but left untreated or diagnosed in later stages, these cancers are deadly.

Infertility _____

_____

Key Point:
• The causes of infertility may include uterine or cervical abnormalities, tubal occlusion or scarring, a hormonal imbalance, or psychological factors.

Sexually Transmitted Diseases _____

_____

Key Point:
• Since STDs are easily transmitted, all STDs must be reported to the local health department by the medical office.

AIDS _____

_____

Key Points:
• AIDS is an infectious disease that overwhelms the body's immune system.
• Although new treatments prolong the HIV-positive individual's life, there currently is no cure, however research to find more effective treatments and a possible cure is ongoing.

Syphilis _____

_____

Key Point:
• The cause of syphilis is a microorganism known as *Treponema pallidum,* a spriochete.

Chlamydia _____

Key Point:
• Chlamydia infections cause urethritis in men, cervicitis in women, and lymphogranuloma venereum in both, all caused by the organism *Chlamydia trachomatis.*

Condylomata Acuminata _____

Key Point:
• Condylomata acuminata is a viral infection of the genital area causing the growth of soft, papillary warts that appear in a wide variety of places, including the vulva, vagina, cervix, and perineum.

Gonorrhea _____

Key Point:
• Gonorrhea is the second most common STD and is caused by a gram-negative diplococcus, *Neisseria gonorrhoeae.*

Herpes Genitalis _____

Key Point:
• Herpes genitalis is caused by the herpes simplex virus 2 (HSV2), and is characterized by painful vesicular lesions in the vaginal, vulvar, or anorectal area.

Vulvovaginitis, Salpingitis, and Pelvic Inflammatory Disease _____

Key Term: culdocentesis
Key Points:
• Although vulvovaginitis, salpingitis, and pelvic inflammatory disease can be caused by any type of microorganism, these disorders are commonly caused by sexually transmitted infections.
• Salpingitis is a bacterial infection of the fallopian tubes that is most often transmitted by sexual intercourse.

☐ **LEARNING OBJECTIVE 2:** List and describe common gynecological disorders.

Common Diagnostic and Therapeutic Procedures _____

The Gynecological Examination

Key Point:
• As part of the gynecological examination, the physician examines the patient's breasts, performs a pelvic examination, and obtains a Pap smear.

Colposcopy

Key Point:
• Colposcopy is visual examination of the vaginal and cervical surfaces using a stereoscopic microscope called a colposcope.

Hysterosalpingography

Key Term: hysterosalpingogram
Key Point:
• Hysterosalpingography is a diagnostic procedure in which the uterus and uterine tubes are radiographed after injection of a contrast medium.

Dilation and Curettage

Key Term: abortion
Key Point:
• Dilation and curettage (D & C) may be performed to remove uterine tissue for diagnostic testing, to remove endometrial tissue, to prevent or treat menorrhagia, or to remove retained products of conception after a spontaneous abortion or miscarriage.

Obstetric Care

Diagnosis of Pregnancy

Key Terms: gravid; human chorionic gonadotropin (HCG); Braxton-Hicks contractions; Goodell's sign; Chadwick's sign
Key Point:
• Many patients suspect that they are gravid, or pregnant, because they have signs, however early signs of pregnancy may indicate other disorders and therefore are considered presumptive until a conclusive diagnostic procedure is done.

First Prenatal Visit _____

_____

Key Point:
• The first examination is done to establish a detailed base-line of the patient's physical condition and includes a confirmation of pregnancy, a complete history and physical, determination of the estimated date of delivery, assessment of gestational age, identification of risk factors, and patient education.

Parity Versus Gravidity _____

_____

Key Terms: parity; gravidity; gravida; nulligravida; primigravida; nullipara; primipara; multipara

Subsequent Prenatal Visits _____

_____

_____

Onset of Labor _____

_____

Key Term: lightening
Key Points:
• Labor is the physiological process leading to expelling the fetus from the uterus.
• The actual onset of labor is characterized by regular uterine contractions that become more intense and more frequent with time.

The Cesarean Section _____

_____

_____

Postpartum Care _____

_____

Key Terms: puerperium; lochia
Key Points:
• The postpartum period, the puerperium, runs from childbirth until involution, when the reproductive structures return to normal.
• The time for the first postpartum visit depends on the type of delivery and the patient's condition when discharged from the hospital.

☐ **LEARNING OBJECTIVE 3:** Explain the diagnostic and therapeutic procedures associated with the female reproductive system.

☐ **LEARNING OBJECTIVE 4:** Identify your role in the care of gynecological patients.

☐ **LEARNING OBJECTIVE 5:** Describe the components of prenatal and postpartum patient care.

Obstetric Disorders _____

_____

_____

Ectopic Pregnancy _____

_____

Key Point:
- Gestation in which a fertilized ovum implants somewhere other than in the uterine cavity is an ectopic pregnancy.

Hyperemesis Gravidarum _____

_____

Key Point:
- Nausea and vomiting, commonly called morning sickness, are expected during early pregnancy and usually can be treated with small frequent meals, adequate hydration, and reassurance.

Abortion _____

_____

Key Points:
- One of the common disorders of pregnancy is first-trimester spontaneous abortion, also called an early pregnancy loss or miscarriage.
- A spontaneous abortion is defined as the loss of pregnancy before the fetus is viable.

Preeclampsia and Eclampsia _____

_____

Key Term: proteinuria
Key Points:
- Preeclampsia is characterized by **proteinuria**, edema of the lower extremities, and hypertension after the 20th week of gestation.
- In eclampsia, the clinical signs of preeclampsia are still present but become more extreme.

Placenta Previa and Abruptio Placentae _____

_____

Key Points:
- Placenta previa is a condition in which the placenta is implanted either partially or completely over the internal cervical os, making delivery of the fetus before the placenta difficult.
- The premature separation or detachment of the placenta from the uterus is abruptio placentae.

☐ **LEARNING OBJECTIVE 6:** List and describe common obstetric disorders.

Common Obstetric Tests and Procedures _____

_____

_____

Pregnancy Tests _____

_____

_____

Alpha-Fetoprotein _____

_____

Key Term: amniocentesis
Key Points:
- Levels of alpha-fetoprotein (AFP) are obtained from maternal serum to screen the fetus for defects in the neural tube, a part of the fetus that develops into the brain and spinal cord.
- Amniocentesis is insertion of a needle through the abdomen and into the gravid uterus to remove fluid from the amniotic sac.

Fetal Ultrasonography _____

_____

Key Point:
- An ultrasound of the fetus is performed using high-frequency sound waves to create an image of internal structures.

Contraction Stress Test and Nonstress Test

Key Points:
- A contraction stress test (CST) is performed in the third trimester to determine how the fetus will tolerate uterine contractions.
- The nonstress test (NST) is a noninvasive obstetric procedure used to evaluate the fetal heart tones and movement in relation to spontaneous uterine contractions.

☐ **LEARNING OBJECTIVE 7:** Explain common obstetric tests and procedures and identify your role in caring for obstetric patients.

Contraception

Key Point:
- The decision to practice contraception and the selection of an appropriate method involves many factors, including the patient's religious, cultural, and personal beliefs.

☐ **LEARNING OBJECTIVE 8:** Identify the various methods of contraception.

Menopause

Key Term: oligomenorrhea
Key Point:
- Menopause, also called the climacteric period, is the stage of life during which ovulation ceases because of decreasing ovarian function.

☐ **LEARNING OBJECTIVE 9:** Describe menopause.

Content Review

FOUNDATIONAL KNOWLEDGE

Gynecological Disorders

1. Complete this chart, which shows common gynecological disorders, their signs and symptoms, and possible treatments.

Disorder	Signs and Symptoms	Treatment
Dysfunctional uterine bleeding	**a.**	Hormone therapy, contraceptives, curettage, hysterectomy
Premenstrual syndrome	Severe physical, psychological, and behavioral signs and symptoms during the 7 to 10 days before menses	**b.**
Endometriosis	**c.**	Hormone and drug therapy, laparoscopic excision, hysterectomy, bilateral salpingo-oophorectomy
Uterine prolapse and displacement	Pelvic pressure, dyspareunia, urinary problems, constipation	**d.**
Leiomyomas	**e.**	Monitoring, myomectomy, hysterectomy
f.	Anovulation, irregular menses or amenorrhea, hirsutism	Hormone therapy, oral contraceptives
Infertility	Inability to conceive	**g.**

2. Some ovarian cysts are functional, while others are problematic. Give an example of each.

3. How is premenstrual dysphoric disorder (PMDD) diagnosed and treated?

4. What is the difference between HIV and AIDS?

5. Match each of the following sexually transmitted diseases (STDs) with its corresponding cause.

STD

a. AIDS ＿＿
b. Syphilis ＿＿
c. Chlamydia ＿＿
d. Condylomata acuminata ＿＿
e. Gonorrhea ＿＿
f. Herpes genitalis ＿＿

Cause

1. Herpes simplex virus 2 (HSV2)
2. Human papilloma virus (HPV)
3. *Treponema pallidum*
4. *Chlamydia trachomatis*
5. Human immunodeficiency virus (HIV)
6. *Neisseria gonorrhoeae*

Medical Assistants in the OB/Gyn Office

6. Which of the following is your responsibility concerning the care of a gynecological and obstetric patient? Circle all that apply.

   a. Give the patient instructions prior to her pelvic examination, such as refraining from douching, intercourse, and applying vaginal medication for 24 hours before her exam.

   b. Warm the speculum prior to the pelvic exam.

   c. Perform a breast examination.

   d. Instruct the patient to change into an examining gown.

   e. Inform patient of the effectiveness of different birth control methods.

   f. Confirm whether a patient is gravid.

   g. Decide whether a patient should go to the medical office, or go to the hospital after displaying signs and/or symptoms of labor.

   h. Determine if the patient's medical history includes any over-the-counter medications known to be harmful to a developing fetus.

7. A pregnant patient is listed as gr iv, pret 0, ab 2, p i. What does this listing describe?

   _____

   _____

8. What is a cesarean section, and what are the reasons to have one performed?

   _____

   _____

9. Which muscles are strengthened by Kegel exercises? How can these exercises benefit a patient?

   _____

   _____

10. Complete this chart, which shows common diagnostic and therapeutic procedures and their purposes.

Procedure	Description	Purpose
Pelvic examination	a.	To identify or diagnose any abnormal conditions
Breast examination	Examination of the breast and surrounding tissue; performed with the hands	b.
Papanicolaou (Pap) test	c.	To detect signs of cervical cancer
Colposcopy	Visual examination of the vaginal and cervical surfaces using a stereoscopic microscope called a colposcope	d.
e.	Injection of a contrast medium into the uterus and fallopian tubes followed by a radiograph, using a hysterosalpingogram	To determine the configuration of the uterus and the patency of the fallopian tubes for patients with infertility
Dilation and curettage	f.	To remove uterine tissue for diagnostic testing, to remove endocrine tissue, to prevent or treat menorrhagia, or to remove retained products of conception after a spontaneous abortion or miscarriage

Getting Ready for Baby

11. A patient has just learned she is pregnant. What will you tell her to expect during her first prenatal visit? How often will you schedule the patient's subsequent prenatal visits?

_____

_____

12. Match each of the following stages of lochia with its correct description.

Lochia Stage	Description
a. Lochia rubra _____	**1.** Thin, brownish discharge lasting about 3 to 4 days after the previous stage
b. Lochia serosa _____	**2.** Blood-tinged discharge within 6 days of delivery
c. Lochia alba _____	**3.** White discharge that has no evidence of blood that can last up to week 6

13. Identify the obstetric disorder associated with the following signs and symptoms.

a. Nausea and vomiting (morning sickness) that has escalated to an unrelenting level, resulting in dehydration, electrolyte imbalance, and weight loss. _____

b. The premature separation or detachment of the placenta from the uterus. _____

c. Hypertension that is directly related to pregnancy and can be classified as either preeclampsia or eclampsia. _____

d. The loss of pregnancy before the fetus is viable; preceded by vaginal bleeding, uterine cramps, and lower back pain. _____

e. A fertilized ovum that has implanted somewhere other than the uterine cavity, such as the fallopian tubes, the abdomen, the ovaries, and the cervical os, causing breast enlargement or tenderness, nausea, pelvic pain, syncope, abdominal symptoms, painful sexual intercourse, and irregular menstrual bleeding. _____

14. After a patient's AFP (alpha-fetoprotein) levels were found to be abnormal, the physician has recommended the patient for an amniocentesis and a fetal ultrasonography to be performed at the medical office. What are your responsibilities concerning these procedures?

_____

_____

15. What signs differentiate true labor from false labor?

_____

_____

16. During the first prenatal visit, you will be responsible for instructing the patient to contact the physician if she experiences certain alarming signs or symptoms. Below, eliminate the signs or symptoms that should not be included in the list. Then, explain why these signs and/or symptoms should not be included in the list.

• Vaginal bleeding or spotting

• Persistent vomiting

• Weight gain

• Increased appetite

• Fever or chills

• Dysuria

• Frequent urination

• Unusual food cravings

• Abdominal or uterine cramping

• Leaking amniotic fluid

- Alteration in fetal movement
- Depressed mood
- Dizziness or blurred vision

_____

_____

Birth Control

17. Review the list of contraceptive methods. Then place a check mark in the appropriate box to indicate the category.

Methods	Surgical	Hormonal	Barrier	Other
a. The pill				
b. Vasectomy				
c. Male condom				
d. Spermicide				
e. Injection				
f. The patch				
g. Emergency contraception				
h. Female condom				
i. The ring				
j. Diaphragm/spermicide				
k. Fertility awareness				
l. IUD				

Understanding Menopause

18. What should a patient nearing the age range of 45 to 50 be told to expect during menopause?

_____

_____

19. Match the following key terms to their definitions.

Key Terms

a. abortion _____

b. amenorrhea _____

c. amniocentesis _____

d. Braxton-Hicks _____

e. Chadwick's sign _____

f. colpocleisis _____

g. culdocentesis _____

h. cystocele _____

i. dysmenorrhea _____

j. dyspareunia _____

Definitions

1. a woman who has never given birth to a viable fetus

2. softening of the cervix early in pregnancy

3. the presence of large amounts of protein in the urine; usually a sign of renal dysfunction

4. herniation of the rectum into the vaginal area

5. surgical puncture and aspiration of fluid from the vaginal cul-de-sac for diagnosis or therapy

6. when inserted into the vagina, device that supports the uterus

7. sign of early pregnancy in which the vaginal, cervical, and vulvar tissues develop a bluish violet color

8. herniation of the urinary bladder into the vagina

k. Goodell's sign _____

l. hirsutism _____

m. human chorionic gonadotropin (HCG) _____

n. hysterosalpingogram _____

o. menorrhagia _____

p. menarche _____

q. metrorrhagia _____

r. multipara _____

s. nullipara _____

t. pessary _____

u. polymenorrhea _____

v. primipara _____

w. proteinuria _____

x. puerperium _____

y. rectocele _____

z. salpingo-oophorectomy _____

9. period of time (about 6 weeks) from childbirth until reproductive structures return to normal

10. hormone secreted by the placenta and found in the urine and blood of a pregnant female

11. irregular uterine bleeding

12. puncture of the amniotic sac to remove fluid for testing

13. termination of pregnancy or products of conception prior to fetal viability and/or 20 weeks' gestation

14. condition of not menstruating

15. painful coitus or sexual intercourse

16. a woman who has given birth to one viable infant

17. abnormally frequent menstrual periods

18. surgery to occlude the vagina

19. a woman who has given birth to more than one fetus

20. surgical excision of both the fallopian tube and the ovary

21. sporadic uterine contractions during pregnancy

22. painful menstruation

23. abnormal or excessive hair growth in women

24. radiograph of the uterus and fallopian tubes after injection with a contrast medium

25. onset of first menstruation

26. excessive bleeding during menstruation

20. True or False? Determine whether the following statements are true or false. If false, explain why.

a. A woman's first Pap test and pelvic examination should be performed about 3 years after her first sexual intercourse or by age 21, whichever comes first, as recommended by the American College of Obstetricians and Gynecologists (ACOG).

_____

_____

b. A pelvic examination is performed for a pregnant patient during each prenatal visit to the obstetrician's office.

_____

_____

c. The presence of Braxton-Hicks contractions is a conclusive sign of pregnancy and leads to a formal diagnosis of pregnancy.

_____

_____

d. The date on which the patient last had sexual intercourse is used to calculate the expected date of delivery.

_____

_____

APPLICATION

Critical Thinking Practice

1. A patient at your medical office tested positive for a sexually transmitted disease (STD). What steps will you take after this positive identification of an STD? Describe each of your responsibilities in connection with this diagnosis.

_____

_____

2. While working at a gynecological/obstetrics office, you receive a frantic phone call from a pregnant patient who is experiencing vaginal bleeding, uterine cramps, and lower back pain. You put the patient on hold in order to consult the physician, but you learn that the physician has just been called to the hospital for a delivery. What information should you give the patient?

_____

_____

Patient Education

1. Your 34-year-old patient is concerned about gynecological cancers because there are cases of breast cancer and cervical cancer in her family history. What can you recommend the patient do to ensure early detection of any gynecological problems? Describe these procedures to her in a way that will ease her anxieties.

_____

_____

Documentation

1. Your patient Mrs. Park has arrived at the office for her first prenatal visit. As you are recording her history, you learn that Mrs. Park is pregnant for the third time. Her first pregnancy spontaneously aborted. Her second pregnancy resulted in a premature delivery of triplets, 2 females and 1 male. How would you record this information for the physician's review?

_____

_____

Active Learning

1. With so many prenatal tests, procedures, and appointments at the physician's office, a pregnant patient can feel overwhelmed. Create a packet that can be distributed to a patient during the first prenatal visit. Include the schedule of prenatal visits and the procedures that will be done at each of these visits. Also include important information for the patient to consult throughout the duration of the pregnancy; especially include a list of signs and symptoms that may indicate a problematic condition.

2. Using the Internet or library, research the prevalence of sexually transmitted diseases in the United States or, if possible, your city and state. Compare current statistics to those from 5, 10, and 15 years ago. Use this information to create a patient education pamphlet for young adults. Include information on how teenagers and young adults can protect themselves from STDs and where to turn for help if they suspect they have contracted an STD. Be sure to use a professional, nonjudgmental tone when educating about STDs; passing negative judgment may distort your message.

3. Using a model, demonstrate the procedure for performing a breast self-examination for another student or family member or friend. Ask for feedback from your audience regarding your clarity, thoroughness, and professionalism. Practice the demonstration until you are confident about explaining all steps of the procedure.

Professional Journal

REFLECT

(Prompts and Ideas: Have you or a loved one ever been pregnant? What do you wish you had known before and after the delivery? How were you or your loved one treated by medical staff during prenatal and postpartum visits? Did you feel that the staff made the prenatal care as anxiety-free and problem-free as possible?)

_____

_____

_____

_____

_____

_____

_____

PONDER AND SOLVE

1. A 20-year-old female patient has made an appointment with the physician because she believes that she has PMDD, which she blames for her failing grades and damaged personal relationships. When you meet with the patient to assess her medical history, she asks you to write a note to her professors excusing her from any missed assignments. What should you do next?

_____

_____

_____

_____

_____

_____

_____

2. You are working in a gynecologic and obstetric office. The physician, Dr. Gordon, is away from the office caring for a patient until late afternoon. While pulling patient's files for the day's appointments, you overhear a coworker, a fellow medical office assistant, answering a telephone call from a patient. After asking the patient several questions, your coworker tells the patient that she should proceed immediately to the hospital emergency room. You know that the office policy is to page Dr. Gordon with any patient inquiries, and, if he is not available, to refer patients to Dr. Gordon's colleague, Dr. Reese. Your coworker has not followed office policy. What would you say to your coworker? What should you do next?

_____

_____

_____

_____

_____

_____

_____

EXPERIENCE

Skills related to this chapter include:

1. Instruct the Patient on the Breast Self-Examination (Procedure 35-1).
2. Assist with the Pelvic Examination and Pap Smear (Procedure 35-2).
3. Assist with Colposcopy and Cervical Biopsy (Procedure 35-3).

Record any common mistakes, lessons learned, and/or tips you discovered during your experience of practicing and demonstrating these skills.

_____

_____

_____

_____

_____

_____

_____

Skill Practice

PERFORMANCE OBJECTIVES:

1. Instruct the patient on the breast self-examination (Procedure 35-1).
2. Assist with the pelvic examination and Pap smear (Procedure 35-2).
3. Assist with colposcopy and cervical biopsy (Procedure 35-3).

Name _____ Date _____ Time _____

Procedure 35-1:	INSTRUCT THE PATIENT ON THE BREAST SELF-EXAMINATION

EQUIPMENT/SUPPLIES: Patient education instruction sheet, if available; breast examination model, if available

STANDARDS: Given the needed equipment and a place to work, the student will perform this skill with _____% accuracy in a total of _____ minutes. *(Your instructor will tell you what the percentage and time limits will be before you begin practicing.)*

KEY: 4 = Satisfactory 0 = Unsatisfactory NA = This step is not counted

PROCEDURE STEPS	SELF	PARTNER	INSTRUCTOR
1. Wash your hands.	☐	☐	☐
2. Explain the purpose and frequency of examining the breasts.	☐	☐	☐
3. Describe three positions necessary for the patient to examine the breasts: in front of a mirror, in the shower, and while lying down.	☐	☐	☐
4. In front of a mirror: **a.** Disrobe and inspect the breasts with her arms at sides and with arms raised above her head. **b.** Look for any changes in contour, swelling, dimpling of the skin, or changes in the nipple.	☐	☐	☐
5. In the shower: **a.** Feel each breast with hands over wet skin using the flat part of the first three fingers. **b.** Check for any lumps, hard knots, or thickenings. **c.** Use right hand to lightly press over all areas of left breast. **d.** Use left hand to examine right breast.	☐	☐	☐
6. Lying down: **a.** Place a pillow or folded towel under the right shoulder and place right hand behind head to examine the right breast. **b.** With left hand, use flat part of the fingers to palpate the breast tissue. **c.** Begin at the outermost top of the right breast. **d.** Work in a small circular motion around the breast in a clockwise rotation.	☐	☐	☐
7. Encourage patient to palpate the breast carefully moving her fingers inward toward the nipple and palpating every part of the breast including the nipple.	☐	☐	☐
8. Repeat the procedure for the left breast. Place a pillow or folded towel under the left shoulder with the left hand behind the head.	☐	☐	☐
9. Gently squeeze each nipple between the thumb and index finger. **a.** Report any clear or bloody discharge to the physician. **b.** Promptly report any abnormalities found in the breast self-examination to the physician.	☐	☐	☐
10. Document the patient education.	☐	☐	☐

CALCULATION

Total Possible Points: _____
Total Points Earned: _____ Multiplied by 100 = _____ Divided by Total Possible Points = _____%

Pass   **Fail**
☐   ☐   Comments:

Student's signature _____ Date _____
Partner's signature _____ Date _____
Instructor's signature _____ Date _____

Name_____ Date _____ Time _____

Procedure 35-2:	ASSIST WITH THE PELVIC EXAMINATION AND PAP SMEAR

EQUIPMENT/SUPPLIES: Patient gown and drape, appropriate size vaginal speculum, cotton-tipped applicators, water-soluble lubricant, examination gloves, examination light, tissues. *Materials for Pap smear:* Cervical spatula and/or brush, glass slides, fixative solution, laboratory request form, identification labels OR the materials required according to the laboratory, biohazard container.

STANDARDS: Given the needed equipment and a place to work, the student will perform this skill with _____% accuracy in a total of _____ minutes. *(Your instructor will tell you what the percentage and time limits will be before you begin practicing.)*

KEY: 4 = Satisfactory   0 = Unsatisfactory   NA = This step is not counted

PROCEDURE STEPS	SELF	PARTNER	INSTRUCTOR
1. Wash your hands.	☐	☐	☐
2. Assemble the equipment and supplies. 　**a.** Warm vaginal speculum by running under warm water. 　**b.** Do not use lubricant on the vaginal speculum before insertion.	☐	☐	☐
3. Label each slide with date and type of specimen on the frosted end with a pencil.	☐	☐	☐
4. Greet and identify the patient. Explain the procedure.	☐	☐	☐
5. Ask the patient to empty her bladder and, if necessary, collect a urine specimen.	☐	☐	☐
6. Provide a gown and drape and ask patient to disrobe from the waist down.	☐	☐	☐
7. Position patient in the dorsal lithotomy position—buttocks at bottom edge of table.	☐	☐	☐
8. Adjust drape to cover patient's abdomen and knees—expose the genitalia.	☐	☐	☐
9. Adjust light over the genitalia for maximum visibility.	☐	☐	☐
10. Assist physician with the examination as needed.	☐	☐	☐
11. Put on examination gloves. 　**a.** Hold microscope slides while the physician obtains and makes the smears. 　**b.** Spray or cover each slide with fixative solution.	☐	☐	☐
12. Have a basin or other container ready to receive the now-contaminated speculum.	☐	☐	☐
13. Apply lubricant across the physician's two fingers.	☐	☐	☐
14. Encourage the patient to relax during the bimanual examination as needed.	☐	☐	☐
15. After the examination, assist the patient in sliding up to the top of the examination table and remove both feet at the same time from the stirrups.	☐	☐	☐

PROCEDURE STEPS	SELF	PARTNER	INSTRUCTOR

16. Offer the patient tissues to remove excess lubricant.
   a. Assist her to a sitting position if necessary.
   b. Watch for signs of vertigo.
   c. Ask the patient to get dressed and assist as needed.
   d. Provide for privacy as the patient dresses.
	☐	☐	☐

17. Reinforce any physician instructions regarding follow-up appointments needed. **a.** Advise patient on the procedure for obtaining results from the Pap smear.	☐	☐	☐
18. Properly care for or dispose of equipment and clean the examination room.	☐	☐	☐
19. Wash your hands.	☐	☐	☐
20. Document your responsibilities during the procedure.	☐	☐	☐

CALCULATION

Total Possible Points: _____
Total Points Earned: _____ Multiplied by 100 = _____ Divided by Total Possible Points = _____%

Pass   **Fail**
☐   ☐   Comments:

Student's signature _____ Date _____
Partner's signature _____ Date _____
Instructor's signature _____ Date _____

Name_____ Date _____ Time _____

Procedure 35-3:	ASSIST WITH COLPOSCOPY AND CERVICAL BIOPSY

EQUIPMENT/SUPPLIES: Patient gown and drape, vaginal speculum, colposcope, specimen container with preservative (10% formalin), sterile gloves, appropriate size sterile cotton-tipped applicators, sterile normal saline solution, sterile 3% acetic acid, sterile povidone-iodine (Betadine), silver nitrate sticks or ferric subsulfate (Monsel's solution), sterile biopsy forceps or punch biopsy instrument, sterile uterine curet, sterile uterine dressing forceps, sterile 4 × 4 gauze pad, sterile towel, sterile endocervical curet, sterile uterine tenaculum, sanitary napkin, examination gloves, examination light, tissues, biohazard container.

STANDARDS: Given the needed equipment and a place to work, the student will perform this skill with _____% accuracy in a total of _____ minutes. *(Your instructor will tell you what the percentage and time limits will be before you begin practicing.)*

KEY: 4 = Satisfactory   0 = Unsatisfactory   NA = This step is not counted

PROCEDURE STEPS	SELF	PARTNER	INSTRUCTOR
1. Wash your hands.	☐	☐	☐
2. Verify that the patient has signed the consent form.	☐	☐	☐
3. Assemble the equipment and supplies.	☐	☐	☐
4. Check the light on the colposcope.	☐	☐	☐
5. Set up the sterile field without contaminating it.	☐	☐	☐
6. Pour sterile normal saline and acetic acid into their respective sterile containers.	☐	☐	☐
7. Cover the field with a sterile drape.	☐	☐	☐
8. Greet and identify the patient. Explain the procedure.	☐	☐	☐
9. When the physician is ready to proceed with the procedure: **a.** Assist the patient into the dorsal lithotomy position. **b.** Put on sterile gloves after positioning the patient if necessary.	☐	☐	☐
10. Hand the physician: **a.** The applicator immersed in normal saline. **b.** Followed by the applicator immersed in acetic acid. **c.** The applicator with the antiseptic solution (Betadine).	☐	☐	☐
11. If you did not apply sterile gloves to assist the physician: **a.** Apply clean examination gloves. **b.** Accept the biopsy specimen into a container of 10% formalin preservative.	☐	☐	☐
12. Provide the physician with Monsel's solution or silver nitrate sticks.	☐	☐	☐

PROCEDURE STEPS	SELF	PARTNER	INSTRUCTOR

13. When the physician is finished with the procedure:
   a. Assist the patient from the stirrups and into a sitting position.
   b. Explain to the patient that a small amount of bleeding may occur.
   c. Have a sanitary napkin available for the patient.
   d. Ask the patient to get dressed and assist as needed.
   e. Provide for privacy as the patient dresses.
   f. Reinforce any physician instructions regarding follow-up appointments.
   g. Advise the patient on how to obtain the biopsy results.
	☐	☐	☐

14. Label the specimen container with the patient's name and date.
   a. Prepare the laboratory request.
   b. Transport the specimen and form to the laboratory.
	☐	☐	☐

15. Properly care for, or dispose of, equipment and clean the examination room.	☐	☐	☐
16. Wash your hands.	☐	☐	☐
17. Document your responsibilities during the procedure.	☐	☐	☐

CALCULATION

Total Possible Points: _____
Total Points Earned: _____ Multiplied by 100 = _____ Divided by Total Possible Points = _____%

Pass   **Fail**
☐   ☐

Comments:

Student's signature _____ Date _____
Partner's signature _____ Date _____
Instructor's signature _____ Date _____

Work Product 1

Document appropriately.

Jane Kovach is a 28-year-old female on a routine visit. She is scheduled to see Dr. Smith for a pelvic examination and Pap smear. You assist in the procedure, and a sample is collected and sent to the laboratory. Based on the laboratory results, Ms. Kovach is asked to return 1 week later for a colposcopy and cervical biopsy. You also assist in these procedures. If you are currently working in a medical office, use a blank paper patient chart from the office. If this is not available to you, use the lines below. Record the pelvic examination, Pap smear, colposcopy, and cervical biopsy in the chart.

_____

_____

_____

_____

Chapter Self-Assessment Quiz

1. Within 24 hours before a gynecological examination, a patient should avoid:

   a. showering.

   b. using vaginal medication.

   c. taking a home pregnancy test.

   d. performing a breast self-examination.

   e. beginning a new method of contraception.

2. A cesarean section is used to:

   a. diagnose gynecological cancers.

   b. screen the fetus for defects in the neural tube.

   c. analyze fluid from the amniotic sac for nervous system disorders.

   d. deliver an infant when vaginal delivery is not possible or advisable.

   e. stabilize an infant that was delivered before the 37th week of pregnancy.

3. Morning sickness that has escalated to a serious condition is known as:

   a. eclampsia.

   b. endometriosis.

   c. abruptio placentae.

   d. hyperemesis gravidarum.

   e. endometriosis.

4. A pessary may be used to treat:

   a. leiomyomas.

   b. ovarian cysts.

   c. endometriosis.

   d. uterine prolapse.

   e. ectopic pregnancy.

5. The most common sexually transmitted disease in the United States is:

   a. syphilis.

   b. gonorrhea.

   c. chlamydia.

   d. herpes genitalis.

   e. AIDS.

6. Which of the following methods of contraception works hormonally and is worn on the skin for three out of four weeks to prevent ovulation?

   a. Pill

   b. Ring

   c. Patch

   d. Condom

   e. Spermicide

7. Which of the following is a presumptive sign of pregnancy?

　　a. Goodell's sign

　　b. Fetal heart tone

　　c. Nausea and vomiting

　　d. HCG in urine and blood

　　e. Visualization of the fetus

8. A contraction stress test (CST) should be performed in the:

　　a. hospital.

　　b. patient's home.

　　c. obstetrician's office.

　　d. gynecologist's office.

　　e. laboratory.

9. A hysterosalpingography is used to determine:

　　a. the location and severity of cervical lesions.

　　b. whether the patient will abort or miscarry a fetus.

　　c. the presence of abnormal cells associated with cervical cancer.

　　d. the position of the uterus and the patency of the fallopian tubes.

　　e. the presence of sexually transmitted disease.

Scenario: Your patient is a pregnant 32-year-old woman in her 22nd week of gestation. She is complaining of edema, headaches, blurred vision, and vomiting. After laboratory results confirm proteinuria, the physician concludes that the patient has preeclampsia.

10. Which of the following should you advise the patient to increase in her diet?

　　a. Protein

　　b. Sodium

　　c. Calcium

　　d. Folic acid

　　e. Iron

11. What more severe condition could result if her present condition does not improve?

　　a. Epilepsy

　　b. Eclampsia

　　c. Posteclampsia

　　d. Premature labor

　　e. Hyperemesis gravidarum

End Scenario

12. An undiagnosed ectopic pregnancy could lead to:

　　a. polymenorrhea.

　　b. salpingo-oophorectomy.

　　c. herniation of the ovaries.

　　d. displacement of the uterus.

　　e. rupture of the fallopian tube.

13. How should the lochia appear immediately and for up to six days after delivery?

　　a. White

　　b. Red

　　c. Green

　　d. Yellow

　　e. Clear

14. The onset of eclampsia is marked by:

　　a. seizures.

　　b. vomiting.

　　c. hypertension.

　　d. premature labor.

　　e. contractions.

15. A woman who is pregnant for the first time is:

　　a. nulligravida.

　　b. primigravida.

　　c. nullipara.

　　d. primipara.

　　e. multipara.

16. If animal research indicates no fetal risk concerning the use of a medication but no human studies have been completed, the medication can be found in which category of drugs?

　　a. Category A

　　b. Category B

　　c. Category C

　　d. Category D

　　e. Category X

17. The onset of first menses is called:
    a. menarche.
    b. menses.
    c. menorrhagia.
    d. metrorrhagia.
    e. polymenorrhea.

18. Surgery to occlude the vagina is called:
    a. colporrhaphy.
    b. laparoscopy.
    c. ultrasound.
    d. pessary.
    e. colpocleisis.

19. The height of the fundus is determined each visit by:
    a. ultrasound.
    b. blood work.
    c. urinalysis.
    d. fetal heart monitor.
    e. palpation.

20. Elevated AFP levels in a pregnant woman may indicate:
    a. nervous system deformities.
    b. preeclampsia.
    c. hyperemesis gravidarum.
    d. placenta previa.
    e. uterine contractions.

Chapter Checklist

☐ Read textbook chapter and take notes within the Chapter Notes outline. Answer the Learning Objectives as you reach them in the content, and then check them off.

☐ Work the Content Review questions—both Foundational Knowledge and Application.

☐ Perform the Active Learning exercise(s).

☐ Complete Professional Journal entries.

☐ Complete Skill Practice Activity(s) using Competency Evaluation Forms and Work Products, when appropriate.

☐ Take the Chapter Self-Assessment Quiz.

☐ Insert all appropriate pages into your Portfolio.

Learning Objectives

1. Spell and define the key terms.

2. Identify abnormal conditions of the thyroid, pancreas, adrenal, and pituitary glands.

3. Describe the tests commonly used to diagnose disorders of these endocrine system glands.

4. Explain your role in working with patients with endocrine systems disorders.

Chapter Notes

Note: Bold-faced headings are the major headings in the text chapter; headings in regular font are lower-level headings (i.e., the content is subordinate to, or falls "under," the major headings). Make sure you understand the key terms used in the chapter, as well as the concepts presented as Key Points.

TEXT SUBHEADINGS   **NOTES**

Introduction _____

_____

_____

☐ **LEARNING OBJECTIVE 1:** Spell and define the key terms.

_____

Common Disorders of the Respiratory System _____

Key Terms: hormones; endocrinologist
Key Points:
- Endocrine glands secrete **hormones** directly into the bloodstream for transmission rather than having direct access to target tissues.
- Many disorders of the endocrine system result from an over-secretion or under-secretion of **hormones**.

Disorders of the Thyroid _____

Hyperthyroidism _____

Key Terms: Graves disease; thyrotoxicosis; goiter; exophthalmia
Key Point:
- In addition to elevated blood levels of thyroid hormones (T_3 and T_4), the patient may have an enlarged thyroid gland known as a **goiter** and unusual protrusion of the eyeballs known as **exophthalmia**.

Hypothyroidism _____

Key Term: Hashimoto thyroiditis
Key Points:
- Hypothyroidism results from an under-secretion of thyroid hormones, which may be congenital or acquired.
- Treatment of hypothyroidism regardless of the cause is replacement of thyroid hormones, which must be taken by the patient for the remainder of his or her life.

Disorders of the Pancreas _____

Diabetes Mellitus _____

Key Terms: hyperglycemia; glycosuria
Key Point:
- Dysfunction of the islets of Langerhans cells within the pancreas results in diabetes mellitus, a disorder affecting carbohydrate metabolism.

Type I Diabetes Mellitus

Key Terms: insulin-dependent diabetes mellitus; polydipsia; polyuria; polyphagia
Key Point:
- Type I diabetes mellitus is sometimes referred to as **insulin-dependent diabetes mellitus** and occurs most often in children and young adults.

Type II Diabetes Mellitus

Key Terms: non-insulin diabetes mellitus; pruritus
Key Point:
- Type II diabetes mellitus may be referred to as **non-insulin diabetes mellitus**; however, many patients with this condition do require insulin to control elevated blood glucose levels.

Diabetic Emergencies

Key Terms: ketones; ketoacidosis; hypoglycemia

Disorders of the Adrenal Glands

Addison Disease

Key Term: Addison disease
Key Point:
- Hypoadrenocorticalism, or **Addison disease**, results from a deficiency of hormone secretion (mineralocorticoids and glucocorticoids) from the adrenal cortex.

Cushing Syndrome

Key Terms: Cushing syndrome; hyperplasia
Key Point:
- Hyperadrenocorticalism, also known as **Cushing syndrome**, may be caused by **hyperplasia** of the adrenal cortex or a tumor, resulting in an increased production of ACTH from the pituitary.

Disorders of the Pituitary Gland _____

_____

Gigantism and Acromegaly _____

_____

Key Terms: gigantism; acromegaly
Key Point:
- Hyperpituitarism is marked by an excess production of human growth hormone (HGH) secreted from the anterior lobe of the pituitary gland.

Dwarfism _____

_____

Key Term: dwarfism
Key Point:
- Hypopituitarism is a deficiency of the anterior pituitary hormones, which may be caused by injury, atrophy of the gland, or certain types of tumors.

Diabetes Insipidus _____

_____

Key Term: diabetes insipidus
Key Point:
- **Diabetes insipidus** results from a deficiency of antidiuretic hormone (ADH) secreted by the posterior pituitary gland.

☐ **LEARNING OBJECTIVE 2:** Identify abnormal conditions of the thyroid, pancreas, adrenal, and pituitary glands.

Common Diagnostic and Therapeutic Procedures _____

_____

Key Term: radioimmunoassay
Key Points:
- Your assistance with performing or scheduling these laboratory or other diagnostic procedures is important so that treatment may be initiated as quickly as possible.
- The glycohemoglobin, or hemoglobin A1C, blood test may be ordered by the physician to determine how well the blood glucose has been controlled in a patient with Type I or Type II diabetes mellitus during the previous 2 to 3 months.

☐ **LEARNING OBJECTIVE 3:** Describe the tests commonly used to diagnose disorders of these endocrine system glands.

☐ **LEARNING OBJECTIVE 4:** Explain your role in working with patients with endocrine system disorders.

Content
Review

FOUNDATIONAL KNOWLEDGE

Problems with the Endocrine System

1. Fill in the chart below with the names of the results of hyperpituitarism that occur during childhood or adolescence and at the end of puberty or during adulthood.

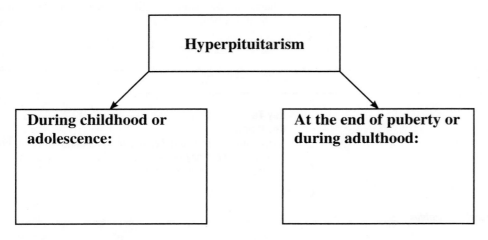

2. When does ketoacidosis occur?

_____

_____

Helping Patients Cope

3. A patient is stunned to learn that she has been diagnosed with type II diabetes mellitus. She is 43 years old and in excellent health. As a personal trainer and nutritionist, she has always taken good care of her body. What potential cause of type II diabetes mellitus might she be overlooking?

_____

_____

4. A patient complains that, lately, his appetite has been ferocious, but he is actually losing weight. He does not understand why this is happening. What do you tell him?

_____

_____

5. Why is it difficult for many sufferers of endocrine disorders to comply with physicians' orders?

_____

_____

6. A patient who has been diagnosed with type II diabetes mellitus explains that a friend told him the disease is sometimes called non-insulin diabetes mellitus. He asks if this means that he will not need to take insulin. Is he correct? Why, or why not?

_____

_____

Insulin and Hormonal Problems

7. Who might be at risk for gestational diabetes mellitus?

_____

_____

8. What is the cause of hypoglycemia?

_____

_____

9. How is Addison disease treated?

_____

_____

Scenario: A young patient appears to be unusually short. The physician has decided to perform tests on her endocrine function.

10. What condition is the physician most likely looking for?

   a. Hyperpituitarism
   b. Hyperadrenocorticalism
   c. Hypopituitarism
   d. Hypoadrenocorticalism

11. The patient is diagnosed with dwarfism, and the patient's mother is extremely distressed, wondering if certain body parts will grow normally while others will not. She also wonders if her daughter could ever grow normally. What could you tell the mother?

_____

_____

End scenario.

12. What do the fasting glucose test and glucose tolerance test for diabetes mellitus have in common?

_____

_____

13. What is the purpose of the A1C blood test?

_____

_____

14. Which deficiency is associated with diabetes insipidus?

   a. Insulin
   b. Blood glucose
   c. Antidiuretic hormone
   d. Human growth hormone

15. Cushing syndrome and Addison disease are both disorders of which gland?

_____

_____

16. Why is it important that patients with diseases of the endocrine system wear a medical alert bracelet or necklace?

_____

_____

17. What hormone is probably excessively present in the blood of a patient with hyperpigmentation?

_____

_____

18. Read the following list of symptoms. Are these symptoms representative of hyperglycemia or hypoglycemia?

Pale complexion
Moist skin
Shallow respirations
Rapid, bounding pulse
Subnormal blood glucose levels

_____

_____

19. Match the following key terms to their definitions.

Key Terms

a. acromegaly _____
b. Addison disease _____
c. Cushing syndrome _____
d. diabetes insipidus _____
e. dwarfism _____
f. endocrinologist _____
g. exophthalmia _____
h. gigantism _____
i. glycosuria _____
j. goiter _____
k. Graves disease _____
l. Hashimoto thyroiditis _____
m. hormones _____
n. hyperglycemia _____
o. hyperplasia _____
p. hypoglycemia _____
q. insulin-dependent diabetes mellitus _____
r. ketoacidosis _____
s. ketones _____
t. non-insulin diabetes mellitus _____
u. polydipsia _____
v. polyphagia _____

Definitions

1. an enlargement of the thyroid gland

2. a substance that is produced by an endocrine gland and travels through the blood to a distant organ or gland where it acts to modify the structure or function of that gland or organ

3. an adrenal gland disorder that results in an increased production of ACTH from the pituitary glands

4. excess quantities of thyroid hormone in tissues

5. excessive proliferation of normal cells in the normal tissue arrangement of an organism

6. the end products of fat metabolism

7. itching

8. pronounced hyperthyroidism with signs of enlarged thyroid and exophthalmos

9. a type of diabetes in which patients do not require insulin to control blood sugar

10. a deficiency in insulin production that leads to an inability to metabolize carbohydrates

11. partial or complete failure of the adrenal cortex functions, causing general physical deterioration

12. the presence of glucose in the urine

13. a disease of the immune system in which the tissue of the thyroid gland is replaced with fibrous tissue

14. excessive thirst

15. abnormal underdevelopment of the body with extreme shortness but normal proportion; achondroplastic dwarfism is an inherited growth disorder characterized by shortened limbs and a large head but almost normal trunk proportions

16. acidosis accompanied by an accumulation of ketones in the body

w. polyuria _____

x. pruritus _____

y. radioimmunoassay _____

z. thyrotoxicosis _____

17. excessive size and stature caused most frequently by hypersecretion of the human growth hormone

18. deficiency of sugar in the blood

19. an unusual protrusion of the eyeballs as a result of a thyroid disorder

20. a disorder of metabolism characterized by polyuria and polydipsia; caused by a deficiency in ADH or an inability of the kidneys to respond to ADH

21. excessive excretion and elimination of urine

22. hyperfunction of the anterior pituitary gland near the end of puberty that results in increased bone width

23. the introduction of radioactive substances in the body to determine the concentration of a substance in the serum, usually the concentration of antigens, antibodies, or proteins

24. a doctor who diagnoses and treats disorders of the endocrine system and its hormone-secreting glands

25. abnormal hunger

26. an increase in blood sugar, as in diabetes mellitus

20. True or False? Determine whether the following statements are true or false. If false, explain why.

a. Endocrine glands are unlike other glands in the body because they are ductless.

_____

_____

b. Hashimoto thyroiditis is a disease of the endocrine system.

_____

_____

c. Type I diabetes mellitus occurs only in children and young adults.

_____

_____

d. Addison disease has no effect on the pituitary gland.

_____

_____

APPLICATION

Critical Thinking Practice

1. A patient is worried that a thyroid functions test requires the use of radioactive material. Explain, to the best of your ability, how the test works and why there is no need to be concerned about radiation. If necessary, do additional research on thyroid functions tests to prepare your answer.

_____

_____

2. After an examination, a pregnant patient asks why the physician performed a test on her blood glucose level. She says she does not have diabetes. Explain why the physician chose to do the test.

_____

_____

Patient Education

1. Write out an exercise regimen for a 60-year-old who has just been diagnosed with type II diabetes mellitus.

_____

_____

Documentation

1. Now, write a narrative note describing the regimen and your explanation to the patient from the question above to be included in the patient's chart.

_____

_____

Active Learning

1. A variety of antidiabetic drugs exist. Select one and research its intended effects. Explain how it can be used to manage a patient's diabetes and its role in a diabetes management program.

2. Make a list of common foods for a diabetes sufferer to avoid. Then create a poster to display in the office highlighting your findings. Be sure to stress the importance of proper nutrition.

3. Glucose meters have changed a great deal over the last decade. Research these improvements and assess ways in which they could be further improved. Draw up plans for the ideal glucose meter that would be the most patient-friendly. Then create a presentation for your new model.

Professional Journal

REFLECT

(Prompts and Ideas: Do you know someone who suffers/suffered from diabetes? How is life different for that person on a daily basis?)

_____

_____

_____

_____

_____

_____

_____

PONDER AND SOLVE

1. Young children are sometimes afflicted with diabetes mellitus. This can be difficult for both the child and the family. What is your perspective of the medical assistant's role in this situation?

_____

_____

_____

_____

_____

_____

_____

2. A patient with hyperthyroidism says she would prefer not to be treated because she has few negative symptoms, and the increased metabolic rate helps keep her thin. How would you respond to this?

_____

_____

_____

_____

_____

_____

_____

_____

EXPERIENCE

Skills related to this chapter include:

1. Manage a Patient with a Diabetic Emergency (Procedure 36-1).

Record any common mistakes, lessons learned, and/or tips you discovered during your experience of practicing and demonstrating these skills:

_____

_____

_____

_____

_____

_____

_____

Skill Practice

PERFORMANCE OBJECTIVES:

1. Manage a patient with a diabetic emergency (Procedure 36-1).

Name _____ Date _____ Time _____

Procedure 36-1:	**MANAGE A PATIENT WITH A DIABETIC EMERGENCY**

EQUIPMENT/SUPPLIES: Gloves, blood glucose monitor and strips, fruit juice or oral glucose tablets

STANDARDS: Given the needed equipment and a place to work, the student will perform this skill with _____% accuracy in a total of _____ minutes. *(Your instructor will tell you what the percentage and time limits will be before you begin practicing.)*

KEY: 4 = Satisfactory   0 = Unsatisfactory   NA = This step is not counted

PROCEDURE STEPS	SELF	PARTNER	INSTRUCTOR
1. Wash your hands.	☐	☐	☐
2. Recognize the signs and symptoms of hyperglycemia and hypoglycemia.	☐	☐	☐
3. Identify the patient and escort him/her into the examination room.	☐	☐	☐
4. Determine if the patient has been previously diagnosed with diabetes mellitus.	☐	☐	☐
5. Ask the patient if he or she has eaten today or taken any medication.	☐	☐	☐
6. Notify the physician about the patient and perform a capillary stick for a blood glucose as directed.	☐	☐	☐
7. Notify the physician with the results of the blood glucose and treat the patient as ordered by the physician. **a.** Administer insulin subcutaneously to a patient with hyperglycemia. **b.** Administer a quick-acting sugar, such as an oral glucose tablet or fruit juice, for a patient with hypoglycemia.	☐	☐	☐
8. Be prepared to notify EMS as directed by the physician if the symptoms do not improve or worsen.	☐	☐	☐
9. Document any observations and treatments given.	☐	☐	☐

CALCULATION

Total Possible Points: _____
Total Points Earned: _____ Multiplied by 100 = _____ Divided by Total Possible Points = _____%

Pass   **Fail**
☐   ☐   Comments:

Student's signature _____ Date _____
Partner's signature _____ Date _____
Instructor's signature _____ Date _____

Work Product 1

Document appropriately.

John Suiker is an athletic 38-year-old male scheduled for a routine visit. He arrives disoriented and appears to be drunk and unsteady on his feet. He presents with pale and moist skin, rapid bounding pulse, and shallow breathing. You notify the physician, Dr. Burns, of the patient's condition and she orders an immediate blood glucose test. The patient's blood glucose is 48 mg/dL. The patient is still conscious, so you provide him with fruit juice, which he accepts. Recovery is immediate.

If you are currently working in a medical office, use a blank paper patient chart from the office. If this is not available to you, use the space below to record the incident in the chart.

_____

_____

_____

_____

Chapter Self-Assessment Quiz

1. A patient with hypothyroidism must take hormone replacements:
   a. for as many years as he has had the disease.
   b. until the conclusion of puberty.
   c. for his entire life.
   d. until middle age.
   e. for 10 years.

2. Diabetics often need supplemental insulin to:
   a. test blood glucose levels.
   b. reverse vascular changes.
   c. reduce the presence of ketones.
   d. restore pancreatic function.
   e. control blood glucose levels.

3. One symptom of ketoacidosis is:
   a. shallow respirations.
   b. low blood glucose levels.
   c. overhydration.
   d. abdominal pain.
   e. pale, moist skin.

4. Diabetes mellitus affects metabolism of which type of molecule?
   a. Neurotransmitters
   b. Carbohydrates
   c. Hormones
   d. Vitamins
   e. Lipids

5. One symptom of type 1 diabetes mellitus is:
   a. excessive urination.
   b. extreme fatigue.
   c. loss of appetite.
   d. weight gain.
   e. a goiter.

6. Hyperpigmentation of the skin might be an indication of:
   a. Cushing syndrome.
   b. Hashimoto thyroiditis.
   c. Graves disease.
   d. Addison disease.
   e. diabetes insipidus.

7. To control gestational diabetes, a blood glucose specimen should be taken from a pregnant woman between:
   a. 28 and 32 weeks of gestation.
   b. 24 and 28 weeks of gestation.
   c. 20 and 24 weeks of gestation.
   d. 16 and 20 weeks of gestation.
   e. 12 and 16 weeks of gestation.

8. Cushing syndrome sufferers may experience accelerated:
   a. Addison disease.
   b. endocarditis.
   c. osteoporosis.
   d. arthritis.
   e. dementia.

9. Acromegaly results primarily in:
   a. an increase in bone width.
   b. muscular atrophy.
   c. an increase in bone length.
   d. muscular hypertrophy.
   e. an increase in bone density.

10. Growth can be stimulated for children with dwarfism by:
    a. repairs in the pituitary gland.
    b. administration of growth hormone.
    c. psychotherapy.
    d. increased physical activity.
    e. a high-protein diet.

11. Diabetes inspidus results from a deficiency of:
    a. adrenocorticotropic hormone.
    b. anterior pituitary hormones.
    c. human growth hormone.
    d. antidiuretic hormone.
    e. thyroid hormones.

12. Insulin shock could be a result of:
    a. Cushing syndrome.
    b. Addison disease.
    c. Graves disease.
    d. hyperglycemia.
    e. hypoglycemia.

13. Diabetes mellitus patients need to care for their feet because:
    a. they regularly develop skin problems.
    b. their peripheral circulation may be poor.
    c. they suffer severe joint pain.
    d. they have weak calves.
    e. foot pain occurs.

14. Exophthalmia is a protrusion of the:
    a. thyroid gland.
    b. pancreas.
    c. gall bladder.
    d. eyeballs.
    e. liver.

15. Patients taking corticosteroids may be at risk for:
    a. Cushing disease.
    b. Addison disease.
    c. type II diabetes mellitus.
    d. Graves disease.
    e. Hashimoto thyroiditis.

16. The A1C test determines how well blood glucose has been controlled during the previous:
    a. 2 to 3 hours.
    b. 2 to 3 days.
    c. 2 to 3 weeks.
    d. 2 to 3 months.
    e. 2 to 3 years.

17. Gigantism is a disorder of the:
    a. adrenal glands.
    b. pancreas.
    c. liver.
    d. thyroid.
    e. pituitary gland.

18. A thyroid scan relies on a radioactive isotope of what element?
    a. Iodine
    b. Barium
    c. Indium
    d. Bismuth
    e. Iridium

19. Addison disease is a disorder of the:
    a. pituitary gland.
    b. pancreas.
    c. thyroid.
    d. adrenal gland.
    e. salivary glands.

20. Both Graves disease and goiters are examples of:
    a. hypothyroidism.
    b. hypoglycemia.
    c. hyperthyroidism.
    d. hyperglycemia.
    e. hypertension.

CHAPTER

37 Pediatrics

Chapter Checklist

- ☐ Read textbook chapter and take notes within the Chapter Notes outline. Answer the Learning Objectives as you reach them in the content, and then check them off.
- ☐ Work the Content Review questions—both Foundational Knowledge and Application.
- ☐ Perform the Active Learning exercise(s).

- ☐ Complete Professional Journal entries.
- ☐ Complete Skill Practice Activity(s) using Competency Evaluation Forms and Work Products, when appropriate.
- ☐ Take the Chapter Self-Assessment Quiz.
- ☐ Insert all appropriate pages into your Portfolio.

Learning Objectives

1. Spell and define the key terms.
2. List safety precautions for the pediatric office.
3. List types and schedule of immunizations.
4. Explain the difference between a well-child and a sick-child visit.
5. Describe the types of feelings a child might have during an office visit.
6. Describe the role of the parent during the office visit.

7. List and explain how to record the anthropometric measurements obtained in a pediatric visit.
8. Identify two injection sites to use on an infant and two used on a child.
9. List the names, symptoms, and treatment for common pediatric illnesses.

Chapter Notes

Note: Bold-faced headings are the major headings in the text chapter; headings in regular font are lower-level headings (i.e., the content is subordinate to, or falls "under," the major headings). Make sure you understand the key terms used in the chapter, as well as the concepts presented as Key Points.

TEXT SUBHEADINGS   **NOTES**

Introduction _____

_____

_____

☐ **LEARNING OBJECTIVE 1:** Spell and define the key terms.

_____

The Pediatric Practice

Key Terms: psychosocial; congenital anomalies; pediatrician; neonatologist
Key Point:
• Pediatrics is the medical specialty devoted to the care of infants, children, and adolescents.

Safety

Key Points:
• Safety should be a prime concern for choosing toys and equipment for a pediatric office.
• Keep all medical equipment out of a child's reach, and never leave a young child alone in the examining room.

☐ **LEARNING OBJECTIVE 2:** List safety precautions for the pediatric office.

Types of Pediatric Office Visits

The Well-Child Office Visit

Key Terms: well-child visit; immunizations
Key Points:
• **Well-child visits** are regularly scheduled office visits whose goal is to maintain the child's optimum health.
• In addition to the reflexes, the physician observes for development appropriate for the age of the infant or child.
• Immunization schedules are developed by the American Academy of Pediatrics (AAP) and the Centers for Disease Control and Prevention, and they change periodically as new vaccines become available.
• If you are responsible for administering vaccines, you must read all package inserts and become familiar with the correct administration and possible adverse effects before administering the medication.

☐ **LEARNING OBJECTIVE 3:** List types and schedule of immunizations.

The Sick-Child Office Visit

Key Term: sick-child visit
Key Point:
- A **sick-child visit** occurs whenever an infant or child requires medical treatment for signs or symptoms of illness or injury.

☐ **LEARNING OBJECTIVE 4:** Explain the difference between a well-child and a sick-child visit.

Child Development

Psychological Aspects of Care

Key Points:
- Understanding a child's psychological needs and development helps you provide safe and effective care.
- As a professional medical assistant, you can reassure patients and family members by demonstrating your understanding of the child's feelings and displaying a kind and gentle manner.

Physiological Aspects of Care

Key Points:
- To anticipate age-appropriate behavior and to provide proper psychological support and physical care, you must have a broad knowledge of child growth and development patterns.
- During regular visits to the pediatrician, the infant is tested for infantile automatisms—reflexes found in the newborn that disappear later in childhood.

☐ **LEARNING OBJECTIVE 5:** Describe the types of feelings a child might have during an office visit.

Role of the Parent

Key Terms: restrain; autonomous
Key Point:
- Encourage parents to remain with young children and to assist in care when appropriate.

☐ **LEARNING OBJECTIVE 6:** Describe the role of the parent during the office visit.

The Pediatric Physical Examination

Key Point:
• Involve the parents as much as possible during the examination and keep them in the infant or child's view to reduce anxiety for both the patient and the parent.

The Pediatric History

Key Point:
• During the early years, it is important to know the prenatal history including details of the mother's pregnancy, labor, and delivery.

Obtaining and Recording Measurements and Vital Signs

Key Point:
• Weight is the most frequently obtained measurement in pediatrics, often needed by the physician to assess nutritional status and determine medication dosages.

☐ **LEARNING OBJECTIVE 7:** List and explain how to record the anthropometric measurements obtained in a pediatric visit.

Pediatric Vital Signs

Temperature

Key Point:
• A child's temperature may be measured by the axillary, oral, rectal, tympanic, or temporal artery method.

Pulse and Respirations _____

_____

Key Points:
- The pulse of children under 2 years of age should be assessed apically.
- Expect the child's heart rate to be considerably higher than an adult's.
- Because infants breathe using the abdominal muscles more than the chest, observe abdominal movements and count for 1 full minute.

Blood Pressure _____

_____

Key Point:
- Because of their soft, nonresistant vessels and smaller bodies, children have lower blood pressure than adults.

Administering Medications _____

_____

Key Point:
- To prevent errors, always check drug dosage calculations for an infant or child with another staff member.

Oral Medications _____

_____

Key Term: aspiration
Key Point:
- Many children will suck medication from a syringe easily and safely.

Injections _____

_____

Key Point:
- Although it is important for the child to know that an injection is about to be given, you can prevent some anxiety by not letting the child see the syringe.

☐ **LEARNING OBJECTIVE 8:** Identify two injection sites to use on an infant and two used on a child.

Collecting a Urine Specimen

Key Point:
• Because infants and small children cannot void into a specimen container on command, if a urine specimen is needed, you must use a collection device.

Understanding Child Abuse

Key Points:
• Abuse is thought to be the second most common cause of death in children under age 5 years.

Pediatric Illnesses and Disorders

Key Points:
• Because children do not have a well-developed immune system, they are particularly susceptible to viruses and bacterial infections.
• All parents should be advised never to give aspirin to young children with a viral fever, since aspirin has been associated with Reye syndrome.

Impetigo

Key Point:
• A common skin disorder in children is impetigo, a contagious bacterial infection that may be caused by either the Staphylococcus or Streptococcus bacteria.

Meningitis

Key Point:
• Inflammation of the meninges covering the spinal cord and the brain, meningitis can result from either a bacterial or a viral infection.

Encephalitis _____

_____

Key Point:
- Encephalitis is inflammation of the brain that frequently results from a viral infection following chicken pox, measles, or mumps.

Tetanus _____

_____

Key Point:
- Tetanus, commonly called lockjaw, is an infection of nervous tissue caused by the tetanus bacillus, *Clostridium tetani*, which lives in the intestinal tract of animals and is excreted in their feces.

Cerebral Palsy _____

_____

Key Point:
- Cerebral palsy is a term for a group of neuromuscular disorders that result from central nervous system damage sustained during the prenatal, neonatal, or postnatal period of development.

Croup _____

_____

Key Point:
- This disease is caused by a viral infection of the larynx resulting in swelling and narrowing of the airway.

Epiglottitis _____

_____

Key Point:
- A child diagnosed with epiglottitis in the medical office must be transported immediately to the hospital, since the first priority is maintaining and possibly establishing an airway.

Cystic Fibrosis

Key Points:

- Cystic fibrosis is an inherited disease that affects the exocrine glands of the body, changing their secretions and making the mucus extremely thick and sticky.
- Children with this disease are prone to repeated respiratory infections because of the difficulty in clearing the mucus from their airways.

Asthma

Key Point:

- In children, asthma attacks may be triggered by exposure to an allergen in the environment such as mold or dust, an inhaled irritant such as cigarette smoke, or upper respiratory infection.

Otitis Media

Key Point:

- Otitis media, an inflammation or infection of the middle ear, is frequently caused by an upper respiratory infection (URI) in infants and children.

Tonsillitis

Key Point:

- Pharyngitis, or a sore throat, may be caused by inflammation of the tissues of the throat and/or the tonsils.

Obesity

Key Points:

- According to the American Academy of Pediatrics (AAP), obesity in children has become an epidemic.
- Since children develop eating habits early in life and take these habits into adulthood, you should teach parents about eating in moderation and increasing physical activity as a means to reduce the weight of an overweight child or prevent abnormal gains in weight.

Attention Deficit Hyperactivity Disorder _____

Key Points:
- Attention deficit hyperactivity disorder (ADHD) is a condition of the brain affecting boys more frequently than girls and causing difficulty in controlling behavior.
- In addition to inattention and hyperactivity, children with ADHD are often impulsive and behave irrationally to others, even after being repeatedly warned about a specific behavior, dangerous or not.

☐ **LEARNING OBJECTIVE 9:** List the names, symptoms, and treatment for common pediatric illnesses.

Content Review

FOUNDATIONAL KNOWLEDGE

Safety First

1. Decide if the following statements are true or false. If false, rewrite the statement so that it accurately reflects the proper procedures for a pediatric waiting room and examination room.

   a. It's common practice to leave a child alone in the examination room when talking with his or her parents.

   _____

   b. Infant scales should always be placed on the floor next to the adult scale.

   _____

   c. It is a violation of HIPAA to have two separate waiting rooms for sick children and well children.

   _____

   d. There should be no toys in the waiting room because they may help spread germs.

   _____

   e. Children outgrow child-sized furniture too quickly, so it is not a worthwhile investment.

   _____

   f. Many childhood diseases are highly contagious and can be controlled by stringent handwashing measures.

   _____

2. What does the Federal Child Abuse Prevention and Treatment Act mandate?

   _____

   _____

Immunizations

3. Review the immunization schedule in your textbook. Then answer the questions below.

   a. How many doses of the rotavirus vaccine are given? When?

   _____

b. How many immunizations do children receive at four months? Which ones?

_____

c. When do children start receiving a yearly influenza vaccination?

_____

d. How many doses of the hepatitis B vaccine are administered?

_____

4. What is the VIS? Why do you give the parent or caregiver of a child a copy?

_____

_____

Well Child or Sick Child?

5. Why do sick-child visits occur frequently during early childhood?

_____

_____

6. What is the difference between a well-child and a sick-child visit?

_____

_____

7. Complete the chart below with information about childhood reflexes. Briefly describe each response and note the age it generally disappears.

Reflex	Response	Age When It Generally Disappears
a. Sucking or rooting		
b. Moro or startle		
c. Grasp		
d. Tonic neck or fencing		
e. Placing or stepping		
f. Babinski		

Feelings

8. List five feelings a child might have during an office visit.

a. _____

b. _____

c. _____

d. _____

e. _____

Mom and Dad Are Here, Too

9. What role does a parent or caregiver play in the child's exam?

_____

_____

All the Right Signs

10. What are the five different ways to test a child's temperature?

a. _____

b. _____

c. _____

d. _____

e. _____

11. Match each pulse-rate range with the appropriate age.

Age	Rate/Minute
a. newborn _____	**1.** 80–150
b. 3 months to 2 years _____	**2.** 60–100
c. 2 years to 10 years _____	**3.** 100–180
d. 10 years and older _____	**4.** 65–130

Injections and Medication

12. Fill in the boxes with one injection site used on an infant and one used on a child.

a. Injection site for infant	
b. Injection site for child over age of two years	

13. How is a child's medication dosage calculated?

_____

_____

14. What are the seven "rights" of drug administration?

a. _____

b. _____

c. _____

c. _____

e. _____

f. _____

g. _____

Common Childhood Illnesses

15. Why is epiglottitis considered more serious than croup?

_____

_____

16. Fill in the web with six symptoms of meningitis.

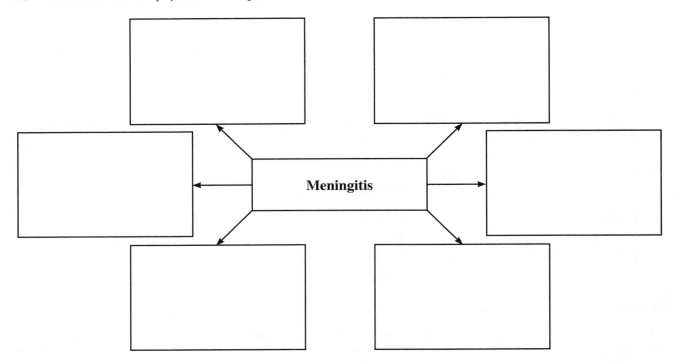

17. If a child has been reported as being easily distracted, forgetful, extremely talkative, impulsive, and showing a dislike for school activities, does the child have ADHD?

_____

_____

18. A worried mother calls in because her newborn baby is vomiting. She wants to know if she should bring her baby into the office for examination. What do you tell her?

_____

_____

19. Match the following key terms to their definitions.

Key Terms

a. aspiration _____

b. autonomous _____

c. congenital anomaly _____

d. immunization _____

e. neonatologist _____

f. pediatrician _____

g. pediatrics _____

h. psychosocial _____

Definitions

1. to control or confine movement

2. a physician who specializes in the care and treatment of newborns

3. a viral infection manifested by the characteristic rash of successive crops of vesicles that scab before resolution; also called chicken pox

4. a physician who specializes in the care of infants, children, and adolescents

5. a visit to the medical office for the administration of immunizations and evaluation of growth and development

6. drawing in or out by suction, as in breathing objects into the respiratory tract or suctioning substances from a site

i. restrain _____

j. sick-child visit _____

k. varicella zoster _____

l. well-child visit _____

7. an abnormality, either structural or functional, present at birth

8. a pediatric visit for the treatment of illness or injury

9. a specialty of medicine that deals with the care of infants, children, and adolescents

10. existing or functioning independently

11. relating to mental and emotional aspects of social encounters

12. the act or process of rendering an individual immune to specific disease

20. True or False? Determine whether the following statements are true or false. If false, explain why.

a. Immunization schedules change every 5 years.

_____

b. A child's heartbeat is much slower than an adult's heart rate.

_____

c. Asthma is a respiratory problem that usually develops after puberty.

_____

d. Minors do not need to be informed of what you're going to do.

_____

APPLICATION

Critical Thinking Practice

1. A mother calls in, saying her 15-month-old daughter has been fussy and tugging at her ear. There is no fever, but the girl has been tired and had a cold a few days before. What do you tell her to do?

_____

_____

2. A young boy, accompanied by his mother, greets you in the examination room and starts asking all kinds of questions about things you do. He enjoys helping you test his reflexes and reading the vision chart, but he firmly refuses to cooperate when you try to give him a shot. What can you or his mother do to get him settled down enough to give him the shot?

_____

_____

Patient Education

1. A 16-year-old boy has been diagnosed as obese, and his parents have come in to find out what they can do to help their son achieve a healthy weight. The physician wants the boy to exercise at a local gym and to return in 6 months to check his progress. Write instructions that will help the boy and his parents start a healthier lifestyle.

_____

_____

Documentation

1. How would you document the above scenario on the boy's chart? Be sure to document the interaction, as well as the education that was provided during his visit and any scheduled follow-up appointments.

_____

_____

Active Learning

1. The physician has asked that you make a poster for the waiting room that shows important hygienic tips for children, such as washing hands, covering the mouth while sneezing, etc. Come up with a list of five hygienic tips that could be illustrated and design the poster. Use clip art and images so that children who are too young to read can understand the concepts being displayed.

2. Sometimes books are a great way to help a child relax and to educate them at the same time. Look online or go to a local library to find a book that deals with going to the doctor's office or health in general. Share it with the class and discuss the age range you might read this to, and why.

3. The pediatric waiting room should have a variety of toys, magazines, and books for all of the children seen in a practice, from babies through teenagers. Create a plan for appropriate waiting room supplies to satisfy the variety of children seen at a practice. Look online, in catalogues, and in stores for toys and books that might be good for a safe and friendly environment. Next, create a chart of ten books, five toys, and five magazines that you would like to include. Include information about which age group could use each item, the estimated cost for each item, and why you think that it is important to include each item.

Professional Journal

REFLECT

(Prompts and Ideas: It's natural for children to occasionally be frightened by the doctor's office. Do you remember a doctor's visit from your childhood that was particularly frightening or stressful? How was the situation taken care of? How would you address a similar situation if it arose?)

_____

_____

_____

_____

_____

PONDER AND SOLVE

1. A young child has come in with a broken arm. During the examination, you notice the child also has several scrapes and bruises on his legs and feet as well. His mother says he got them from playing outdoors. Do you report this as child abuse to the physician? If not, what do you do?

_____

_____

_____

_____

_____

2. Spanking children for misbehaving is sometimes considered child abuse. However, the parents who spank their children say that they were spanked when they were young, and they believe it is the best way to safely punish bad behavior. They also say that children who are not spanked become spoiled and difficult to control. What do you think? Is it your duty to report spanking as child abuse?

_____

_____

_____

_____

_____

_____

_____

EXPERIENCE

Skills related to this chapter include:

1. Obtain an Infant's Length and Weight (Procedure 37-1).
2. Obtain the Head and Chest Circumference (Procedure 37-2).
3. Apply a Urinary Collection Device (Procedure 37-3).

Record any common mistakes, lessons learned, and/or tips you discovered during your experience of practicing and demonstrating these skills.

_____

_____

_____

_____

_____

_____

_____

Skill Practice

PERFORMANCE OBJECTIVES:

1. Obtain an infant's length and weight (Procedure 37-1).
2. Obtain the head and chest circumference (Procedure 37-2).
3. Apply a urinary collection device (Procedure 37-3).

Name _____ Date _____ Time _____

Procedure 37-1:	OBTAIN AN INFANT'S LENGTH AND WEIGHT

EQUIPMENT/SUPPLIES: Examining table with clean paper, tape measure, infant scale, protective paper for the scale, appropriate growth chart

STANDARDS: Given the needed equipment and a place to work, the student will perform this skill with _____% accuracy in a total of _____ minutes. *(Your instructor will tell you what the percentage and time limits will be before you begin practicing.)*

KEY: 4 = Satisfactory   0 = Unsatisfactory   NA = This step is not counted

PROCEDURE STEPS	SELF	PARTNER	INSTRUCTOR
1. Wash your hands.	☐	☐	☐
2. Explain the procedure to the parent. Ask parent to remove the infant's clothing except for the diaper.	☐	☐	☐
3. Place the child on a firm examination table covered with clean table paper.	☐	☐	☐
4. Fully extend the child's body by holding the head in the midline.	☐	☐	☐
5. Grasp the knees and press flat onto the table gently but firmly.	☐	☐	☐
6. Make a mark on table paper with pen at the top of the head and heel of the feet.	☐	☐	☐
7. Measure between marks in either inches or centimeters.	☐	☐	☐
8. Record the child's length on the growth chart and in the patient's chart.	☐	☐	☐
9. Either carry the infant or have the parent carry the infant to the scale.	☐	☐	☐
10. Place a protective paper on the scale and balance the scale.	☐	☐	☐
11. Remove the diaper just before laying the infant on the scale.	☐	☐	☐
12. Place the child gently on the scale. Keep one of your hands over or near the child on the scale at all times.	☐	☐	☐
13. Balance the scale quickly but carefully.	☐	☐	☐
14. Pick infant up and instruct the parent to replace the diaper if removed.	☐	☐	☐
15. Record the infant's weight on the growth chart and in the patient chart.	☐	☐	☐
16. Wash your hands.	☐	☐	☐

CALCULATION

Total Possible Points: _____

Total Points Earned: _____ Multiplied by 100 = _____ Divided by Total Possible Points = _____%

Pass **Fail**

☐   ☐   Comments:

Student's signature _____ Date _____

Partner's signature _____ Date _____

Instructor's signature _____ Date _____

Name _____ Date _____ Time _____

Procedure 37-2: OBTAIN THE HEAD AND CHEST CIRCUMFERENCE

EQUIPMENT/SUPPLIES: Paper or cloth measuring tape, growth chart

STANDARDS: Given the needed equipment and a place to work, the student will perform this skill with _____% accuracy in a total of _____ minutes. *(Your instructor will tell you what the percentage and time limits will be before you begin practicing.)*

KEY: 4 = Satisfactory   0 = Unsatisfactory   NA = This step is not counted

PROCEDURE STEPS	SELF	PARTNER	INSTRUCTOR
1. Wash your hands.	☐	☐	☐
2. Place the infant in the supine position on the examination table or ask the parent to hold.	☐	☐	☐
3. Measure around the head above the eyebrow and posteriorly at the largest part of the occiput.	☐	☐	☐
4. Record the child's head circumference on the growth chart.	☐	☐	☐
5. With clothing removed from chest, measure around the chest at the nipple line, keeping the measuring tape at the same level anteriorly and posteriorly.	☐	☐	☐
6. Record the child's chest circumference on the growth chart.	☐	☐	☐
7. Wash your hands.	☐	☐	☐

CALCULATION

Total Possible Points: _____
Total Points Earned: _____ Multiplied by 100 = _____ Divided by Total Possible Points = _____%

Pass   **Fail**
☐   ☐   Comments:

Student's signature _____ Date _____
Partner's signature _____ Date _____
Instructor's signature _____ Date _____

Name_____ Date _____ Time _____

Procedure 37-3:	**APPLY A URINARY COLLECTION DEVICE**

EQUIPMENT/SUPPLIES: Gloves, personal antiseptic wipes, pediatric urine collection bag, completed laboratory request slip, biohazard transport container

STANDARDS: Given the needed equipment and a place to work, the student will perform this skill with _____% accuracy in a total of _____ minutes. *(Your instructor will tell you what the percentage and time limits will be before you begin practicing.)*

KEY: 4 = Satisfactory   0 = Unsatisfactory   NA = This step is not counted

PROCEDURE STEPS	SELF	PARTNER	INSTRUCTOR
1. Wash your hands and assemble the equipment and supplies.	☐	☐	☐
2. Explain the procedure to the child's parents.	☐	☐	☐
3. Place the child in a supine position. Ask for help from the parents as needed.	☐	☐	☐
4. After putting on gloves, clean the genitalia with the antiseptic wipes: **a.** For females: (1) Cleanse front to back with separate wipes for each downward stroke on the outer labia. (2) The last clean wipe should be used between the inner labia. **b.** For males: (1) Retract the foreskin if the baby has not been circumcised. (2) Cleanse the meatus in an ever-widening circle. (3) Discard the wipe and repeat the procedure. (4) Return the foreskin to its proper position.	☐	☐	☐
5. Holding the collection device: **a.** Remove the upper portion of the paper backing and press it around the mons pubis. **b.** Remove the second section and press it against the perineum. **c.** Loosely attach the diaper.	☐	☐	☐
6. Give the baby fluids unless contraindicated and check the diaper frequently.	☐	☐	☐
7. When the child has voided, remove the device, clean the skin of residual adhesive, and rediaper.	☐	☐	☐
8. Prepare the specimen for transport to the laboratory.	☐	☐	☐
9. Remove your gloves and wash your hands.	☐	☐	☐
10. Record the procedure.	☐	☐	☐

CALCULATION

Total Possible Points: _____
Total Points Earned: _____ Multiplied by 100 = _____ Divided by Total Possible Points = _____%

Pass   **Fail**

☐   ☐   Comments:

Student's signature _____ Date _____
Partner's signature _____ Date _____
Instructor's signature _____ Date _____

Work Product 1

Document appropriately.

Rose Ryan is a 24-month-old girl visiting your office for a well-child visit. The physician directs you to obtain her length, weight, and head and chest circumference. You find the child measures 92 cm tall and weighs 15 kg. Her head circumference is 50 cm and her chest circumference is 52 cm. Document these procedures. If you are currently working in a medical office, use a blank paper patient chart from the office. If this is not available to you, use the space below to record the procedure in the chart.

_____

_____

_____

Chapter Self-Assessment Quiz

1. The top priority in a pediatrics office is:
   a. organization.
   b. safety.
   c. efficiency.
   d. location.
   e. size.

2. In a pediatrician's waiting room, it's most important that the toys are:
   a. trendy.
   b. interesting to all age groups.
   c. large enough to share.
   d. washable.
   e. educational.

3. Which method of taking a temperature is most readily accepted by children of all ages?
   a. Axillary
   b. Oral
   c. Rectal
   d. Tympanic
   e. Touch

4. One symptom of meningitis is:
   a. dysuria.
   b. disorientation.
   c. coughing.
   d. stiff neck.
   e. chills.

5. Which of the following has been associated with Reye syndrome?
   a. Pyloric stenosis
   b. Aspirin
   c. Cerebral palsy
   d. Phenylalanine hydroxylase
   e. Otitis media

6. Which of the following is something that is routinely done at a child's wellness exam?
   a. Blood test
   b. Urine test
   c. Immunization
   d. Radiography
   e. Measurements

7. To minimize a child's anxiety during a visit, you should:
   a. avoid talking to the child.
   b. speak directly to the parent.
   c. be gentle but firm.
   d. ask the child to be quiet.
   e. spend as little time in the room as possible.

8. Which of the following statements is true?
   a. The reflexes an infant has disappear by three months of age.
   b. A pediatrician is responsible for a child's physical and mental health.
   c. Disinfectants should be kept in patient rooms on high shelves.
   d. Vaccination Information Statements may be provided upon request.
   e. The DDST measures all physical and mental aspects of a child.

9. One warning sign of child abuse is a child who:

    a. comes in with scraped knees.

    b. shrinks away as you approach.

    c. has a poor growth pattern.

    d. has a bloody nose.

    e. screams when you administer a shot.

10. What might make the examination more fun for a 4- or 5-year-old child?

    a. Allowing the child to crawl on the floor

    b. Answering all the questions he or she asks

    c. Showing the child medical pictures

    d. Letting the child listen to his or her heartbeat

    e. Asking the parent to assist with the exam

Scenario: A child comes in for a well-child visit and begins to panic when she hears she will need to get a vaccination.

11. What should you do?

    a. Let another assistant give her the shot.

    b. Ask the parent or caregiver to calm her down.

    c. Show her the needle ahead of time.

    d. Tell her gently that it won't hurt at all.

    e. Hide the needle until you give her the shot.

12. After you administer the medication, the girl becomes sullen and withdrawn. What is the best way to address this behavior?

    a. Leave and allow her mother to comfort her.

    b. Praise and comfort her before you leave.

    c. Ask her if the shot was really that bad.

    d. Promise it won't hurt so much next time.

    e. Laugh and say it was just a little shot.

End Scenario

13. Which of the following disorders has symptoms that may become obvious only with the passage of time?

    a. Meningitis

    b. Croup

    c. Epiglottitis

    d. Cerebral palsy

    e. Pyloric stenosis

14. Children are more likely to develop ear infections than adults because they have:

    a. an immature nervous system.

    b. short and straight Eustachian tubes.

    c. decreased resistance to diseases.

    d. more exposure to bacteria.

    e. poor handwashing skills.

15. Which infant reflex is a result of the cheek being stroked?

    a. Rooting

    b. Moro

    c. Stepping

    d. Fencing

    e. Babinski

16. Children have lower blood pressure than adults because:

    a. they cannot sit still for long periods of time.

    b. they require a smaller cuff for measurements.

    c. their heart does not pump as quickly as adults' hearts.

    d. their vessels are softer and less resistant.

    e. you must use a standard sphygmomanometer.

17. At what age does a child's respiratory rate slow to that of an adult's?

    a. 0–1 year

    b. 1–5 years

    c. 5–10 years

    d. 10–15 years

    e. 15–20 years

18. Which of the following can help a physician test an infant for pyloric stenosis?

    a. Blood tests

    b. Urine tests

    c. Parental history

    d. Percentile comparisons

    e. Weight

19. Which of the following disorders cannot be cured at this time?

    a. Meningitis

    b. Impetigo

    c. Tetanus

    d. Cystic fibrosis

    e. Cerebral palsy

20. A sharp barking cough is a symptom of:

    a. meningitis.

    b. croup.

    c. tetanus.

    d. encephalitis.

    e. impetigo.

Geriatrics

☐ Read textbook chapter and take notes within the Chapter Notes outline. Answer the Learning Objectives as you reach them in the content, and then check them off.

☐ Work the Content Review questions—both Foundational Knowledge and Application.

☐ Perform the Active Learning exercise(s).

☐ Complete Professional Journal entries.

☐ Complete Skill Practice Activity(s) using Competency Evaluation Forms and Work Products, when appropriate.

☐ Take the Chapter Self-Assessment Quiz.

☐ Insert all appropriate pages into your Portfolio.

1. Spell and define the key terms.
2. Explain how aging affects thought processes.
3. Describe methods to increase compliance with health maintenance programs among the elderly.
4. Discuss communication problems that may occur with the elderly and list steps to maintain open communication.
5. Recognize and describe the coping mechanisms used by the elderly to deal with multiple losses.

6. Explain the types of long-term care facilities available.
7. Name the risk factors and signs of elder abuse.
8. Describe the effects of aging on the way the body processes medication.
9. Discuss the responsibility of medical assistants with regard to teaching elderly patients about medication.
10. List and describe physical changes and diseases common to the aging process.

Note: Bold-faced headings are the major headings in the text chapter; headings in regular font are lower-level headings (i.e., the content is subordinate to, or falls "under," the major headings). Make sure you understand the key terms used in the chapter, as well as the concepts presented as Key Points.

TEXT SUBHEADINGS   **NOTES**

Introduction _____

_____

☐ **LEARNING OBJECTIVE 1:** Spell and define the key terms.

_____

Concepts of Aging

Key Terms: gerontologists; senility; dementia
Key Points:
- The branch of medicine that deals with the elderly population is geriatrics, and while some physicians today are treating only geriatric patients, any physician in family practice or internal medicine will take care of the elderly.
- Stereotyping the elderly is a subtle and usually unconscious way to disassociate ourselves from the prospect of growing old.
- While some memory loss and difficulty with thought processes are inevitable as a result of aging, memory loss in the elderly is often the result of various disease processes and medications.

☐ **LEARNING OBJECTIVE 2:** Explain how aging affects thought processes.

Reinforcing Medical Compliance in the Elderly

Key Points:
- A patient who has good rapport with the office staff is likely to be truthful about the need for memory aids, and compliance may be increased.
- It is important that each time a patient visits the medical office, you ask for a complete account of all medications being taken, including prescribed and over-the-counter medications, herbal supplements, and vitamins.

☐ **LEARNING OBJECTIVE 3:** Describe methods to increase compliance with health maintenance programs among the elderly.

Reinforcing Mental Health in the Elderly

Key Point:
- Adjusting to pain or disability is often easier than adjusting to loss of social interaction or dependency.

☐ **LEARNING OBJECTIVE 4:** Discuss communication problems that may occur with the elderly and list steps to maintain open communication.

Coping with Aging _____

_____

Key Point:
- You can help patients to cope with stress by listening to their fears and concerns, respecting their right to have these feelings, and helping them to reduce the stressors in their lives.

Alcoholism _____

_____

Key Term: potentiation
Key Points:
- Some elderly, like adults coping with other losses, turn to alcohol as a way to escape dealing with the various losses associated with aging.
- As often as necessary, you should reinforce with elderly patients and their caregivers the effects of alcohol on mental processes and undesirable interactions with medications.

Suicide _____

_____

Key Point:
- Unlike suicide among younger people, suicide among the elderly is likely to be well planned and successful.

☐ **LEARNING OBJECTIVE 5:** Recognize and describe the coping mechanisms used by the elderly to deal with multiple losses.

Long-Term Care _____

_____

Key Term: activities of daily living
Key Point:
- Although many elderly are able to live in their own homes, some enter long-term care facilities if they cannot return to health and independence.

☐ **LEARNING OBJECTIVE 6:** Explain the types of long-term care facilities available.

Elder Abuse _____

Key Points:
- Although elder abuse is not as widely publicized as child abuse, it is thought to be almost as prevalent.
- Elder abuse and neglect may take several forms, but family members (adult children and spouses) are the typical perpetrators.

☐ **LEARNING OBJECTIVE 7:** Name the risk factors and signs of elder abuse.

Medications and the Elderly _____

Key Term: biotransform
Key Points:
- At the same time that elderly patients need more medications for various disorders, the body is coping with the stress of illness, disease, or injury along with slowing of many bodily functions.
- All of these decreases in body systems can result in possible toxic effects of medications in the elderly.

☐ **LEARNING OBJECTIVE 8:** Describe the effects of aging on the way the body processes medication.

☐ **LEARNING OBJECTIVE 9:** Discuss the responsibility of medical assistants with regard to teaching elderly patients about medication.

Systemic Changes in the Elderly _____

Key Terms: lentigines; keratoses; kyphosis; osteoporosis; degenerative joint disease; vertigo; syncope; Kegel exercises; dysphagia; presbyopia; cataracts; glaucoma; presbycusis
Key Point:
- Although longevity is considered largely hereditary, environmental factors play a significant part in how long and how well we will live.

Diseases of the Elderly _____

Parkinson Disease

Key Term: bradykinesia

Key Points:

- Parkinson disease is a slow, progressive neurological disorder affecting specific cells of the brain that produce the neurotransmitter dopamine.
- The diagnosis of Parkinson disease is usually made by excluding other causes, however testing may show decreased levels of dopamine in the urine.
- Treatment is symptomatic, supportive, and palliative.
- Parkinson's patients retain their mental and cognitive functions unless an organic brain disturbance is also present.

Alzheimer Disease

Key Points:

- Roughly half of the cases of dementia in the elderly are due to Alzheimer disease.
- Alzheimer disease has seven recognized stages.
- Home care agencies usually offer respite care, which can be vitally important for caregivers, who need to maintain their own mental and physical health.

☐ **LEARNING OBJECTIVE 10:** List and describe physical changes and diseases common to the aging process.

Maintaining Optimum Health

Exercise

Key Point:

- Older patients should begin an exercise program only after a thorough physical examination and should follow the physician's recommendation.

Diet _____

_____

Key Points:
- Many elderly patients have difficulty maintaining good nutrition.
- Although activity levels, hence calorie requirements, are lower among the elderly, vitamin and mineral requirements do not decrease with age.

Safety _____

_____

_____

Content Review

FOUNDATIONAL KNOWLEDGE

Reinforcing Medical Compliance

1. Some elderly patients suffer from memory loss, which may make it difficult for them to remember to take their medications. As a medical assistant, it is important to give these patients tools to help them remember and maintain their medication regimens. List five ways you can help elderly patients remember their medication regimens.

a. _____

b. _____

c. _____

d. _____

e. _____

2. You ask Mr. Walton if he is taking his blood pressure medication and he tells you that he is. Later, the physician comes to you and tells you that Mr. Walton has been taking three pills a day instead of just one. How could this situation be avoided with other elderly patients?

_____

_____

3. Which of the following are common reasons for elderly patients not taking their medications correctly? Circle all that apply.

a. Financial difficulties

b. To attract attention

c. Forgetfulness

d. Tiring of the constraints of taking long-term medication

e. Deliberate defiance

4. Mrs. Kim is 89 years old and suffers from memory lapses. It is apparent that she is both frustrated and lonely. List three ways that you can maintain good communication with her and help her express her feelings.

   a. _____

   b. _____

   c. _____

5. Mrs. Driscoll is an 84-year-old female with poor eyesight who suffers from forgetfulness. She needs to take two different types of medication three times a day. List four ways that you could help ensure that Mrs. Driscoll adheres to her medication regimen.

   a. _____

   b. _____

   c. _____

   d. _____

Dealing with Grief and Loss

6. Elderly patients whose health and economic situation are unstable may experience feelings of grief and loss. These feelings can be about both specific and nonspecific aspects of their lives. Fill in the chart below, listing five specific and nonspecific losses that elderly patients may find difficult to cope with.

Specific Losses	Nonspecific Losses

7. Mrs. Dawson is a widow who lives in a long-term care facility. Her family is worried that she has recently become withdrawn and uncommunicative. Before her husband died, Mrs. Dawson led an active life and took a large role in running the household. What advice would you give to Mrs. Dawson's family to help her cope with the loss of her spouse and her independence?

   _____

   _____

8. Patients who react negatively to moving to a long-term care facility can show signs of grief. List five symptoms that could indicate that a patient is suffering from a sense of loss.

   a. _____

   b. _____

   c. _____

   d. _____

   e. _____

Battling Unhealthy Coping Mechanisms

9. Sometimes an elderly patient will turn to alcohol as a way of coping. The effects of drinking alcohol can often be mistaken for other ailments. List three conditions that exhibit symptoms similar to the influence of alcohol.

   a. _____

   b. _____

   c. _____

10. Suicide is a risk for elderly patients, especially those who have recently lost a spouse to death or divorce. Which of the following warning signs indicate that an elderly patient is contemplating suicide? Circle all that apply.

    a. Giving away favored objects

    b. Increased interest in family affairs

    c. Secretive behavior

    d. Increased anger, hostility, or isolation

    e. Increased forgetfulness

    f. Increased alcohol or drug use

    g. Loss of interest in matters of health

11. Match the following types of long-term care facilities with the correct descriptions.

Types of Facilities

a. Group homes or assisted living facilities _____

b. Long-term care facilities _____

c. Skilled-nursing facilities _____

Descriptions

1. Facilities for those who need help with most areas of personal care and moderate medical supervision

2. Facilities for those who are gravely or terminally ill and need constant supervision

3. Facilities for those who can tend to their own activities of daily living but need companionship and light supervision for safety

12. Read the following case studies. Using your knowledge of the causes of elder abuse decide which patient falls into the highest risk category for abuse.

    a. Mr. Simpson is an 89-year-old widower who lives alone. He is still fairly active and is able to carry out most daily activities by himself. He has a daughter and a son, who take turns visiting him every week and doing his shopping and laundry for him. Mr. Simpson takes medication for high blood pressure and angina.

    b. Mrs. Lewis is an 83-year-old patient who lives in a long-term care facility. She suffers from mild senile dementia, which her family sometimes finds frustrating, but is learning to cope with. Mrs. Lewis has a home health aide and private nurse to help her carry out activities of daily living. She sleeps for most of the day.

    c. Mrs. Beddowes is a 90-year-old widow who lives with her son. She suffers from senile dementia, incontinence, and insomnia. Her family members cannot afford to place her in a long-term care facility, so they share the responsibility of taking care of her. However, most of the responsibility falls onto her son, who helps Mrs. Beddowes carry out most activities of daily living.

    d. Mr. Williams is an 81-year-old patient who lives in an assisted living facility. He was recently widowed and is having difficulty coming to terms with his wife's death. Mr. Williams used to be extremely active, but has recently become withdrawn and has started drinking heavily. He has two daughters who visit him regularly.

Watch for Abuse

13. Which of the following indicate that a patient is suffering from elder abuse? Circle all that apply.

    a. Disturbed sleep patterns

    b. Signs of restraint on the wrists or ankles

    c. Large, deep pressure ulcers

    d. Incontinence

    e. Poor hygiene or poor nutrition

    f. Untreated injury or condition

    g. Dehydration not caused by disease

The Aging Body

14. The passage below describes how medications affect the body of an elderly person. However, some of the important terms are missing. Read the passage and fill in the correct words from the box below.

The _____ system no longer moves medications along as efficiently because _____ has slowed. The _____ system does not absorb dissolved medication from the _____ or the _____ and deliver it to the target tissue as quickly. The _____ does not _____ medication as quickly, causing medications to remain in the body longer than desirable and possibly add to the cumulative effect. Finally, the _____ receive less blood, so less medication is filtered and removed from the body. These decreases in body system function can result in possible _____ of medications in the elderly.

| circulatory system | gastrointestinal system | intestines | biotransform | kidneys |
| toxic effects | | liver | peristalsis | injection site |

15. Which of the following are symptoms of Parkinson disease? Circle all that apply.

a. Muscle rigidity

b. Increased anger

c. Involuntary tremors

d. Difficulty walking

e. Loss of memory

f. Dysphagia and drooling

g. Expressionless face and infrequent blinking

16. Decide whether each of the following suggestions is appropriate for a patient with Parkinson disease or for a patient with Alzheimer disease. Place a check mark in the appropriate box.

Suggestion	Patient with Parkinson Disease	Patient with Alzheimer Disease
a. Speak calmly and without condescension.		
b. Do not argue with the patient.		
c. Tell the patient to take small bites and chew each mouthful carefully before swallowing.		
d. Encourage the patient to use no-spill cups, plates with high sides, and special utensils.		
e. Free the home from rugs and loose cords that may cause tripping.		
f. Speak in short, simple, direct sentences and explain one action at a time.		
g. Listen to the patient and stimulate his intelligence.		
h. Remind the patient who you are and what you must do.		

17. List three reasons why an elderly patient can have difficulty maintaining good nutrition.

a. _____

b. _____

c. _____

18. Mr. Gonzalez is an 85-year-old patient who lives alone. He is still fairly active and is able to carry out most activities of daily living by himself. However, members of his family have expressed some concerns that he is lonely and that they are not able to visit him as often as they would like. What options could you discuss with the family?

_____

_____

19. Match the following key terms to their definitions.

Key Terms

a. activities of daily living (ADL) _____

b. biotransform _____

c. bradykinesia _____

d. cataracts _____

e. cerebrovascular accident (CVA) _____

f. compliance _____

g. degenerative joint disease (DJD) _____

h. dementia _____

i. dysphagia _____

j. gerontologist _____

k. glaucoma _____

l. Kegel exercises _____

m. keratosis (senile) _____

n. kyphosis (dowager's hump) _____

o. lentigines _____

p. osteoporosis _____

q. potentiation _____

r. presbycucis _____

s. presbyopia _____

t. senility _____

u. syncope _____

v. transient ischemic attack (TIA) _____

w. vertigo _____

Definitions

1. a specialist who studies aging

2. general mental deterioration associated with old age

3. to convert the molecules of a substance from one form to another, as in medications within the body

4. a sensation of whirling of oneself or the environment, dizziness

5. abnormally slow voluntary movements

6. a sudden fall in blood pressure or cerebral hypoxia resulting in loss of consciousness

7. progressive organic mental deterioration with loss of intellectual function

8. a skin condition characterized by overgrowth and thickening

9. difficulty speaking

10. an abnormal porosity of the bone, most often found in the elderly, predisposing the affected bony tissue to fracture

11. an acute episode of cerebrovascular insufficiency, usually a result of narrowing of an artery by atherosclerotic plaques, emboli, or vasospasm; usually passes quickly but should be considered a warning for predisposition to cerebrovascular accidents

12. a progressive loss of transparency of the lens of the eye, resulting in opacity and loss of sight

13. describes the actions of two drugs taken together in which the combined effects are greater than the sum of the independent effects

14. a vision change (farsightedness) associated with aging

15. isometric exercises in which the muscles of the pelvic floor are voluntarily contracted and relaxed while urinating

16. brown skin macules occurring after prolonged exposure to the sun; freckles

17. a loss of hearing associated with aging

18. an abnormally deep dorsal curvature of the thoracic spine; also known as humpback or hunchback

19. activities usually performed in the course of the day, i.e., bathing, dressing, feeding oneself

20. also known as osteoarthritis; arthritis characterized by degeneration of the bony structure of the joints, usually noninflammatory

21. willingness of a patient to follow a prescribed course of treatment

22. ischemia of the brain due to an occlusion of the blood vessels supplying the brain, resulting in varying degrees of debilitation

23. an abnormal increase in the fluid of the eye, usually as a result of obstructed outflow, resulting in degeneration of the intraocular components and blindness

20. True or False? Determine whether the following statements are true or false. If false, explain why.

a. Newspaper word puzzles are just a temporary distraction to help entertain elderly people.

_____

_____

b. Attempts to commit suicide by elderly people are usually just a cry for help.

_____

_____

c. If a patient has an advance directive on file somewhere other than the medical office, it should be noted in her medical record.

_____

_____

d. Most elderly abuse is committed by workers in long-term care facilities.

_____

_____

APPLICATION

Critical Thinking Practice

1. Your patient is a 90-year-old male with various age-associated health problems. He has been recently diagnosed with dementia, but during his recent visits to the physician's office you have smelled alcohol on his breath. List three things that you would do.

_____

_____

2. Your patient is an 82-year-old female who suffers from mild hearing loss. She recently lost her husband and has been making frequent appointments at the physician's office for minor complaints. You suspect that the patient is lonely and is visiting the office for company and human interaction. Explain what you would do.

_____

_____

Patient Education

1. Your patient is an 80-year-old female who has recently lost a noticeable amount of weight. She tells you that she has not been very hungry lately and has not felt like eating very much. Write a list of nutritional guidelines for her to follow and explain why they are important.

_____

_____

Documentation
1. A 78-year-old patient visits the physician's office to ask about treatment for arthritis in his knees. While you are talking to the patient, you notice that his hearing has decreased considerably since the last time he was in the physician's office. How would you document this information in the patient's chart?

_____

_____

Active Learning

1. Research the latest information about Alzheimer disease on the Internet. Produce an informative poster to display in a physician's waiting room, educating people about the early warning signs of Alzheimers. Include information about the stages of Alzheimers and what friends and families can expect if a loved one develops the disease.

2. Research different support groups and activity groups in your local area aimed at people over the age of 60. Compile a booklet including descriptions of the different support groups and activity groups, with contact information for each and a brief description of what the group does. Keep copies of the booklet in the physician's office to hand out to patients over the age of 60 and their families.

3. Visit one of the local community resource centers that you listed in your booklet from the question above. Talk to some of the people who run the programs and some of the senior citizens who participate in them. Write a one-page reaction paper describing the program and your experience there.

Professional Journal

REFLECT

(Prompts and Ideas: Do you have any elderly relatives? How are they coping with the aging process? Do they always have their medication regimen clearly explained to them by their physician? What could be done to make their life easier? Who is primarily responsible for their welfare? Do any outside agencies assist them?)

_____

_____

_____

_____

_____

PONDER AND SOLVE

1. Your patient is a 91-year-old male with Alzheimer disease. After his appointment with the physician, you overhear his family trying to get him into the car. The patient has forgotten where he is and refuses to leave the physician's office. His daughter loses her temper and shouts at her father loudly until he complies. What would you do? Explain your actions.

_____

_____

_____

_____

_____

2. You overhear a coworker asking a 77-year-old patient about her medical history. When the patient tells your coworker that she is taking gingko to improve her memory, your coworker tells her that she needs to know only about actual medications. What would you say to your coworker?

_____

_____

_____

_____

_____

Chapter Self-Assessment Quiz

1. Which of the following statements is true about elderly patients who require long-term medication?

   a. If elderly patients take their medication every day, they are unlikely to forget a dosage.

   b. Compliance over a long period of time can become problematic in elderly patients.

   c. With a chronic illness, an elderly patient can neglect to take his medication for a few weeks with no side effects.

   d. Patients who take their medication for a long period of time will eventually notice a significant improvement.

   e. Elderly patients will eventually become immune to long-term medication.

2. Which of these conditions can sometimes be improved by taking the herbal supplement gingko?

   a. Arthritis

   b. Parkinson disease

   c. Loss of appetite

   d. Poor concentration

   e. Alzheimer disease

3. The purpose of an advance directive is to:

   a. divide a person's possessions in the event of death.

   b. inform the physician of any allergies that an individual has to specific medications.

   c. outline a person's wishes should he become unable to communicate decisions about end-of-life care.

   d. transfer a patient's medical records between physicians' offices.

   e. order a physician not to resuscitate a patient under any circumstances.

4. Which of these is a task performed by a home health aide?

   a. Light housecleaning

   b. Refilling prescriptions

   c. Reorganizing bulky furniture

   d. Writing daily task lists and reminders

   e. Keeping the elderly person occupied

5. Which of these is a good place to find information about respite care for elderly relatives?

   a. Local newspaper

   b. Television advertisement

   c. Community senior citizen program

   d. Local business directory

   e. Library bulletin board

6. What is an example of passive neglect of an elderly patient?

   a. Withholding medication from the patient

   b. Locking the patient in a room

   c. Overmedicating the patient to make her easier to care for

   d. Isolating the patient from friends and family

   e. Forgetting to give the patient regular baths

7. Which of the following statements is true about the aging process?

   a. Longevity is based entirely on environmental factors.

   b. People who have dangerous occupations will not live as long as people who do not.

   c. Longevity is hereditary, so it does not make a difference how you live your life.

   d. Longevity is largely hereditary, but environmental factors play a significant role.

   e. An obese, physically inactive smoker will have a shorter lifespan than a healthy nonsmoker.

8. What is the best way to deal with a patient who is hearing impaired?

    a. Raise your voice until the patient can hear you.

    b. Give written instructions whenever possible.

    c. Talk to the patient with your back to the light.

    d. Talk directly into the patient's ear.

    e. Find a coworker who is able to communicate using sign language.

Scenario: A 55-year-old patient comes into the physician's office and tells you that he thinks he is suffering from Parkinson disease.

9. The patient would be diagnosed by:

    a. taking a blood test.

    b. performing dexterity tasks.

    c. excluding other causes.

    d. undergoing an MRI scan.

    e. testing his reflexes.

10. How would you explain deep brain stimulation to the patient?

    a. It increases the levels of dopamine in the brain.

    b. It lowers a person's acetylcholine levels.

    c. It blocks the impulses that cause tremors.

    d. It controls a person's stress and anxiety levels.

    e. It acts as a muscle relaxant and prevents rigidity.

11. What would you tell the patient about Levodopa?

    a. It has no serious side effects.

    b. It remains effective for the entire length of the disease.

    c. It can cause headaches and migraines.

    d. It should not be taken with alcohol.

    e. It may aggravate stomach ulcers.

End Scenario

12. When elderly patients are beginning a new exercise regime, it is a good idea for them to:

    a. rest when they get tired.

    b. start with a brisk 30-minute jog.

    c. keep to the same weekly routine.

    d. exercise alone so they are not distracted.

    e. work through any initial pain or discomfort.

13. Which of the following statements is true about the nutritional requirements of elderly patients?

    a. Elderly patients need less food and water than younger patients because the elderly are not as active.

    b. It is easier for elderly patients to maintain good nutrition because they have more time to prepare meals.

    c. Vitamin and mineral requirements are lower in elderly patients than in younger patients.

    d. Elderly patients should eat smaller, more frequent meals to aid digestion.

    e. Elderly patients can replace meals with liquid dietary supplements without damaging their health.

14. A caregiver can help increase safety in the home of an elderly patient by:

    a. installing handrails in the bathtub and near the commode.

    b. placing childproof locks on the kitchen cupboards.

    c. encouraging the patient to exercise regularly.

    d. covering highly polished floors with scatter rugs.

    e. keeping the patient's medicine in a locked bathroom cabinet.

15. What action should you take if you suspect a caregiver of elderly abuse?

    a. Try to separate the caregiver from the patient for the examination.

    b. Tell the caregiver you will be reporting her to the authorities.

    c. Question the patient about suspicious injuries until she tells you the truth.

    d. Call the police while the patient is in the examination room.

    e. Wait to inform the physician of your suspicions until you are sure they are correct.

16. What does the acronym HOH mean in a patient's chart?

    a. Has ordinary hearing

    b. Head of household

    c. Has own home

    d. Hard on health

    e. Hard of hearing

17. Another name for the herbal supplement gingko is:

   a. folic acid.

   b. kew tree.

   c. aloe vera.

   d. green tea.

   e. milk thistle.

18. What is the best advice to give a patient who is having difficulty swallowing medication?

   a. Grind the medication into powder.

   b. Ask the pharmacist for smaller pills.

   c. Put the medication on the back of the tongue and drink water with a straw.

   d. Lie down and swallow the medication with a lot of water.

   e. Dissolve the medication in a hot drink.

19. A physician who specializes in disorders that affect the aging population is called a(n):

   a. gastroenterologist.

   b. gerontologist.

   c. oncologist.

   d. otorhinolaryngologist.

   e. rheumatologist.

20. An eye condition that causes increased intraocular pressure and intolerance to light is:

   a. cataracts.

   b. kyphosis.

   c. bradykinesia.

   d. osteoporosis.

   e. glaucoma.

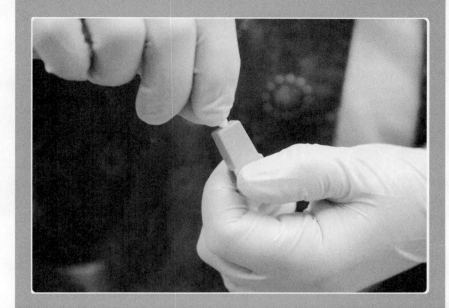

PART

IV

The Clinical
Laboratory

Fundamentals of Laboratory Procedures

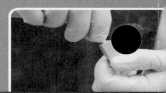

CHAPTER

39 Introduction to the Clinical Laboratory

Chapter Checklist

☐ Read textbook chapter and take notes within the Chapter Notes outline. Answer the Learning Objectives as you reach them in the content, and then check them off.

☐ Work the Content Review questions—both Foundational Knowledge and Application.

☐ Perform the Active Learning exercise(s).

☐ Complete Professional Journal entries.

☐ Complete Skill Practice Activity(s) using Competency Evaluation Forms and Work Products, when appropriate.

☐ Take the Chapter Self-Assessment Quiz.

☐ Insert all appropriate pages into your Portfolio.

Learning Objectives

1. Spell and define the key terms.
2. List reasons for laboratory testing.
3. Outline the medical assistant's responsibility in the clinical laboratory.
4. Name the kinds of laboratories where medical assistants work and the functions of each.
5. Name the types of departments found in most large laboratories and give their purposes.

6. List the types of personnel in laboratories and describe their jobs.
7. Explain how to use a package insert to determine the procedure for a laboratory test.
8. List the equipment found in most small laboratories and give the purpose of each.
9. List and describe the parts of a microscope.

Chapter Notes

Note: Bold-faced headings are the major headings in the text chapter; headings in regular font are lower-level headings (i.e., the content is subordinate to, or falls "under," the major headings). Make sure you understand the key terms used in the chapter, as well as the concepts presented as Key Points.

TEXT SUBHEADINGS	NOTES

Introduction _____

Key Terms: normal values; specimens; Clinical Laboratory Improvement Amendments (CLIA); quality assurance (QA); quality control (QC)

Key Points:

- Laboratory staff analyzes blood, urine, and other body samples to facilitate identification of diseases and disorders.
- Laboratory testing is most commonly used for the following:
  - Detecting and diagnosing disease
  - Following the progress of a disease and its response to treatment
  - Meeting legal requirements (e.g., drug testing, a marriage license)
  - Monitoring a patient's medication and treatment
  - Determining the levels of essential substances in the body
  - Identifying the cause of an infection
  - Determining a baseline value
  - Preventing disease

☐ **LEARNING OBJECTIVE 1:** Spell and define the key terms.

☐ **LEARNING OBJECTIVE 2:** List reasons for laboratory testing.

☐ **LEARNING OBJECTIVE 3:** Outline the medical assistant's responsibility in the clinical laboratory.

Types of Laboratories _____

Key Point:

- Three types of laboratories significant to the medical assistant are reference, hospital, and physician office laboratories (POLs). Hospital and reference laboratories may perform hundreds of specialized tests and may process thousands of specimens per day. In contrast, POLs perform only a few types of tests on a limited number of patients.

Reference Laboratory _____

Key Term: aliquots

Hospital Laboratory _____

Physician Office Laboratory _____

_____

Key Points:
- The most common type of laboratory is the POL, which may vary greatly in size and diversity.
- Medical assistants may perform all of these tasks, only if a physician monitors QC and abnormal results.

☐ **LEARNING OBJECTIVE 4:** Name the kinds of laboratories where medical assistants work and the functions of each.

Laboratory Departments _____

_____

Key Point:
- Most large laboratories are divided into departments.

Hematology _____

_____

Key Term: hematology
Key Point:
- The **hematology** department performs tests on blood and blood-forming tissues.

Coagulation _____

_____

Key Terms: coagulation; anticoagulant
Key Point:
- Often a part of the hematology department, **coagulation** testing entails evaluating how well the body's blood clotting process is performing.

Clinical Chemistry _____

_____

Key Term: clinical chemistry
Key Point:
- The **clinical chemistry** department measures chemical substances in blood or serum. These substances may include hormones, enzymes, electrolytes, gases, medicines and drugs, sugars, proteins, fats, and waste products.

Toxicology

Key Term: toxicology
Key Point:
• **Toxicology** testing entails measuring blood levels of both therapeutic drugs and drugs of abuse.

Urinalysis

Key Term: urinalysis
Key Point:
• The most common **urinalysis** assay is the complete **urinalysis** (UA), an evaluation of the physical, chemical, and microscopic properties of urine. CLIA approves Medical Assistants to perform the physical and chemical evaluations of urine.

Immunohematology

Key Term: immunohematology
Key Point:
• The **immunohematology** department performs blood typing and compatibility testing of patient's blood with blood products for transfusion purposes.

Immunology

Key Term: immunology
Key Point:
• Testing in the **immunology** department is based on the reactions of antibodies formed against certain diseases in the presence of proteins called antigens.

Microbiology

Key Term: microbiology
Key Point:
• The **microbiology** department identifies the various microorganisms that cause disease.

Anatomical and Surgical Pathology _____

Key Point:
• The anatomical and surgical pathology department studies tissue and body fluid specimens from aspirations, autopsies, biopsies, organ removal, and other procedures to identify or evaluate the effects of cancer and other diseases.

Histology _____

Key Term: histology

Cytology and Cytogenetics _____

Key Terms: cytology; cytogenetics

☐ **LEARNING OBJECTIVE 5:** Name the types of departments found in most large laboratories and give their purposes.

Laboratory Personnel _____

☐ **LEARNING OBJECTIVE 6:** List the types of personnel in laboratories and describe their jobs.

Physician Office Laboratory Testing _____

Key Points:
• Many tests can be performed in an office laboratory that meet the standards set forth in the Clinical Laboratory Improvement Amendments and in modifications of the original amendment (discussed in Chapter 42).
• The best source of information for safe and accurate testing is the package insert shipped inside the test kit or the instrument reagents and QC instructions specific for various office test instruments.

☐ **LEARNING OBJECTIVE 7:** Explain how to use a package insert to determine the procedure for a laboratory test.

Laboratory Request Forms _____

Laboratory Test Panels _____

_____

Key Term: panels
Key Point:
• To effectively evaluate disease processes or organ systems, laboratory tests are organized into standard groups or **panels**.

Laboratory Equipment _____

_____

_____

Cell Counter _____

_____

Key Point:
• A cell counter is an automated analyzer used to count and size blood cells.

Microscope _____

_____

Key Point:
• Microscopes are delicate, expensive instruments. To ensure that the microscope used in your clinical laboratory is kept in good working order, you must handle it properly (Box 39-4) and maintain it according to the manufacturer's standards (Procedure 39-1).

Chemistry Analyzers _____

_____

Key Point:
• Like cell counters, traditional chemistry analyzers vary from simple instruments that perform one or a few tests and require manual operation to complex analyzers that perform 30 or more tests per sample and are operated by computer.

Centrifuges _____

_____

Key Points:
• A centrifuge swings its contents in a circle to separate liquids into their component parts.
• Tubes must always be balanced in the centrifuge.

Incubator _____

_____

_____

Refrigerators and Freezers _____

_____

_____

☐ **LEARNING OBJECTIVE 8:** List the equipment found in most small laboratories and give the purpose of each.

☐ **LEARNING OBJECTIVE 9:** List and describe the parts of a microscope.

Content Review

FOUNDATIONAL KNOWLEDGE

All About Lab Testing

1. List eight reasons for laboratory testing.

   a. _____

   b. _____

   c. _____

   d. _____

   e. _____

   f. _____

   g. _____

   h. _____

2. Review the list of responsibilities below. Then place a check mark in the appropriate box to indicate if the medical assistant is responsible for performing these tasks in the clinical laboratory.

Task	Yes	No
a. Obtaining a quality specimen		
b. Accompanying patients to lab testing at other sites		
c. Performing common lab tests in compliance with CLIA		
d. Arranging for appropriate transport if the specimen is to be analyzed at another site		
e. Explaining lab results to patients		
f. Documenting and maintaining a quality assurance program		
g. Sharing test results with family members		
h. Informing patients of proper procedure or preparation		
i. Maintaining laboratory instruments and equipment		

3. Fill in the table below with three kinds of laboratories where medical assistants work and the function of each one.

Type of Lab	Function
a.	
b.	
c.	

Who's Who in the Lab

4. List four job titles you might have if you work as a medical assistant in a hospital.

a. _____

b. _____

c. _____

d. _____

5. Each of the medical assistants below needs a lab test completed for a patient. Review the task that must be performed and then decide which laboratory department should handle each task.

a. Ericka needs to send in blood for a complete blood count. _____

b. Kwon needs to find out more about the chemical properties of a patient's urine. _____

c. Darren has to send a patient to the lab for glucose testing. _____

d. Carlton needs to send a patient to have a test to evaluate her blood-clotting time. _____

e. The physician asks Mariah to submit a patient's blood to test it for the presence of illegal drugs. _____

f. Don needs to rule out a diagnosis of infectious mononucleosis. _____

6. Which department is commonly called the blood bank? List two places where you may find this department.

_____

_____

7. A patient has had a mole removed, and the physician wants to have a biopsy done to make sure it is noncancerous. To which department in a reference laboratory would you send the specimen?

_____

_____

8. What is cytology, and how is it used?

_____

_____

9. Match the job title with the correct job description for laboratory personnel.

Job Titles

a. pathologist _____
b. chief technologist _____
c. medical technologist _____
d. medical laboratory technician _____
e. laboratory assistant _____
f. phlebotomist _____
g. histologist _____
h. cytologist _____
i. specimen processor _____

Job Descriptions

1. supervise the day-to-day operations of a laboratory
2. perform specimen testing within limits defined by CLIA
3. process and evaluate tissue samples
4. draw blood and process blood and other samples
5. accept shipments of specimens and centrifuges, and separate, or otherwise process, the samples to prepare them for testing
6. perform all levels of testing
7. collect and process specimens and perform certain waived and moderately complex testing
8. examine cells under the microscope to look for abnormal changes
9. study disease processes

Lab Tests and Tips

10. How does a package insert determine the procedure for a laboratory test?

_____

_____

11. Why are quality control and machine maintenance so important?

_____

_____

12. List five panels defined by the American Medical Association.

a. _____

b. _____

c. _____

d. _____

e. _____

13. Explain the difference between dry and wet reagent technology. Why is wet considered better?

_____

_____

14. What are three blood products that are prepared, stored, and dispensed in the immunohematology department?

a. _____

b. _____

c. _____

15. What are laboratory request forms?

_____

_____

16. The physician you work for is beginning his practice and has asked you to purchase whatever lab equipment the office will need. List six pieces of equipment found in most small laboratories and their functions in the chart below.

Equipment	Function

17. Describe the function of the parts of the microscope listed below.

a. The frame _____

b. The coarse adjustment knob _____

c. The fine adjustment knob _____

d. The stage _____

e. The condenser _____

f. The diaphragm _____

18. The centrifuge has just completed spinning a specimen with an anticoagulant. Look at the image below and label the different sections of the sample inside.

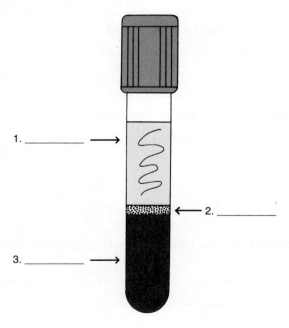

1. _____ →

← 2. _____

3. _____ →

19. Match the following key terms to their definitions.

Key Terms

a. aliquot _____

b. anticoagulant _____

c. clinical chemistry _____

Definitions

1. the study of the antigen-antibody reaction, including the study of auto-immunity

2. study of the function and disorders of the blood

3. anything that prevents or delays the clotting of the blood

d. Clinical Laboratory Improvement Amendments (CLIA) _____

e. coagulation _____

f. cytogenetics _____

g. cytology _____

h. hematology _____

i. histology _____

j. immunohematology _____

k. immunology _____

l. microbiology _____

m. normal values _____

n. panels _____

o. quality assurance (QA) _____

p. quality control (QC) _____

q. specimens _____

r. toxicology _____

s. urinalysis _____

4. an evaluation of health care services as compared with accepted standards

5. an acceptable range as established for an age, a population, or a sex; variations usually indicate a disorder

6. the lab department that measures chemical substances in blood or serum

7. portion of specimens used for testing

8. the change from a liquid to a solid or semi-solid mass

9. study of the genetic structure of cells to test for chromosome deficiencies related to genetic disease

10. the study of the microscopic structure and organization of cells

11. the study of the body's immune system and its functions and disorders

12. guidelines established by Congress in 1988 to standardize and improve laboratory testing

13. the study of microscopic organisms

14. a standard group of laboratory tests

15. study of cells

16. examination of the physical, chemical, and microscopic properties of urine

17. method to evaluate the proper performance of testing procedures, supplies, or equipment in a laboratory

18. the laboratory department that tests blood levels of both therapeutic and illegal drugs

19. a small portion of anything used to evaluate the nature of the whole

20. True or False? Determine whether the following statements are true or false. If false, explain why.

a. A medical office can perform any test, but most prefer to send its samples to an offsite facility.

_____

b. Patient confidentiality does not need to be maintained if a specimen is sent offsite for further analysis.

_____

c. All of a specimen is used when you are conducting a test.

_____

d. Departments might be divided into subdivisions and contain smaller departments within the larger body.

_____

APPLICATION

Critical Thinking Practice

1. The physician wants to run a few tests using a patient's serum. Describe the steps you will need to take to get the proper specimen from the patient.

_____

_____

2. A pregnant woman comes in and asks what tests can be run to ensure that her baby does not have any genetic diseases. What kind of tests could you run? What kind of specimen would you obtain, and where would you send it to be tested?

_____

_____

Patient Education

1. You will be collecting a blood sample for HIV testing. Many states require that you give counseling to the patient before and after the test. Write a brief summary of what might be said to the patient, both before and after you run the test.

_____

_____

Documentation
1. How would you document a blood specimen and prepare it to be sent out for testing?

_____

_____

Active Learning

1. In large laboratories, there may be several departments running different types of tests. Within these departments, there are specialists who are highly trained to run specific types of tests and to analyze the results. Choose a department and find a position that interests you. Outline the basic job description, as well as any skills or special training you might need to fill that position.

2. The microscope is an essential instrument used in the lab. Working with a partner, practice using a microscope to gain familiarity with this tool. Make three slides that you can look at under the microscope.

3. Patient confidentiality is always an important part of your job, but so is safety. Research your state's rules and regulations in regard to the rights of a patient and the rights of the public. For instance, is someone with HIV/AIDS required by law to report his condition to his employer? What about other illnesses? After you have run a test and found a patient who tested positive for a specific disease, what are the obligations of your office in dealing with this?

Professional
Journal

REFLECT

(Prompts and Ideas: Safety should always be a concern when dealing with specimens. When obtaining an HIV patient's samples, you must be particularly careful. How would you react if you were told to obtain a specimen from an HIV or AIDS patient? What could you do or say to make sure that the patient is not alienated while maintaining your own safety?)

_____

_____

_____

_____

_____

_____

_____

PONDER AND SOLVE

1. Your friend has to have a drug test for her new job. She knows that her sample will be sent through a lab's toxicology department to determine if there are any drugs in her system. She admits to you that she smoked marijuana last week, and she's worried about failing the drug test. Her sister has offered to take the test for her. What should you tell your friend?

_____

_____

_____

_____

_____

_____

_____

2. You have just finished analyzing the test results of a urinalysis, and the results came back positive for pregnancy. The specimen belongs to a 15-year-old girl who came in with her mother for a regular physical. How would you handle the situation?

_____

_____

_____

_____

_____

_____

_____

EXPERIENCE

Skills related to this chapter include:

1. Caring for a Microscope (Procedure 39-1).

Record any common mistakes, lessons learned, and/or tips you discovered during your experience of practicing and demonstrating these skills.

_____

_____

_____

_____

_____

_____

_____

_____

Skill Practice

PERFORMANCE OBJECTIVES:

1. Care for the microscope (Procedure 39-1).

Name_____   Date _____   Time _____

Procedure 39-1:   CARING FOR A MICROSCOPE

EQUIPMENT: Lens paper, lens cleaner, gauze, mild soap solution, microscope, hand disinfectant, surface disinfectant

STANDARDS: Given the needed equipment and a place to work, the student will perform this skill with _____% accuracy in a total of _____ minutes. *(Your instructor will tell you what the percentage and time limits will be before you begin practicing.)*

KEY: 4 = Satisfactory   0 = Unsatisfactory   NA = This step is not counted

PROCEDURE STEPS	SELF	PARTNER	INSTRUCTOR
1. Wash your hands.	☐	☐	☐
2. Assemble the equipment.	☐	☐	☐
3. If you need to move the microscope, carry it in both hands, one holding the base and the other holding the arm.	☐	☐	☐
4. Clean the optical areas following these steps: **a.** Place a drop or two of lens cleaner on a piece of lens paper. **b.** Wipe each eyepiece thoroughly with the lens paper. Do not touch the optical areas with your fingers. Wipe each eyepiece with lens paper and lens cleaner. **c.** Wipe each objective lens, starting with the lowest power and continuing to the highest power (usually an oil immersion lens). If the lens paper appears to have dirt or oil on it, use a clean section of the lens paper or a new piece of lens paper with cleaner. Wipe each objective lens with lens paper and lens cleaner. Clean oil objective last so you do not carry its oil to the other objective lenses. **d.** Using a new piece of dry lens paper, wipe each eyepiece and objective lens so that no cleaner remains. **e.** With a new piece of lens paper moistened with lens cleaner, clean the condenser and illuminator optics. Clean and dry the condenser and illuminator optics.	☐	☐	☐
5. Clean the areas other than the optics: **a.** Moisten gauze with mild soap solution or use an alcohol wipe and wipe all areas other than the optics, including the stage, base, and adjustment knobs. **b.** Moisten another gauze with water and rinse the washed areas.	☐	☐	☐
6. To store the cleaned microscope, ensure that the light source is turned off. Rotate the nosepiece so that the low-power objective is pointed down toward the stage. Cover the microscope with the plastic dust cover that came with it or a small trash bag.	☐	☐	☐
7. Document microscope cleaning on the microscope maintenance log sheet (sample instrument log sheet).	☐	☐	☐

CALCULATION

Total Possible Points: _____
Total Points Earned: _____ Multiplied by 100 = _____ Divided by Total Possible Points = _____%

Pass   **Fail**

☐   ☐   Comments:

Student's signature _____ Date _____
Partner's signature _____ Date _____
Instructor's signature _____ Date _____

Work Product 1

Perform routine maintenance of clinical equipment.

Clean a microscope in your medical office or one provided by your school according to the manufacturer's directions and Procedure 39-1. Attach a copy of the checklist for the steps performed to this sheet.

Work Product 2

Document appropriately.

If you are currently working in a medical office, use an instrument log sheet from the office. If this is not available to you, use the sample instrument log sheet below. Document cleaning the microscope above on the microscope maintenance log sheet.

**Third Street
Physician's Office, Inc.**
123 Main Street
Baltimore, MD 21201
410-895-6214

Equipment Inventory

Item Description	Item Number or Code	Purchase Date	Condition	Comments	Expected New Purchase Date	Cost if Purchased This Year

Chapter Self-Assessment Quiz

1. The best place to keep a microscope in a medical office is in:
   a. a section set aside from the office waiting room.
   b. a separate, less trafficked section of the laboratory.
   c. the physician's office, preferably upon his desk.
   d. one of the examining rooms, on one of the counter-tops.
   e. an office that does not require frequent use of the microscope.

2. The purpose of the immunology department is to:
   a. identify microscopic organisms that cause disease.
   b. perform tests on blood and blood-forming tissues.
   c. perform blood typing and compatibility testing.
   d. study the microscopic structure of tissue.
   e. study the reactions of antibodies and antigens.

3. One responsibility of a specimen processor at a reference laboratory is to:
   a. prepare aliquots if indicated.
   b. obtain specimens from patients.
   c. troubleshoot problems by telephone.
   d. provide information about the test to patients.
   e. contact patients and relay test results.

4. When using a microscope and viewing a lower-powered objective, you can focus the image using the:
   a. nosepiece.
   b. fine adjustment knob.
   c. coarse adjustment knob.
   d. light source.
   e. diaphragm.

5. Most lab tests results are available in:
   a. less than an hour.
   b. 1 to 6 hours.
   c. 6 to 12 hours.
   d. 24 to 48 hours.
   e. a week.

Scenario: A patient comes in, and the physician requests a urinalysis be run.

6. What is the first thing you need to do to obtain a sample?
   a. Tell the patient the name of the test.
   b. Explain how to obtain the specimen.
   c. Approximate the time it will take for results.
   d. Give the patient the specimen cup.
   e. Make a note on the patient's chart of the test.

7. Once you have obtained the specimen, the next step is to:
   a. divide the specimen into aliquots.
   b. prepare the specimen for transport.
   c. clearly label the specimen container.
   d. write a laboratory request form.
   e. store specimen in refrigerator or freezer.

8. If the specimen needs to be sent out for further testing, what information can be omitted from the laboratory request form?
   a. Patient's date of birth and gender
   b. Physician's contact information
   c. Checklist of test or tests to be performed
   d. Date and time of collection
   e. History of tests performed in the past

End Scenario

9. What information found on the package insert might be shared with the patient?
   a. Procedure
   b. Test principles
   c. Reagents needed
   d. Expected values
   e. Interferences

10. Which of the following tasks can a histologist perform?
    a. Accept and process specimens
    b. Perform all levels of testing
    c. Perform certain levels of testing
    d. Obtain specimen samples
    e. Evaluate specific samples

11. A Pap test specimen would be sent to which department for analysis?

    a. Histology

    b. Cytology

    c. Immunohematology

    d. Microbiology

    e. Clinical chemistry

12. How must a centrifuge be set up in order to work properly?

    a. Tubes must be equidistant.

    b. All tubes must have the same substance.

    c. Only one tube may be spun at a time.

    d. The lid must be down at all times.

    e. Spin must alternate every 30 minutes.

13. Specimens sent to clinical chemistry might be tested for which chemical substance?

    a. Cryoprecipitate

    b. RhoGAM

    c. Electrolytes

    d. Bacteria

    e. Chromosomes

14. The best place to find the most accurate information about a test is:

    a. on the package insert.

    b. from the physician.

    c. from a qualified CLIA administrator.

    d. on a patient's chart.

    e. in the HCPCS booklets.

15. The part of the microscope that concentrates the light rays to focus on the slide is the:

    a. diaphragm.

    b. light source.

    c. nosepiece.

    d. condenser.

    e. stage.

16. What is the purpose of spinning specimens on the centrifuge?

    a. The spinning mixes the reagents and specimen.

    b. The centrifugal force separates the components.

    c. The force oxidizes the specimen contents.

    d. Some reagents only react to high-gravity environments.

    e. The spin helps with filtration of waste.

17. Which of the following is a federal regulation for the transportation of biohazardous materials?

    a. Completely filled out laboratory request form

    b. Packaged to withstand rough handling

    c. Temperature-controlled container

    d. Clearly labeled shipping container

    e. Leak-proof secondary transport container

18. It's important for a laboratory to contain an incubator because warm temperatures:

    a. are required for some microorganisms to thrive.

    b. help reagents create reactions.

    c. sterilize the specimen before testing.

    d. accelerate the coagulation process.

    e. make the materials easier to work with.

19. Which of the following should be placed in a separate, noncontrolled environment?

    a. Urine specimens

    b. Blood specimens

    c. Edible items

    d. Reagents

    e. Medication

20. A common test performed in a POL is:

    a. a urine pregnancy test.

    b. a blood glucose level test.

    c. HIV test.

    d. a biopsy.

    e. measuring the blood's ability to clot.

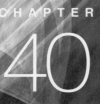

40 CLIA Compliance and Laboratory Safety

Chapter Checklist

☐ Read textbook chapter and take notes within the Chapter Notes outline. Answer the Learning Objectives as you reach them in the content, and then check them off.

☐ Work the Content Review questions—both Foundational Knowledge and Application.

☐ Perform the Active Learning exercise(s).

☐ Complete Professional Journal entries.

☐ Complete Skill Practice Activity(s) using Competency Evaluation Forms and Work Products, when appropriate.

☐ Take the Chapter Self-Assessment Quiz.

☐ Insert all appropriate pages into your Portfolio.

Learning Objectives

1. Spell and define the key terms.
2. Explain the significance of the Clinical Laboratory Improvement Amendments and how to follow their regulations to ensure quality control.
3. Using CLIA guidelines, identify laboratory tests that are and are not within the scope of practice for a medical assistant.
4. Define panic values and document the proper notification to the health care professional.
5. Identify results that require follow-up and document action in chart.
6. Identify how to handle all test results whether normal or abnormal and document on a flow sheet.
7. Identify and use quality control methods.
8. Define OSHA and state its purpose.
9. List the laboratory safety guidelines.

Chapter Notes

Note: Bold-faced headings are the major headings in the text chapter; headings in regular font are lower-level headings (i.e., the content is subordinate to, or falls "under," the major headings). Make sure you understand the key terms used in the chapter, as well as the concepts presented as Key Points.

TEXT SUBHEADINGS   **NOTES**

Introduction _____

_____

☐ **LEARNING OBJECTIVE 1:** Spell and define the key terms.

_____

Clinical Laboratory Improvement Amendments _____

_____

_____

Laws Governing the Clinical Laboratory

Key Term: Clinical Laboratory Improvement Amendments

Key Points:

• With the goals of standardizing laboratory testing and enforcing quality protocols, Congress originally passed the Clinical Laboratory Improvement Amendments (CLIA) in 1988 to establish regulations governing any facility that performs testing for the diagnosis, prevention, or treatment of human disease or for assessment of patients' health status. While final modification of the amendments was made on January 24, 2003, with an effective date of April 24, 2003, the amendments maintain their original name, CLIA '88.

• Standards were developed to cover all laboratories from large regional laboratories to the smallest Physician Office Laboratory (POL). The Centers for Medicare and Medicaid Services (CMS) regulate all laboratory testing (except research) performed on humans in the United States through CLIA.

☐ **LEARNING OBJECTIVE 2:** Explain the significance of the Clinical Laboratory Improvement Amendments and how to follow their regulations to ensure quality control.

Levels of Testing

Key Point:

• CLIA regulations established the three levels of testing discussed next based on the complexity of the testing method.

Waived Tests

Key Points:

• Waived tests are low-complexity tests that require minimal judgment or interpretation. They include many tests simple enough for the patient to perform at home (e.g., dipstick urinalysis and glucose monitoring). If these are the only types of tests performed on site, the laboratory can apply for a certificate of waiver (CLIA Waiver Registration), but it still must follow all manufacturers' recommendations for each piece of equipment or product used for testing.

• Many additional tests, including rapid strep kits, have waived methodologies available, but the Food and Drug Administration (FDA) has not provided waived status to every manufacturer. The most up-to-date listing of available waived tests can be found on the CMS website.

Moderate-Complexity Tests _____

Key Point:
• PPM can be performed only by a physician or dentist or by a nurse midwife, nurse practitioner, or physician assistant under the direct supervision of a physician.

High-Complexity Tests _____

Key Points:
• If the level of testing to be performed is in question, it must be considered high complexity until its level can be designated by CMS. CMS publishes a list of all tests in the moderate-complexity category. States may establish stricter rules than those set by the governing body, but they may not adopt less strict rules.
• Laboratory personnel must also meet the educational levels set forth by CLIA. These guidelines and their updates can be found in the Federal Register. The Federal Register is the official daily publication for rules, proposed rules, and notices of Federal agencies and organizations, as well as executive orders and other presidential documents. Access the Federal Register through this website: http://www.gpoaccess.gov/fr/index.html.
• As a source of CLIA '88 compliance support for POLs, the Commission on Office Laboratory Accreditation (COLA) was established. COLA was subsequently granted deemed status under CLIA. The Joint Commission on Accreditation of Healthcare Organizations (JCAHO) also recognized COLA's laboratory accreditation program and granted it deemed status under JCAHO standards. COLA works to support the health care industry by providing knowledge and resources for maintaining quality laboratory operations.

☐ **LEARNING OBJECTIVE 3:** Using CLIA guidelines, identify laboratory tests that are and are not within the scope of practice for a medical assistant.

Laboratory Standards _____

Laboratory Quality Assurance

Key Term: quality assurance (QA)
Key Points:
- **Quality assurance** (QA) is a plan for ensuring the quality of all areas of the laboratory's technical and support functions.
- The laboratory's policy and procedure manual should cover recommendations for continuing education for the laboratory personnel and evaluation methods for ensuring that workers are competent. The qualifications and responsibilities of all laboratory workers are specified by CLIA, with education and training requirements for all levels of personnel. Employers must ascertain the educational background of employees, provide opportunities for continuing education, and conduct or provide for proficiency testing. This information must be documented and available for inspection by CLIA representatives.

Patient Test Management

Key Point:
- A written system must be in place to ensure that the specimens are properly maintained and identified and that the results are accurately recorded and reported. Policies must be written for standards of patient care and employee conduct. Each test performed will be evaluated for safety, reliability, and diagnostic indication for its performance.

CLIA Standards for Laboratory Procedure Manuals

Key Term: laboratory procedure manual
Key Points:
- The **Laboratory Procedure Manual** is the primary reference in operating the POL. CLIA regulations require each laboratory to have its own procedure manual describing how to perform every test in the laboratory.
- Laboratories performing moderate complexity testing, such as using cell counters for Complete Blood Counts, must have procedures for performing these tests and reporting the patient results, calibrating the instrument, quality control, and for resolving problems.

Screen and Follow-Up Test Results

Key Terms: normal values; panic values; reportable range
Key Points:
- The Medical Assistant's responsibilities do not stop with being familiar with the laboratory tests performed in a specific office laboratory. Key information needed to screen and follow-up any report will be documented on the report (Procedure 40-1).
- The **normal values** (normal range or reference interval) for the test or tests included in the report will be listed. They are the test results usually seen in a healthy population.
- **Panic values** are also known as alert values or critical limits. Critical limits define the boundaries of the life-threatening values of laboratory test results. See Box 40-2 for results considered to be panic values in some offices. Urgent clinician notification of critical results is a responsibility of the laboratory. Documentation of the proper notification of such test results to the health care professional responsible for the patient is essential.
- For the tests performed in the POL, the medical assistant must know how to reference the **reportable range** of each assay reported from that laboratory. The reportable range is the very lowest and highest value the manufacturer has documented the test can determine. Manufacturers provide these ranges in their package inserts and instrument manuals.

☐ **LEARNING OBJECTIVE 4:** Define panic values and document the proper notification to the health care professional.

☐ **LEARNING OBJECTIVE 5:** Identify results that require follow-up and document action in chart.

Using Flow Sheets to Improve Patient Care

Key Term: flow sheet
Key Point:
- A **flow sheet** is a form that gathers all the important data regarding a patient's condition. The flow sheet stays in the patient's chart and serves as a reminder of care and a record of whether care expectations have been met.

☐ **LEARNING OBJECTIVE 6:** Identify how to handle all test results whether normal or abnormal and document on a flow sheet.

Quality Control _____

Key Terms: quality control (QC); Clinical and Laboratory Standards Institute (CLSI)

Key Points:
- A comprehensive **quality control** program monitors each phase of the laboratory process, including specimen collection, specimen processing, testing, and reporting results. The programs also monitor reagents, instruments, and personnel in addition to actual test performance. Each laboratory must have its own written policies and procedures that include instructions to ensure that all QC standards for monitoring the accuracy and quality of each test are in place for all levels of testing the laboratory conducts.
- The performance of these controls must be recorded in the QC log.
- The **Clinical and Laboratory Standards Institute** (CLSI) establishes rules to ensure the safety, standards, and integrity of all testing performed on human specimens.

Methods of Quality Control _____

QC for Qualitative Methods _____

Key Point:
- To satisfy CLIA requirements for quality control, the actual testing personnel must run, review for acceptability, and document the results produced by positive and negative controls at a frequency established by the reagent manufacturer. Corrective action must be taken and documented for unacceptable QC results.

QC for Quantitative Methods _____

Key Terms: shifts; trends

Key Point:
- The basic tool for manually recording quantitative quality control is the Levey-Jennings QC Chart (Figure 40-3). Using the chart builds a picture of how your test is performing over time. Monitoring the charts for shifts and trends will warn you that a test may not be performing optimally. A laboratory test is exhibiting a **shift** when QC results make an obvious change in performance levels. A laboratory test is exhibiting a **trend** when results progressively increase or decrease over time.

☐ **LEARNING OBJECTIVE 7:** Identify and use quality control methods.

Proficiency Testing

Key Point:
• To continue testing and maintain Medicare eligibility, all laboratories, even those conducting only waived tests, must participate in three proficiency tests a year and must be available for at least one on-site inspection.

Reagent Management

Key Point:
• CLIA requires each laboratory to have a procedure to test new reagents (or kit lots) for acceptability before using them to perform patient's tests. Specifically, new reagent lots must be compared to previously used reagent lots to ensure comparability between the newly received lots and lots that have already been in use. Documentation of this verification process is required.

Instrument Calibration and Maintenance

Key Term: calibration
Key Point:
• Instruments are designed to produce results within a documented reportable range. If the QC results are not within the stated reference range, the instrument's **calibration** (standardization) should be checked by the manufacturer's instructions, and patients' and QC specimens should be retested.

Laboratory Safety

Key Term: material safety data sheet (MSDS)
Key Point:
• Chemical hazards can be minimized by labeling all chemicals with the **material safety data sheet (MSDS)** information. MSDS are obtained from the manufacturer and provide the manufacturer's instructions for storage, handling, and disposal of the chemical. They describe the risks associated with the product and indicate steps necessary to prevent exposure. An up-to-date volume of MSDS for all chemicals used in the laboratory is the focal part of the facility's chemical hygiene plan. The plan should also include chemical safety protocols specific to that facility.

Occupational Safety and Health Administration

Key Terms: Occupational Safety and Health Administration (OSHA); aerosol; Chemical Hygiene Plan

Key Points:

- **OSHA** is a federal agency in the U.S. Department of Labor that monitors and protects the health and safety of workers. OSHA standards are federal regulations that protect workers by eliminating or minimizing chemical, physical, and biological hazards and preventing accidents. OSHA standards supersede all other regulatory agency requirements. Two OSHA standards of particular importance to medical laboratories are the Occupational Exposure to Blood-borne Pathogens Standard and the Hazardous Communication (HazCom) Standard, or the "right to know law."

- The OSHA Blood-borne Pathogens Standard (review the use of standard precautions in Chapter 2). requires all medical employers to provide training for their employees in techniques that will protect them from occupational exposure to infectious agents, including blood-borne pathogens. Safety manuals must be available or incorporated into the policies and procedures manual to guide employees in correct procedures and emergency protocols.

- OSHA specifically mandates a written **Chemical Hygiene Plan** (CHP) be written by office management and made available to employees exposed to chemical hazards. A chemical hygiene plan is a part of the HazCom standard and must address these concerns.

☐ **LEARNING OBJECTIVE 8:** Define OSHA and state its purpose.

Safety Guidelines

Key Point:

- These guidelines are some of the most important safety factors required in all laboratories. Follow them carefully to protect yourself, your coworkers, and your patients.

☐ **LEARNING OBJECTIVE 9:** List the laboratory safety guidelines.

Incident Reports

Key Point:

- When there is an occurrence in the medical setting for which liability could be considered, an incident report should be completed.

Content Review

FOUNDATIONAL KNOWLEDGE

Brushing up on CLIA

1. CLIA works to support the health care industry by providing knowledge and resources for maintaining quality laboratory operations. List four areas that CLIA regulations set standards for.

   a. _____

   b. _____

   c. _____

   d. _____

2. Explain the significance of waived tests.

   _____

   _____

3. Review the list of laboratory tests below and place a check mark to indicate whether it is eligible for a CLIA waiver.

Test	Eligible	Ineligible
a. Non-automated copper sulfate testing for hemoglobin		
b. Gram staining		
c. Manual white blood cell count differentials without identification of atypical cells		
d. Fecal leukocyte examinations		
e. Centrifuged microhematocrits		
f. Histopathology		
g. Ovulation testing in packets with color comparison charts		

4. If you don't know the complexity level of a laboratory test, what level should you assume?

   _____

   _____

5. Which laboratory functions are monitored by a quality assurance plan?

   _____

   _____

Don't Panic!

6. Explain the difference between normal values and panic values in the chart below.

Normal Values	Panic Values

7. Fill in the chart to show the critical values for some common laboratory tests.

Lab Test	Critical Values	
	Low	**High**
a. Serum glucose		
b. Serum sodium		
c. White blood cell count		
d. Platelet count		
e. Partial Thromboplastin Time		

8. The test result for a patient's laboratory test is 44 units. The manufacturer of the test lists the reportable range of the test as 70–600. What should you list as the test result?

_____

Go With the Flow

9. Every office should have its own procedure for handling all normal and abnormal test results. What are three steps that should be included in this procedure?

a. _____

b. _____

c. _____

10. Describe the difference between a flow sheet and a patient history.

_____

_____

Controlling Quality

11. In the context of laboratory medical testing, what is the purpose of a control?

_____

_____

12. Explain the difference between qualitative and quantitative tests.

_____

_____

Lab Safety

13. What is the purpose of OSHA?

_____

_____

14. Name two OSHA standards that are important to medical laboratories.

a. _____

b. _____

15. Place a check mark in the correct box to indicate those items that may be used as personal protective equipment in the lab.

Types of Equipment	Yes	No
a. Gloves		
b. Ear plugs		
c. Gas mask		
d. Apron		
e. Work boots		
f. Contact lenses		
g. Goggles		
h. Glasses with side shields		
i. Mask		
j. Lab coat		
k. Reflective vest		
l. Face shield		
m. Soft helmet		
n. Gown		

16. A bottle of sodium hydroxide, a common alkali, has the diamond-shaped symbol of the National Fire Protection Association printed on it. The number "3" is printed in the blue quadrant. What does this number indicate?

_____

_____

17. Why is it important to keep an up-to-date volume of material safety data sheets in the office?

_____

_____

18. Read the following scenarios. Then decide if lab-safety guidelines are properly followed. If not, explain why.

a. Marco has to run three lab tests that need to be completed within the hour. However, it's time for his lunch break. To ensure that the tests are completed on time, he brings an energy drink into the lab and saves his lunch for later.

_____

_____

b. Hilel uses a glass beaker for a lab test. Then she realizes she needs the same equipment for her next test. So, she cleans the beaker with soap and water and dries it well. Then she reuses the glass beaker for the next test.

_____

_____

c. Jackson can't find the specific chemical he needs for a lab test. His coworker points out a container in the lab, but when Jackson picks it up, he finds the label is illegible. He checks with his coworker and she says she's positive that it's the correct chemical. With her reassurance, he uses the chemical to run the test.

_____

_____

19. Match the following key terms to their definitions.

Key Terms

a. aerosol _____

b. calibration _____

c. Chemical Hygiene Plan (CHP) _____

d. Clinical Laboratory Improvement Amendments (CLIA) _____

e. Clinical and Laboratory Standards Institute (CLSI) _____

f. flow sheet _____

g. laboratory procedure manual _____

h. material safety data sheet (MSDS) _____

i. normal values _____

j. Occupational Safety and Health Administration (OSHA) _____

k. panic values _____

l. quality assurance (QA) _____

m. quality control (QC) _____

n. reportable range _____

o. shift _____

p. trend _____

Definitions

1. normal values

2. suspended particles in gas or air

3. color-coded sheets that allow information to be recorded in graphic or tabular form for easy retrieval

4. reportable range

5. measurement for size or volume, as in calibrations on a syringe or pipette

6. quality assurance

7. a plan required by OSHA incorporating chemical-safety protocols

8. a set of laws that establish regulations governing any facility that performs testing for the diagnosis, prevention, or treatment of human disease or for assessment of patients' health status

9. agency that establishes rules to ensure the safety, standards, and integrity of all testing performed on human specimens

10. the federal agency that oversees working conditions

11. a reference guideline that describes how to perform every test in the laboratory; required in every lab

12. an obvious change in performance levels

13. a detailed record of all hazardous substances kept within a site

14. progressive change in performance levels over time

15. values representing the boundaries of the life-threatening laboratory test results

16. method to evaluate the proper performance of testing procedures, supplies, or equipment in a laboratory

20. True or False? Determine whether the following statements are true or false. If false, explain why.

a. Laboratories performing only waived tests need not undergo proficiency tests.

_____

_____

b. All specimens studied in the laboratory should be considered hazardous and must be treated as such.

_____

_____

c. Changes to the laboratory procedure manual can be approved by any laboratory employee.

_____

_____

d. Laboratories that provide free testing need not comply with CLIA guidelines.

_____

_____

APPLICATION

Critical Thinking Practice

1. The Levey-Jennings QC Chart for a test commonly performed in your office appears to suggest that the test is producing progressively higher results. How would you go about researching this phenomenon? What information should you present to the physician?

   _____

   _____

2. In order to test a specimen, you are required to use a corrosive reageant. Explain how you will prepare to perform the test.

   _____

   _____

Patient Education

1. You are explaining the results of a test to a patient. In one instance, a result is listed as "<20 mg/dL" and the patient wants to know why the actual result is not listed. One result is listed as critically low. Explain what this means to the patient.

   _____

   _____

Documentation

1. You receive laboratory reports from the reference laboratory. The results for Marsha Long's came in at 600 mg/dL. This is higher than the normal results. Document these results and any follow-up in the patient's chart.

   _____

   _____

Active Learning

1. Choose three hazardous materials that you may encounter in a lab, including chemicals, cleaning supplies, and disinfectants. Then locate the material safety data sheet for each item. Make a copy of each MSDS and then make a short list of the most essential information that you would like to remember about each item.

2. Each state has laws for reporting communicable diseases. Research the conditions that must be reported to your city or county health department. Then make a list that could be incorporated into your laboratory's procedure manual.

3. You are taking a job at a new laboratory and your supervisor has asked you to create a list of the personal protective equipment that must be ordered to protect workers in the lab. First create a list of the items that you need to purchase. Then research the costs of each item on your list. Create a spreadsheet showing the items and the unit cost as well as the quantity that you should order for the first shipment.

Professional Journal

REFLECT

(Prompts and Ideas: Lab safety is a critical issue when working in a laboratory. Do you have any concerns for your own safety when working in a lab? What can you do to protect yourself?)

_____

_____

_____

_____

_____

_____

_____

PONDER AND SOLVE

1. A test is showing systematically low results; that is, in each case, the result is proportionately lower than expected. The results are precise, but inaccurate. What must you do to ensure proper results?

_____

_____

_____

_____

_____

_____

_____

2. Your coworkers have suggested that CLIA guidelines are not significant in the case of waived tests. Why might they feel this way? Why are they wrong?

_____

_____

_____

_____

_____

_____

_____

EXPERIENCE

Skills related to this chapter include:

1. Screen and Follow-up Test Results and Document Laboratory Results Appropriately (Procedure 40-1).
2. Perform Routine Maintenance of Clinical Equipment (Procedure 40-2).
3. Quality Control Monitoring Using a QC Chart (Procedure 40-3).

Record any common mistakes, lessons learned, and/or tips you discovered during your experience of practicing and demonstrating these skills:

_____

_____

_____

_____

_____

_____

_____

Skill Practice

PERFORMANCE OBJECTIVES:

1. Screen and follow-up test results and document laboratory results appropriately (Procedure 40-1).
2. Perform routine maintenance of clinical equipment (Procedure 40-2).
3. Use methods of quality control (Procedure 40-3).

Name_____   Date _____   Time _____

Procedure 40-1:	SCREEN AND FOLLOW-UP TEST RESULTS AND DOCUMENT LABORATORY RESULTS APPROPRIATELY

EQUIPMENT/SUPPLIES: Patient laboratory results, Critical Values List for office, patient's chart, telephone (as needed)

STANDARDS: Given the needed equipment and a place to work, the student will perform this skill with _____% accuracy in a total of _____ minutes. *(Your instructor will tell you what the percentage and time limits will be before you begin practicing.)*

KEY: 4 = Satisfactory   0 = Unsatisfactory   NA = This step is not counted

PROCEDURE STEPS	SELF	PARTNER	INSTRUCTOR
1. Review laboratory reports received from reference laboratory.	☐	☐	☐
2. Note which reports may be placed directly on the patient's chart and which require immediate notification due to critical results.	☐	☐	☐
3. Notify the physician of the result. Take any immediate instructions from the physician.	☐	☐	☐
4. Follow instructions and document notification and follow-up.	☐	☐	☐
5. Chart remaining reports appropriately.	☐	☐	☐

CALCULATION

Total Possible Points: _____
Total Points Earned: _____ Multiplied by 100 = _____ Divided by Total Possible Points = _____%

Pass   **Fail**
☐   ☐   Comments:

Student's signature _____ Date _____
Partner's signature _____ Date _____
Instructor's signature _____ Date _____

Name _____ Date _____ Time _____

Procedure 40-2: PERFORM ROUTINE MAINTENANCE OF CLINICAL EQUIPMENT

EQUIPMENT: Laboratory instrument to be maintained, instrument manual from manufacturer, instrument maintenance log, maintenance supplies as indicated in the instrument manual, personal protective equipment, hand sanitizer, surface sanitizer, contaminated waste container

STANDARDS: Given the needed equipment and a place to work, the student will perform this skill with _____% accuracy in a total of _____ minutes. *(Your instructor will tell you what the percentage and time limits will be before you begin practicing.)*

KEY: 4 = Satisfactory   0 = Unsatisfactory   NA = This step is not counted

PROCEDURE STEPS	SELF	PARTNER	INSTRUCTOR
1. Wash your hands. Put on gloves.	☐	☐	☐
2. Read or review the maintenance section of the instrument manual.	☐	☐	☐
3. Follow the manufacturer's step-by-step instructions for maintaining the instrument.	☐	☐	☐
4. Turn on the instrument and ensure that it is calibrated.	☐	☐	☐
5. Perform the test on the quality control material. Record results. Determine whether QC is within control limits. If yes, proceed with patient testing. If no, take corrective action and recheck controls. Document corrective action. Proceed with patient testing when acceptable QC results are obtained.	☐	☐	☐
6. Document maintenance procedures performed in instrument maintenance log.	☐	☐	☐
7. Properly care for or dispose of equipment and supplies.	☐	☐	☐
8. Clean the work area. Remove personal protective equipment, and wash your hands.	☐	☐	☐

CALCULATION

Total Possible Points: _____
Total Points Earned: _____ Multiplied by 100 = _____ Divided by Total Possible Points = _____%

Pass   **Fail**
☐   ☐   Comments:

Chart Documentation

_____

_____

Student signature _____ Date _____
Partner signature _____ Date _____
Instructor signature _____ Date _____

Name _____ Date _____ Time _____

Procedure 40-3:	QUALITY CONTROL MONITORING USING A QC CHART

EQUIPMENT: Instrument test results, quality control charts

STANDARDS: Given the needed equipment and a place to work, the student will perform this skill with _____% accuracy in a total of _____ minutes. *(Your instructor will tell you what the percentage and time limits will be before you begin practicing.)*

KEY: 4 = Satisfactory   0 = Unsatisfactory   NA = This step is not counted

PROCEDURE STEPS	SELF	PARTNER	INSTRUCTOR
1. Assemble the charts and data.	☐	☐	☐
2. On the QC chart, plot the control results obtained for the test run.	☐	☐	☐
3. Evaluate chart for acceptability of results.	☐	☐	☐
4. If results are within accepted limits, report patient results.	☐	☐	☐
5. If results are not within accepted limits, do not report patient results. Troubleshoot the test. Repeat testing on the patient and control specimens.	☐	☐	☐
6. If results are within accepted limits, report patient results. Document corrective action and acceptable control results.	☐	☐	☐
7. If results are not within accepted limits, notify the physician of test malfunction. Arrange to have patient specimen referred for testing or store the specimen appropriately until repairs can be made.	☐	☐	☐
8. Troubleshoot within manufacturer's guidelines for operator troubleshooting. Document in the maintenance log. If this is not successful, arrange repairs for the instrument. Document any manufacturer supplied repairs in the maintenance log.	☐	☐	☐
9. Keep physician informed of testing status.	☐	☐	☐
10. Before returning the instrument to service, validate calibration and quality control. Document appropriately.	☐	☐	☐

CALCULATION

Total Possible Points: _____
Total Points Earned: _____ Multiplied by 100 = _____ Divided by Total Possible Points = _____%

Pass   **Fail**
☐   ☐   Comments:

Chart Documentation

_____

_____

Student's signature _____ Date _____
Partner's signature _____ Date _____
Instructor's signature _____ Date _____

Work Product 1

Use methods of quality control.

HCG pregnancy tests are qualitative tests, giving either a positive or a negative result. The manufacturer of the HCG test your office uses requires that controls be run for each lot of the test. You receive a shipment of "PREGNANCY TEST - URINE (HCG-omatic)," manufactured by "Acme Medical Products" and purchased from American Science & Surplus. The positive control is lot #QCC-1000P, and the negative control is lot #QCC-1000N. Using these controls give positive and negative results, respectively. The actual test kit is lot #HCG-1234R. Controls and tests all have an expiration date of June 2015.

You administer these HCG tests to five patients. The first two patients have a positive result. The third patient has a negative result. The fourth patient has a weak positive result, which fails the QC and is administered a second time to get a positive result. A fifth patient tests negative.

Record this information using the QC control log sample below.

QUALITATIVE QC LOG SHEET FOR _____								
RECORD LOT NUMBER IF DIFFERENT FROM LAST LOT NUMBER.								
TEST DATE	KIT LOT	POSITIVE CONTROL LOT #	NEGATIVE CONTROL LOT #	POSITIVE CONTROL RESULT	NEGATIVE CONTROL RESULT	OK TO USE?	IF NO, CORRECTIVE ACTION	INITIALS

Work Product 2

Document appropriately.

You administer an HCG pregnancy test to Marie Coyote. She has a weak positive result, which fails the QC so you must administer the test again. The second time the test shows a positive result. You refer the patient to LabTest to have some initial blood tests before her next appointment. If you are currently working in a medical office, use a blank paper patient chart from the office. If this is not available to you, use the space below to document the results of her HCG pregnancy tests and QC results below.

_____

_____

_____

_____

Chapter Self-Assessment Quiz

1. What body regulates non-research laboratory testing in the United States?

  a. The Centers for Disease Control and Prevention

  b. The Centers for Medicare and Medicaid Services

  c. The Food and Drug Administration

  d. The Department of Labor

  e. Congress

2. Which result is within the reportable range 200 μg /l − 450 μg /l?

  a. 360 mg/l

  b. 500 μg /l

  c. 190 μg /l

  d. 265 μg /l

  e. 300 mg/l

3. A laboratory must have a written quality assurance policy that:

  a. is communicated to all staff.

  b. is stored neared the site of use.

  c. includes all HazCom requiremements.

  d. includes all MSDSs supplied by the manufacturers.

  e. is updated once a week.

4. Which belongs in a POL Quality Assurance Plan?

  a. Laboratory standards

  b. Accreditation policies

  c. Patient test management

  d. Quality control

  e. Prescription information

5. A pronounced and immediate change in test performance is known as a:

  a. control.

  b. trend.

  c. reagent.

  d. flow.

  e. shift.

6. What might the white quadrant of the National Fire Safety Association diamond indicate?

  a. Health hazard

  b. Fire hazard

  c. Reaction hazard

  d. Biological hazard

  e. Natural hazard

7. An aerosol is:

  a. a group of particles suspended in gas or air.

  b. a liquid required for many tests.

  c. a flammable material.

  d. a polymer used in many labs.

  e. a jelly-like substance.

8. OSHA is a federal agency within the:

  a. Department of the Interior.

  b. Department of Health and Human Services.

  c. Department of Labor.

  d. Department of Commerce.

  e. Department of the Treasury.

9. All hazardous chemicals must be:

   a. placed on top shelves out of a patient's reach.

   b. placed near a sink in case a person's skin is exposed.

   c. labeled with a warning and statement of the hazard.

   d. used only by medical professionals while wearing heavy boots.

   e. stored away from sunlight.

10. What must you do immediately in the event of biohazard exposure?

    a. Alert local public health officials.

    b. Report to your supervisor.

    c. Go to the emergency room.

    d. Perform a self-examination.

    e. Dispose of your clothing.

11. If you draw blood from the wrong patient, you should fill out a(n):

    a. flow sheet.

    b. insurance claim.

    c. lab procedure manual.

    d. incident report.

    e. test report.

12. The best source of normal values for the POL is:

    a. the Physician's Desk Reference.

    b. the manufacturer's packaging insert.

    c. the ICD-9 CM.

    d. the Laboratory Procedure Manual.

    e. the CLIA certificate.

13. CLIA waivers are available for:

    a. fecal occult blood packets.

    b. Gram staining.

    c. microscopic urinalysis.

    d. urine and throat cultures.

    e. centrifuged microhematocrits.

14. Procedure for proper maintenance of specimens falls under which category of a POL Quality Assurance Plan?

    a. Patient test management

    b. Quality control

    c. Proficiency testing

    d. Reagent management

    e. Instrument calibration and maintenance

15. The presence of a panic value in test results indicates:

    a. an outbreak of a contagious virus.

    b. imminent death of the patient.

    c. general good health.

    d. a potentially life-threatening situation.

    e. negligence on the part of the laboratory.

16. The QC log is used to:

    a. document quality control procedures.

    b. report quality control procedures to CMA.

    c. describe consequences of failed quality control.

    d. present quality control statistics to laboratory inspectors.

    e. record the performance of quality controls.

17. Who provides quality control instructions for a given test?

    a. FDA

    b. CLSI

    c. Laboratory director

    d. Manufacturer

    e. OSHA

18. Proficiency testing occurs:

    a. once a year.

    b. twice a year.

    c. three times a year.

    d. four times a year.

    e. five times a year.

19. What document describes the appropriate methods for performing every test offered by a laboratory?

    a. Quality assurance plan

    b. CLIA certificate

    c. Laboratory Procedure Manual

    d. Flow sheet

    e. Material safety data sheet

20. One example of a moderate-complexity test is:

    a. urine and throat cultures.

    b. fecal occult blood packets.

    c. non-automated copper sulfate test for hemoglobin.

    d. urine pregnancy testing kits.

    e. manual cell counts.

Chapter Checklist

☐ Read textbook chapter and take notes within the Chapter Notes outline. Answer the Learning Objectives as you reach them in the content, and then check them off.

☐ Work the Content Review questions—both Foundational Knowledge and Application.

☐ Perform the Active Learning exercise(s).

☐ Complete Professional Journal entries.

☐ Complete Skill Practice Activity(s) using Competency Evaluation Forms and Work Products, when appropriate.

☐ Take the Chapter Self-Assessment Quiz.

☐ Insert all appropriate pages into your Portfolio.

Learning Objectives

1. Spell and define the key terms.
2. List precautions to be observed when drawing blood.
3. Identify equipment and supplies used to obtain a routine venous specimen.
4. List the major anticoagulants, their color codes, and the suggested order in which they are filled from a venipuncture.
5. Identify equipment and supplies used to obtain a routine capillary skin puncture.

6. Explain the importance of correct patient identification and complete specimen and requisition labeling.
7. Describe the location, selection, and preparation of the blood collection sites for veins.
8. Describe the location, selection, and preparation of the blood collection sites for capillaries.
9. Describe care for a puncture site after blood has been drawn.

Chapter Notes

Note: Bold-faced headings are the major headings in the text chapter; headings in regular font are lower-level headings (i.e., the content is subordinate to, or falls "under," the major headings). Make sure you understand the key terms used in the chapter, as well as the concepts presented as Key Points.

TEXT SUBHEADINGS   **NOTES**

Introduction _____

Key Terms: barrier precautions; prophylaxis
Key Points:
- The quality of a laboratory test result is only as good as the quality of the specimen collected for testing. The quality of the specimen starts with the phlebotomist's attention to several factors.
- You must perform blood collection in the safest manner possible. Blood is a biohazardous material, so it should be handled with standard precautions and appropriate **barrier precautions**, physical products or equipment used specifically for the purpose of protecting the patient and the healthcare worker from exposure to potentially infectious material.
- Needlestick injuries contribute to the overall burden of health care worker injuries.

☐ **LEARNING OBJECTIVE 1:** Spell and define the key terms.

☐ **LEARNING OBJECTIVE 2:** List precautions to be observed when drawing blood.

General Phlebotomy Equipment _____

Blood Drawing Station _____

Gloves _____

Key Points:
- Guidelines from the CDC and the Occupational Safety and Health Administration (OSHA) require that gloves be worn during phlebotomy procedures. A new pair of gloves must be used for each patient and removed when the procedure is finished. Nonsterile, disposable latex, nitrile, vinyl, or polyethylene gloves are acceptable.
- Standard precautions require handwashing after glove removal.
- Some users have allergic responses to glove powder. Powder in latex gloves can also facilitate suspension of latex particles in the air, posing danger to those with latex allergy. Gloves are available powder free and/or latex free. Best practice for the medical assistant is to ask the patient if he or she has a latex allergy, prior to starting the phlebotomy procedure. The phlebotomist can avoid gloves, tourniquets, and band-aids containing latex before exposing the patient.

Antiseptics _____

Key Term: antiseptics
Key Point:
• The most commonly used **antiseptic** for routine blood collection is 70% isopropyl alcohol.

Spill Kit Supplies and Instructions _____

Key Point:
• When cleaning blood spills, you should wear disposable gloves of sufficient sturdiness that they will not tear while you clean. If the gloves develop holes, tears, or splits, remove them, wash hands immediately, and put on fresh gloves. Disposable gloves must never be washed or reused.

Gauze Pads _____

Bandages _____

Key Points:
• If a patient is allergic to adhesive bandages, use paper, cloth, or knitted tape over a folded gauze square. Do not use a bandage on infants under 2 years of age because of the danger of aspiration and suffocation.
• Latex-free bandages are available in case of latex allergy.

Sharps Containers _____

Key Term: sharps container

☐ **LEARNING OBJECTIVE 3:** Identify equipment and supplies used to obtain a routine venous specimen.

Venipuncture Equipment _____

Tourniquets

Key Terms: hemoconcentration; hemolysis
Key Point:
- It can easily be released with one hand, does not cut into the patient's arm, and is inexpensive enough that a new tourniquet can be used for each patient. The maximum time limit for leaving the tourniquet in place is one minute. Extending the time limit can alter test results by causing **hemoconcentration** (decrease of the fluid content of blood) and by causing **hemolysis** (rupturing of red blood cells causing release of intracellular contents into the plasma).

Needles

Key Terms: bevel; gauge
Key Points:
- Due to the frequency of phlebotomist exposure to communicable disease by needlestick, OSHA requires needles to have safety features to minimize accidental needlesticks. Manufacturers provide needles with various features to facilitate this requirement. Users can select products that both meet requirements and provide ease of use.
- The larger the **gauge** number, the smaller the diameter of the needle (e.g., 20 gauge is larger than 25 gauge).

Blood Collection Systems

Key Term: evacuated tube
Key Point:
- The primary blood collection system most commonly used today for venipuncture is the vacuum or **evacuated tube** system.

Evacuated Tube System

Key Term: multisample needle
Key Point:
- The tube fills until the vacuum is exhausted, so that a tube that has lost all or part of its vacuum will not fill completely, if at all.

Tube Additives

Key Terms: anticoagulant; gel separator

Key Points:

- Different laboratory tests require different types of blood specimens.
- The clotting process takes 30–60 minutes at 22–25°C. The specimen should be allowed to complete the clotting process prior to being centrifuged for separation of the serum from the clot and is required to attain the optimum specimen.
- It is necessary to use the correct **anticoagulant** because improper anticoagulant use can alter test results. It is also necessary to fill the tube until the vacuum is exhausted. Under-filled tubes will alter patient test results due to over-dilution of the specimen by the tube additive.

Order of Draw

Key Term: order of draw

Key Points:

- A designated **order of draw** is recommended to avoid contamination of nonadditive tubes by additive tubes, cross-contamination between different types of additive tubes, contamination with tissue thromboplastin, and microbial contamination.
- The protocol for your facility should be the order you use.

☐ **LEARNING OBJECTIVE 4:** List the major anticoagulants, their color codes, and the suggested order in which they are filled from a venipuncture.

Syringe System

Key Point:

- A syringe is helpful with fragile veins because the vacuum can be applied slowly and gently, rather than all at once as with vacuum tubes.

Winged Infusion Set _____

_____

Key Term: luer adapter
Key Points:
- It is preferred in geriatric and pediatric phlebotomy because the tubing length allows more flexibility for patients who cannot keep still and those whose limbs may be not be able to extend adequately enough to accommodate the needle holder and stationary needle.
- Blood specimens for laboratory testing should be drawn with gauge 22 needles or larger (smaller gauge number).
- During withdrawal of the specimen into the collection device, the red blood cells endure tremendous pressure. The combination of the pull of the vacuum with the small bore of the needle can result in more pressure than the cell structure can withstand causing red blood cells to rupture.
- Hemolysis contamination of the plasma can result in significant inaccuracies in test results.

Capillary Puncture (Microcollection) Equipment _____

_____

Key Point:
- The equipment used to collect the specimen depends on the patient's age and condition, and on the test being performed.

Puncture Devices _____

_____

Microhematocrit Tubes _____

_____

Microcollection Containers _____

_____

Filter Paper Test Requisitions _____

_____

Warming Devices _____

_____

Key Point:
- Important especially for heel sticks, warmers increase blood flow before the skin is punctured.

☐ **LEARNING OBJECTIVE 5:** Identify equipment and supplies used to obtain a routine capillary skin puncture.

Phlebotomy Quality Control

Key Points:
- Many factors must be addressed to ensure specimen quality. Phlebotomy errors may cause serious harm to patients. Quality control consists of methods practiced in every capillary puncture or venipuncture to optimize the quality of each specimen.
- Quality Control begins with a thorough specimen collection manual that specifies the instructions for collecting every type of specimen. The phlebotomist must meet the written standards at all times.

☐ **LEARNING OBJECTIVE 6:** Explain the importance of correct patient identification and complete specimen and requisition labeling.

Patient Preparation

Key Term: syncope
Key Points:
- Always believe patients who say they faint during venipuncture. Have these patients lie down during the procedure. This reduces the chance of **syncope** (fainting), and if the patient does faint, he or she will not fall. If the patient is sitting and feels faint or mentions feeling weak, have him or her lower the head and take deep breaths. Call for assistance without leaving the patient unattended.
- Specimens should be labeled before the patient exits the facility using the collection protocol for that facility.

Performing a Venipuncture with a Multisample Needle or a Winged Infusion Set

Key Term: antecubital space
Key Points:
- The commonly used vein for venipuncture is the median cubital vein.

Selection of the Venipuncture Site _____

Key Term: palpate
Key Points:
- Begin the procedure by washing your hands and putting on gloves. Equipment and supplies should be assembled near the phlebotomy chair. The tourniquet should be placed 3 to 4 inches above the planned venipuncture site and secured with a half-bow knot.
- Do not allow the patient to open and close the fist because it will cause hemoconcentration (pooling of blood components) and lead to erroneous test results.
- While some veins are visible, the best choice for venipuncture is found by touch.
- Do not slap arm when trying to locate a vein as this can cause bruising.
- If no suitable antecubital vein is found in either arm, check hand veins and finally wrist veins. Massaging the arm from wrist to elbow increases blood flow and makes veins more palpable. Warming the site with a warm towel can produce the same effect.

Special Concerns Using the Winged Infusion System _____

Key Points:
- To avoid specimen contamination by transferring additives with the winged infusion system, hold the collection tube horizontally or slightly lowered. To enhance the use of the winged infusion set, use the smallest evacuated collection tube. This puts less pressure on small, fragile veins.
- A drawback in using the winged infusion system is that in some sets the bevel cut is more blunt than the multi-sample needle resulting in more painful punctures. Because the needle part of the system is much shorter than the multi-sample needle, it cannot reach deeper veins.
- Several studies have shown that winged sets cause increased numbers of needlesticks to phlebotomists. After withdrawing the needle from the patient, it tends to hang loose on the end of the tubing offering less control than the multi-sample needle. Phlebotomists should use extra caution and activate the safety device as quickly as possible.
- Due to their limitations, winged sets should be used only for small, fragile veins in pediatrics and geriatrics.

Venipuncture Using The Evacuated Tube _____

Key Point:
- Comply with your facility's protocol for the allowed number of attempts to obtain a specimen. A common number of attempts is two.

Complications of Venipuncture

Key Term: hematoma
Key Points:
- The most common complication of venipuncture is **hematoma** formation caused by blood leaking into the tissues during or after venipuncture.
- If a hematoma begins to form during the venipuncture, release the tourniquet immediately, withdraw the needle, and hold pressure on the site for at least 2 minutes.
- Accidental puncture of an artery is recognized by the blood's bright red color and the pulsing of the specimen into the tube. In this case, it is important to hold pressure over the site for a full 5 minutes after the needle is removed.

☐ **LEARNING OBJECTIVE 7:** Describe the location, selection, and preparation of the blood collection sites for veins.

Performing a Capillary Puncture

Key Point:
- However, some results are more accurate on venipuncture specimens than on capillary specimens. The phlebotomist must be aware of these tests in choosing the appropriate procedure for the patient. Tests that cannot be performed on skin puncture specimens include erythrocyte sedimentation rate methods, coagulation studies on plasma, cultures, and tests that require large blood volumes.

Selection of the Capillary Puncture Site

Key Point:
- Recommended sites are the fleshy pad of the third or fourth finger of the patient's nondominant hand only. For finger puncture sites, it is best to have the hand below the heart. For infant heel punctures in children under 1 year of age, the CLSI (described earlier in this chapter) set the standard of a maximum of 2 mm for heel punctures to avoid hitting bone.

Complications of Capillary Puncture _____

Key Points:
- The capillary puncture activates the body's clotting system to stop the bleeding as soon as the skin is punctured. If an anticoagulated specimen is required, it should be drawn first to get an adequate volume before the blood begins to clot.
- Avoid excessive squeezing of the fingertip or heel because the red blood cells will rupture and contaminate the specimen.

☐ **LEARNING OBJECTIVE 8:** Describe the location, selection, and preparation of the blood collection sites for capillaries.

☐ **LEARNING OBJECTIVE 9.** Describe care for a puncture site after blood has been drawn.

Content Review

FOUNDATIONAL KNOWLEDGE

Phlebotomy 101

1. Give a description and purpose for the following phlebotomy equipment.

Equipment	Description	Purpose
a. Blood drawing station		
b. Gloves		
c. Antiseptics		
d. Spill kit supplies and instructions		
e. Gauze pads		
f. Bandages		
g. Sharps containers		

2. Name the four steps for avoiding hemoconcentration.

a. _____

b. _____

c. _____

d. _____

All About Venipuncture

3. Give a description and purpose of the following venipuncture equipment.

Equipment	Description	Purpose
a. Tourniquet		
b. Needle		
c. Blood Collection System		
d. Tube Additives		

4. Following an order of draw enables you to avoid:

    a. contamination of nonadditive tubes.

    b. contamination with tissue thromboplastin.

    c. microbial contamination.

    d. all of the above

5. Review the list of characteristics in the box below. Then decide if it is a characteristic that describes a syringe system or winged infusion set and place in the appropriate box in the chart.

Syringe System	Winged Infusion Set

Characteristics

- Helpful with fragile veins
- Preferred in geriatric and pediatric phlebotomy
- Comes with attachments to be used
- Pulling on plunger creates a vacuum in the barrel
- Requires a collection of blood to a collection tube
- Allows more flexibility for patient who can not stay still

6. Name six ways in which you can reduce the risk of phlebotomy liability.

    a. _____

    b. _____

    c. _____

    d. _____

    e. _____

    f. _____

7. What is a warming device? What is its purpose in capillary puncture?

_____

_____

8. Circle the tasks below that are considered quality-control methods in specimen collection.

   a. Selection of the venipuncture or capillary puncture site

   b. Type of collection and amount of specimen to be collected

   c. Collecting samples only before 12 PM

   d. Types and amounts of preservatives and anticoagulants

   e. Patient posture

   f. Duration of tourniquet use

   g. Actual time of specimen collection

   h. Choosing the correct equipment

   i. Order of draw

   j. Need for special handling between time of collection and time received by the laboratory

   k. Providing the patient with juice before draw

9. Jordan, your 5-year-old patient, is afraid to have a skin puncture. She is extremely agitated and her mother is having a difficult time trying to get her to sit still. Gloria, the phlebotomist, decides to have the parent restrain the child by firmly holding the child's finger very still. Gloria notices that the screaming child's hands are cold and clammy. With gloves on, Gloria quickly performs the skin puncture, capturing every drop. Identify the mistakes Gloria made in preparing the patient and list possible effects.

10. Give definitions for and explain the importance of the following dietary restrictions.

   a. Fasting:

   b. NPO:

11. List the six contraindications in choosing a specific site for venipuncture.

   a.

   b.

   c.

   d.

   e.

   f.

12. What should you do if a hematoma begins to form during venipuncture?

13. List the four contraindications in choosing a specific site for capillary puncture.

   a.

   b.

   c.

   d.

14. Match the order of draw with rationale for collection order.

a. Heparin tubes	**1.** Minimizes chance of microbial contamination
b. Coagulation tubes	**2.** Prevents contamination by additives in other tubes
c. (EDTA) tubes	**3.** Second or third position in order of draw; prevents tissue thromboplastin contamination; must be the first additive tube in the order because all other additive tubes affect coagulation tests
d. Blood cultures	**4.** Prevents contamination additives in other tubes; comes after coagulation tests because silica particles activate clotting and affect coagulation tests; carryover of silica into subsequent tubes can be overridden by the anticoagulant in them
e. (PSTs)	**5.** Contains heparin, which affects coagulation tests and interferes in collection of serum specimens; causes the least interference in tests other than coagulation tests
f. Oxalate/fluoride tubes	**6.** Same as PST
g. Serum separator gel tubes	**7.** Causes more carryover problems than any other additive; elevates sodium and potassium levels; chelates and decreases calcium and iron levels; elevates prothrombin time and partial thromboplastin time results
h. Plain (nonadditive) tubes	**8.** Sodium fluoride and potassium oxalate elevate sodium and potassium levels, respectively; comes after hematology tubes because oxalate damages cell membranes and causes abnormal red blood cell morphology

15. Fill in the blanks on situations that may trigger hematoma formation.

   a. The vein is _____ or too _____ for the needle.

   b. The needle _____ all the way through the _____.

   c. The needle is only _____ inserted into the vein.

   d. _____ or _____ probing is used to find the vein.

   e. The needle is _____ while the _____ is still on.

   f. _____ is not adequately _____ after venipuncture.

16. Name eight sources of error in venipuncture procedure.

   a. _____

   b. _____

   c. _____

   d. _____

   e. _____

   f. _____

   g. _____

   h. _____

17. Which of the following is a source of error in skin puncture?

   a. Puncturing an infant's heel

   b. Failing to add Betadine to the specimen

   c. Failing to use the first drop of blood

   d. Excessive massaging of puncture site

18. Decide if the following instructions apply to evacuated tube/winged infusion, capillary puncture, or both. Place a check mark in the appropriate box.

	Evacuated Tube/ Winged Infusion	Capillary Puncture	Both
a. Check the requisition slip.			
b. Make sure the site is warm and not cyanotic or edematous.			
c. Check the expiration date on tubes.			
d. Ask the patient the last time he ate or drank anything other than water.			
e. Hold the patient's finger or heel firmly.			
f. Touch only the tip of the collection device to the drop of blood.			
g. Instruct the patient to sit with a well-supported arm.			
h. Release the tourniquet after palpating the vein.			
i. Do not shake the tube.			
j. Cap microcollection tubes.			
k. Obtain the first drop of blood and wipe it away with dry gauze.			
l. Instruct the patient not to lift heavy objects for one hour.			
m. Make a swift, firm puncture.			
n. Test, transfer, or store specimen according to the medical office policy.			
o. Check the puncture site for bleeding.			

19. Match the following key terms to their definitions.

Key Terms

a. antecubital space _____
b. anticoagulant _____
c. antiseptic _____
d. barrier precautions _____
e. bevel _____
f. evacuated tube _____
g. gauge _____
h. gel separator _____
i. hematoma _____
j. hemoconcentration _____
k. hemolysis _____
l. luer adapter _____
m. multisample needle _____
n. order of draw _____
o. palpate _____
p. prophylaxis _____
q. sharps container _____
r. syncope _____

Definitions

1. protective treatment for the prevention of disease once exposure has occurred
2. physical products or equipment used specifically for the purpose of protecting the patient and the health care worker from exposure to potentially infectious material
3. any substance that inhibits the growth of bacteria; used on skin before any procedure that breaks the integumentary barrier
4. special puncture-resistant, leak-proof, disposable receptacles used to dispose of used needles
5. a condition in which the plasma portion of the blood filters into the tissues causing an increase in nonfilterable blood components
6. rupture of erythrocytes with the release of hemoglobin into the plasma or serum causing the specimen to appear pink or red in color
7. the point of the needle that has been cut on a slant for ease of entry
8. a standard for measuring the diameter of the lumen of a needle
9. premeasured vaccum tube that receives the patient's blood during the venipuncture procedure
10. a special blood-drawing needle used with an evacuated tube system that allows the user to collect more than one tube of blood without contaminating the tubes or holder
11. anything that prevents or delays clotting of blood

12. a nonreacting substance located in an evacuated tube that forms a physical barrier between the cells and serum or plasma after the specimen has been centrifuged

13. a device for connecting a syringe or evacuated holder to the needle to promote a secure fit

14. sudden fall in blood pressure or cerebral hypoxia resulting in loss of consciousness

15. inner surface of the bend of the elbow where the major veins for venipuncture are located

16. to examine by feel or touch

17. blood clot that forms at an injury site

18. the special sequence in which multiple specimen tubes are collected

20. True or False? Determine whether the following statements are true or false. If false, explain why.

a. Winged sets cause increased numbers of needlesticks to phlebotomists.

_____

b. For finger-puncture sites, it is best to have the hand below the heart.

_____

c. Never believe patients when they say they faint during venipuncture.

_____

d. Warmers decrease blood flow before the skin is punctured.

_____

APPLICATION

Critical Thinking Practice

1. You have a patient who says that he always becomes nervous at the sight of his own blood, but has never fainted before. You ask the patient to lie down during the procedure. Your patient is fine with the needle insertion, but as soon as he sees the sight of his own blood, he passes out. What should you do?

_____

_____

2. It is your first time performing a skin puncture on the heel of an infant, and as much as the father tries to comfort his baby, the baby won't stop crying or hold still. How would you handle this situation?

_____

_____

Patient Education

1. An elderly patient comes in for a venipuncture procedure. You insert the needle at a narrow angle because of the shallowness of the patient's veins. However, your patient's vein "rolls" during this procedure and after removing the needle, your patient begins to develop a huge hematoma. How do you treat your patient's condition and console your patient, who has become very anxious?

_____

_____

Documentation

1. Write a narrative note that describes the procedure in the exercise above. Include all necessary details, as this will be included in the patient's chart.

_____

_____

Active Learning

1. Make an information chart on preventing needle sticks, detailing safe needle procedures and how to avoid punctures. Include in the chart preventative vaccinations that can help keep phlebotomists safe from blood-borne pathogens.

2. Create a sequence chart for the physician's office that pictorially represents order-of-draw color coding and outlines CLSI guidelines and protocols.

3. Familiarize yourself with phlebotomy equipment and draw a diagram of your blood-drawing station; detail on your diagram where supplies are kept. Think in terms of safety about where your blood station should be positioned in the office. Think about how the organization of your station will assist you in phlebotomy procedures and minimize the likelihood of accidents.

Professional Journal

REFLECT

(Prompts and Ideas: Have you ever known anyone with a fear of needles? What would you say to him to lessen his fears? If you had a patient with a fear of needles, what kind of body language and verbal language would you use to comfort and reassure him?)

_____

_____

_____

_____

_____

_____

_____

PONDER AND SOLVE

1. After drawing blood with a winged set, you inadvertently poke yourself with the needle. How would you handle this situation?

_____

_____

_____

_____

_____

_____

2. Your last patient of the day, a young child accompanied by her mother, accidentally knocks over your collection tubes that were within her reach as you were disposing of sharps. How would you handle this situation?

_____

_____

_____

_____

_____

_____

_____

EXPERIENCE

Skills related to this chapter include:

1. Obtaining a Blood Specimen by Evacuated Tube or Winged Infusion Set (Procedure 41-1).

2. Obtaining a Blood Specimen by Capillary Puncture (Procedure 41-2).

Record any common mistakes, lessons learned, and/or tips you discovered during your experience of practicing and demonstrating these skills.

_____

_____

_____

_____

_____

_____

_____

Skill Practice

PERFORMANCE OBJECTIVES:

1. Obtain a blood specimen by evacuated tube or winged infusion set (Procedure 41-1).

2. Obtain a blood specimen by capillary puncture (Procedure 41-2).

Name _____ Date _____ Time _____

Procedure 41-1:	OBTAINING A BLOOD SPECIMEN BY EVACUATED TUBE OR WINGED INFUSION SET

EQUIPMENT/SUPPLIES: Multisample needle and adaptor or winged infusion set, evacuated tubes, tourniquet, sterile gauze pads, bandages, sharps container, 70% alcohol pad, permanent marker or pen, appropriate personal protective equipment (e.g., gloves, impervious gown, face shield)

STANDARDS: Given the needed equipment and a place to work, the student will perform this skill with _____% accuracy in a total of _____ minutes. *(Your instructor will tell you what the percentage and time limits will be before you begin practicing.)*

KEY: 4 = Satisfactory   0 = Unsatisfactory   NA = This step is not counted

PROCEDURE STEPS	SELF	PARTNER	INSTRUCTOR
1. Check the requisition slip to determine the tests ordered and specimen requirements.	☐	☐	☐
2. Wash your hands.	☐	☐	☐
3. Assemble the equipment. Check the expiration date on the tubes.	☐	☐	☐
4. Greet and identify the patient. Explain the procedure. Ask for and answer any questions.	☐	☐	☐
5. If a fasting specimen is required, ask the patient the last time he or she ate or drank anything other than water.	☐	☐	☐
6. Put on nonsterile latex or vinyl gloves. Use other personal protective equipment as defined by facility policy.	☐	☐	☐
7. <u>For evacuated tube collection</u>: Break the seal of the needle cover and thread the sleeved needle into the adaptor, using the needle cover as a wrench. <u>For winged infusion set collection</u>: Extend the tubing. Thread the sleeved needle into the adaptor. <u>For both methods</u>: Tap the tubes that contain additives to ensure that the additive is dislodged from the stopper and wall of the tube. Insert the tube into the adaptor until the needle slightly enters the stopper. Do not push the top of the tube stopper beyond the indentation mark. If the tube retracts slightly, leave it in the retracted position.	☐	☐	☐
8. Instruct the patient to sit with a well-supported arm.	☐	☐	☐
9. Apply the tourniquet around the patient's arm 3–4 inches above the elbow. **a.** Apply the tourniquet snuggly, but not too tightly. **b.** Secure the tourniquet by using the half-bow knot. **c.** Make sure the tails of the tourniquet extend upward to avoid contaminating the venipuncture site. **d.** Ask the patient to make a fist and hold it, but not to pump the fist.	☐	☐	☐
10. Select a vein by palpating. Use your gloved index finger to trace the path of the vein and judge its depth.	☐	☐	☐

PROCEDURE STEPS	SELF	PARTNER	INSTRUCTOR
11. Release tourniquet after palpating the vein if it has been left on for more than one minute. Have patient release fist.	☐	☐	☐
12. Cleanse the venipuncture site with an alcohol pad, starting in the center of puncture site and working outward in a circular motion. Allow the site to dry or dry the site with sterile gauze. Do not touch the area after cleansing.	☐	☐	☐
13. If blood being drawn for culture will be used in diagnosing a septic condition, make sure the specimen is sterile. To do this, apply alcohol to the area for 2 full minutes. Then apply a 2% iodine solution in ever-widening circles. Never move the wipes back over areas that have been cleaned; use a new wipe for each sweep across the area.	☐	☐	☐
14. Reapply the tourniquet if it was removed after palpation. Ask patient to make a fist.	☐	☐	☐
15. Remove the needle cover. Hold the needle assembly in your dominant hand, thumb on top of the adaptor and fingers under it. Grasp the patient's arm with the other hand, using your thumb to draw the skin taut over the site. This anchors the vein about 1–2 inches below the puncture site and helps keep it in place during needle insertion.	☐	☐	☐
16. With the bevel up, line up the needle with the vein approximately one-quarter to half an inch below the site where the vein is to be entered. At a 15- to 30-degree angle, rapidly and smoothly insert the needle through the skin. Use a lesser angle for winged infusion set collections. Place two fingers on the flanges of the adapter and with the thumb push the tube onto the needle inside the adapter. Allow the tube to fill to capacity. Release the tourniquet and allow the patient to release the fist. When blood flow ceases, remove the tube from the adapter by gripping the tube with your nondominant hand and placing your thumb against the flange during removal. Twist and gently pull out the tube. Steady the needle in the vein. Avoid pulling up or pressing down on the needle while it is in the vein. Insert any other necessary tubes into adapter and allow each to fill to capacity.	☐	☐	☐
17. With the tourniquet released, remove the tube from the adapter before removing the needle from the arm.	☐	☐	☐
18. Place a sterile gauze pad over the puncture site at the time of needle withdrawal. Do not apply any pressure to the site until the needle is completely removed. **a.** After the needle is removed, immediately activate the safety device and apply pressure or have the patient apply direct pressure for 3–5 minutes. Do not bend the arm at the elbow.	☐	☐	☐
19. If the vacuum tubes contain an anticoagulant, they must be mixed immediately by gently inverting the tube 8–10 times. Do not shake the tube.	☐	☐	☐
20. Label the tubes with patient information as defined in facility protocol.	☐	☐	☐
21. Check the puncture site for bleeding. Apply a dressing, a clean 2 × 2 gauze pad folded in quarters, and hold in place by an adhesive bandage or 3-inch strip of tape.	☐	☐	☐
22. Thank the patient. Instruct the patient to leave the bandage in place at least 15 minutes and not to carry a heavy object (such as a purse) or lift heavy objects with that arm for 1 hour.	☐	☐	☐

23. Properly care for or dispose of all equipment and supplies. Clean the work area. Remove personal protective equipment and wash your hands.	☐	☐	☐
24. Test, transfer, or store the blood specimen according to the medical office policy.	☐	☐	☐
25. Record the procedure.	☐	☐	☐

CALCULATION

Total Possible Points: _____
Total Points Earned: _____ Multiplied by 100 = _____ Divided by Total Possible Points = _____%

Pass   **Fail**
☐   ☐   Comments:

Student signature _____ Date _____
Partner signature _____ Date _____
Instructor signature _____ Date _____

Name_____ Date_____ Time_____

Procedure 41-2:	OBTAINING A BLOOD SPECIMEN BY CAPILLARY PUNCTURE

EQUIPMENT/SUPPLIES: Skin puncture device, 70% alcohol pads, 2×2 gauze pads, microcollection tubes or containers, heel-warming device if needed, small band-aids, pen or permanent marker and personal protective equipment (e.g., gloves, impervious gown, face shield)

STANDARDS: Given the needed equipment and a place to work, the student will perform this skill with _____% accuracy in a total of _____ minutes. *(Your instructor will tell you what the percentage and time limits will be before you begin practicing.)*

KEY: 4 = Satisfactory   0 = Unsatisfactory   NA = This step is not counted

PROCEDURE STEPS	SELF	PARTNER	INSTRUCTOR
1. Check the requisition slip to determine the tests ordered and specimen requirements.	☐	☐	☐
2. Wash your hands.	☐	☐	☐
3. Assemble the equipment.	☐	☐	☐
4. Greet and identify the patient. Explain the procedure. Ask for and answer any questions.	☐	☐	☐
5. Put on gloves.	☐	☐	☐
6. Select the puncture site (the lateral portion of the tip of the middle or ring finger of the nondominant hand or lateral curved surface of the heel of an infant). The puncture should be made in the fleshy central portion of the second or third finger, slightly to the side of center, and perpendicular to the grooves of the fingerprint. Perform heel puncture only on the plantar surface of the heel, medial to an imaginary line extending from the middle of the great toe to the heel, and lateral to an imaginary line drawn from between the fourth and fifth toes to the heel. Use the appropriate puncture device for the site selected.	☐	☐	☐
7. Make sure the site chosen is warm and not cyanotic or edematous. Gently massage the finger from the base to the tip or massage the infant's heel.	☐	☐	☐
8. Grasp the finger firmly between your nondominant index finger and thumb, or grasp the infant's heel firmly with your index finger wrapped around the foot and your thumb wrapped around the ankle. Cleanse the selected area with 70% isopropyl alcohol and allow to air dry.	☐	☐	☐
9. Hold the patient's finger or heel firmly and make a swift, firm puncture. Perform the puncture perpendicular to the whorls of the fingerprint or footprint. Dispose of the used puncture device in a sharps container.	☐	☐	☐

10. Optain the first drop of blood.
  a. Wipe away the first drop of blood with dry gauze.
  b. Apply pressure toward the site but do not milk the site.
	☐	☐	☐

11. Collect the specimen in the chosen container or slide. Touch only the tip of the collection device to the drop of blood. Blood flow is encouraged if the puncture site is held downward and gentle pressure is applied near the site. Cap microcollection tubes with the caps provided and mix the additives by gently tilting or inverting the tubes 8–10 times.	☐	☐	☐

PROCEDURE STEPS	SELF	PARTNER	INSTRUCTOR
12. When collection is complete, apply clean gauze to the site with pressure. Hold pressure or have the patient hold pressure until bleeding stops. Label the containers with the proper information. Do not apply a dressing to a skin puncture of an infant under 2 years of age. Never release a patient until the bleeding has stopped.	☐	☐	☐
13. Thank the patient. Instruct the patient to leave the bandage in place at least 15 minutes.	☐	☐	☐
14. Properly care for or dispose of equipment and supplies. Clean the work area. Remove gloves and wash your hands.	☐	☐	☐
15. Test, transfer, or store the specimen according to the medical office policy.	☐	☐	☐
16. Record the procedure.	☐	☐	☐

CALCULATION

Total Possible Points: _____

Total Points Earned: _____ Multiplied by 100 = _____ Divided by Total Possible Points = _____%

Pass **Fail**
☐   ☐

Comments:

Student signature _____ Date _____
Partner signature _____ Date _____
Instructor signature _____ Date _____

Work Product 1

Document appropriately.

Nicole Patton is a 35-year-old female inpatient receiving both a Lovenox injection and oral Coumadin. You are directed to obtain blood specimens by evacuated tube for platelet count, prothrombin time, and partial thromboplastin time tests. If you are currently working in a medical office, use a blank paper patient chart from the office. If this is not available to you, use the space below to record the procedure in the chart.

_____

_____

_____

_____

_____

_____

Chapter Self-Assessment Quiz

1. When obtaining a blood specimen for a winged infusion set you need all of the following except:
   a. evacuated tubes.
   b. tourniquet.
   c. gauze pads.
   d. skin puncture device.
   e. permanent marker.

2. A source of error in venipuncture is:
   a. puncturing wrong area of infant heel.
   b. inserting needle bevel side down.
   c. prolonged tourniquet application.
   d. pulling back on syringe plunger too forcefully.
   e. failure to release tourniquet prior to needle withdrawal.

3. When your patient is feeling faint during venipuncture, you should do all of the following except:
   a. remove the tourniquet and withdraw the needle.
   b. divert attention from the procedure.
   c. have patient raise head and breathe deeply.
   d. loosen a tight collar or tie.
   e. apply a cold compress or washcloth.

4. To avoid hemoconcentration the phlebotomist should:
   a. ensure the tourniquet is not too tight.
   b. have patient make a fist.
   c. use occluded veins.
   d. draw blood from the heel.
   e. use needle with a small diameter.

5. If you accidentally puncture an artery, you should:
   a. hold pressure over the site for a full five minutes.
   b. use a cold compress to reduce pain.
   c. perform a capillary puncture.
   d. use a multi-sample needle instead.
   e. use a flatter angle when inserting needle.

6. What is the difference between NPO and fasting?
   a. Fasting is no food and NPO is no water.
   b. Fasting and NPO are basically the same.
   c. Fasting allows the patient to drink water while NPO does not.
   d. NPO requires that the patient drinks water while fasting does not.
   e. Fasting is for surgery and NPO is for getting true test results.

7. Aseptic techniques to prevent infection of the venipuncture site include:

   a. using sterile gloves.

   b. wearing a lab coat.

   c. using a gel separator.

   d. not opening bandages ahead of time.

   e. not speaking while you draw blood.

8. When collecting a blood sample from the fingers, you should use:

   a. the thumb.

   b. the second finger.

   c. the fifth finger.

   d. all fingers.

   e. the third and fourth fingers.

9. You should not draw blood using a small-gauge needle because:

   a. there is a greater likelihood of it breaking off in the vein.

   b. blood cells will rupture, causing hemolysis of the specimen.

   c. the luer adaptor will not fit venipuncture cuffs.

   d. the small needles are awkward to hold and manipulate.

   e. the small needles do not allow you to collect enough blood.

10. Which of the following may trigger hematoma formation?

   a. Pressure is applied after venipuncture.

   b. The needle is removed after the tourniquet is removed.

   c. The needle penetrates all the way through the vein.

   d. The needle is fully inserted into the vein.

   e. The patient has not properly followed preparation instructions.

11. If you are exposed to blood by needlestick, it is necessary to:

   a. wash the needle with hot soap and water.

   b. flush splashes to the nose, mouth, or skin with water.

   c. determine the type of needle involved in the injury.

   d. alert the patient.

   e. activate the safety device on the needle.

12. Gloves that are dusted with powder may:

   a. contaminate blood tests collected by capillary puncture.

   b. transfer disease from patient to patient.

   c. inhibit the growth of bacteria.

   d. cause an allergic reaction in the patient.

   e. hold up better than regular latex gloves.

13. The purpose of antiseptics is to:

   a. hold needles.

   b. clean biohazardous spills.

   c. inhibit the growth of bacteria.

   d. promote anticoagulation.

   e. prevent hematomas.

14. The most commonly used antiseptic for routine blood collection is:

   a. 70% isopropyl alcohol.

   b. povidone iodine.

   c. 0.5% chlorhexidine gluconate.

   d. benzalkonium chloride.

   e. sodium chloride.

15. The end of the needle that pierces the vein is cut into a slant called a:

   a. bevel.

   b. hub.

   c. gauge.

   d. shaft.

   e. adapter.

16. Gauze pads are used to:

   a. cover the venipuncture site once the bleeding has stopped.

   b. prevent blood clots at the venipuncture site.

   c. handle used needles.

   d. hold pressure on the venipuncture site following removal of the needle.

   e. reduce the spread of blood-borne pathogens.

17. Which tubes must be first in the order of the draw?

   a. Oxalate/fluoride tubes

   b. Coagulation tubes

   c. Heparin tubes

   d. Serum separator tubes (SSTs)

   e. Plain tubes

18. Which of the following is true of ethylenediaminetetraacetic acid (EDTA) tubes?

   a. They cause the least interference in test.

   b. They should be filled after hematology tubes.

   c. They are the same as PSTs.

   d. They minimize the chance of microbial contamination.

   e. They elevate sodium and potassium levels.

19. What safety features are available for the holder used with the evacuated tube system?

    a. Shields that cover the needle, or devices that retract the needle into the holder

    b. A self-locking cover for recapping the needle

    c. A gripper to clamp the holder to the Vacutainer tube, preventing slippage

    d. Orange color as a reminder to discard in biohazard container

    e. A beveled point on only one end

20. What example explains the best advantage of using the evacuated tube system?

    a. Multiple tubes may be filled from a single venipuncture.

    b. The tubes are color coded according to the tests to be done.

    c. The vacuum draws the blood into the tubes.

    d. It is a universal system, used in all phlebotomy laboratories around the country.

    e. It is the least painful way to draw blood from a patient.

42 Hematology

Chapter Checklist

☐ Read textbook chapter and take notes within the Chapter Notes outline. Answer the Learning Objectives as you reach them in the content, and then check them off.

☐ Work the Content Review questions—both Foundational Knowledge and Application.

☐ Perform the Active Learning exercise(s).

☐ Complete Professional Journal entries.

☐ Complete Skill Practice Activity(s) using Competency Evaluation Forms and Work Products, when appropriate.

☐ Take the Chapter Self-Assessment Quiz.

☐ Insert all appropriate pages into your portfolio.

Learning Objectives

1. Spell and define the key terms.
2. Explain hemostasis.
3. Explain the three general types of blood cells.
4. List the parameters measured in the complete blood count and their normal ranges.
5. List the leukocytes seen normally in the blood and their functions.
6. State the conditions associated with selected abnormal erythrocyte findings.
7. Describe the purpose of testing for the erythrocyte sedimentation rate.
8. List and describe the tests that measure the body's ability to form a fibrin clot.
9. Explain how to determine the prothrombin time and partial thromboplastin time.

Chapter Notes

Note: Bold-faced headings are the major headings in the text chapter; headings in regular font are lower-level headings (i.e., the content is subordinate to, or falls "under," the major headings). Make sure you understand the key terms used in the chapter, as well as the concepts presented as Key Points.

TEXT SUBHEADINGS   **NOTES**

Introduction _____

Key Term: hemostasis
Key Points:
• The hematology laboratory analyzes the blood cells, their quantities, and their characteristics for diagnosis and management of many conditions.
• In addition, hematology includes the study of **hemostasis**, or the ability of the patient's blood to form and dissolve a clot. Thus, the hematology laboratory is helpful in evaluating individuals who have difficulty forming a clot and those who form clots spontaneously within their blood vessels.

☐ **LEARNING OBJECTIVE 1:** Spell and define the key terms.

☐ **LEARNING OBJECTIVE 2:** Explain hemostasis.

Formation of Blood Cells _____

Key Terms: erythrocytes; leukocytes; thrombocytes; hematopoiesis
Key Points:
• Blood is made up of fluid (plasma) and three general types of cells, **erythrocytes** (red blood cells or RBCs), **leukocytes** (white blood cells or WBCs), and **thrombocytes** (platelets).
• Blood cells are formed in the bone marrow.
• **Hematopoiesis** (blood cell production) starts with very young, immature cells within the bone marrow that eventually divide and differentiate (acquire distinct or individual characteristics and mature).

☐ **LEARNING OBJECTIVE 3:** Explain the three general types of blood cells.

Pathophysiology and Hematological Testing _____

Key Term: complete blood count
Key Point:
• Common hematological tests include the **complete blood count** (CBC), erythrocyte sedimentation rate (ESR or sed rate), and coagulation tests.

Complete Blood Count

Key Point:
- The CBC, or hemogram, is one of the most frequently ordered tests in the laboratory. It consists of a number of parameters, including these:
  - WBC count and differential
  - RBC count
  - Hemoglobin (Hgb) determination
  - Hematocrit (Hct) determination
  - Mean cell volume (MCV)
  - Mean corpuscular hemoglobin (MCH)
  - Mean corpuscular hemoglobin concentration (MCHC)
  - Platelet count

☐ **LEARNING OBJECTIVE 4:** List the parameters measured in the complete blood count and their normal ranges.

White Blood Cell Count and Differential

Key Terms: granulocytes; lymphocytes; monocytes
Key Points:
- WBCs (leukocytes) provide the main line of defense against foreign invaders such as bacteria and viruses.
- The normal range for a WBC count is 4300 to 10,800/mm^3.
- The WBC differential determines the amounts of various WBC types in the peripheral blood.
- These cell types fall into three general categories: **granulocytes** (subdivided into neutrophils, eosinophils, and basophils and so called because of granules in their cytoplasm that have distinctive staining characteristics); **lymphocytes**; and **monocytes**. Each of the three has a distinct purpose in fighting infection.

☐ **LEARNING OBJECTIVE 5:** List the leukocytes seen normally in the blood and their functions.

Neutrophils

Key Terms: neutrophils; folate
Key Point:
- **Neutrophils**—also called polymorphonuclear neutrophils, polys, segmented neutrophils, or segs—are the most abundant leukocytes and are the main granulocyte.

Lymphocytes _____

_____

Key Point:
• Lymphocytes (lymphs) are the second most numerous WBC. The main function of lymphocytes is to recognize that a particular cell or particle is foreign to the body and to make antibodies specific to its destruction.

Monocytes _____

_____

Key Point:
• Monocytes (monos) are the third most abundant leuko-cytes. Like neutrophils, monocytes phagocytize foreign material.

Eosinophils _____

_____

Key Term: eosinophils

Basophils _____

_____

Key Term: basophils

Red Blood Cell Count _____

_____

Key Terms: erythropoietin; morphology; anisocytosis; poikilocytosis
Key Points:
• RBCs (erythrocytes) transport gases (mainly oxygen and carbon dioxide) between the lungs and the tissues. Their special structure, a biconcave disk containing hemoglobin, lets them readily exchange gases in the tissues and lung fields.
• RBCs are made in the bone marrow along with all other blood cells. Their production is influenced by the hormone **erythropoietin**, which is released from the kidneys.

Hemoglobin _____

_____

Key Terms: hemoglobin; sickle cell anemia
Key Point:
• **Hemoglobin** is the functioning unit of the red blood cell.

Hematocrit _____

_____

Key Term: hematocrit
Key Point:
• The **hematocrit** is the percentage of RBCs in whole blood.

Erythrocyte Indices _____

_____

Key Term: erythrocyte indices
Key Point:
• Three measurements are included in the **erythrocyte indices**: mean cell volume (MCV), mean cell hemoglobin (MCH), and mean cell hemoglobin concentration (MCHC). These measurements indicate the size of the RBC and how much hemoglobin the RBC holds. Erythrocyte indices are significant in diagnosing and treating the anemias.

☐ **LEARNING OBJECTIVE 6:** State the conditions associated with selected abnormal erythrocyte findings.

Mean Cell Volume _____

_____

_____

Mean Cell Hemoglobin and Mean Cell Hemoglobin Concentration _____

_____

_____

Platelet Count _____

_____

Key Point:
• Platelets (thrombocytes), like other blood cells, are made in the bone marrow. However, they are not actually cells but cell fragments that adhere to damaged endothelium. Platelets are essential to hemostasis because they not only aid in sealing wounds and stopping bleeding until a clot can form but also help initiate the clotting factors to form the more stable fibrin clot.

Erythrocyte Sedimentation Rate

Key Term: erythrocyte sedimentation rate
Key Points:
- The **erythrocyte sedimentation rate** (ESR) measures the rate in millimeters per hour at which RBCs settle out in a tube.
- The normal range for men is 0 to 10 mm/hour, and for women, 0 to 20 mm/hour. Elevations in ESR values are not specific for any disorder but indicate either inflammation or any other condition that causes increased or altered proteins in the blood (e.g., rheumatoid arthritis). The more rapidly the RBCs fall in the column, the greater the degree of inflammation.

☐ **LEARNING OBJECTIVE 7:** Describe the purpose of testing for the erythrocyte sedimentation rate.

Coagulation (Hemostasis) Tests

Key Point:
- Coagulation tests measure the ability of whole blood to form a clot.

☐ **LEARNING OBJECTIVE 8:** List and describe the tests that measure the body's ability to form a fibrin clot.

Prothrombin Time

Key Term: thromboplastin
Key Point:
- The PT is the primary monitor of coumarin anticoagulant therapy. The PT is reported along with its corresponding International Normalized Ratio (INR) to standardize results.

Partial Thromboplastin Time

Key Point:
- PTT may be prolonged in certain factor deficiencies, especially those that cause hemophilia. Heparin (anticoagulant) therapy also prolongs the PTT. Thus, it is used to monitor dosages.

☐ **LEARNING OBJECTIVE 9:** Explain how to determine the prothrombin time and partial thromboplastin time.

Content Review

FOUNDATIONAL KNOWLEDGE

1. Blood Is Thicker than Water

When a blood vessel is damaged, there are several different steps necessary for its repair. Match these steps to their correct descriptions on the right.

a. Vasoconstriction	**1.** The vein constricts to reduce blood loss.
b. Platelet plug formation	**2.** Proteins slowly dissolve the fibrin clot as the surrounding endothelial tissue of the blood vessel wall replicates to repair the damage.
c. Fibrin clot formation	**3.** When activated, the clotting factors form an insoluble clot at the wound site.
d. Clot lysis and vascular repair	**4.** Platelets adhere to the wound and form a plug, temporarily slowing or stopping the blood flow.

2. Red, White, and Purplish Blue

Fill in the table below to show the common name, the medical term, and function of the different cells found in blood.

Common Name	Medical Term	Function
a. Red blood cells (RBCs)		
b. White blood cells (WBCs)		
c. Platelets		

3. Seeing Red

What are the six parameters in a CBC measuring red blood cells and hemoglobin? List their normal ranges.

Parameters	Normal Ranges
a.	
b.	
c.	
d.	
e.	
f.	

4. What are the six parameters in a CBC measuring white blood cells? List their normal ranges.

Parameters	Normal Ranges
a.	
b.	
c.	
d.	
e.	
f.	

5. Sticky Business

A CBC also measures coagulating factors. Name this test and list its normal range.

_____

_____

Likely Leukocytes

6. Name the five primary types of leukocytes according to their functions.

a. _____ phagocytize (ingest) foreign material and aid the destruction of foreign particles by antibodies.

b. _____ release histamines and control inflammation and damage of tissues in the body.

c. _____ phagocytize (ingest) invading organisms.

d. _____ recognize foreign cells or particles and make antibodies specific to their destruction.

e. _____ produce histamines and respond to parasitic infections.

Feeling Weak

7. Name the condition indicated by the following abnormalities.

a. Hemoglobin (Hgb) <13 g/dL (men) _____

b. Hemocrit <45% (men) _____

c. MCV <80 fL _____

d. MCV >95 fL _____

e. MCH >31 picograms _____

f. MCH <27 picograms _____

g. MCHC <32 g/dL _____

h. MCHC >36 g/dL _____

8. Name the condition indicated by the following abnormalities.

a. Pale RBCs with more area of central pallor. _____

b. RBCs appear to have less or no area of central pallor. _____

c. Some RBCs have a blue color. _____

d. RBCs are smaller than usual. _____

e. RBCs are larger than normal. _____

f. RBCs are distinctly oval in shape. _____

g. Target cells—RBCs resemble a target with light and dark rings. _____

h. RBCs are fragmented. _____

i. RBCs show no area of central pallor. _____

j. RBCs have small, regular spicules (sharp points). _____

9. Settling Matters

What condition is monitored using the Erythrocyte Sedimentation Rate?

_____

_____

10. What are the correct guidelines for performing an Erythrocyte Sedimentation Rate test? Place a check mark in the appropriate box to indicate yes or no.

	Yes	No
a. Test should be started at least 2 hours after specimen collection.		
b. Shake the sample before beginning the test.		
c. Calcium and thromboplastin are added at the start of the test.		
d. The blood column must contain no bubbles.		
e. The tube must remain completely vertical during testing.		
f. The test can be done more quickly using a centrifuge.		
g. The sedimentation rack must be away from all drafts and direct sunlight.		
h. Test results should be read at exactly 30 minutes.		
i. The normal range for women is 0 to 10 mm/hour, and for men, 0 to 20 mm/hour.		
j. Test should be conducted at room temperature.		

Coagulation

11. Two postoperative patients are receiving anticoagulant therapy. Patient A is receiving heparin, and patient B is receiving coumadin. Name and describe the different hemostasis tests given to monitor these two patients.

    a. _____

    b. _____

12. Two postoperative patients are receiving anticoagulant therapy. Patient A is receiving heparin, and patient B is receiving coumadin. How are results reported in the different tests given to monitor patient A and patient B?

    a. _____

    b. _____

Bloodwork

13. A patient comes in with rapidly developing abdominal pain. His bloodwork shows a "shift to the left." Describe what a "shift to the left" is and what it indicates.

    _____

    _____

14. A patient has a high number of lymphocytes in her bloodwork. What does this imply?

    _____

    _____

15. How is hemoglobin organized? Arrange and explain the relationships between the structures listed below.

    heme
    hemoglobin
    iron
    globins

    _____

    _____

16. A virus enters the body through the respiratory system. The body has encountered and combated this virus before. What type of cell carries the memory of this virus and how does it begin the counterattack?

_____

_____

17. List four early warning signs of folate deficiency.

a. _____

b. _____

c. _____

d. _____

18. What two factors besides arthritis can affect an ESR?

a. _____

b. _____

19. Match the following key terms to their definitions.

Key Terms

a. anisocytosis _____
b. basophils _____
c. complete blood count _____
d. eosinophils _____
e. erythrocyte _____
f. erythocyte indices _____
g. erythrocyte sedimentation rate _____
h. erythropoietin _____
i. folate _____
j. granulocytes _____
k. hematocrit _____
l. hematopoiesis _____
m. hemoglobin _____
n. hemostasis _____
o. leukocyte _____
p. lymphocyte _____
q. monocyte _____
r. morphology _____
s. neutrophils _____
t. poikilocytosis _____
u. sickle cell anemia _____
v. thrombocytes _____
w. thromboplastin _____

Definitions

1. a set of measurements that indicate the size and hemoglobin content of red blood cells
2. a complex substance found in the blood and tissue that aids the clotting process
3. the least numerous of the white blood cells, comprising less than one percent of the white blood cell population
4. the percentage of red blood cells in whole blood
5. a series of tests measuring red blood cells, white blood cells, platelets, and hemoglobin
6. granular leukocytes whose granules are beadlike and stain bright orange-red with the eosin acid stain
7. description of the physical characteristics of blood cells
8. the time in millimeters per hour at which red blood cells settle out in a tube
9. abnormal variations in the shapes of red blood cells
10. blood abnormality in which red blood cells are not equal in size
11. blood cell production
12. the largest of the leukocytes making up from one percent to seven percent of the white blood cell population
13. a condition in which the patient has both copies of the gene for hemoglobin S; the red cells become sickle shaped and nonflexible causing obstruction of small vessels and capillaries
14. a nongranular leukocyte that is the second most numerous of the white blood cells
15. a substance that helps the enzymes that build structures, such as blood cells
16. white blood cells that have visible granules when stained
17. a hormone produced mainly by the kidney in response to lowered oxygen levels; stimulates the production of red blood cells to increase blood oxygen levels
18. an iron protein pigment found in red blood cells that carries oxygen and carbon dioxide in the bloodstream
19. process that results in control of bleeding after an injury
20. white blood cell
21. red blood cell
22. platelets or cell fragments which form the first stage of clotting
23. normally the most numerous of the white blood cells, averaging 65 percent of the total white blood cell count

20. True or False? Determine whether the following statements are true or false. If false, explain why.

    a. Thrombocytosis is associated with increased bleeding.

_____

_____

    b. The Wintrobe method of calculating erythrocyte sedimentation rate is safer.

_____

_____

    c. Liver disorders reduce the mean corpuscular volume.

_____

_____

    d. Turnips are a good source of iron.

_____

_____

APPLICATION

Critical Thinking Practice

1. Men over age 35 and alcoholics frequently have difficulty absorbing vitamin B. What symptoms would you expect to see in an older male who drinks, and how could these be best addressed?

_____

_____

2. A trauma patient arrives in the hospital with extensive bleeding and internal injuries. The next day you are asked to run lab tests on this patient's bloodwork. How do you expect her results to differ from those of a healthy patient?

_____

_____

Patient Education

1. Your patient is a 40-year-old male who has anemia resulting from a folate deficiency. Write a sheet of instructions that clearly explains the nature of his illness and what corrective measures he has to take.

Documentation

1. You perform an ESR test on an elderly male patient with rheumatoid arthritis. You measure a rate of 16 mL/hour. How would you document the results of this test in the patient's chart?

_____

_____

Active Learning

1. Research medical literature on iron and folate deficiencies. Then research the same topics in popular literature on the Internet and as found in health food stores. Compare these two sources. Do they contradict each other? How do their recommendations differ?

2. Research literature on sickle cell anemia and its treatments. Prepare a one-page patient brochure describing your findings.

3. White blood cells are the body's defense against foreign substances and objects that enter the bloodstream. However, there are cancers, diseases, and other ailments that attack the white blood cells and their production. Working with a partner, research one of these diseases. How many people are reported to have this disease? Is there current treatment or therapy? How is gene therapy affecting the research for this disease? What are some of the cures that are being developed to stop these diseases and to rebuild the immune system? After you have gathered the information, prepare a report on this disease to present to the class.

Professional Journal

REFLECT

(Prompts and Ideas: Do you or someone you know have a blood disorder? Does it require a special diet or medication? How would it feel to need to have your blood drawn and tested frequently?)

_____

_____

_____

_____

_____

_____

PONDER AND SOLVE

1. A patient's uncle is diagnosed with a bone marrow disease, and the entire family is being tested to find possible donors. The patient wants to help her uncle, but she has heard that getting a bone marrow biopsy is a very painful experience. What can you tell her to put her more at ease about the procedure?

_____

_____

_____

_____

_____

_____

2. A young boy has just tested positive for sickle cell anemia. What important information can you tell his parents? How do you explain the disease to a young child?

_____

_____

_____

_____

_____

_____

_____

EXPERIENCE

Skills related to this chapter include:

1. Making a Peripheral Blood Smear (Procedure 42-1).
2. Staining a Peripheral Blood Smear (Procedure 42-2).
3. Performing a Hemoglobin Determination (Procedure 42-3).
4. Performing a Microhematocrit Determination (Procedure 42-4).
5. Westergren Erythrocyte Sedimentation Rate (Procedure 42-5).

Record any common mistakes, lessons learned, and/or tips you discovered during your experience of practicing and demonstrating these skills.

_____

_____

_____

_____

_____

_____

_____

Skill Practice

PERFORMANCE OBJECTIVES:

1. Make a peripheral blood smear (Procedure 42-1).
2. Stain a peripheral blood smear (Procedure 42-2).
3. Perform a hemoglobin determination (Procedure 42-3).
4. Perform a microhematocrit determination (Procedure 42-4).
5. Determine a Westergren erythrocyte sedimentation rate (Procedure 42-5).

Name _____ Date _____ Time _____

Procedure 42-1:	MAKING A PERIPHERAL BLOOD SMEAR

EQUIPMENT/SUPPLIES: Clean glass slides with frosted ends, pencil, well-mixed whole blood specimen, transfer pipette, hand disinfectant, surface disinfectant, gloves, biohazard container

STANDARDS: Given the needed equipment and a place to work, the student will perform this skill with _____% accuracy in a total of _____ minutes. *(Your instructor will tell you what the percentage and time limits will be before you begin practicing.)*

KEY: 4 = Satisfactory   0 = Unsatisfactory   NA = This step is not counted

PROCEDURE STEPS	SELF	PARTNER	INSTRUCTOR
1. Wash your hands. Put on personal protective equipment.	☐	☐	☐
2. Assemble the equipment and supplies.	☐	☐	☐
3. Obtain a recently made dried blood smear.	☐	☐	☐
4. Place the slide on a stain rack blood side up.	☐	☐	☐
5. Place staining solution(s) onto slide according to manufacturer's instructions.	☐	☐	☐
6. Holding the slide with tweezers, gently rinse the slide with water. Wipe off the back of the slide with gauze. Stand the slide upright and allow it to dry.	☐	☐	☐
7. Properly care for or dispose of equipment and supplies. Clean the work area. Remove gloves and wash your hands. *Note:* Some manufacturers provide a simple one-step method that consists of dipping the smear in a staining solution, then rinsing. Directions provided by the manufacturer vary with the specific test.	☐	☐	☐

CALCULATION

Total Possible Points: _____
Total Points Earned: _____ Multiplied by 100 = _____ Divided by Total Possible Points = _____%

Pass   **Fail**
☐   ☐   Comments:

Chart Documentation _____
Student signature _____ Date _____
Partner signature _____ Date _____
Instructor signature _____ Date _____

Name _____ Date _____ Time _____

Procedure 42-2:	**STAINING A PERIPHERAL BLOOD SMEAR**

EQUIPMENT/SUPPLIES: Staining rack, Wright's stain materials, prepared slide, tweezers, hand disinfectant, surface disinfectant, gloves

STANDARDS: Given the needed equipment and a place to work, the student will perform this skill with _____% accuracy in a total of _____ minutes. *(Your instructor will tell you what the percentage and time limits will be before you begin practicing.)*

KEY: 4 = Satisfactory   0 = Unsatisfactory   NA = This step is not counted

PROCEDURE STEPS	SELF	PARTNER	INSTRUCTOR
1. Wash your hands. Put on personal protective equipment.	☐	☐	☐
2. Assemble the equipment and supplies.	☐	☐	☐
3. Obtain a recently made dried blood smear.	☐	☐	☐
4. Place the slide on a stain rack blood side up.	☐	☐	☐
5. Place staining solution(s) onto slide according to manufacturer's instructions.	☐	☐	☐
6. Holding the slide with tweezers, gently rinse the slide with water. Wipe off the back of the slide with gauze. Stand the slide upright and allow it to dry.	☐	☐	☐
7. Properly care for or dispose of equipment and supplies. Clean the work area. Remove gloves and wash your hands. *Note:* Some manufacturers provide a simple one-step method that consists of dipping the smear in a staining solution, then rinsing. Directions provided by the manufacturer vary with the specific test.	☐	☐	☐

CALCULATION

Total Possible Points: _____
Total Points Earned: _____ Multiplied by 100 = _____ Divided by Total Possible Points = _____%

Pass   **Fail**
☐   ☐ | Comments: |

Chart Documentation _____
Student signature _____ Date _____
Partner signature _____ Date _____
Instructor signature _____ Date _____

Name _____   Date _____   Time _____

Procedure 42-3:	PERFORMING A HEMOGLOBIN DETERMINATION

EQUIPMENT/SUPPLIES: Hemoglobin meter, applicator sticks, whole blood, hand disinfectant, surface disinfectant, gloves, biohazard container

NOTE: These are generic instructions for using a hemoglobin meter. Refer to the manufacturer's instructions shipped with the meter for instructions specific for the instrument in use.)

STANDARDS: Given the needed equipment and a place to work, the student will perform this skill with _____% accuracy in a total of _____ minutes. *(Your instructor will tell you what the percentage and time limits will be before you begin practicing.)*

KEY: 4 = Satisfactory   0 = Unsatisfactory   NA = This step is not counted

PROCEDURE STEPS	SELF	PARTNER	INSTRUCTOR
1. Wash your hands. Put on personal protective equipment.	☐	☐	☐
2. Assemble the equipment and supplies.	☐	☐	☐
3. Review instrument manual for your hemoglobin meter. Turn meter on and validate quality control before testing patient specimen.	☐	☐	☐
4. Obtain an EDTA (lavender-top tube) blood specimen from the patient, following procedures in Chapter 41.	☐	☐	☐
5. Place well-mixed whole blood into the hemoglobin meter chamber as described by the manufacturer.	☐	☐	☐
6. Slide the chamber into the hemoglobin meter.	☐	☐	☐
7. Record the hemoglobin level from the digital readout.	☐	☐	☐
8. Clean the work area with surface disinfectant. Dispose of equipment and supplies appropriately. Remove gloves and wash your hands. *Note:* This procedure may vary with the instrument.	☐	☐	☐

CALCULATION

Total Possible Points: _____
Total Points Earned: _____ Multiplied by 100 = _____ Divided by Total Possible Points = _____%

Pass   **Fail**
☐   ☐   Comments:

Chart Documentation _____
Student signature _____ Date _____
Partner signature _____ Date _____
Instructor signature _____ Date _____

Name _____ Date _____ Time _____

Procedure 42-4:	PERFORMING A MICROHEMATOCRIT DETERMINATION

EQUIPMENT/SUPPLIES: Microcollection tubes, sealing clay, microhematocrit centrifuge, microhematocrit reading device, hand disinfectant, surface disinfectant, gloves, biohazard container, sharps container

STANDARDS: Given the needed equipment and a place to work, the student will perform this skill with _____% accuracy in a total of _____ minutes. *(Your instructor will tell you what the percentage and time limits will be before you begin practicing.)*

KEY: 4 = Satisfactory   0 = Unsatisfactory   NA = This step is not counted

PROCEDURE STEPS	SELF	PARTNER	INSTRUCTOR
1. Wash your hands. Put on personal protective equipment.	☐	☐	☐
2. Assemble the equipment and supplies.	☐	☐	☐
3. Draw blood into the capillary tube by one of two methods: **a.** Directly from a capillary puncture (see Chapter 41) in which the tip of the capillary tube is touched to the blood at the wound and allowed to fill to three-quarters or the indicated mark. **b.** From a well-mixed EDTA tube of whole blood; again, the tip is touched to the blood and allowed to fill three-quarters of the tube.	☐	☐	☐
4. Place the forefinger over the top of the tube, wipe excess blood off the sides, and push the bottom into the sealing clay.	☐	☐	☐
5. Draw a second specimen in the same manner.	☐	☐	☐
6. Place the tubes, clay-sealed end out, in the radial grooves of the microhematocrit centrifuge opposite each other. Put the lid on the grooved area and tighten by turning the knob clockwise. Close the centrifuge lid. Spin for 5 minutes or as directed by the centrifuge manufacturer.	☐	☐	☐
7. Remove the tubes from the centrifuge and read the results; instructions are printed on the device. Results should be within 5% of each other. Take the average and report as a percentage.	☐	☐	☐
8. Dispose of the microhematocrit tubes in a biohazard container. Properly care for or dispose of other equipment and supplies. Clean the work area. Remove gloves and wash your hands. *Note:* Some microhematocrit centrifuges have the scale printed in the machine at the radial grooves.	☐	☐	☐

CALCULATION

Total Possible Points: _____
Total Points Earned: _____ Multiplied by 100 = _____ Divided by Total Possible Points = _____%

Pass	**Fail**
☐	☐

Comments:

Chart Documentation _____

Student signature _____ Date _____

Partner signature _____ Date _____

Instructor signature _____ Date _____

Name _____ Date _____ Time _____

Procedure 42-5:	WESTERN ERYTHROCYTE SEDIMENTATION RATE

EQUIPMENT/SUPPLIES: Hand disinfectant, gloves, EDTA blood sample less than 2 hours old, ESR kit, sedimentation rack, pipette, timer, surface disinfectant, biohazard disposal container, sharps container

STANDARDS: Given the needed equipment and a place to work, the student will perform this skill with _____% accuracy in a total of _____ minutes. *(Your instructor will tell you what the percentage and time limits will be before you begin practicing.)*

KEY:　　4 = Satisfactory　　　　0 = Unsatisfactory　　　　NA = This step is not counted

PROCEDURE STEPS	SELF	PARTNER	INSTRUCTOR
1. Wash your hands. Put on personal protective equipment.	☐	☐	☐
2. Assemble the equipment and supplies.	☐	☐	☐
3. Gently mix EDTA lavender-stoppered anticoagulation tube for 2 minutes.	☐	☐	☐
4. Using a vial from the ESR kit and a pipette, fill vial to the indicated mark. Replace stopper and invert vial several times to mix.	☐	☐	☐
5. Using an ESR calibrated pipette from the kit, insert the pipette through the tube's stopper with a twist and push down slowly but firmly until the pipette meets the bottom of the vial. The pipette will autozero with the excess flowing into the holding area. If the blood column does not reach the autozero point, discard used materials and start again at step 4.	☐	☐	☐
6. Place the tube in a holder that will keep the tube vertical.	☐	☐	☐
7. Wait exactly 1 hour; use a timer for accuracy. Keep the tube straight upright and undisturbed during the hour.	☐	☐	☐
8. Record the level of the top of the RBCs after 1 hour. Normal results for men are 0–10 mL/hour; for women, 0–15 mL/hour.	☐	☐	☐
9. Properly care for or dispose of equipment and supplies. Clean the work area. Remove gloves, gown, and face shield. Wash your hands.	☐	☐	☐

CALCULATION

Total Possible Points: _____
Total Points Earned: _____ Multiplied by 100 = _____ Divided by Total Possible Points = _____%

Pass　　**Fail**
☐　　　　☐　　| Comments: |

Chart Documentation _____
Student signature _____ Date _____
Partner signature _____ Date _____
Instructor signature _____ Date _____

Work Product 1

Perform hematology testing.

Make and stain a peripheral blood smear, perform a hemoglobin determination and a microhematocrit determination, and determine the Westergren erythrocyte sedimentation rate of blood samples provided or using samples you have drawn from a patient. Record the test results in the space below.

_____

_____

_____

_____

Work Product 2

Use methods of quality control.

You encounter a problem with the microhematocrit centrifuge while performing a manual microhematocrit determination. Fill in the log to show that proper quality control procedures were used to address the problem with the instrument.

Instrument History Record

Model No: _____	**Instrument:** _____
Date Purchased: _____	**Serial Number:** _____
Manufacturer: _____	**Cost** _____
_____	
Telephone: _____	**State** _____ **Zip:** _____
Dealer: _____	**Contact Person** _____
_____	
Telephone: _____	**State** _____ **Zip:** _____
Warranty: _____	**Expiration Date** _____
_____	

Technical Service Representative _____

Date	Comments	Who Was Contacted	Action Taken

Work Product 3

Document appropriately.

Manuel Gonzalez is a 30-year-old male undergoing a CBC. You are directed to make and stain a peripheral blood smear, perform a hemoglobin determination and a microhematocrit determination, and determine the Westergren erythrocyte sedimentation rate for this patient. WBC is $4300/mm^3$, neutrophils are 60% with no hypersegmented or stab neutrophils. Lymphocytes compose 35% of the count, monos 3%, and eos 2%. RBC count is 5 million/mm^3. You measure hemoglobin at 15 g/dL, and hematocrit at 50%. ESR is 5 mm/hour.

If you are currently working in a medical office, use a blank paper patient chart from the office. If this is not available to you, use the space below to record the procedure and results in the chart.

_____

_____

_____

_____

Work Product 4

Screen and follow-up test results.

Use the information from Work Product 3 to write a letter to Manuel Gonzalez to inform him about his test results. Print the letter and attach it to this sheet.

Chapter Self-Assessment Quiz

1. Hematopoiesis is:
   a. the ability of a person's blood to form a clot.
   b. creation of new blood cells.
   c. the proportion of red blood cells to plasma.
   d. a protein released by the kidneys to stimulate red blood cell creation.
   e. the shape of red blood cells.

2. Leukocytosis is most likely caused by:
   a. chemical toxicity.
   b. inflammation.
   c. nutritional deficiencies.
   d. chronic infection.
   e. anticoagulant therapy.

3. What indicates a vitamin B_{12} deficiency?
   a. The presence of bands
   b. Neutrophils with more than 5 lobes in their nuclei
   c. High numbers of lymphocytes
   d. Erythrocytes which lack a nucleus
   e. Microcytosis or a mean cell volume (MCV) less than 80 fL

4. Which white blood cells produce antibodies?
   a. Neutrophils
   b. Lymphocytes
   c. Monocytes
   d. Eosinophils
   e. Basophils

5. Oval-shaped erythrocytes indicate:

    a. B_{12} (folate) deficiency.

    b. bacterial infection.

    c. liver impairment.

    d. sickle cell anemia.

    e. viral infection.

6. Which food is a good natural source of folate?

    a. Chicken

    b. Leafy green vegetables

    c. Liver

    d. Oysters

    e. Root vegetables

7. A parasitic infection is indicated by increased numbers of which leukocyte?

    a. Neutrophils

    b. Lymphocytes

    c. Monocytes

    d. Eosinophils

    e. Basophils

8. Which condition could be caused by chemotherapy?

    a. Anemia

    b. Folate deficiency

    c. Leukocytosis

    d. Monocytosis

    e. Thrombocytopenia

9. One symptom of vitamin K deficiency is:

    a. left shift.

    b. macrocytosis.

    c. prolonged ESR.

    d. prolonged PT.

    e. thrombocytosis.

10. ESR tests should be read:

    a. after 1 minute.

    b. at 15 minutes.

    c. at 30 minutes.

    d. at 60 minutes.

    e. at any time; the exact time is not important.

11. Which of the following is true of thrombocytosis?

    a. It indicates bacterial infection.

    b. It indicates bleeding.

    c. It is benign.

    d. It results from nutritional deficiency.

    e. It is a warning sign of embolism.

12. Microcytosis indicates:

    a. B_{12} deficiency.

    b. the presence of gamma globins.

    c. liver disorders.

    d. iron deficiency.

    e. sickle cell anemia.

13. Patients with iron deficiencies should be encouraged to eat:

    a. dairy.

    b. fish.

    c. fruit.

    d. liver.

    e. tofu.

14. Erythropoiesis is driven by chemical signals from:

    a. the brain.

    b. the kidneys.

    c. the liver.

    d. the marrow.

    e. the spleen.

Scenario: A patient comes to the office complaining of chronic fatigue.

15. What is the most direct measurement of the blood's ability to deliver oxygen available in the CBC?

    a. RBC count

    b. Hemoglobin (Hgb) determination

    c. Hematocrit (Hct) determination

    d. Mean cell volume (MCV)

    e. Mean corpuscular hemoglobin (MCH)

16. What would indicate that the patient's problem is hereditary?

    a. Erythropoiesis

    b. Hemostasis

    c. Hematocrit

    d. Microcytosis

    e. Poikilocytosis

End Scenario

17. Increased numbers of which leukocyte correspond to allergies and asthma?

    a. Neutrophils

    b. Lymphocytes

    c. Monocytes

    d. Eosinophils

    e. Basophils

18. Which is a normal platelet count for women?

   a. 4300 to 10,800/mm^3

   b. 200,000 to 400,000/mm^3

   c. 4.2 to 5.4 million/mm^3

   d. 4.6 to 6.2 million/mm^3

   e. 27 to 31 million/mm^3

19. Which is the normal RBC count for women?

   a. 4300 to 10,800/mm^3

   b. 200,000 to 400,000/mm^3

   c. 4.2 to 5.4 million/mm^3

   d. 4.6 to 6.2 million/mm^3

   e. 27 to 31 million/mm^3

20. Which is the normal WBC count for men?

   a. 4300 to 10,800/mm^3

   b. 200,000 to 400,000/mm^3

   c. 4.2 to 5.4 million/mm3

   d. 4.6 to 6.2 million/mm^3

   e. 27 to 31 million/mm^3

43 Urinalysis

Chapter Checklist

- [ ] Read textbook chapter and take notes within the Chapter Notes outline. Answer the Learning Objectives as you reach them in the content, and then check them off.
- [ ] Work the Content Review questions—both Foundational Knowledge and Application.
- [ ] Perform the Active Learning exercise(s).

- [ ] Complete Professional Journal entries.
- [ ] Complete Skill Practice Activity(s) using Competency Evaluation Forms and Work Products, when appropriate.
- [ ] Take the Chapter Self-Assessment Quiz.
- [ ] Insert all appropriate pages into your Portfolio.

Learning Objectives

1. Spell and define the key terms.
2. Describe the methods of urine collection.
3. List and explain the physical and chemical properties of urine.

4. List confirmatory tests available and describe their use.
5. List and describe the components that can be found in urine sediment and describe their relationships to chemical findings.

Chapter Notes

Note: Bold-faced headings are the major headings in the text chapter; headings in regular font are lower-level headings (i.e., the content is subordinate to, or falls "under," the major headings). Make sure you understand the key terms used in the chapter, as well as the concepts presented as Key Points.

TEXT SUBHEADINGS   **NOTES**

Introduction _____

_____

Key Points:
- A urinalysis is a physical and chemical examination of urine to assess renal function and other possible problems. Because so many urinalyses are done in the office laboratory, proficiency in this skill is essential for the medical assistant.
- The medical assistant may prepare urine sediment for microscopic examination (Procedure 43-5). The microscopic examination may be performed by the physician under the CLIA category Physician-Performed Microscopy.

☐ **LEARNING OBJECTIVE 1:** Spell and define the key terms.

Specimen Collection Methods _____

_____

Key Points:
- Proper collection of a urine specimen varies with the test to be performed. Unless otherwise specified by the physician, a freshly voided specimen is all that is necessary. This is called a random urine. The patient voids the urine into a clean, dry container. To diagnose a urinary tract infection (UTI), the specimen is collected either as clean-catch midstream or by catheter and submitted to the laboratory in a sterile container with a lid.
- All cultures require the specimen not be contaminated during the preliminary testing process.
- Once the urine is collected, many of its elements deteriorate within 1 hour. If testing cannot be performed within this time, the specimen is refrigerated at 4°C to 8°C for up to 4 hours.
- The timing of collection is sometimes an important consideration. First-morning urine specimens are the most concentrated and are useful for many tests that are more easily determined with concentrated components (e.g., pregnancy testing); 2-hour postprandial (after a meal) specimens are used for glucose testing.

Random Specimen _____

_____

_____

First Morning Void _____

_____

_____

Postprandial Specimen _____

_____

_____

Clean-Catch Midstream Urine Specimen _____

_____

Key Points:
• A clean-catch midstream urine is the most commonly ordered random specimen. It is useful when the physician suspects an infection, because any microorganisms present after this collection will be from the urinary tract and not from contamination such as the perineal area. This specimen can be used for a culture if nothing has been allowed to contaminate the urine, such as a pipette or reagent strip. Collection is done after the urinary meatus and surrounding skin have been cleansed. The urine is voided into a sterile container.

Clean-Catch _____

_____

_____

Midstream _____

_____

_____

24-Hour Collection _____

_____

Key Term: diurnal variation
Key Point:
• Because some substances such as proteins are excreted with diurnal variation, variation during a 24-hour period, a 24-hour collection is a better indicator of values than a random specimen. To obtain this kind of specimen, the patient collects all voided urine within a 24-hour period (Procedure 43-2). Providing an information sheet with written instructions for collecting a 24-hour urine specimen helps ensure the patient's compliance.

Other Specified Number of Hours _____

_____

_____

Bladder Catheterization _____

_____

_____

Suprapubic Aspiration _____

_____

_____

Drug Testing _____

_____

_____

Chain-of-Custody _____

_____

Key Point:
- The term **chain-of-custody** indicates the ability to guarantee the identity and integrity of a specimen from collection, through all steps of transport and processing, to the reporting of the test results. The chain-of-custody process is used to maintain and document the history of the specimen and ensures that the sample has been in possession of, or secured by, a responsibile person at all times. It should eliminate doubt about sample identification or that the sample has been tampered with. The chain-of-custody document should include the name or initials of the individual collecting the specimen, each person who subsequently has custody of it, and the date the specimen was collected or transferred. A secure chain-of-custody leads to the production of a legally defensible test report.

Patient Preparation _____

_____

☐ **LEARNING OBJECTIVE 2:** Describe the methods of urine collection.

Physical Properties of Urine _____

_____

Key Point:
- The physical properties include the urine's color, appearance (such as clarity or turbidity), specific gravity, and odor.

Color _____

_____

Key Point:
- Urine color can be affected by many things: diet, drugs, diseases, and the concentration of the urine. The normal color of urine is a pale straw color to dark yellow. The yellow color is due to the pigment urochrome.

Clarity _____

_____

Key Point:
• Normal, freshly voided urine is usually clear (transparent). Haziness or turbidity (cloudiness) indicates the presence of particulate matter.

Specific Gravity _____

_____

Key Term: specific gravity
Key Points:
• The **specific gravity** reflects the concentration of a urine specimen. The weight of the urine is compared to the weight of water. Normal urine is slightly heavier than water. If you were to compare the weight of distilled water to itself, the specific gravity of the water would be 1.000.
• The specific gravity pad on the reagent strip takes a drop of urine, and the color change is compared to a chart to determine the value. This allows specific gravity to be determined in combination with the other chemical assays on the reagent strip and is the most common and efficient method of measurement.

Chemical Properties of Urine _____

_____

Key Term: quantitative

pH _____

_____

Key Point:
• Expected values for urine pH can range from 5.0 (acidic) to 8.0 (slightly basic). The typical value for freshly voided urine is slightly acidic at 6.0. While acidic urine is normal, it also occurs with a high-protein diet and uncontrolled diabetes. Alkaline urine (above 7.0) can occur after meals and with a vegetarian diet, certain renal diseases, and urinary tract infection.

Glucose

Key Terms: threshold; glycosuria
Key Point:
• Glucose is filtered and reabsorbed in the kidneys. If plasma renal **threshold** levels exceed 180 g/dL, not all of the glucose will be reabsorbed, and detectable amounts of it will be present in the urine. This can vary and requires measuring the actual blood level for a diagnostic assessment. The amount of glucose in urine corresponds to plasma levels; normal urine does not contain glucose.

Ketones

Key Term: ketones
Key Point:
• **Ketones** are a group of chemicals produced during fat metabolism. In normal circumstances, energy is derived primarily from carbohydrate metabolism. In conditions of insufficient carbohydrates, as in starvation, low-carbohydrate diets, and inadequately managed diabetes, fats are used by the body for energy and ketones are produced.

Proteins

Key Term: proteinuria
Key Point:
• **Proteinuria** (increased amounts of protein in the urine) is an important indicator of renal disease.

Blood

Key Term: hemoglobinuria
Key Point:
• The reagent strip reacts to hemoglobin, which is the primary constituent of red cells. **Hemoglobinuria** may occur with transfusion reaction, chemical toxicity, or burn.

Bilirubin _____

Key Points:
- Bilirubin is formed during breakdown of hemoglobin. It is processed in the liver before being excreted into the intestines. Urine contains very low levels of bilirubin, reflecting the usual low serum levels.
- Important note: Bilirubin is a highly unstable substance and will break down with exposure to light. Specimens must be shielded from light and processed as soon as possible to avoid deterioration of the specimen.

Urobilinogen _____

Key Term: urobilinogen
Key Points:
- When bilirubin is secreted into the intestines in the bile, bacterial action converts it to **urobilinogen**. Some of this is reabsorbed into the bloodstream and excreted by the kidneys. The remaining urobilinogen leaves the body in the feces.
- Small amounts of urobilinogen are normally found in urine, usually 0.1 to 1.0 mg/dL.

Nitrite _____

Key Term: nitrite
Key Point:
- Some types of bacteria that infect the urinary tract have an enzyme that can reduce nitrate to **nitrite**. This factor is used to assess the presence of bacteria in urine. If these types of bacteria are present, nitrates will be converted to nitrites, and the resulting pink color development can be observed on the reagent pad.

Leukocyte Esterase _____

Key Term: leukocyte esterase
Key Point:
- Leukocytes in the urine indicate a urinary tract infection.

☐ **LEARNING OBJECTIVE 3:** List and explain the physical and chemical properties of urine.

Confirmatory Testing _____

Key Point:
• Confirmation of positive reagent strip reactions (e.g., bilirubin, protein) is sometimes part of laboratory protocol as defined by the facility where the test is performed. Box 43-2 lists several types of confirmation tests. Check your Laboratory Procedure Manual for the confirmation testing used in your laboratory.

Copper Reduction Test _____

Key Point:
• Its use is significant to children aged 2 years or less to screen for galactosuria. (Galactosuria, or increased level of galactose in the blood and urine, is a condition in newborns lacking an enzyme that metabolizes galactose.)

Nitroprusside Test _____

Precipitation Test _____

Key Term: sulfosalicylic acid

Diazo Test _____

☐ **LEARNING OBJECTIVE 4:** List confirmatory tests available and describe their use.

Urine Sediment _____

Key Terms: sediment; supernatant
Key Point:
• The microscopic examination of urine can corroborate the findings of the urinalysis and may produce additional data with diagnostic value. Cells and other structures are noted and counted during a microscopic examination. Microscopic examination of urine is not a CLIA-waived procedure.

Structures Found in Urine Sediment

Key Point:
- The following structures may appear in the urine: red blood cells, white blood cells, bacteria, epithelial cells, crystals, casts, and others.

Red Blood Cells

Key Point:
- The presence of red cells in urine, as stated previously, can occur with a number of conditions, including renal damage.

White Blood Cells

Key Point:
- Leukocytes in the sediment indicate a urinary tract infection.

Bacteria

Key Point:
- Bacteria are always present on the skin but not usually in the bladder. Urine normally does not contain bacteria if a clean-catch specimen is collected properly. The presence of significant amounts (more than a trace) of bacteria in a urine specimen is considered an indication of a urinary tract infection.

Epithelial Cells

Key Point:
- Epithelial cells cover the skin and organs and line pathways, such as the digestive and urinary tracts. Their shapes vary according to their location of origin. Epithelial cells normally slough off and are found in the urine, but increased amounts can indicate an irritation, such as inflammation somewhere in the urinary system. The three types of epithelial cells in the urine are squamous, transitional, and renal. Squamous epithelial cells cover external skin surfaces and are considered a normal finding in urine, since urine comes in contact with skin during urination. Transitional epithelial cells line the bladder and are seen with infections of the lower urinary tract, such as cystitis. Renal epithelial cells line the nephrons and are seen with infections and inflammations of the upper urinary tract.

Crystals _____

Key Point:
• The three most common crystals found in urine sediment—calcium oxalate, uric acid (both of which occur in urine with a pH below 7.0), and triple phosphate (found in urine above pH 7.0)—are not independently pathological. Uric acid crystals can, however, be seen with fever, leukemia, or gout. Crystals can contribute to the formation of stones in the urinary tract.

Casts _____

Key Point:
• Cast formation occurs in the tubules of the nephron.

Other Structures _____

☐ **LEARNING OBJECTIVE 5:** List and describe the components that can be found in urine sediment and describe their relationships to chemical findings.

Content Review

FOUNDATIONAL KNOWLEDGE

Specimen Collection

1. Match the following types of specimen collection methods with the correct description.

Collection Method

a. Random specimen _____
b. First morning void _____
c. Postprandial specimen _____
d. Clean-catch midstream urine specimen _____
e. Suprapubic aspiration _____
f. 24-hour collection _____

Description

1. A specimen that is collected two hours after a patient consumes a meal
2. A specimen that is voided into a sterile container after the urinary meatus and surrounding skin have been cleansed
3. A specimen that is formed over a 6–8 hour period
4. A specimen voided into a clean, dry container
5. A specimen consisting of all urine voided over a 24-hour period
6. A specimen that is taken directly from the bladder using a needle

2. A patient provides a sample of urine for testing. You know that everyone in the medical office is extremely busy and that it will not get tested for at least three hours. What should you do with the sample?

_____

_____

3. Complete the web diagram below to show what happens to urine after an hour outside of the body.

```
┌──────────────────────────┐                          ┌──────────────────────────┐
│  _____      │                          │  _____     │
│  _____      │                          │  _____     │
│  _____      │                          │  _____     │
│  _____      │                          │  _____     │
│  _____      │                          │  _____     │
└──────────────────────────┘                          └──────────────────────────┘
                    ↖                              ↗
                    ┌──────────────────────────┐
                    │  Changes in Urine Samples │
                    │      after One Hour        │
                    └──────────────────────────┘
                    ↙                              ↘
┌──────────────────────────┐                          ┌──────────────────────────┐
│  _____      │                          │  _____     │
│  _____      │                          │  _____     │
│  _____      │                          │  _____     │
│  _____      │                          │  _____     │
│  _____      │                          │  _____     │
└──────────────────────────┘                          └──────────────────────────┘
```

4. A female patient visits the physician's office and tells you that she thinks she is pregnant. You tell her that it is possible to confirm this by taking a urine sample. Which collection method would make it easiest for you to determine the result? Explain your answer.

_____

_____

5. List five drugs that can be detected in a urine test.

a. _____

b. _____

c. _____

d. _____

e. _____

6. Chain-of-Custody

The chain-of-custody process is used to ensure that all urine specimens are identifiable and have not been tampered with. Read the scenarios in the table below and decide whether the correct chain-of-custody procedure has taken place. Place a check mark in the appropriate box.

Scenario	Correct Procedure Used	Possibility of Contamination
a. A patient faxes you her identification in advance to save time at the reception desk.		
b. A patient enters the bathroom to give a urine sample wearing jeans and a T-shirt.		
c. A patient selects his own sealed collection container from the cupboard.		
d. A patient empties her pockets before entering the bathroom to give a urine sample while carrying a bottle of water.		
e. A patient enters the bathroom to give a urine sample wearing cargo pants, a sweater, and a baseball cap.		
f. A patient washes and dries his hands before entering the bathroom to give a urine sample.		
g. A patient has forgotten her ID, but an employer representative verifies that she is the correct person.		

Physical and Chemical Properties of Urine

7. List four things that can affect the color of urine.

   a. _____

   b. _____

   c. _____

   d. _____

8. A severely underweight 15-year-old girl comes into the physician's office to give a urine sample. The test reveals that there are ketones in the patient's urine. Explain why this may be the case.

   _____

   _____

9. Read the descriptions of five of Dr. Philbin's patients. From your knowledge of chemical and physical properties of urine, match each patient with the correct diagnosis.

Patient Description

a. Mr. Himmel is a 45-year-old father who is suffering from a stomach upset. His urine sample has a high specific gravity and is a deep yellow color. _____

b. Mrs. Lincoln is a 33-year-old receptionist. Her urine sample is alkaline and contains leukocytes and a small amount of blood. _____

c. Mr. Ackton is a 60-year-old gardener. His urine sample is dark yellow and contains bilirubin. _____

d. Mrs. Franklin is a 75-year-old widow. Her urine sample has a high specific gravity, contains a high level of glucose, and is very acidic. _____

e. Mrs. Taylor is a 29-year-old surgeon who has little time to exercise. She has a large quantity of protein in her urine. _____

Diagnosis

1. Urinary tract infection
2. Diabetes mellitus
3. Pregnancy
4. Dehydration
5. Hepatitis

10. When blood is found in the urine, it can be an indication of several conditions. Read the following list and circle all of the disorders that may cause blood to appear in urine.

    a. Renal disorder

    b. Diabetes

    c. Neoplasms

    d. Urinary tract infection

    e. Appendicitis

    f. Trauma to the urinary tract

11. You are testing a urine sample for its physical properties. While you are checking for clarity, you hold the sample in front of a piece of lined white paper. There is a small amount of turbidity, but the black lines can still be seen through the specimen. Which term would you use to describe the specimen?

    a. Clear

    b. Hazy

    c. Cloudy

12. List three things that can cause urine to become more alkaline.

    a. _____

    b. _____

    c. _____

It's Confirmed. . .

13. Match each of the following types of confirmation tests with its correct description.

Type of Test	Description
a. Copper reduction method _____	**1.** A test to confirm a protein on the regeant strip
b. Nitroprusside test _____	**2.** A test that uses a tablet to detect bilirubin
c. Precipitation test _____	**3.** A test used to detect any reducing sugar
d. Diazo test _____	**4.** A reaction test used to detect ketones

14. A urine sample has tested positive for protein. What procedure would be used to confirm the reagent strip reaction? Explain how the procedure works.

_____

_____

Searching the Sediment

15. List six structures that can appear in urine sediment.

    a. _____

    b. _____

    c. _____

    d. _____

    e. _____

    f. _____

16. The following passage is about the collection of urine sediment. However, some of the important terms are missing. Insert the correct words from the box below the passage into the missing spaces.

Urine sediment is prepared by _____ urine and saving the button of cells and other _____ matter that collects in the bottom of the tube. This button is _____ in the residual _____ (urine above the sediment when the tube of urine is centrifuged), and a drop of this suspension is placed on a _____ and viewed with a _____. Making a _____ concentrates all the structures in the urine so that it is unlikely that any _____ will be missed.

supernatant	particulate	slide	components
centrifuging	sediment button	resuspend	microscope

17. Match the following types of epithelial cells that can be found in urine with their correct description.

Epithelial Cells

a. Squamous _____

b. Transitional _____

c. Renal _____

Description

1. Cells that line the bladder and are seen with infections of the lower urinary tract

2. Cells that line the nephrons and are seen with infections of the upper urinary tract

3. Cells that cover external skin surfaces

18. All in a Day's Work

As a medical assistant, you'll probably be asked to assist in the urinalysis procedure. Study the list of tasks below and decide which duties you would be responsible for, and which would be completed by someone else. Place a check in the "Yes" box for tasks you would complete yourself and in the "No" box for tasks that would be completed by another member of the team.

Task	Yes	No
a. Prepare urine sediment for microscopic examination.		
b. Instruct patient on how to provide urine sample.		
c. Perform microscopic examination of urine sediment.		
d. Ensure that urine is tested or refrigerated within the correct time period.		
e. Use suprapubic aspiration to collect a urine sample.		
f. Perform confirmatory tests on urine samples.		
g. Label specimens for clear identification.		
h. Assemble equipment needed for urinalysis procedures.		

19. Match the following key terms to their definitions.

Key Terms

a. bilirubinuria _____

b. diurnal variation _____

c. glycosuria _____

d. hemoglobinuria _____

e. ketones _____

f. leukocyte esterase _____

g. nitrite _____

h. proteinuria _____

i. quantitative _____

j. sediment _____

k. specific gravity _____

l. sulfosalicylic acid _____

m. supernatant _____

n. threshold _____

o. urobilinogen _____

Definitions

1. variation in the urine during a 24-hour period

2. density of a liquid, such as urine, compared with water

3. the measuring of an amount

4. concentration of a substance in the blood above which it will begin to appear in the urine

5. the presence of glucose in the urine

6. the end products of fat metabolism

7. the presence of large quantities of protein in the urine; usually a sign of renal dysfunction

8. presence of free hemoglobin in urine

9. bilirubin in the urine

10. a compound formed when bilirubin is secreted into the intestines in bile and converted by bacterial action

11. a radical formed from the reduction of nitrate that is used to assess the presence of bacteria in urine

12. a test used to detect the presence of white blood cells in urine

13. an acid used to test for protein

14. insoluble material prepared by centrifuging urine and saving particulate matter at the bottom of the tube

15. urine above the sediment when the tube of urine is centrifuged

20. True or False? Determine whether the following statements are true or false? If false, explain why.

a. A physician always performs a bladder catheterization.

_____

b. If a urine specimen tests negative for drugs, it will be tested a second time to make certain.

_____

c. Normal, freshly voided urine is usually clear.

_____

d. Urine with low specific gravity is concentrated.

_____

APPLICATION

Critical Thinking Practice

1. During an initial urine test, a specimen tests positive for ketones. The physician asks you to perform a confirmatory test on the specimen to make sure the diagnosis is correct. Explain what you would do to confirm the presence of ketones in urine and what you would expect to happen if the test is positive.

_____

_____

2. A patient gives a urine sample at 11 AM and the physician asks you to perform a urinalysis on the specimen. Before you can analyze the sample, there is an emergency situation in the office and you become distracted. At 2 PM you remember that the specimen has still not been analyzed and it is in a container that is not refrigerated. What should you do? Explain your answer.

_____

_____

Patient Education

1. One of your patients needs to provide a 24-hour urine collection. She has never done it before and is unsure how to carry out the procedure. Write the patient a list of instructions, explaining what she should do in order to provide an accurate specimen.

Documentation

1. You instruct a patient how to perform a clean-catch midstream urine specimen. When you test the sample, you discover that the urine is cloudy, with a pH level of 7.5 and contains traces of red blood cells, nitrites, and leukocytes. How would you document this information on the patient's chart?

_____

_____

Active Learning

1. Research the guidelines for drug testing in the workplace. Write a simple one-page guide for employees informing them about the standard procedures for providing a urine specimen for a drug test. Include information about what will be expected of them throughout the procedure and what will happen to ensure confidentiality and accuracy of results.

2. Use the clean-catch midstream urine specimen collection method to obtain a sample of your own urine. Test the physical properties of your sample. Can you detect anything about your physical health from your specimen? Document the information as you would in a patient's chart.

3. Identify common features that patients can take note of in their own urine (e.g., dark color = possible dehydration). Make a brochure to raise patients' awareness of how their physical health can be reflected in the color and clarity of their urine.

Professional Journal

REFLECT

(Prompts and Ideas: Have you been asked to provide a urine specimen for a drug test? Was the procedure clearly explained to you? Did you receive your results promptly? Was there anything about the procedure that you did not understand?)

_____

_____

_____

_____

_____

_____

PONDER AND SOLVE

1. A patient provides a urine sample at 9 AM. The sample is refrigerated until it can be tested. At 3 PM, your coworker tells you that she is going to test the specimen. She says that the results will be accurate because the sample has been refrigerated. What do you say to your coworker?

_____

_____

_____

_____

_____

_____

2. A patient asks you what types of drugs can be detected in urine. Two weeks later, the same patient comes into the office to provide a urine specimen. He appears to be acting suspiciously and you think you see him pick up a bottle before entering the bathroom. What should you do next?

_____

_____

_____

_____

_____

_____

_____

EXPERIENCE

Skills related to this chapter include:

1. Obtaining a Clean-catch Midstream Urine Specimen (Procedure 43-1).
2. Obtaining a 24-hour Urine Specimen (Procedure 43-2).
3. Determining Color and Clarity of Urine (Procedure 43-3).
4. Chemical Reagent Strip Analysis (Procedure 43-4).
5. Preparing Urine Sediment (Procedure 43-5).

Record any common mistakes, lessons learned, and/or tips you discovered during your experience of practicing and demonstrating these skills.

_____

_____

_____

_____

_____

_____

_____

Skill Practice

PERFORMANCE OBJECTIVES:

1. Explain to and/or assist a patient in obtaining a clean-catch midstream urine specimen (Procedure 43-1).
2. Explain the method of obtaining a 24-hour urine collection (Procedure 43-2).
3. Determine color and clarity of urine (Procedure 43-3).
4. Accurately interpret chemical reagent strip reactions (Procedure 43-4).
5. Prepare urine sediment for microscopic examination (Procedure 43-5).

Name_____ Date _____ Time _____

Procedure 43-1:	OBTAINING A CLEAN-CATCH MIDSTREAM URINE SPECIMEN

EQUIPMENT/SUPPLIES: Sterile urine container labeled with patient's name, cleansing towelettes (2 for males, 3 for females), gloves if you are to assist patient, hand sanitizer

STANDARDS: Given the needed equipment and a place to work, the student will perform this skill with _____% accuracy in a total of _____ minutes. *(Your instructor will tell you what the percentage and time limits will be before you begin practicing.)*

KEY:　　4 = Satisfactory　　　0 = Unsatisfactory　　　NA = This step is not counted

PROCEDURE STEPS	SELF	PARTNER	INSTRUCTOR
1. Wash your hands. Put on personal protective equipment.	☐	☐	☐
2. Assemble the equipment and supplies.	☐	☐	☐
3. Identify the patient and explain the procedure. Ask for and answer any questions.	☐	☐	☐
4. If the patient is to perform the procedure, provide the necessary supplies.	☐	☐	☐
5. Have the patient perform the procedure.	☐	☐	☐
a. Instruct the male patient:			
(1) If uncircumcised, expose the glans penis by retracting the foreskin, then clean the meatus with an antiseptic wipe. The glans should be cleaned in a circular motion away from the meatus. A new wipe should be used for each cleaning sweep.			
(2) Keeping the foreskin retracted, initially void a few seconds into the toilet or urinal.			
(3) Bring the sterile container into the urine stream and collect a sufficient amount (about 30–60 mL). Instruct the patient to avoid touching the inside of the container with the penis.			
(4) Finish voiding into the toilet or urinal.			
b. Instruct the female patient:			
(1) Kneel or squat over a bedpan or toilet bowl. Spread the labia minora widely to expose the meatus. Using an antiseptic wipe, cleanse on either side of the meatus, then the meatus itself. Use a wipe only once in a sweep from the anterior to the posterior surfaces, then discard it.			
(2) Keeping the labia separated, initially void a few seconds into the toilet.			
(3) Bring the sterile container into the urine stream and collect a sufficient amount (about 30–60 mL).			
(4) Finish voiding into the toilet or bedpan.			
6. Cap the filled container and place it in a designated area.	☐	☐	☐
7. Transport the specimen in a biohazard container for testing.	☐	☐	☐
8. Properly care for or dispose of equipment and supplies. Clean the work area. Remove gloves and wash your hands.	☐	☐	☐

CALCULATION

Total Possible Points: _____

Total Points Earned: _____ Multiplied by 100 = _____ Divided by Total Possible Points = _____%

Pass   **Fail**

☐   ☐   Comments:

Student signature _____ Date _____
Partner signature _____ Date _____
Instructor signature _____ Date _____

Name_____ Date _____ Time _____

Procedure 43-2:	OBTAINING A 24-HOUR URINE SPECIMEN

EQUIPMENT/SUPPLIES: Patient's labeled 24-hour urine container (some patients require more than one container), preservatives required for the specific test, chemical hazard labels, graduated cylinder that holds at least 1 L, serological or volumetric pipettes, clean random urine container, fresh 10% bleach solution, gloves, hand disinfectant, surface disinfectant

STANDARDS: Given the needed equipment and a place to work, the student will perform this skill with _____% accuracy in a total of _____ minutes. *(Your instructor will tell you what the percentage and time limits will be before you begin practicing.)*

KEY: 4 = Satisfactory   0 = Unsatisfactory   NA = This step is not counted

PROCEDURE STEPS	SELF	PARTNER	INSTRUCTOR
1. Wash your hands.	☐	☐	☐
2. Assemble the equipment.	☐	☐	☐
3. Identify the type of 24-hour urine collection requested and check for any special requirements, such as any acid or preservative that should be added. Label the container appropriately.	☐	☐	☐
4. Add to the 24-hour urine container the correct amount of acid or preservative using a serological or volumetric pipette.	☐	☐	☐
5. Use the provided label or make a label with spaces for the patient's name, beginning time and date, and ending time and date so that the patient can fill in the appropriate information.	☐	☐	☐
6. Instruct the patient to collect a 24-hour urine sample as follows: **a.** Void into the toilet, and note this time and date as beginning. **b.** After the first voiding, collect each voiding and add it to the urine container for the next 24 hours. **c.** Precisely 24 hours after beginning collection, empty the bladder even if there is no urge to void and add this final volume of urine to the container. **d.** Note on the label the ending time and date.	☐	☐	☐
7. Explain to the patient that depending on the test requested, the 24-hour urine may have to be refrigerated the entire time. Instruct the patient to return the specimen to you as soon as possible after collection is complete.	☐	☐	☐
8. Record in the patient's chart that supplies and instructions were given to collect a 24-hour urine specimen and the test that was requested.	☐	☐	☐
9. When you receive the specimen, verify beginning and ending times and dates before the patient leaves. Check for any acids or preservatives to be added before the specimen goes to the testing laboratory.	☐	☐	☐
10. Put on gloves.	☐	☐	☐
11. Pour the urine into a cylinder to record the volume. Pour an aliquot of the urine into a clean container to be sent to the laboratory. (Label the specimen with the patient's identification.) Record the volume of the urine collection and the amount of any acid or preservative added on the sample container and on the laboratory requisition. If permitted, you may dispose of the remainder of the urine.	☐	☐	☐

PROCEDURE STEPS	SELF	PARTNER	INSTRUCTOR
12. Record the volume on the patient's test requisition and chart.	☐	☐	☐
13. Clean the cylinder with fresh 10% bleach solution, then rinse with water. Let it air dry. If you are using a disposable container, be sure to dispose of it in the proper biohazard container.	☐	☐	☐
14. Clean the work area and dispose of waste properly. Remove protective equipment and wash your hands. *Note*: Some containers come with the preservative already added. In either case, be sure the patient is instructed not to discard preservative and not to allow it to be handled. *Warning!* Use caution when handling acids and other hazardous materials. Be familiar with the material safety data sheets for each chemical in your site.	☐	☐	☐

CALCULATION

Total Possible Points: _____
Total Points Earned: _____ Multiplied by 100 = _____ Divided by Total Possible Points = _____%

Pass   **Fail**
☐   ☐   Comments:

Student signature _____ Date _____
Partner signature _____ Date _____
Instructor signature _____ Date _____

Name _____ Date _____ Time _____

Procedure 43-3:	DETERMINING COLOR AND CLARITY OF URINE

EQUIPMENT/SUPPLIES: Gloves, impervious gown, 10% bleach solution, patient's labeled urine specimen, clear tube, usually a centrifuge, white paper scored with black lines, hand disinfectant, surface disinfectant

STANDARDS: Given the needed equipment and a place to work, the student will perform this skill with _____% accuracy in a total of _____ minutes. *(Your instructor will tell you what the percentage and time limits will be before you begin practicing.)*

KEY: 4 = Satisfactory   0 = Unsatisfactory   NA = This step is not counted

PROCEDURE STEPS	SELF	PARTNER	INSTRUCTOR
1. Wash your hands.	☐	☐	☐
2. Assemble the equipment.	☐	☐	☐
3. Put on personal protective equipment.	☐	☐	☐
4. Verify that the names on the specimen container and the report form are the same.	☐	☐	☐
5. Pour about 10 mL of urine into the tube.	☐	☐	☐
6. In bright light against a white background, examine the color. The most common colors are straw (very pale yellow), yellow, dark yellow, and amber (brown-yellow).	☐	☐	☐
7. Determine clarity. Hold the tube in front of the white paper scored with black lines. If you see the lines clearly (not obscured), record as clear. If you see the lines but they are not well delineated, record as hazy. If you cannot see the lines at all, record as cloudy.	☐	☐	☐
8. Properly care for or dispose of equipment and supplies. Clean the work area using a surface disinfectant. Remove personal protective equipment. Wash your hands. *Notes*: Rapid determination of color and clarity is necessary because some urine turns cloudy if left standing. Bilirubin, which may be found in urine in certain conditions, breaks down when exposed to light. Protect the specimen from light if urinalysis is ordered but testing is delayed. If further testing is to be done but is delayed more than an hour, refrigerate the specimen to avoid alteration of chemistry.	☐	☐	☐

CALCULATION

Total Possible Points: _____
Total Points Earned: _____ Multiplied by 100 = _____ Divided by Total Possible Points = _____%

Pass   **Fail**
☐   ☐ | Comments: |

Student signature _____ Date _____
Partner signature _____ Date _____
Instructor signature _____ Date _____

Name_____ Date_____ Time_____

Procedure 43-4:	CHEMICAL REAGENT STRIP ANALYSIS

EQUIPMENT/SUPPLIES: Patient's labeled urine specimen, chemical strip (such as Multistix or Chemstrip), manufacturer's color comparison chart, stopwatch or timer, personal protective equipment, hand disinfectant, surface disinfectant

STANDARDS: Given the needed equipment and a place to work, the student will perform this skill with _____% accuracy in a total of _____ minutes. *(Your instructor will tell you what the percentage and time limits will be before you begin practicing.)*

KEY: 4 = Satisfactory   0 = Unsatisfactory   NA = This step is not counted

PROCEDURE STEPS	SELF	PARTNER	INSTRUCTOR
1. Wash your hands.	☐	☐	☐
2. Assemble the equipment.	☐	☐	☐
3. Put on personal protective equipment.	☐	☐	☐
4. Verify that the names on the specimen container and the report form are the same.	☐	☐	☐
5. Mix the patient's urine by gently swirling the covered container.	☐	☐	☐
6. Remove the reagent strip from its container and replace the lid to prevent deterioration of strips by humidity.	☐	☐	☐
7. Immerse the reagent strip in the urine completely, then immediately remove it, sliding the edge of the strip along the lip of the container to remove excess urine.	☐	☐	☐
8. Start your stopwatch or timer immediately.	☐	☐	☐
9. Compare the reagent pads to the color chart, determining results at the intervals stated by the manufacturer. Example: Glucose is read at 30 seconds. To determine results, examine that pad 30 seconds post dipping and compare with color chart for glucose.	☐	☐	☐
10. Read all reactions at the times indicated and record the results.	☐	☐	☐
11. Discard the reagent strips in the proper receptacle. Discard urine unless more testing is required.	☐	☐	☐
12. Clean the work area with surface disinfectant. Remove personal protective equipment. Wash your hands. *Warning*: Do not remove the desiccant packet in the strip container; it ensures that minimal moisture affects the strips. The desiccant is toxic and should be discarded appropriately after all of the strips have been used. *Notes*: The manufacturer's color comparison chart is assigned a lot number that must match the lot number of the strips used for testing. Record this in the quality assurance (QA/QC) log. False-positive and false-negative results are possible. Review the manufacturer's package insert accompanying the strips to learn about factors that may give false results and how to avoid them. Aspirin may cause false-positive ketones. Document any medications the patient is taking. If the patient is taking Pyridium, do not use a reagent strip for testing, because the medication will interfere with the color. Outdated materials give inaccurate results. If the expiration date has passed, discard the materials.	☐	☐	☐

CALCULATION

Total Possible Points: _____
Total Points Earned: _____ Multiplied by 100 = _____ Divided by Total Possible Points = _____%

Pass   **Fail**
☐   ☐   Comments:

Student signature _____ Date _____
Partner signature _____ Date _____
Instructor signature _____ Date _____

Name_____ Date_____ Time_____

Procedure 43-5:   PREPARING URINE SEDIMENT

EQUIPMENT/SUPPLIES: Patient's labeled urine specimen, urine centrifuge tubes, transfer pipette, centrifuge (1,500–2,000 rpm), personal protective equipment, hand disinfectant, surface disinfectant

STANDARDS: Given the needed equipment and a place to work, the student will perform this skill with _____% accuracy in a total of _____ minutes. *(Your instructor will tell you what the percentage and time limits will be before you begin practicing.)*

KEY: 4 = Satisfactory   0 = Unsatisfactory   NA = This step is not counted

PROCEDURE STEPS	SELF	PARTNER	INSTRUCTOR
1. Wash your hands.	☐	☐	☐
2. Assemble the equipment.	☐	☐	☐
3. Put on personal protective equipment.	☐	☐	☐
4. Verify that the names on the specimen container and the report form are the same.	☐	☐	☐
5. Swirl specimen to mix. Pour 10 mL of well-mixed urine into a labeled centrifuge tube or standard system tube. Cap the tube with a plastic cap or Parafilm.	☐	☐	☐
6. Centrifuge the sample at 1500 rpm for 5 minutes.	☐	☐	☐
7. When the centrifuge has stopped, remove the tubes. Make sure no tests are to be performed first on the supernatant. Remove the caps and pour off the supernatant, leaving 0.5–1.0 mL of it. Suspend the sediment again by aspirating up and down with a transfer pipette, or follow manufacturer's directions for a standardized system.	☐	☐	☐
8. Properly care for and dispose of equipment and supplies. Clean the work area with surface disinfectant. Remove personal protective equipment. Wash your hands. *Notes:* If the urine is to be tested by chemical reagent strip, perform the dip test before spinning the urine. Preparing a urine specimen of less than 3 mL for sediment is not recommended because that is not enough urine to create a true sediment. However, some patients cannot provide a large amount of urine. In such cases, document the volume on the chart under sediment to ensure proper interpretation of results. Centrifuge maintenance requires periodic checks to ensure that the speed and timing are correct. Document this information on the maintenance log.	☐	☐	☐

CALCULATION

Total Possible Points: _____
Total Points Earned: _____ Multiplied by 100 = _____ Divided by Total Possible Points = _____%

Pass   **Fail**
☐   ☐   Comments:

Student signature _____ Date _____
Partner signature _____ Date _____
Instructor signature _____ Date _____

Chapter Self-Assessment Quiz

1. What color will be observed on the reagent pad if nitrites are present in urine?

  a. Blue

  b. Pink

  c. Red

  d. Yellow

  e. Green

2. How many tests are required to prove a positive drug result in a urine sample?

  a. One

  b. Two

  c. Three

  d. Four

  e. Five

3. Why is a 24-hour collection a better indicator of values than a random specimen?

  a. Some substances are excreted with diurnal variation.

  b. Some bacteria do not develop fully for 24 hours.

  c. A 24-hour collection gives the physician a more accurate idea of the patient's diet.

  d. The higher the volume of urine tested, the more accurate the result.

  e. Some substances are excreted only at night.

4. The most common method of urine collection is:

  a. suprapubic aspiration.

  b. clean-catch midstream.

  c. random specimen.

  d. first morning void.

  e. postprandial specimen.

5. Which official body approves the drug test used to analyze urine samples?

  a. Clinical Laboratory Improvement Amendments

  b. Centers for Medicare & Medicaid Services

  c. Occupational Safety and Health Administration

  d. Food and Drug Administration

  e. Drug and Alcohol Testing Industry Association

6. Which of these conditions may cause a patient's urine to smell sweet?

  a. Urinary tract infection

  b. Kidney infection

  c. Diabetes

  d. Dehydration

  e. Yeast infection

7. What is the specific gravity of a normal urine specimen?

  a. 0.900–1.000

  b. 1.001–1.035

  c. 1.100–1.135

  d. 1.500–1.635

  e. 2.000–2.001

8. Why is a urinometer no longer used in a laboratory to test specific gravity?

  a. It requires a large volume of urine.

  b. It is not as accurate as other equipment.

  c. It is too expensive to use frequently.

  d. It takes longer to process a sample than other equipment.

  e. It takes up too much space in the laboratory.

9. What is the expected pH range for urine?

  a. 3.0–6.0

  b. 4.0–7.0

  c. 5.0–8.0

  d. 6.0–9.0

  e. 7.0–10.0

10. Increased numbers of epithelial cells in urine may indicate:

  a. there is an irritation, such as inflammation, somewhere in the urinary system.

  b. the patient is overly hydrated.

  c. the patient is pregnant.

  d. the urine sample has sat for too long before examination.

  e. the testing was not performed correctly.

11. Which of the following statements is true about bilirubin?

    a. Bilirubin is formed in the kidneys.

    b. Bilirubin is a dark red pigment.

    c. Normal urine will contain a small amount of bilirubin.

    d. Bilirubin will break down with exposure to light.

    e. Bilirubin in the urine usually results from a urinary tract infection.

12. Which group of people are most at risk of developing galactosuria?

    a. Teenagers

    b. Newborns

    c. Pregnant women

    d. Elderly men

    e. Elderly women

13. A patient with uric acid crystals in their urine possibly has:

    a. leukemia.

    b. a urinary tract infection.

    c. hepatitis.

    d. a renal disorder.

    e. gallbladder cancer.

14. A patient who has been asked to provide a 24-hour specimen should:

    a. keep the urine at room temperature.

    b. collect urine only after mealtimes.

    c. gently shake the container after each specimen is added.

    d. drink more water than usual during the collection period.

    e. avoid drinking soda or alcohol during the collection period.

15. Which of these should be included on a chain-of-custody document?

    a. The results of the urine test

    b. The patient's name, address, date of birth, and social security number

    c. Instructions for providing a specimen

    d. The date the specimen was collected or transferred

    e. The volume of urine in the specimen

16. Which biological pigment gives urine its color?

    a. Melanin

    b. Hemoglobin

    c. Myoglobin

    d. Beta-carotene

    e. Urochrome

17. Why is a urine test preferable to a blood test for a routine drug test?

    a. It is more accurate.

    b. It is less expensive.

    c. There is less risk of contamination.

    d. It requires less equipment.

    e. A urine specimen will stay fresh longer than a blood sample.

18. Strenuous physical exercise may cause:

    a. elevated quantities of protein in urine.

    b. decreased amounts of epithelial cells.

    c. increased numbers of ketones.

    d. urine to be hazy.

    e. a low concentration of phosphates.

19. Cast formation occurs in the:

    a. liver.

    b. small intestine.

    c. bladder.

    d. pathways of the digestive tract.

    e. tubules of the nephron.

20. Sulfosalicylic acid added to normal urine would cause the urine to:

    a. turn orange.

    b. remain clear.

    c. become cloudy.

    d. turn pink.

    e. form crystals.

44 Microbiology and Immunology

Chapter Checklist

- ☐ Read textbook chapter and take notes within the Chapter Notes outline. Answer the Learning Objectives as you reach them in the content, and then check them off.
- ☐ Work the Content Review questions—both Foundational Knowledge and Application.
- ☐ Perform the Active Learning exercise(s).

- ☐ Complete Professional Journal entries.
- ☐ Complete Skill Practice Activity(s) using Competency Evaluation Forms and Work Products, when appropriate.
- ☐ Take the Chapter Self-Assessment Quiz.
- ☐ Insert all appropriate pages into your Portfolio.

Learning Objectives

1. Spell and define the key terms.
2. List and describe primary microorganisms.
3. Describe how bacteria are named.
4. Identify various bacterial illustrations.
5. Describe the classifications of rickettsiae, chlamydiae, fungi, protozoa, and metazoa.
6. Describe the medical assistant's responsibilities in microbiological testing.
7. List the most common types of microbiological specimens collected in the physician's office laboratory.
8. State the factors necessary for microbial growth.

9. Describe the different types of media used for microbial testing.
10. List the steps used in caring for media plates.
11. List each step in Gram staining and state the purpose of each step.
12. State the purpose of sensitivity testing and give the meaning of sensitive and resistant results.
13. Describe the antigen-antibody reaction.
14. Explain the storage and handling of test kits.
15. List and describe immunology tests most commonly encountered through the medical office.

Chapter Notes

Note: Bold-faced headings are the major headings in the text chapter; headings in regular font are lower-level headings (i.e., the content is subordinate to, or falls "under," the major headings). Make sure you understand the key terms used in the chapter, as well as the concepts presented as Key Points.

TEXT SUBHEADINGS   **NOTES**

Introduction _____

_____

Key Terms: pathogens; normal flora; nosocomial infections; aerobes; anaerobes

Key Points:

• Microbiology means the study of small life, too small to be seen without a microscope.

• **Pathogens**, microorganisms likely to cause disease, are those that thrive at temperatures between 96°F and 101°F in a fairly neutral environment. Many **normal flora** (bacteria that are not pathogens) live and thrive on the human body without causing disease. As a medical assistant, to protect yourself, the physician, patients, and all coworkers from **nosocomial infections** (infections acquired in a medical setting), you need to be aware of the organisms present around us and their potential for causing disease.

• Bacteria require the following five elements for survival: nutrients, warmth, moisture, darkness, and oxygen (**aerobes**) or lack of oxygen (**anaerobes**). The human body provides all five elements. These same five elements are simulated in the microbiology laboratory with the use of culture media, incubators, and techniques to control the specimen's exposure to oxygen.

☐ **LEARNING OBJECTIVE 1:** Spell and define the key terms.

Microbiological Life Forms _____

_____

_____

Bacteria _____

_____

Key Terms: bacteriology; cocci; morphology; bacilli

Key Point:

• **Bacteriology** is the study of bacteria. Organisms have both a genus and species name. The genus is always spelled with a capital letter, and the species begins with a lowercase letter (*Staphylococcus aureus*). In print the name is in italics or underlined.

Rickettsiae and Chlamydiae _____

_____

_____

Fungi _____

_____

Key Term: mycology

Molds _____
_____
_____

Yeasts _____
_____
_____

Viruses _____
_____

Key Term: virology
_____

Protozoa _____
_____

Key Term: parasitology
_____

Metazoa _____
_____

☐ **LEARNING OBJECTIVE 2:** List and describe primary microorganisms.

☐ **LEARNING OBJECTIVE 3:** Describe how bacteria are named.

☐ **LEARNING OBJECTIVE 4:** Identify various bacterial illustrations.

☐ **LEARNING OBJECTIVE 5:** Describe the classifications of rickettsiae, chlamydiae, fungi, protozoa, and metazoa.

Specimen Collection and Handling _____

Key Point:
- As a medical assistant, you may be responsible for collecting most of the specimens in the medical office. To ensure that the office or reference laboratory receives a sample that will indicate the disease process for which the specimen was collected, you must collect the specimen from the appropriate site using the proper method. You also must handle the specimen so that it will yield accurate findings.

☐ **LEARNING OBJECTIVE 6:** Describe the medical assistant's responsibilities in microbiological testing.

☐ **LEARNING OBJECTIVE 7:** List the most common types of microbiological specimens collected in the physician's office laboratory.

Types of Specimens _____

_____

_____

Types of Culture Media _____

_____

Key Term: media

☐ **LEARNING OBJECTIVE 8:** State the factors necessary for microbial growth.

☐ **LEARNING OBJECTIVE 9:** Describe the different types of media used for microbial testing.

Caring for the Media _____

_____

Key Point:
• Agar must be refrigerated until needed, then warmed to room temperature before use. A cold plate or tube will kill many microorganisms, most of which require a warmer temperature for growth.

☐ **LEARNING OBJECTIVE 10:** List the steps used in caring for media plates.

Transporting the Specimen _____

_____

Key Points:
• Care must be taken to transport or process the specimen as soon as possible so the organisms do not die.
• Special care must be taken in filling out all identification slips and information.
• For the most reliable results, laboratory tests should be performed on fresh specimens within 1 hour after collection. When this is not possible, the specimen must be stored properly to preserve the physical and chemical properties necessary for accurate diagnosis. Specimens should never be subjected to extreme temperature changes.

Microscopic Examination of Microorganisms _____

_____

_____

Smears and Slides _____

_____

Identification by Staining _____

_____

_____

☐ **LEARNING OBJECTIVE 11:** List each step in Gram staining and state the purpose of each step.

Inoculation _____

_____

_____

Sensitivity Testing _____

_____

Key Term: sensitivity testing

_____

☐ **LEARNING OBJECTIVE 12:** State the purpose of sensitivity testing and give the meaning of sensitive and resistant results.

Antigens and Antibodies _____

_____

Key Terms: antigens; antibodies; specificity, sensitivity
Key Points:
- **Antigens** are substances recognized as foreign to the body that cause the body to initiate a defense response, including the production of antibodies. Pathogenic microbes are among the substances recognized by the body as antigens. **Antibodies** are proteins produced by the body in response to a specific antigen that bind to that specific antigen. Antibodies float freely in the bloodstream and are found in serum. Each antibody combines with (in most instances) only one antigen; this is called **specificity**. It allows laboratory personnel to test the exact substance desired without interference from any other substance in serum.
- Because an antibody has a particularly strong attraction for its antigen, little antigen needs to be present in a sample for the antibody to find it; this is referred to as **sensitivity**. A test is very sensitive if it can determine the presence of a substance even if only a small amount is present.

_____

☐ **LEARNING OBJECTIVE 13:** Describe the antigen-antibody reaction.

Immunology Testing Principles _____

_____

_____

Reagent and Kit Storage and Handling _____

_____

Key Point:
• Reagents from kits with different lot numbers should not be used together. The manufacturer will not guarantee that they will work correctly when components from different lots are mixed. Reagents should never be used past their expiration date.

☐ **LEARNING OBJECTIVE 14:** Explain the storage and handling of test kits.

Immunology Tests _____

_____

_____

Infectious Mononucleosis _____

_____

_____

Pregnancy Test _____

_____

_____

Group A Streptococcus _____

_____

_____

☐ **LEARNING OBJECTIVE 15:** List and describe immunology tests most commonly encountered through the medical office.

Immunohematology _____

_____

_____

ABO Group _____

_____

_____

Rh Type _____

_____

_____

Content Review

FOUNDATIONAL KNOWLEDGE

Get To Know Your Microorganisms

1. List five primary microorganisms and briefly describe each one.

a. _____

b. _____

c. _____

d. _____

e. _____

2. Match each type of bacteria with the correct morphology.

Type	Morphology
a. staphylococci _____	**1.** rod-shaped, end-to-end chains
b. streptococci _____	**2.** round, grapelike clusters
c. coccobacilli _____	**3.** rigid, curved rods (comma-shaped)
d. streptobacilli _____	**4.** rod-shaped and somewhat oval
e. vibrios _____	**5.** round chain formations

3. Bacteria can be categorized based on shape and appearance, or their morphology. Take a look at the illustration below and determine what kind of bacteria are shown. Draw a circle around the following types of bacteria and then label them correctly.

a. single cocci

b. diplococci

c. staphylococci

d. streptobacilli

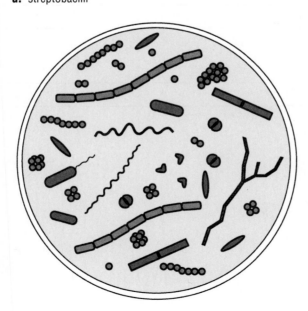

4. Match each of the following classifications of metazoa with the damage it can cause.

Metazoa	**Possible Damage**
a. helminths _____	**1.** liver fluke and tapeworm infestation
b. nematodes _____	**2.** bites or stings
c. arthropods _____	**3.** intestinal obstruction

5. Why are viruses so difficult to cure?

_____

_____

Microbiological Testing in the Medical Office

6. List three responsibilities in microbiological testing that you can assume as a medical assistant.

a. _____

b. _____

c. _____

7. List six common microbiological specimens that are collected in a physician's office laboratory.

a. _____

b. _____

c. _____

d. _____

e. _____

f. _____

Helping Microorganisms Grow

8. Microorganisms require certain factors in order to grow properly. How does an incubator assist in the process of microbial growth?

_____

_____

9. What is the typical media used for microbial testing?

_____

_____

10. You must pay special attention to how you handle and care for media plates in the lab. Below is a list of possible steps to take when caring for media plates. Place a check mark in the appropriate box to indicate if the action shows good practice in caring for media plates.

Action	Yes	No
a. Store the plates in the refrigerator with the side containing the medium on the bottom.		
b. Store the plates in the plastic wrapper to keep the medium moist.		
c. Discard any medium that has dried or cracked.		
d. Avoid using disposable plastic Petri plates to keep contamination at a minimum.		
e. Date each sleeve of Petri plates when a shipment arrives.		
f. Rotate the media in the refrigerator so that the oldest is in front and used first.		
g. Check and record the temperature in the refrigerator once a week.		

Gram Staining

11. You are responsible for staining a microorganism. Below is a list of the steps for Gram staining. However, some of them are missing. Fill in the missing steps in this process in the blank spaces below.

1. _____

2. Assemble the equipment.

3. _____

4. Put on personal protective equipment.

5. Place the slide on the staining rack with the smear side up.

6. _____

7. Hold the slide with slide forceps.

    a. Tilt the slide to an angle of about 45 degrees to drain the excess dye.

    b. Rinse the slide with distilled water for about 5 seconds and drain off excess water.

8. _____

9. Using the forceps, tilt the slide at a 45 degree angle to drain iodine solution. With the slide tilted, rinse the slide with distilled water from the wash bottle for about 5 to 10 seconds. Slowly and gently wash with the alcohol-acetone solution until no more stain runs off.

10. _____

11. _____

12. Drain the excess counterstain from the slide by tilting it at a 45 degree angle. Rinse the slide with distilled water for 5 seconds to remove the counterstain. Gently blot the smear dry with bibulous paper. Take care not to disturb the smeared specimen. Wipe the back of the slide clear of any solution. It may be placed between the pages of a bibulous paper pad and gently pressed to remove excess moisture.

13. _____

14. Document the procedure.

15. _____

12. One of the steps in the Gram-staining process requires that you flood the slide with Gram iodine for 60 seconds. What is the purpose of this action?

_____

_____

Antigens and Antibodies

13. How do antibodies and antigens interact with one another?

_____

_____

14. How does sensitivity testing relate to the antigen-antibody relationship? What does a sensitive result mean? What does a resistant result mean?

_____

_____

15. List three steps you should follow when storing and handling test kits.

a. _____

b. _____

c. _____

Immunology and Immunohematology

16. List the three most common immunology tests you can expect to encounter in the medical office.

a. _____

b. _____

c. _____

17. What is the ABO group? What do the letters mean?

_____

_____

18. A pregnant woman is found to be Rh positive. The baby's father is Rh negative. Will the mother need to receive the RhoGAM injection to protect her unborn child?

_____

_____

19. Match the following key terms with their definitions.

Key Terms	Definitions
a. aerobe _____	1. rod-shaped or cylindrical organisms
b. anaerobe _____	2. an illness acquired in a medical setting, generally in a hospital setting but may also refer to the medical office
c. antibody _____	3. studies performed to check if an organism is susceptible to a certain substance
d. antigen _____	4. bacterium that does not require oxygen for growth and reproduction
e. bacilli _____	5. disease-causing microorganisms

f. bacteriology _____

g. cocci _____

h. media _____

i. morphology _____

j. mycology _____

k. normal flora _____

l. nosocomial infection _____

m. parasitology _____

n. pathogens _____

o. sensitivity _____

p. sensitivity testing _____

q. specificity _____

r. virology _____

6. protein markers on cells that cause formation of antibodies and react specifically with those antibodies

7. an environment created for microorganism growth

8. relating to a definite result

9. the structural and physical characteristics of something, such as bacteria or blood cells

10. microorganism that requires oxygen to live and reproduce

11. the science and study of bacteria

12. the science and study of parasites

13. microorganisms normally found in the body

14. susceptibility to a certain substance

15. complex glycoprotein produced by B lymphocytes in response to antigen

16. the science and study of fungi

17. bacteria that have a spherical shape

18. the study and science of viruses

20. True or False? Determine whether the following statements are true or false. If false, explain why.

a. Antibodies react to only one type of antigen.

_____

_____

b. If there is a zone of inhibition around an antibiotic disk, this means the disk failed to halt the growth of the bacteria.

_____

_____

c. Most bacteria are variations of cocci bacteria.

_____

_____

d. All microorganisms can be seen with the aid of a bright-field microscope.

_____

_____

APPLICATION

Critical Thinking Practice

1. A patient comes in complaining of a sore throat, and the physician wants to run a few tests. She asks you to run a strep test. List the steps you would take to obtain the specimen, and the procedure for preparing a slide for the physician to examine.

_____

_____

2. You prepared several plates yesterday afternoon and put them in the incubator overnight. Upon examining them today you find that about half of the plates continued their growth, whereas others had growth of varying degrees. Two plates in particular seemed to have little to no growth. What can you conclude from these results?

_____

_____

Patient Education

1. The physician wants you to schedule a fecal occult blood testing. She asks you to set up an appointment with the patient and to instruct him on preparation for the test. Write a page of instructions for the patient, including dieting instructions and any medications he might need to take or cease taking before and after the procedure.

Documentation

1. Write a narrative note about the interaction in the previous question to include in the patient's chart.

_____

_____

_____

_____

_____

_____

Active Learning

1. Children have been told that it's important to wash their hands after playing and before they eat, but many do not understand why. With a partner, create a poster that illustrates the different microorganisms that kids might come in contact with when they're outside. You may want to include an image of the microorganism, as well as a brief description of where you find it, what it does, what the symptoms are, and how to treat it. Try to keep it child-friendly as well as informative.

2. When working with transfusions, it is imperative to know your patient's blood type. Many times, however, the patient may not be aware of his own blood type. Create a survey and ask at least 15 different people if they know their blood type. Find out your own blood type, if you don't already know. Then, look on websites for organizations such as the Red Cross to see what material they have on the subject. Create a chart that shows which blood types can be blood donors for the various blood types.

3. Many soaps and cleaning products today are antibacterial, meaning that they work to kill bacteria. People use these antibacterial products to wash and sanitize their hands as well as their homes, especially the kitchen and bathroom. Some studies have shown that the rise in popularity of antibacterial products may be creating strains of bacteria that are resistant to antibiotics. Perform research on this topic and work with a partner to debate the safety and necessity of antibacterial products. Present your debate to the class.

Professional Journal

REFLECT

(Prompts and Ideas: Working in a lab, you may be exposed to a variety of bacteria and bloodborne pathogens. Does this cause any anxiety for you? How can you prepare yourself to work safely under these conditions?)

_____

_____

_____

_____

_____

_____

PONDER AND SOLVE

1. A pregnant woman comes into the office, and test results indicate that she is Rh negative and her baby is Rh positive. She has received the RhoGAM injection, but she is still worried that the baby might have complications regardless of the shot. What can you say to calm her worries, and how would you explain the injection's effect on her child?

_____

_____

_____

_____

_____

_____

2. A test's result has come back positive, and you inform the physician of this result. However, upon further examination of the test kit, you discover that the kit expired several days ago. Do you tell the physician about this, do you rerun the test with whatever left over specimen you have, or do you simply call the patient with the test results? Why?

_____

_____

_____

_____

_____

_____

_____

EXPERIENCE

Skills related to this chapter include:

1. Collecting a Throat Specimen (Procedure 44-1).
2. Collecting a Nasopharyngeal Specimen (Procedure 44-2).
3. Collecting a Wound Specimen (Procedure 44-3).

4. Collecting a Sputum Specimen (Procedure 44-4).
5. Collecting Stool for Culture (Procedure 44-5).
6. Collecting Blood for Culture (Procedure 44-6).
7. Collecting Genital Specimens for Culture (Procedure 44-7).
8. Preparing a Smear for Microscopic Evaluation (Procedure 44-8).
9. Performing a Gram Stain (Procedure 44-9).
10. Inoculating a Culture (Procedure 44-10).
11. Testing a Stool Specimen for Occult Blood—Guaiac Method (Procedure 44-11).
12. Mononucleosis Testing (Procedure 44-12).
13. HCG Pregnancy Test (Procedure 44-13).
14. Rapid Group A Strep Testing (Procedure 44-14).

Record any common mistakes, lessons learned, and/or tips you discovered during your experience of practicing and demonstrating these skills:

_____

_____

_____

_____

_____

_____

_____

Skill Practice

PERFORMANCE OBJECTIVES:

1. Collect throat specimens (Procedure 44-1).
2. Collect nasopharyngeal specimens (Procedure 44-2).
3. Collect wound specimens (Procedure 44-3).
4. Collect sputum specimens (Procedure 44-4).
5. Collect stool specimens (Procedure 44-5).
6. Collect blood specimens for culture (Procedure 44-6).
7. Collect genital specimens (Procedure 44-7).
8. Prepare a smear for microscopic evaluation (Procedure 44-9).
9. Perform a Gram stain (Procedure 44-10).
10. Inoculate a culture (Procedure 44-11).
11. Test stool specimen for occult blood (Procedure 44-8).
12. Perform mononucleosis testing (Procedure 44-12).
13. Perform HCG pregnancy testing (Procedure 44-13).
14. Perform rapid group A strep testing (Procedure 44-14).

Name _____ Date _____ Time _____

Procedure 44-1:   COLLECTING A THROAT SPECIMEN

EQUIPMENT/SUPPLIES: Tongue blade, light source, sterile specimen container and swab, personal protective equipment, hand sanitizer, surface sanitizer and biohazard transport bag (if to be sent to the laboratory for analysis)

STANDARDS: Given the needed equipment and a place to work, the student will perform this skill with _____% accuracy in a total of _____ minutes. *(Your instructor will tell you what the percentage and time limits will be before you begin practicing.)*

KEY: 4 = Satisfactory   0 = Unsatisfactory   NA = This step is not counted

PROCEDURE STEPS	SELF	PARTNER	INSTRUCTOR
1. Wash your hands. Put on personal protective equipment.	☐	☐	☐
2. Assemble the equipment and supplies.	☐	☐	☐
3. Greet and identify the patient. Explain the procedure. Ask for and answer any questions.	☐	☐	☐
4. Have the patient sit with a light source directed at the throat.	☐	☐	☐
5. Carefully remove the sterile swab from the container. If performing both the rapid strep and culture or confirming negative results with a culture, swab with 2 swabs held together.	☐	☐	☐
6. Have the patient say "Ah" as you press down on the midpoint of the tongue with the tongue depressor.	☐	☐	☐
7. Swab the mucous membranes, especially the tonsillar area, the crypts, and the posterior pharynx in a "figure 8" motion. Turn the swab to expose all of its surfaces to the membranes. Avoid touching tongue, teeth, sides of mouth, and uvula.	☐	☐	☐
8. Maintain the tongue depressor position while withdrawing the swab from the patient's mouth.	☐	☐	☐
9. Follow the instructions on the specimen container for transferring the swab or processing the specimen in the office using a commercial kit. Label the specimen with the patient's name, the date and time of collection, and the origin of the material.	☐	☐	☐
10. Properly dispose of the equipment and supplies in a biohazard waste container. Remove personal protective equipment and wash your hands.	☐	☐	☐
11. Route the specimen or store it appropriately until routing can be completed.	☐	☐	☐
12. Document the procedure.	☐	☐	☐
13. Sanitize the work area.	☐	☐	☐

CALCULATION

Total Possible Points: _____

Total Points Earned: _____ Multiplied by 100 = _____ Divided by Total Possible Points = _____%

Pass **Fail**

☐ ☐ Comments:

Student signature _____ Date _____

Partner signature _____ Date _____

Instructor signature _____ Date _____

Name _____ Date _____ Time _____

| Procedure 44-2: | COLLECTING A NASOPHARYNGEAL SPECIMEN |

EQUIPMENT/SUPPLIES: Penlight, tongue blade, sterile flexible wire swab, transport media, personal protective equipment, hand sanitizer, surface sanitizer and biohazard transport bag (if to be sent to the laboratory for analysis)

STANDARDS: Given the needed equipment and a place to work, the student will perform this skill with _____% accuracy in a total of _____ minutes. *(Your instructor will tell you what the percentage and time limits will be before you begin practicing.)*

KEY: 4 = Satisfactory   0 = Unsatisfactory   NA = This step is not counted

PROCEDURE STEPS	SELF	PARTNER	INSTRUCTOR
1. Wash your hands. Put on personal protective equipment.	☐	☐	☐
2. Assemble the equipment and supplies.	☐	☐	☐
3. Greet and identify the patient. Explain the procedure. Ask for and answer any questions.	☐	☐	☐
4. Position the patient with his head tilted back.	☐	☐	☐
5. Using a penlight and a tongue blade, inspect the nasopharyngeal area.	☐	☐	☐
6. Gently pass the swab through the nostril and into the nasopharynx, keeping the swab near the septum and floor of the nose. Rotate the swab quickly, remove it, and place it in the transport media. Do not let the swab touch the sides of the patient's nostril or his tongue to prevent specimen contamination.	☐	☐	☐
7. Label the specimen with the patient's name, the date and time of collection, and the origin of specimen.	☐	☐	☐
8. Properly dispose of the equipment and supplies in a biohazard waste container. Remove personal protective equipment and wash your hands.	☐	☐	☐
9. Route the specimen or store it appropriately until routing can be completed.	☐	☐	☐
10. Document the procedure.	☐	☐	☐
11. Sanitize the work area.	☐	☐	☐

CALCULATION

Total Possible Points: _____
Total Points Earned: _____ Multiplied by 100 = _____ Divided by Total Possible Points = _____%

Pass   **Fail**
☐   ☐   Comments:

Student signature _____ Date _____
Partner signature _____ Date _____
Instructor signature _____ Date _____

Name _____ Date _____ Time _____

Procedure 44-3:	COLLECTING A WOUND SPECIMEN

EQUIPMENT/SUPPLIES: Sterile swab, transport media, personal protective equipment, hand sanitizer, surface sanitizer and biohazard transport bag (if to be sent to the laboratory for analysis)

STANDARDS: Given the needed equipment and a place to work, the student will perform this skill with _____% accuracy in a total of _____ minutes. *(Your instructor will tell you what the percentage and time limits will be before you begin practicing.)*

KEY: 4 = Satisfactory   0 = Unsatisfactory   NA = This step is not counted

PROCEDURE STEPS	SELF	PARTNER	INSTRUCTOR
1. Wash your hands. Put on personal protective equipment.	☐	☐	☐
2. Assemble the equipment and supplies.	☐	☐	☐
3. Greet and identify the patient. Explain the procedure. Ask for and answer any questions.	☐	☐	☐
4. If dressing is present, remove it and dispose of it in biohazard container. Assess the wound by observing color, odor, and amount of exudate.	☐	☐	☐
5. Use the sterile swab to sample the exudate. Saturate swab with exudate.	☐	☐	☐
6. Avoid skin edge around wound.	☐	☐	☐
7. Place swab back into container and crush ampule of transport medium.	☐	☐	☐
8. Label the specimen with the patient's name, the date and time of collection, and the origin of specimen.	☐	☐	☐
9. Route the specimen or store it appropriately until routing can be completed.	☐	☐	☐
10. Clean the wound and apply a sterile dressing using sterile technique.	☐	☐	☐
11. Properly dispose of the equipment and supplies in a biohazard waste container. Remove personal protective equipment and wash your hands.	☐	☐	☐
12. Document the procedure.	☐	☐	☐
13. Sanitize the work area.	☐	☐	☐

CALCULATION

Total Possible Points: _____

Total Points Earned: _____ Multiplied by 100 = _____ Divided by Total Possible Points = _____%

Pass   **Fail**

☐   ☐   Comments:

Student signature _____ Date _____
Partner signature _____ Date _____
Instructor signature _____ Date _____

Name _____ Date _____ Time _____

Procedure 44-4:	**COLLECTING A SPUTUM SPECIMEN**

EQUIPMENT/SUPPLIES: Sterile specimen container, personal protective equipment, hand sanitizer, surface sanitizer, and biohazard transport bag

STANDARDS: Given the needed equipment and a place to work, the student will perform this skill with _____% accuracy in a total of _____ minutes. *(Your instructor will tell you what the percentage and time limits will be before you begin practicing.)*

KEY: 4 = Satisfactory   0 = Unsatisfactory   NA = This step is not counted

PROCEDURE STEPS	SELF	PARTNER	INSTRUCTOR
1. Wash your hands. Put on personal protective equipment.	☐	☐	☐
2. Assemble the equipment and supplies.	☐	☐	☐
3. Greet and identify the patient. Explain the procedure. Ask for and answer any questions.	☐	☐	☐
4. Instruct patient to rinse mouth with water.	☐	☐	☐
5. Ask the patient to cough deeply, using the abdominal muscles as well as the accessory muscles to bring secretions from the lungs and not just the upper airways.	☐	☐	☐
6. Ask the patient to expectorate directly into the specimen container without touching the inside and without getting sputum on the outsides of the container. About 5–10 mL is sufficient for most sputum studies.	☐	☐	☐
7. Handle the specimen container according to standard precautions. Cap the container immediately and put it into the biohazard bag for transport to the laboratory. Fill out a laboratory requisition slip to accompany the specimen.	☐	☐	☐
8. Label the specimen with the patient's name, the date and time of collection, and the origin of specimen.	☐	☐	☐
9. Route the specimen to the laboratory.	☐	☐	☐
10. Properly dispose of the equipment and supplies in a biohazard waste container. Remove personal protective equipment and wash your hands.	☐	☐	☐
11. Document the procedure.	☐	☐	☐
12. Sanitize the work area.	☐	☐	☐

CALCULATION

Total Possible Points: _____
Total Points Earned: _____ Multiplied by 100 = _____ Divided by Total Possible Points = _____%

Pass   **Fail**

☐   ☐   Comments:

Student signature _____ Date _____
Partner signature _____ Date _____
Instructor signature _____ Date _____

Name_____ Date _____ Time _____

Procedure 44-5:   COLLECTING STOOL FOR CULTURE

EQUIPMENT/SUPPLIES: Specimen container dependent on test ordered (Sterile container or Para-Pak collection system for C&S or ova & parasites, test kit or slide for occult blood testing: See Laboratory Procedure Manual), tongue blade or wooden spatula, personal protective equipment, hand sanitizer, surface sanitizer and biohazard transport bag

STANDARDS: Given the needed equipment and a place to work, the student will perform this skill with _____% accuracy in a total of _____ minutes. *(Your instructor will tell you what the percentage and time limits will be before you begin practicing.)*

KEY: 4 = Satisfactory   0 = Unsatisfactory   NA = This step is not counted

PROCEDURE STEPS	SELF	PARTNER	INSTRUCTOR
1. Wash your hands. Put on personal protective equipment.	☐	☐	☐
2. Assemble the equipment and supplies.	☐	☐	☐
3. Greet and identify the patient. Explain the procedure. Ask for and answer any questions.	☐	☐	☐
4. Explain any dietary, medication, or other restrictions necessary for the collection. Instruct patient to defecate into a disposable plastic container or onto plastic wrap placed over the toilet bowl.	☐	☐	☐
5. When obtaining a stool specimen for C&S or ova and parasites, the patient should collect a small amount of the first and last portion of the stool after the bowel movement with the wooden spatula or tongue blade and place it in the specimen container without contaminating the outside of the container. Fill Para-Pak until fluid reaches "fill" line.	☐	☐	☐
6. Handle the specimen container according to standard precautions. Cap the container immediately and put it into the biohazard bag for transport to the laboratory. Fill out a laboratory requisition slip to accompany the specimen.	☐	☐	☐
7. Label the specimen with the patient's name, the date and time of collection, and the origin of specimen.	☐	☐	☐
8. Transport the specimen to the laboratory or store the specimen as directed. Refer to Laboratory Procedure Manual since some samples require refrigeration; others are kept at room temperature, and some must be placed in an incubator at a laboratory as soon as possible after collecting.	☐	☐	☐
9. Properly dispose of the equipment and supplies in a biohazard waste container. Remove personal protective equipment and wash your hands.	☐	☐	☐
10. Document the procedure.	☐	☐	☐
11. Sanitize the work area.	☐	☐	☐

CALCULATION

Total Possible Points: _____

Total Points Earned: _____ Multiplied by 100 = _____ Divided by Total Possible Points = _____%

Pass   **Fail**

☐   ☐   Comments:

Student signature _____ Date _____

Partner signature _____ Date _____

Instructor signature _____ Date _____

Name _____ Date _____ Time _____

Procedure 44-6:	**COLLECTING BLOOD FOR CULTURE**

EQUIPMENT/SUPPLIES: Specimen container depends on testing site (yellow-top sodium polyanethol sulfonate Vacutainer tubes or aerobic and anaerobic blood culture bottles), blood culture skin prep packs (or 70% isopropyl alcohol wipes and povidone-iodine solution swabs or towelettes), venipuncture supplies (see Chapter 41), personal protective equipment, hand sanitizer, surface sanitizer

STANDARDS: Given the needed equipment and a place to work, the student will perform this skill with _____% accuracy in a total of _____ minutes. *(Your instructor will tell you what the percentage and time limits will be before you begin practicing.)*

KEY: 4 = Satisfactory   0 = Unsatisfactory   NA = This step is not counted

PROCEDURE STEPS	SELF	PARTNER	INSTRUCTOR
1. Wash your hands. Put on personal protective equipment.	☐	☐	☐
2. Assemble the equipment and supplies.	☐	☐	☐
3. Greet and identify the patient. Explain the procedure. Ask for and answer any questions.	☐	☐	☐
4. Verify that the patient has not initiated antibiotic therapy. If therapy has started, document antibiotic, strength, dose, duration, and time of last dose.	☐	☐	☐
5. Using skin preparation kits or supplies, apply alcohol to venipuncture site and allow to air dry. Apply povidone-iodine prep in progressively increasing concentric circles without wiping back over skin that is already prepped. Let stand at least one minute and allow to air dry. Do not touch skin following preparation.	☐	☐	☐
6. Wipe bottle stoppers with povidone-iodine solution.	☐	☐	☐
7. Perform venipuncture.	☐	☐	☐
8. Fill bottles or tube according to specific laboratory procedure. Invert each 8–10 times as soon as collected. If using culture bottles, fill the aerobic bottle first.	☐	☐	☐
9. Complete venipuncture. Use an isopropyl alcohol wipe to remove residual povidone-iodine from skin. Label the specimen with the patient's name, the date and time of collection, and the origin of specimen.	☐	☐	☐
10. Repeat steps 5–9 at a second venipuncture site within 30 minutes of the first collection.	☐	☐	☐
11. Label the specimens with the patient's name and the date and time of collection.	☐	☐	☐
12. Properly dispose of the equipment and supplies in a biohazard waste container. Remove personal protective equipment and wash your hands.	☐	☐	☐
13. Document the procedure.	☐	☐	☐
14. Sanitize the work area.	☐	☐	☐

CALCULATION

Total Possible Points: _____
Total Points Earned: _____ Multiplied by 100 = _____ Divided by Total Possible Points = _____%

Pass   **Fail**
☐   ☐   Comments:

Student signature _____ Date _____
Partner signature _____ Date _____
Instructor signature _____ Date _____

Name _____ Date _____ Time _____

Procedure 44-7:	COLLECTING GENITAL SPECIMENS FOR CULTURE

EQUIPMENT/SUPPLIES: Specimen container depends on testing requested (bacterial, viral, and Chlamydia specimens require different media), personal protective equipment, hand sanitizer, surface sanitizer

STANDARDS: Given the needed equipment and a place to work, the student will perform this skill with _____% accuracy in a total of _____ minutes. *(Your instructor will tell you what the percentage and time limits will be before you begin practicing.)*

KEY: 4 = Satisfactory   0 = Unsatisfactory   NA = This step is not counted

PROCEDURE STEPS	SELF	PARTNER	INSTRUCTOR
1. Wash your hands. Put on personal protective equipment.	☐	☐	☐
2. Assemble the equipment and supplies, checking expiration dates.	☐	☐	☐
3. Your role will be to assist the physician in the collection and handling of these specimens. Be sure to verbally verify patient identification.	☐	☐	☐
4. Accept specimens from the physician securing them in the appropriate medium; follow the instructions for that particular medium.	☐	☐	☐
5. Label the specimen with the patient's name, the date and time of collection, and the origin of specimen.	☐	☐	☐
6. Repeat steps 4–5 for each specimen.	☐	☐	☐
7. Store specimens per procedure instructions until transport. Transport to testing facility as soon as possible.	☐	☐	☐
8. Properly dispose of the equipment and supplies in a biohazard waste container. Remove personal protective equipment and wash your hands.	☐	☐	☐
9. Document the procedure.	☐	☐	☐
10. Sanitize the work area.	☐	☐	☐

CALCULATION

Total Possible Points: _____
Total Points Earned: _____ Multiplied by 100 = _____ Divided by Total Possible Points = _____%

Pass   **Fail**
☐   ☐   Comments:

Student signature _____ Date _____
Partner signature _____ Date _____
Instructor signature _____ Date _____

Name_____ Date_____ Time_____

Procedure 44-8:	PREPARING A SMEAR FOR MICROSCOPIC EVALUATION

EQUIPMENT/SUPPLIES: Specimen, Bunsen burner, slide forceps, slide, sterile swab or inoculating loop, pencil or diamond-tipped pen, personal protective equipment, hand sanitizer, surface sanitizer, and contaminated waste container

STANDARDS: Given the needed equipment and a place to work, the student will perform this skill with _____% accuracy in a total of _____ minutes. *(Your instructor will tell you what the percentage and time limits will be before you begin practicing.)*

KEY: 4 = Satisfactory   0 = Unsatisfactory   NA = This step is not counted

PROCEDURE STEPS	SELF	PARTNER	INSTRUCTOR
1. Wash your hands. Put on personal protective equipment.	☐	☐	☐
2. Assemble the equipment and supplies, checking expiration dates.	☐	☐	☐
3. Label the slide with the patient's name and the date on the frosted edge with a pencil.	☐	☐	☐
4. Hold the edges of the slide between the thumb and index finger. Starting at the right side of the slide and using a rolling motion of the swab or a sweeping motion of the inoculating loop, gently and evenly spread the material from the specimen over the slide. The material should thinly fill the center of the slide within half an inch of each end.	☐	☐	☐
5. Do not rub the material vigorously over the slide.	☐	☐	☐
6. Dispose of the contaminated swab or inoculating loop in a biohazard container. If you are not using a disposable loop, sterilize it as follows: **a.** Hold the loop in the colorless part of the flame of the Bunsen burner for 10 seconds. **b.** Raise the loop slowly (to avoid splattering the bacteria) to the blue part of the flame until the loop and its connecting wire glow red. **c.** Cool it so the heat will not kill the bacteria that must be allowed to grow. Do not wave the loop in the air because doing so may expose it to contamination. Do not stab the medium with a hot loop to cool; this creates an aerosol.	☐	☐	☐
7. Allow the smear to air dry in a flat position for at least half an hour. Do not blow on the slide or wave it about in the air. Heat should not be applied until the specimen has been allowed to dry. Some specimens (e.g., Pap smear) require a fixative spray.	☐	☐	☐
8. Hold the dried smear slide with the slide forceps. Pass the slide quickly through the flame of a Bunsen burner three or four times. The slide has been fixed properly when the back of the slide feels slightly uncomfortably warm to the back of the gloved hand. It should not feel hot.	☐	☐	☐
9. Properly dispose of the equipment and supplies in a biohazard waste container. Remove personal protective equipment and wash your hands.	☐	☐	☐
10. Document the procedure.	☐	☐	☐
11. Sanitize the work area.	☐	☐	☐

CALCULATION

Total Possible Points: _____

Total Points Earned: _____ Multiplied by 100 = _____ Divided by Total Possible Points = _____%

Pass   **Fail**

☐   ☐   Comments:

Student signature _____ Date _____
Partner signature _____ Date _____
Instructor signature _____ Date _____

Name_____ Date _____ Time _____

Procedure 44-9:	PERFORMING A GRAM STAIN

EQUIPMENT/SUPPLIES: Crystal violet stain, staining rack, Gram iodine solution, wash bottle with distilled water, alcohol-acetone solution, counterstain (e.g., Safranin), absorbent (bibulous) paper pad, specimen smear on glass slide labeled with a pencil or diamond-tipped pen (as prepared in Procedure 44-7), Bunsen burner, slide forceps, stopwatch or timer, personal protective equipment, hand sanitizer, surface sanitizer, and contaminated waste container

STANDARDS: Given the needed equipment and a place to work, the student will perform this skill with _____% accuracy in a total of _____ minutes. *(Your instructor will tell you what the percentage and time limits will be before you begin practicing.)*

KEY: 4 = Satisfactory   0 = Unsatisfactory   NA = This step is not counted

PROCEDURE STEPS	SELF	PARTNER	INSTRUCTOR
1. Wash your hands. Put on personal protective equipment.	☐	☐	☐
2. Assemble the equipment and supplies, checking expiration dates.	☐	☐	☐
3. Make sure the specimen is heat-fixed to the labeled slide and the slide is room temperature (see Procedure 44-7).	☐	☐	☐
4. Place the slide on the staining rack with the smear side up.	☐	☐	☐
5. Flood the smear with crystal violet. Time for 60 seconds.	☐	☐	☐

6. Hold the slide with slide forceps.
   a. Tilt the slide to an angle of about 45 degrees to drain the excess dye.
   b. Rinse the slide with distilled water for about 5 seconds and drain off excess water.
	☐	☐	☐

7. Replace the slide on the slide rack. Flood the slide with Gram iodine solution for 60 seconds.	☐	☐	☐
8. Using the forceps, tilt the slide at a 45-degree angle to drain iodine solution. With the slide tilted, rinse the slide with distilled water from the wash bottle for about 5 to 10 seconds. Slowly and gently wash with the alcohol-acetone solution until no more stain runs off.	☐	☐	☐
9. Immediately rinse the slide with distilled water for 5 seconds and return the slide to the rack.	☐	☐	☐
10. Flood with Safranin or suitable counterstain for 60 seconds.	☐	☐	☐
11. Drain the excess counterstain from the slide by tilting it at a 45-degree angle. Rinse the slide with distilled water for 5 seconds to remove the counterstain. Gently blot the smear dry with bibulous paper. Take care not to disturb the smeared specimen. Wipe the back of the slide clear of any solution. It may be placed between the pages of a bibulous paper pad and gently pressed to remove excess moisture.	☐	☐	☐
12. Properly dispose of the equipment and supplies in a biohazard waste container. Remove personal protective equipment and wash your hands.	☐	☐	☐
13. Document the procedure.	☐	☐	☐
14. Sanitize the work area.	☐	☐	☐

CALCULATION

Total Possible Points: _____

Total Points Earned: _____ Multiplied by 100 = _____ Divided by Total Possible Points = _____%

Pass   **Fail**

☐   ☐

Comments:

Student signature _____ Date _____

Partner signature _____ Date _____

Instructor signature _____ Date _____

Name _____   Date _____   Time _____

Procedure 44-10:   INOCULATING A CULTURE

EQUIPMENT/SUPPLIES: Specimen on a swab or loop, china marker or permanent laboratory marker, sterile or disposable loop, Bunsen burner, labeled Petri dish of culture medium (the patient's name should be on the side of the plate containing the medium, because it is always placed upward to prevent condensation from dripping onto the culture), personal protective equipment, hand sanitizer, surface sanitizer, and contaminated waste container

STANDARDS: Given the needed equipment and a place to work, the student will perform this skill with _____% accuracy in a total of _____ minutes. *(Your instructor will tell you what the percentage and time limits will be before you begin practicing.)*

KEY: 4 = Satisfactory   0 = Unsatisfactory   NA = This step is not counted

PROCEDURE STEPS	SELF	PARTNER	INSTRUCTOR
1. Wash your hands. Put on personal protective equipment.	☐	☐	☐
2. Assemble the equipment and supplies, checking expiration dates.	☐	☐	☐
3. Label the medium side of the plate with the patient's name, identification number, source of specimen, time collected, time inoculated, your initials, and date.	☐	☐	☐
4. Remove the Petri plate from the cover (the Petri plate is always stored with the cover down), and place the cover on the work surface with the opening up. Do not open the cover unnecessarily.	☐	☐	☐
5. Using a rolling and sliding motion, streak the specimen swab clear across half of the plate, starting at the top and working to the center. Dispose of the swab in a biohazard container.	☐	☐	☐
6. Use a disposable loop or sterilize the loop as described in step 6 of Procedure 44-8.	☐	☐	☐
7. Turn the plate a quarter turn from its previous position. Pass the loop a few times in the original inoculum then across the medium approximately a quarter of the surface of the plate. Do not enter the originally streaked area after the first few sweeps.	☐	☐	☐
8. Turn the plate another quarter turn so that now it is 180 degrees to the original smear. Working in the previous manner, draw the loop at right angles through the most recently streaked area. Again, do not enter the originally streaked area after the first few sweeps. *FOR QUANTITATIVE CULTURES:* **a.** Streak the plate with the specimen from side to side across the middle. **b.** Streak the entire plate back and forth across the initial inoculate. This allows bacteria to grow in a way that colonies can be counted.	☐	☐	☐
9. Properly dispose of the equipment and supplies in a biohazard waste container. Remove personal protective equipment and wash your hands.	☐	☐	☐
10. Document the procedure.	☐	☐	☐
11. Sanitize the work area.	☐	☐	☐

CALCULATION

Total Possible Points: _____
Total Points Earned: _____ Multiplied by 100 = _____ Divided by Total Possible Points = _____%

Pass   **Fail**
☐   ☐   Comments:

Student signature _____ Date _____
Partner signature _____ Date _____
Instructor signature _____ Date _____

Name _____ Date _____ Time _____

Procedure 44-11:	TESTING STOOL SPECIMEN FOR OCCULT BLOOD – GUAIAC METHOD

EQUIPMENT/SUPPLIES: Gloves, patient's labeled specimen pack, developer or reagent drops, personal protective equipment, hand sanitizer, surface sanitizer, and contaminated waste container

STANDARDS: Given the needed equipment and a place to work, the student will perform this skill with _____% accuracy in a total of _____ minutes. *(Your instructor will tell you what the percentage and time limits will be before you begin practicing.)*

KEY: 4 = Satisfactory   0 = Unsatisfactory   NA = This step is not counted

PROCEDURE STEPS	SELF	PARTNER	INSTRUCTOR
1. Wash your hands. Put on personal protective equipment.	☐	☐	☐
2. Assemble the equipment and supplies, checking expiration dates.	☐	☐	☐
3. Verify patient identification on the patient's prepared test pack.	☐	☐	☐
4. Open the test window on the back of the pack and apply 1 drop of the developer or testing reagent to each window according to manufacturer's directions. Read the color change within the specified time, usually 60 seconds.	☐	☐	☐
5. Apply 1 drop of developer as directed on the control monitor section or window of the pack. Note whether the quality control results are positive or negative as appropriate. If results are acceptable, patient results may be reported. If results are not acceptable, notify physician.	☐	☐	☐
6. Properly dispose of the test pack and gloves. Wash your hands.	☐	☐	☐
7. Document the procedure.	☐	☐	☐
8. Sanitize the work area.	☐	☐	☐

CALCULATION

Total Possible Points: _____
Total Points Earned: _____ Multiplied by 100 = _____ Divided by Total Possible Points = _____%

Pass   **Fail**
☐   ☐   Comments:

Student signature _____ Date _____
Partner signature _____ Date _____
Instructor signature _____ Date _____

Name _____ Date _____ Time _____

Procedure 44-12:	MONONUCLEOSIS TESTING

EQUIPMENT/SUPPLIES: Patient's labeled specimen (whole blood, plasma, or serum, depending on the kit), CLIA-waived mononucleosis kit (slide or test strip), stopwatch or timer, personal protective equipment, hand sanitizer, surface sanitizer, and contaminated waste container

STANDARDS: Given the needed equipment and a place to work, the student will perform this skill with _____% accuracy in a total of _____ minutes. *(Your instructor will tell you what the percentage and time limits will be before you begin practicing.)*

KEY: 4 = Satisfactory   0 = Unsatisfactory   NA = This step is not counted

PROCEDURE STEPS	SELF	PARTNER	INSTRUCTOR
1. Wash your hands. Put on personal protective equipment.	☐	☐	☐
2. Assemble the equipment and supplies, checking expiration dates.	☐	☐	☐
3. Verify that the names on the specimen container and the laboratory form are the same.	☐	☐	☐
4. Ensure that the materials in the kit and the patient specimen are at room temperature.	☐	☐	☐
5. Label the test pack or test strip (depending on type of kit) with the patient's name, positive control, and negative control. Use one test pack or strip per patient and control.	☐	☐	☐
6. Aspirate the patient's specimen using the transfer pipette and place volume indicated in kit package insert on the sample well of the test pack or dip test strip labeled with the patient's name.	☐	☐	☐
7. Sample the positive and negative controls as directed in step 6.	☐	☐	☐
8. Set timer for incubation period indicated in package insert.	☐	☐	☐
9. Read reaction results at the end of incubation period.	☐	☐	☐
10. Verify the results of the controls before documenting the patient's results. Log controls and patient information on the worksheet.	☐	☐	☐
11. Properly dispose of the equipment and supplies in a biohazard waste container.	☐	☐	☐
12. Remove personal protective equipment and wash your hands.	☐	☐	☐
13. Document the procedure.	☐	☐	☐
14. Sanitize the work area.	☐	☐	☐

CALCULATION

Total Possible Points: _____
Total Points Earned: _____ Multiplied by 100 = _____ Divided by Total Possible Points = _____%

Pass **Fail**
☐   ☐   Comments:

Student signature _____ Date _____
Partner signature _____ Date _____
Instructor signature _____ Date _____

Name_____   Date _____   Time _____

Procedure 44-13:	HCG PREGNANCY TEST

EQUIPMENT/SUPPLIES: Patient's labeled specimen (plasma, serum, or urine depending on the kit), HCG pregnancy kit (test pack and transfer pipettes or test strip; kit contents will vary by manufacturer), HCG positive and negative control (different controls may be needed when testing urine), timer, personal protective equipment, hand sanitizer, surface sanitizer, and contaminated waste container

STANDARDS: Given the needed equipment and a place to work, the student will perform this skill with _____% accuracy in a total of _____ minutes. *(Your instructor will tell you what the percentage and time limits will be before you begin practicing.)*

KEY: 4 = Satisfactory   0 = Unsatisfactory   NA = This step is not counted

PROCEDURE STEPS	SELF	PARTNER	INSTRUCTOR
1. Wash your hands. Put on personal protective equipment.	☐	☐	☐
2. Assemble the equipment and supplies, checking expiration dates.	☐	☐	☐
3. Verify that the names on the specimen container and the laboratory form are the same.	☐	☐	☐
4. Ensure that the materials in the kit and the patient specimen are at room temperature. Note in the patient's information and in the control log whether you are using urine, plasma, or serum.	☐	☐	☐
5. Label the test pack or test strip (depending on type of kit) with the patient's name, positive control, and negative control. Use one test pack or strip per patient and control.	☐	☐	☐
6. Aspirate the patient's specimen using the transfer pipette and place volume indicated in kit package insert on the sample well of the test pack or dip test strip labeled with the patient's name.	☐	☐	☐
7. Sample the positive and negative controls as directed in step 6.	☐	☐	☐
8. Set timer for incubation period indicated in package insert.	☐	☐	☐
9. Read reaction results at the end of incubation period.	☐	☐	☐
10. Verify the results of the controls before documenting the patient's results. Log controls and patient information on the worksheet.	☐	☐	☐
11. Properly dispose of the equipment and supplies in a biohazard waste container.	☐	☐	☐
12. Remove personal protective equipment and wash your hands.	☐	☐	☐
13. Document the procedure.	☐	☐	☐
14. Sanitize the work area.	☐	☐	☐

CALCULATION

Total Possible Points: _____
Total Points Earned: _____ Multiplied by 100 = _____ Divided by Total Possible Points = _____%

Pass   **Fail**
☐   ☐   Comments:

Student signature _____ Date _____
Partner signature _____ Date _____
Instructor signature _____ Date _____

Name _____ Date _____ Time _____

Procedure 44-14:	**RAPID GROUP A STREP TESTING**

EQUIPMENT/SUPPLIES: Patient's labeled throat specimen, group A strep kit (controls may be included, depending on the kit), timer, personal protective equipment, hand sanitizer, surface sanitizer, and contaminated waste container

STANDARDS: Given the needed equipment and a place to work, the student will perform this skill with _____% accuracy in a total of _____ minutes. *(Your instructor will tell you what the percentage and time limits will be before you begin practicing.)*

KEY: 4 = Satisfactory   0 = Unsatisfactory   NA = This step is not counted

PROCEDURE STEPS	SELF	PARTNER	INSTRUCTOR
1. Wash your hands. Put on personal protective equipment.	☐	☐	☐
2. Assemble the equipment and supplies, checking expiration dates.	☐	☐	☐
3. Verify that the names on the specimen container and the laboratory form are the same.	☐	☐	☐
4. Label one extraction tube with the patient's name, one for the positive control, and one for the negative control.	☐	☐	☐
5. Follow the directions for the kit. Add the appropriate reagents and drops to each of the extraction tubes. Avoid splashing, and use the correct number of drops.	☐	☐	☐
6. Insert the patient's swab into the labeled extraction tube.	☐	☐	☐
7. Add the appropriate controls to each of the labeled extraction tubes.	☐	☐	☐
8. Set the timer for the appropriate time to ensure accuracy.	☐	☐	☐
9. Add the appropriate reagent and drops to each of the extraction tubes.	☐	☐	☐
10. Use the swab to mix the reagents. Then press out any excess fluid on the swab against the inside of the tube.	☐	☐	☐
11. Add three drops from the well-mixed extraction tube to the sample window of the strep A test unit or dip the test stick labeled with the patient's name. Do the same for each control.	☐	☐	☐
12. Set the timer for the time indicated in the kit package insert.	☐	☐	☐
13. A positive result appears as a line in the result window within 5 minutes. The strep A test unit or strip has an internal control; if a line appears in the control window, the test is valid.	☐	☐	☐
14. Read a negative result at exactly 5 minutes to avoid a false negative.	☐	☐	☐
15. Verify results of the controls before recording or reporting test results. Log the controls and the patient's information on the worksheet.	☐	☐	☐
16. Properly dispose of the equipment and supplies in a biohazard waste container.	☐	☐	☐
17. Remove personal protective equipment and wash your hands.	☐	☐	☐
18. Document the procedure.	☐	☐	☐
19. Sanitize the work area.	☐	☐	☐

CALCULATION

Total Possible Points: _____
Total Points Earned: _____ Multiplied by 100 = _____ Divided by Total Possible Points = _____%

Pass **Fail**
☐   ☐   Comments:

Student signature _____ Date _____
Partner signature _____ Date _____
Instructor signature _____ Date _____

Work Product 1

Perform immunological testing.

Collect a urine sample and perform HCG pregnancy testing with the appropriate kit. If you are currently working in a medical office, use a blank paper patient chart from the office. If this is not available to you, use the space below to record the procedure and results in the chart.

_____

_____

_____

_____

_____

Work Product 2

Perform microbiology testing.

Collect throat and nasopharyngeal specimens from a patient. Prepare a smear and perform a Gram stain on the sample. If you are currently working in a medical office, use a blank paper patient chart from the office. If this is not available to you, use the space below to record the procedure and results in the chart.

_____

_____

_____

_____

_____

Work Product 3

Document appropriately.

Jackie Evans is a 17-year-old patient complaining of extreme fatigue and sore throat. The physician, Dr. Weeks, directs you to collect a blood sample and perform mononucleosis testing using a whole blood kit. You perform the test, and the results are negative. Following negative results, Dr. Weeks directs you to collect throat specimens. You prepare a smear with a Gram stain and inoculate a culture according to his instructions. If you are currently working in a medical office, use a blank paper patient chart from the office. If this is not available to you, use the space below to record the procedures and results in the chart.

_____

_____

_____

_____

_____

Work Product 4

Use methods of quality control.

Run the immunology or microbiological test of your choice. When performing the test, be sure to sample positive and negative controls to verify that the test is working properly. Next, verify the results of the controls before documenting the patient's results. Log controls and patient information in the space below and attach this sheet to any necessary documents or test results.

If you are currently working in a medical office, use a blank paper patient chart from the office. If this is not available to you, use the space below to record the procedure and results in the chart.

_____

_____

_____

_____

_____

Chapter Self-Assessment Quiz

1. A pregnancy test detects the presence of:

   a. RhoGAM.

   b. protein.

   c. genetic defects.

   d. HCG.

   e. Immune-D serum.

2. When testing anaerobic bacteria, you must add:

   a. a tablet that generates carbon dioxide.

   b. a tablet that produces oxygen.

   c. a stain to colorize the bacteria.

   d. a paper disk with antibiotic.

   e. reagents or other chemicals.

3. Which of the following is caused by diplococci bacteria?

   a. Scarlet fever

   b. Rheumatic fever

   c. Skin infections

   d. Sore throat

   e. Meningitis

4. Which microorganism is not susceptible to antibiotics?

   a. Bacteria

   b. Fungi

   c. Viruses

   d. Protozoa

   e. Metazoa

5. Sensitivity tests monitor the microorganism's sensitivity to:

   a. RhoGAM.

   b. antibiotics.

   c. light.

   d. color.

   e. other microorganisms.

6. Bacilli can be recognized by their:

   a. globular shape.

   b. long, spiral shape.

   c. rigid, spiral shape.

   d. comma-like shape.

   e. rod-like shape.

7. Why are there certain foods that a patient may not ingest before a fecal occult blood test is run?

   a. They change the chemical balance in the sample.

   b. They may irritate the patient's digestive tract.

   c. They could interfere with some of the reagents.

   d. They do not provide enough nutrients to the patient.

   e. They might cause allergic reactions with the test.

8. A test that tests highly sensitive will have:
   a. no remaining organisms.
   b. few remaining organisms.
   c. no new growth of organisms.
   d. slight increase of organisms.
   e. highly increased number of organisms.

9. Which of the following is a characteristic of protozoa?
   a. Not susceptible to antibiotics
   b. Can survive anywhere in the human body
   c. Resemble plants, but can be microscopic
   d. Unicellular parasitic animals
   e. Unicellular simple organisms

10. Antigens are:
    a. proteins the body creates as a defensive measure against foreign substances.
    b. foreign substances that cause the body to initiate a defense response.
    c. reagents used to detect the presence of antibodies in a culture dish.
    d. media used to create an environment suitable for organism growth.
    e. dyes used to stain cells that are prepared for microscope slides.

Scenario: A woman has brought her young son in because he has abdominal cramps, a slight fever, and diarrhea. She mentioned that he has been playing outside for long periods of time for the last few days, and she believes he contracted something from the snake he caught in the woods near their home.

11. The physician checks the boy and thinks he has a case of salmonellosis. Looking under the microscope, the rod-like structures you see confirm that he has picked up:
    a. cocci bacteria.
    b. bacilli bacteria.
    c. a virus.
    d. a protozoan.
    e. a metazoan.

12. Because you know the boy likes to explore the woods, which of the following diseases should you also warn the boy's mother about?
    a. Meningitis
    b. Lyme disease
    c. Athlete's foot
    d. AIDS
    e. Malaria

End Scenario

13. Microbiological inoculation is the:
    a. injection of dead viral strands to create immunity.
    b. introduction of antigens to a body's immune system.
    c. introduction of microorganisms into a culture medium.
    d. introduction of antibodies into a culture medium.
    e. injection of a stain into a microorganism culture.

14. Which of the following is a factor that some bacteria do *not* require for growth?
    a. Darkness
    b. Oxygen
    c. Moisture
    d. Nutrients
    e. Warmth

15. Which of the following allows you to run a test without interference from other substances in the culture?
    a. Blood agar
    b. Serum contents
    c. Counterstain
    d. Specificity
    e. Sensitivity

16. Which is the best time to run a test on a specimen sample?
    a. As quickly as possible
    b. One to two hours after collection
    c. One day after collection
    d. One week after collection
    e. One month after collection

17. Which of the following can lead to a false reading on a test?
    a. Bacteria that need counterstain instead of Gram stain
    b. Kits that were stored in the refrigerator
    c. Culture dishes placed into the incubator
    d. Rh positive blood specimens being tested
    e. A kit previously opened and then resealed

18. You store blood at cool temperatures to:
    a. speed coagulation rate.
    b. slow coagulation rate.
    c. slow physical and chemical changes.
    d. allow specimen to separate into components.
    e. enable reagents to mix with the specimen.

19. What is always the first step in a specimen collection procedure?

   a. Wash your hands.

   b. Assemble materials.

   c. Greet the patient.

   d. Put on personal protective equipment.

   e. Sterilize collection location.

20. Tests using antigen-antibody reactions are:

   a. specific and sensitive.

   b. rarely used because of their cost.

   c. not very reliable.

   d. performed only in hospitals.

   e. susceptible to interference from other substances.

Clinical Chemistry

☐ Read textbook chapter and take notes within the Chapter Notes outline. Answer the Learning Objectives as you reach them in the content, and then check them off.

☐ Work the Content Review questions—both Foundational Knowledge and Application.

☐ Perform the Active Learning exercise(s).

☐ Complete Professional Journal entries.

☐ Complete Skill Practice Activity(s) using Competency Evaluation Forms and Work Products, when appropriate.

☐ Take the Chapter Self-Assessment Quiz.

☐ Insert all appropriate pages into your Portfolio.

1. Spell and define the key terms.
2. List the common electrolytes and explain the relationship of electrolytes to acid-base balance.
3. Describe the nonprotein nitrogenous compounds and name conditions with abnormal values.
4. List and describe the substances commonly tested in liver function assessment.
5. Explain thyroid function and the hormone that regulates the thyroid gland.
6. Describe how an assessment for a myocardial infarction is made with laboratory tests.
7. Describe how pancreatitis is diagnosed with laboratory tests.
8. Describe glucose use and regulation and the purpose of the various glucose tests.
9. Describe the function of cholesterol and other lipids and their correlation to heart disease.

Note: Bold-faced headings are the major headings in the text chapter; headings in regular font are lower-level headings (i.e., the content is subordinate to, or falls "under," the major headings). Make sure you understand the key terms used in the chapter, as well as the concepts presented as Key Points.

TEXT SUBHEADINGS	NOTES

Introduction _____

Key Points:
- Clinical chemistry entails testing for many of the chemical components found in serum, plasma, whole blood, and other body fluids (fluids that accumulate in the body's compartments). The chemical components can be electrically charged atoms called ions (K^+, Na^+, Cl^-), metabolic by-products (urea, creatinine), proteins (albumin, globulin), or hormones (e.g., testosterone and thyroid-stimulating hormone [TSH]). Quantifying the amount of these chemicals can help the physician:
  - Assess organ function (e.g., bilirubin level is an indicator of liver function).
  - Gain a better understanding of the patient's overall health status (e.g., glucose and cholesterol levels can aid in assessing a patient's health).
- Many chemistry tests are grouped according to body system. These are called panels or profiles and are described in Chapter 39.

☐ **LEARNING OBJECTIVE 1:** Spell and define the key terms.

Renal Function _____

Key Point:
- To assess renal function, the physician may order tests for serum measurements of electrolytes, blood urea nitrogen (BUN), creatinine, and other components. These tests, combined with information from urinalysis, can significantly aid in renal assessment.

Electrolytes _____

Key Terms: electrolyte; ion; cation; anion; bicarbonate
Key Points:
- **Electrolytes** are **ions** (chemicals that carry an electrical charge) in blood and body fluids. They may be positively charged (**cations**) or negatively charged (**anions**). Electrolytes conduct electrical impulses across cell membranes to maintain fluid and acid-base balance, aid in the functioning of nerve cells and muscle tissue, and are activators in the blood coagulation process.
- Electrolytes include sodium, potassium, chloride, **bicarbonate** (dissolved carbon dioxide), calcium, magnesium, and phosphorus.

Sodium _____

Key Term: extracellular
Key Point:
- Sodium (chemical symbol Na) is the major cation of the **extracellular** fluid (the fluid outside the cell). Normal serum levels range from 135 to 145 mmol/L. The sodium level depends on intake and output of water and the kidney's ability to regulate the sodium level.

Potassium _____

Key Term: intracellular
Key Point:
- Potassium (chemical symbol K) is the major cation of the **intracellular** fluid (fluid within the cell). Potassium concentration is 20 times greater inside the cell than outside, so, serum levels are much lower than those of sodium: 3.4 to 5.0 mmol/L (Table 45-2). Potassium's major function in the body is with contraction of skeletal and cardiac muscles.

Chloride _____

Key Point:
- Chloride (chemical symbol Cl) is the major anion of the extracellular fluid. The normal range for chloride is 98 to 107 mmol/L. Hypochloremia is a condition in which the serum chloride level is below 98 mmol/L. In hyperchloremia, the serum chloride level is above 107 mmol/L.

Bicarbonate _____

Key Term: bicarbonate
Key Point:
- **Bicarbonate** (chemical symbol HCO_3) is formed when carbon dioxide dissolves in the bloodstream, forming another negatively charged ion in the extracellular fluid. Bicarbonate is the major factor in acid-base balance; increased levels result in alkalosis (the body pH is too basic), and decreased levels may result in acidosis (the body pH is too acidic). Normal venous carbon dioxide levels are 22 to 29 mmol/L.

Magnesium

Key Point:
• Magnesium (chemical symbol Mg) is a cation found in intracellular fluid. Normal magnesium levels range from 1.2 to 2.1 mEq/L. Magnesium has many significant roles in the body, especially in cardiovascular, metabolic, and neuromuscular function. Clinical use of serum magnesium levels is increasing as more information about magnesium is discovered.

Calcium

Key Point:
• Calcium (chemical symbol Ca) is a cation, with normal serum levels ranging from 8.6 to 10.0 mg/dL. Blood levels are regulated by three hormones: parathyroid hormone, vitamin D and calcitonin. Most of the body's calcium is in the bone.

Phosphorus

Key Point:
• Phosphorus (chemical symbol P), the major anion in the intracellular fluid, is the building block for the body's genetic material. Normal phosphorus levels range from 2.7 to 4.5 mg/dL. 80% of the body's phosphorus is in the bone.

☐ **LEARNING OBJECTIVE 2:** List the common electrolytes and explain the relationship of electrolytes to acid-base balance.

Nonprotein Nitrogenous Compounds

Key Point:
• Three nonprotein nitrogenous compounds that can be increased as a consequence of impaired renal function are urea, creatinine, and uric acid.

Urea

Key Point:
• Urea is the major end product of protein and amino acid metabolism. Because urea is formed in the liver and excreted mainly by the kidneys, it can be an indicator for both liver and renal function. Typically urea, measured as BUN, ranges from 7 to 18 mg/dL.

Creatinine

Key Term: creatinine
Key Points:
- **Creatinine** is a breakdown product of creatine, which aids in delivering energy to cells. Normal range for creatinine is 0.5 to 1.2 mg/dL, with normal ranges varying slightly among laboratories. Creatinine is more specific than BUN for assessing renal function.
- A test called creatinine clearance is used to evaluate the filtering ability of the kidney. A 24-hour urine sample is collected for a creatinine clearance, because excretion of creatinine varies throughout the day.
- A key point for the medical assistant to remember is that the test requires a blood specimen be drawn during the 24-hour collection.

Uric Acid

Key Point:
- Uric acid is a metabolic end product of proteins containing purine, so it is highly influenced by diet. For men, the normal range is 3.5 to 7.2 mg/dL, and for women, 2.6 to 6.0 mg/dL. Increased amounts of uric acid are more significant than decreased amounts.

☐ **LEARNING OBJECTIVE 3:** Describe the nonprotein nitrogenous compounds and name conditions with abnormal values.

Liver Function

Key Point:
- The liver is the largest gland of the body and one of the most complex. Among its major functions are the production of bile, metabolism of many compounds used by the body (glucose, fats, proteins, and vitamins), processing of bilirubin, and detoxifying substances in the blood. Alkaline phosphatase (ALP), alanine aminotransferase (ALT), and aspartate aminotransferase (AST) are some of the commonly tested enzymes that help determine liver function, in addition to the measurement of bilirubin, a component of bile.

Bilirubin

Enzymes _____

Key Point:
• Reference ranges for enzyme tests are the most sensitive to deviation among laboratories. In evaluating patient results, be sure to compare them to the reference ranges for the laboratory that performed the test.

Alkaline Phosphatase (ALP) _____

Key Point:
• ALP is present in the bones, liver, intestines, kidneys, and placenta. Circulating ALP is primarily from the liver and bone. Levels of ALP rise in bone and liver disorders. Normal values vary with age.

Alanine Aminotransferase (ALT) and Aspartate Aminotransferase (AST) _____

Key Point:
• ALT and AST are enzymes in the liver. AST is present in many other organs as well. Increased levels of ALT and AST occur with liver disorders. Approximate reference ranges are ALT 6–37 U/L and AST 5–30 U/L.

☐ **LEARNING OBJECTIVE 4:** List and describe the substances commonly tested in liver function assessment.

Thyroid Function _____

Key Point:
• The thyroid gland is controlled by another hormone, TSH, which is produced in the anterior pituitary gland. Normal thyroid function is dependent on a normally functioning hypothalamus and pituitary gland in addition to a healthy thyroid gland.

Thyroid-Stimulating Hormone _____

Key Point:
• In the absence of disease, when additional thyroid hormones are needed, more TSH is secreted to stimulate the thyroid gland. In the same manner, when lesser amounts of the hormones are required, less TSH is secreted and the thyroid gland reduces its production.

☐ **LEARNING OBJECTIVE 5:** Explain thyroid function and the hormone that regulates the thyroid gland.

Cardiac Function

Key Point:
• When a myocardial infarction occurs, the damaged heart muscle releases into the bloodstream large quantities of specific substances referred to as cardiac markers. A single marker that will quickly and accurately assess cardiac function is not available, so the markers are tested in combination with each other. We will consider the two most common markers: CK-MB and troponin.

Creatine Kinase-MB

Key Point:
• The MB fraction rises with myocardial infarction. A high total CK may indicate damage to either the heart or other muscles, but a high CK-MB suggests that the damage was to heart muscle. CK-MB results indicate heart involvement when they are ≥6% of the total CK result.

Troponin

Key Point:
• Troponin is a protein specific to heart muscle, making it a valuable marker in the diagnosis of acute myocardial infarction. Troponin blood levels begin to rise within 4 hours of the onset of myocardial damage and stay elevated for up to 14 days, which means levels can be measured to monitor the effectiveness of thrombolytic therapy in heart attack patients.

☐ **LEARNING OBJECTIVE 6:** Describe how an assessment for a myocardial infarction is made with laboratory tests.

Pancreatic Function

Key Point:
• Amylase and lipase, two of its exocrine system products, are released as excretory enzymes into the intestines to aid in digestion. Insulin and glucagon, hormonal products of its endocrine function, are released into the bloodstream to regulate carbohydrate metabolism.

Pancreatic Enzymes _____

_____

_____

Amylase and Lipase _____

_____

Key Terms: amylase; lipase
Key Point:
- **Amylase** is markedly increased with pancreatitis (inflammation of the pancreas). The salivary glands also produce amylase, which accounts for the elevated levels occurring with inflammatory diseases of the salivary glands, such as mumps. **Lipase** levels also rise with pancreatitis and stay elevated longer than amylase levels.

Pancreatic Hormones _____

_____

_____

Insulin and Glucagon _____

_____

Key Points:
- Glucose is a primary energy source for the body. When foods are metabolized, nutrients including glucose are released. For glucose to be used for stored energy in the form of glycogen, it must be brought into the cells. Two hormones, insulin and glucagon, regulate this process.
- Insulin brings the glucose used for energy into cells for immediate use or for storage.
- The hormone glucagon releases into the bloodstream glucose stored as glycogen, thereby raising glucose levels.

☐ **LEARNING OBJECTIVE 7:** Describe how pancreatitis is diagnosed with laboratory tests.

Glucose _____

_____

Key Point:
- For diagnostic usefulness, the time a blood sample is taken for glucose testing must be related to length of fasting or to the time of the previous meal.

Fasting Glucose _____

_____

Key Term: fast
Key Points:
- A fasting blood sugar (FBS) level can be obtained from the patient after an 8- to 12-hour **fast** (nothing other than water is ingested during the fast).
- A value of 100 mg/dL or above leads to a diagnosis of impaired fasting glucose, included in the term prediabetes. Prediabetes occurs when a person's glucose levels are higher than normal but not yet high enough for a diagnosis of diabetes. Studies indicate that many people in the prediabetic range go on to develop diabetes within 10 years.

Random Glucose _____

_____

Key Point:
- Although a random glucose test is not as diagnostically useful as a fasting test, it is a good screening tool. A random glucose specimen can be drawn anytime during the day.

Two-Hour Postprandial Glucose _____

_____

Key Point:
- A 2-hour postprandial glucose (PP) test is used to screen for diabetes and to monitor insulin therapy of diabetic patients. The patient must eat a high-carbohydrate meal after a 10- to 12-hour fast. Patients who may not be compliant are given a glucose solution to drink as a substitute for the meal. Then, 2 hours after the meal, a blood sample is drawn and glucose is measured. Timing of the specimen collection is extremely important for this test result.

Oral Glucose Tolerance Test _____

_____

Key Points:
- The ADA does not encourage the use of the GTT to diagnose diabetes. For those situations in which it is still used, the procedure should begin with effective patient preparation.
- The criteria proposed by the National Diabetes Data Group and the World Health Organization and endorsed by the American Diabetes Association recommend a diagnosis of diabetes if the fasting glucose level is greater than 110 mg/dL and the 2-hour measurement is equal to or above 155 mg/dL.

Glucose Tolerance Testing in Obstetric Patients _____

Key Point:
• An increase of glucose intolerance has been frequently noted among pregnant patients in the second and third trimesters. Because gestational diabetes can endanger the fetus, the pregnant patient's glucose level must be monitored.

Hemoglobin A1C _____

Key Point:
• Although blood glucose levels are used to detect and monitor diabetic patients, the test of choice for long-term blood glucose regulation is hemoglobin A1C.

☐ **LEARNING OBJECTIVE 8:** Describe glucose use and regulation and the purpose of the various glucose tests.

Lipids and Lipoproteins _____

Key Term: lipoproteins
Key Point:
• Cholesterol and associated lipids (free fatty acids) and **lipoproteins** (substances composed of lipids and proteins) have long been implicated in heart disease. However, these compounds are important building blocks of our bodies and in proper quantities are vital to health maintenance. They are a component of every cell membrane and of the myelin sheath around the nerves. They also cushion and support organs. Testing for these quantities aids the physician in assessing the risk of heart disease.

Cholesterol _____

Low-Density Lipoprotein _____

Key Point:
• Low-density lipoprotein (LDL) is a plasma protein that transports cholesterol from the liver to the walls of large- and medium-sized arteries.

High-Density Lipoprotein _____

_____

Key Point:
- High-density lipoprotein (HDL) is the protein molecule that carries cholesterol from the cell back to the liver to be excreted in bile.

Triglycerides _____

_____

Key Point:
- Triglycerides store energy. They are stored in adipose tissue and muscle and released and metabolized between meals according to the body's energy demands.

☐ **LEARNING OBJECTIVE 9:** Describe the function of cholesterol and other lipids and their correlation to heart disease.

Content Review

FOUNDATIONAL KNOWLEDGE

Electrolytes

1. Circle the extracellular electrolytes.

Potassium	Bicarbonate	Magnesium
Chloride	Sodium	Phosphorus

2. Electrolyte imbalances can cause a variety of conditions. Review the list of electrolyte imbalances below and indicate which electrolyte causes the problem. Then indicate if the abnormality is a result of the electrolyte existing in quantities too high or too low in the bloodstream.

Abnormality	Caused by an Imbalance of this Electrolyte	Too High	Too Low
a. Hyperkalemia			
b. Hyponatremia			
c. Alkalosis			
d. Hypercalcemia			
e. Hypophosphatemia			
f. Acidosis			
g. Hyperchloremia			
h. Hypermagnesemia			

3. How are anions and cations different from one another?

Anions	Cations

Nonprotein Nitrogenous Compounds

4. List and briefly describe the three nonprotein nitrogenous compounds.

a. _____

b. _____

c. _____

Liver Basics

5. What are the four substances commonly tested in liver function assessments?

a. _____

b. _____

c. _____

d. _____

6. What is a cause of decreased BUN levels?

_____

_____

7. What is bilirubin, and how can it indicate liver failure?

_____

_____

The Thyroid

8. What is TSH, and how does it function in the thyroid gland?

_____

_____

9. A 16-year-old girl comes into the office complaining of fatigue, muscle and joint pain, and slight depression. She says she's been gaining weight over the past few months as well, even though she's been exercising and has not changed her diet. Would you expect her TSH levels to be high or low? Why?

_____

_____

Heart-to-Heart

10. Why is troponin an especially valuable marker in the diagnosis of acute myocardial infarction?

_____

_____

Pancreas Problems

11. How do you diagnose pancreatitis?

_____

_____

Testing . . . Testing, One, Two

12. What is the purpose of performing a fasting blood sugar test?

_____

_____

13. When you are testing for glucose, what is the puncture site, and why is it important to wash the surrounding area?

_____

_____

14. Why should you immediately centrifuge a blood sample when performing a glucose test?

_____

_____

15. What are the two hormones that regulate the process of storing glucose as glycogen?

a. _____

b. _____

16. Why is it so important to quantify the amount of the body's chemical components?

_____

_____

Cholesterol—the Good and the Bad

17. How do cholesterol and other lipids correlate to heart disease?

_____

_____

18. Cholesterol has a bad reputation for causing heart disease. However, it's also used as a building block by the body's organs. List four substances in the body that require cholesterol for production.

a. _____

b. _____

c. _____

d. _____

19. Match the following key terms to their definitions.

Key Terms

a. amylase _____

b. anions _____

c. bicarbonate _____

d. cations _____

e. creatinine _____

f. electrolytes _____

g. extracellular _____

h. fast _____

i. intracellular _____

j. ions _____

k. lipase _____

l. lipoproteins _____

Definitions

1. outside the cell

2. the dissolved form of carbon dioxide; it combines with water to make carbonic acid, H_2CO_3.

3. excretory enzyme created in the pancreas and salivary glands to aid in digestion

4. an atom or group of atoms that has become electrically charged by the loss or gain of one or more electrons

5. positively charged ions

6. certain chemical substances dissolved in the blood and having numerous basic functions, such as conducting electrical currents

7. inside the cell

8. a substance made up of a lipid and a protein

9. negatively charged ions

10. a period of time during which a person only ingests water

11. any of several enzymes that begin the breakdown of fats in the digestive tract

12. the substance formed when creatine (an important compound in metabolic processes) is used

20. True or False? Determine whether the following statements are true or false. If false, explain why.

a. Pregnant women are more likely to develop a glucose intolerance in their second and third trimesters, which may be harmful to the fetus.

_____

_____

b. When a person has a myocardial infarction, his creatine kinase levels will significantly drop.

_____

_____

c. Cholesterol testing involves preparing a slide and cultures.

_____

_____

d. It is quicker and more efficient to do clinical chemistry work in a medical office's laboratory than to send the specimens out to a reference laboratory.

_____

_____

APPLICATION

Critical Thinking Practice

1. A patient comes in complaining of increased urination, diarrhea, and sweating. Measurements of the patient's blood levels indicate that he has slight hypernatremia, and the physician wants him to change his eating habits. What suggestions can you give to him on what kinds of foods to avoid?

_____

_____

2. A diabetic patient comes in to the physician's office after accidentally giving herself too much insulin. How can you help to bring her glucose levels back to normal?

_____

_____

Patient Education

1. A 45-year-old patient's blood tests have come back showing high levels of glucose. The physician diagnoses him with diabetes and asks that you instruct the patient on monitoring glucose levels at home. Compile an instruction sheet about diabetes and glucose testing to give the patient, and give some detail to each point.

Documentation
1. Dr. Ashanti asks you to perform a blood cholesterol test on a patient. The results are 282 mg/dL. Write a note to document this test and results in the patient's chart.

_____

_____

Active Learning

1. Many people get confused about the differences between good and bad cholesterol. Design a pamphlet for patients describing both good and bad cholesterol and the roles they play in the body. Include health tips about things patients can do to decrease low-density lipoproteins and increase high-density lipoproteins.

2. Interview three people who have diabetes. Ask them when they found out they had diabetes, how they're working to control their glucose levels, and how it has affected their lifestyle. Share what you learned with the class, and discuss how you might coach a patient recently diagnosed with diabetes.

3. Gestational diabetes can be a worry for many pregnant women. Research gestational diabetes to find out about its effects and what a patient must do if she is diagnosed with this condition. Then create a pamphlet to distribute to pregnant patients that describes the condition and the glucose test that she will take in the second trimester.

Professional Journal

REFLECT

(Prompts and Ideas: There is a tremendous amount of information about dieting and cholesterol in the media. However, at the same time, Americans eat a tremendous amount of junk food. Think about what you eat on a daily basis. Do you take cholesterol and other health factors into account when you eat?)

_____

_____

_____

_____

_____

_____

PONDER AND SOLVE

1. A new patient says there is a history of heart attacks in his family and he wants to know what he can do to prevent it. He is middle aged and slightly overweight; however, he has a healthy diet and exercises regularly. What suggestions can you give to him to help ease his worries, and what encouragement can you give him?

_____

_____

_____

_____

_____

_____

2. A 15-year-old girl's blood levels have come back with increased levels of uric acid. She has recently become a vegetarian, and she eats only salads. Her mother wants her to start eating meat again so that she can get the protein she needs. How would you address the situation without upsetting the mother or the daughter?

_____

_____

_____

_____

_____

_____

EXPERIENCE

Skills related to this chapter include:

1. Blood Glucose Testing (Procedure 45-1).
2. Blood Cholesterol Testing (Procedure 45-2).
3. Perform Routine Maintenance of a Glucose Meter (Procedure 45-3).

Record any common mistakes, lessons learned, and/or tips you discovered during your experience of practicing and demonstrating these skills:

_____

_____

_____

_____

_____

_____

_____

Skill Practice

PERFORMANCE OBJECTIVES:

1. Perform blood glucose testing (Procedure 45-1).
2. Perform blood cholesterol testing (Procedure 45-2).
3. Perform routine maintenance of a glucose meter (Procedure 45-3).

Name_____ Date _____ Time _____

Procedure 45-1:	BLOOD GLUCOSE TESTING

EQUIPMENT/SUPPLIES: Glucose meter, glucose reagent strips, control solutions, capillary puncture device, personal protective equipment, gauze, paper towel, Band-Aid, lancet, alcohol pad, hand sanitizer, surface sanitizer, contaminated waste container

NOTE: These are generic instructions for using a glucose meter. Refer to the manufacturer's instructions shipped with the meter for instructions specific for the instrument in use.

STANDARDS: Given the needed equipment and a place to work, the student will perform this skill with _____% accuracy in a total of _____ minutes. *(Your instructor will tell you what the percentage and time limits will be before you begin practicing.)*

KEY: 4 = Satisfactory   0 = Unsatisfactory   NA = This step is not counted

PROCEDURE STEPS	SELF	PARTNER	INSTRUCTOR
1. Wash your hands. Put on personal protective equipment.	☐	☐	☐
2. Assemble the equipment and supplies.	☐	☐	☐
3. Turn on the instrument, and ensure that it is calibrated.	☐	☐	☐
4. Perform the test on the quality control material. Record results. Determine whether QC is within control limits. If yes, proceed with patient testing. If no, take corrective action and recheck controls. Document corrective action. Proceed with patient testing when acceptable QC results are obtained.	☐	☐	☐
5. Remove one reagent strip, lay it on the paper towel, and recap the container.	☐	☐	☐
6. Greet and identify the patient. Explain the procedure. Ask for and answer any questions.	☐	☐	☐
7. Have the patient wash his or her hands in warm water.	☐	☐	☐
8. Cleanse the selected puncture site (finger) with alcohol.	☐	☐	☐
9. Perform a capillary puncture, following the steps described in Chapter 41, Phlebotomy. Wipe away the first drop of blood.	☐	☐	☐
10. Turn the patient's hand palm down, and gently squeeze the finger to form a large drop of blood.	☐	☐	☐

11. Bring the reagent strip up to the finger and touch the pad to the blood.
  a. Do not touch the finger.
  b. Completely cover the pad or fill the testing chamber with blood.
	☐	☐	☐

12. Insert the reagent strip into the analyzer.
  a. Meanwhile, apply pressure to the puncture wound with gauze.
  b. The meter will continue to incubate the strip and measure the reaction.
	☐	☐	☐

13. The instrument reads the reaction strip and displays the result on the screen in mg/dL.	☐	☐	☐
14. Apply a small Band-Aid to the patient's fingertip.	☐	☐	☐
15. Properly care for or dispose of equipment and supplies.	☐	☐	☐
16. Clean the work area. Remove personal protective equipment and wash your hands.	☐	☐	☐

CALCULATION

Total Possible Points: _____
Total Points Earned: _____ Multiplied by 100 = _____ Divided by Total Possible Points = _____%

Pass   **Fail**

☐   ☐   Comments:

Chart Documentation _____
Student signature _____ Date _____
Partner signature _____ Date _____
Instructor signature _____ Date _____

Name _____ Date _____ Time _____

Procedure 45-2:	BLOOD CHOLESTEROL TESTING

EQUIPMENT/SUPPLIES: Cholesterol meter and supplies or test kit, control solutions, capillary puncture equipment or blood specimen as indicated by manufacturer, personal protective equipment, hand sanitizer, surface sanitizer, contaminated waste container

NOTE: These are generic instructions for using a cholesterol meter or test kit. Refer to the manufacturer's instructions shipped with the testing tool for instructions specific for the instrument in use.

STANDARDS: Given the needed equipment and a place to work, the student will perform this skill with _____% accuracy in a total of _____ minutes. *(Your instructor will tell you what the percentage and time limits will be before you begin practicing.)*

KEY: 4 = Satisfactory   0 = Unsatisfactory   NA = This step is not counted

PROCEDURE STEPS	SELF	PARTNER	INSTRUCTOR
1. Wash your hands. Put on personal protective equipment.	☐	☐	☐
2. Assemble the equipment and supplies.	☐	☐	☐
3. Review instrument manual for your cholesterol meter or test kit.	☐	☐	☐
4. Perform the test on the quality control material. Record results. Determine whether QC is within control limits. If yes, proceed with patient testing. If no, take corrective action and recheck controls. Document corrective action. Proceed with patient testing when acceptable QC results are obtained.	☐	☐	☐
5. Obtain patient specimen per manufacturer's instructions.	☐	☐	☐
6. Perform the testing procedure following the manufacturer's instructions. Record results.	☐	☐	☐
7. Properly care for or dispose of equipment and supplies.	☐	☐	☐
8. Clean the work area. Remove personal protective equipment and wash your hands.	☐	☐	☐

CALCULATION

Total Possible Points: _____
Total Points Earned: _____ Multiplied by 100 = _____ Divided by Total Possible Points = _____%

Pass   **Fail**
☐   ☐   Comments:

Chart Documentation _____
Student signature _____ Date _____
Partner signature _____ Date _____
Instructor signature _____ Date _____

Name_____ Date_____ Time_____

Procedure 45-3:	PERFORM ROUTINE MAINTENANCE OF A GLUCOSE METER

EQUIPMENT: Glucose meter, maintenance and testing supplies, manufacturer's manual for glucose analyzer, control solutions, personal protective equipment, hand sanitizer, surface sanitizer, contaminated waste container

STANDARDS: Given the needed equipment and a place to work, the student will perform this skill with _____% accuracy in a total of _____ minutes. *(Your instructor will tell you what the percentage and time limits will be before you begin practicing.)*

KEY: 4 = Satisfactory   0 = Unsatisfactory   NA = This step is not counted

PROCEDURE STEPS	SELF	PARTNER	INSTRUCTOR
1. Wash your hands. Put on gloves.	☐	☐	☐
2. Assemble the equipment and supplies.	☐	☐	☐
3. Review the instrument manual for your glucose meter.	☐	☐	☐
4. Perform the maintenance procedures listed in the manufacturer's instructions. Document the performance of these procedures in the instrument maintenance log.	☐	☐	☐
5. Perform the test on the quality control material. Record results. Determine whether QC is within control limits. If yes, maintenance was successful and instrument is ready for patient testing. If no, take corrective action and recheck controls. Document corrective action. Instrument is available for patient testing when acceptable QC results are obtained.	☐	☐	☐
6. Properly care for or dispose of equipment and supplies.	☐	☐	☐
7. Clean the work area. Remove personal protective equipment, and wash your hands. *NOTE:* These are generic instructions for performing routine maintenance of a glucose analyzer. Refer to the manufacturer's manual for instructions specific to the particular instrument.	☐	☐	☐

CALCULATION

Total Possible Points: _____
Total Points Earned: _____ Multiplied by 100 = _____ Divided by Total Possible Points = _____%

Pass   **Fail**
☐   ☐   Comments:

Chart Documentation _____
Student signature _____ Date _____
Partner signature _____ Date _____
Instructor signature _____ Date _____

Work Product 1

Perform chemistry testing.

Collect a blood sample from a patient and perform blood glucose testing with the appropriate kit. Document the test in the patient's chart, identifying it properly as random, FBS, PP, or GTT.

If you are currently working in a medical office, use a blank paper patient chart from the office. If this is not available to you, use the space below to record the procedure in the chart.

_____

_____

_____

Work Product 2

Perform routine maintenance of clinical equipment.

Perform routine maintenance of a glucose meter in a medical office or laboratory. Review the manufacturer's instructions for routine maintenance and be sure to follow all steps. Then complete the log below to detail your maintenance on the equipment.

Instrument History Record

Model No: _____   **Instrument:** _____

Date Purchased: _____   **Serial Number:** _____

Manufacturer: _____   **Cost** _____

Telephone: _____   **State** _____ **Zip:** _____

Dealer: _____   **Contact Person** _____

Telephone: _____   **State** _____ **Zip:** _____

Warranty: _____   **Expiration Date** _____

Technical Service Representative _____

Date	Comments	Who Was Contacted	Action Taken

Chapter Self-Assessment Quiz

1. Sodium is used to maintain:
   a. electrolytes.
   b. TSH stimulation.
   c. waste materials.
   d. fluid balance.
   e. blood oxygen.

2. An enzyme is a(n):
   a. cell that speeds up the production of proteins.
   b. protein that quickens chemical reactions.
   c. chemical reaction that ionizes electrolytes.
   d. ion that has an electrical charge.
   e. specialized cell that deals with blood levels.

3. Which of the following is responsible for neuromuscular function?
   a. Sodium
   b. Potassium
   c. Chloride
   d. Bicarbonate
   e. Magnesium

4. Which of the following is formed in the liver?
   a. Urea
   b. TSH
   c. Creatinine
   d. Lipase
   e. Amylase

5. The kidneys are responsible for:
   a. releasing hormones into the bloodstream.
   b. ridding the body of waste products.
   c. producing bile and enzymes.
   d. removing worn-out red blood cells.
   e. regulating carbohydrate metabolism.

6. A patient's blood work shows her amylase levels are found to be high. What other substance should you check to test for pancreatitis?
   a. Hemoglobin
   b. Triglycerides
   c. Potassium
   d. Lipase
   e. Lipoproteins

7. Which of the following is a normal value for the enzyme AST?
   a. 1
   b. 23
   c. 34
   d. 68
   e. 89

8. The function of LDL is to:
   a. transport enzymes to the heart and lungs.
   b. assist in the production of lipoproteins.
   c. store energy in adipose tissue.
   d. move cholesterol from the liver to arteries.
   e. carry cholesterol from the cells to the liver.

9. Chloride, bicarbonate, and electrolytes are all a part of:
   a. cardiac function.
   b. liver function.
   c. renal function.
   d. pancreatic function.
   e. respiratory function.

10. In patients with renal failure, soft tissue calcification is a long-term effect of:
    a. ketoacidosis.
    b. hypokalemia.
    c. alkalosis.
    d. hypocalcemia.
    e. hyperphosphatemia.

11. The purpose of TSH is to:
    a. produce hormones in the thyroid gland.
    b. stimulate the thyroid gland.
    c. balance pH levels in the blood.
    d. provide warning of a system failure.
    e. carry cholesterol into the heart.

12. Women are screened for gestational diabetes:
    a. before they conceive.
    b. during the first month of pregnancy.
    c. during the second trimester.
    d. during the third trimester.
    e. after the baby is born.

13. When blood sugar levels go below 45 mg/dL, a person may experience:

   a. trembling.

   b. vomiting.

   c. diarrhea.

   d. chills.

   e. a high temperature.

14. Patients should fast before glucose tests to:

   a. allow glucose levels to increase.

   b. allow glucose to be processed.

   c. clear the blood of any pathogens.

   d. empty the stomach for testing.

   e. lower other substance levels.

15. A possible cause of waste product buildup in the blood is:

   a. liver failure.

   b. renal failure.

   c. pancreatitis.

   d. hypokalemia.

   e. alkalosis.

16. Alkaline phosphatase is present in the:

   a. heart.

   b. lungs.

   c. intestines.

   d. brain.

   e. muscles.

17. If you are testing for a substance only found in the blood serum, what should you do with a blood specimen?

   a. Use reagent strips to check for serum presence.

   b. Create a slide and analyze it under a microscope.

   c. Put the specimen in the centrifuge to separate.

   d. Allow the specimen a few days to sit and separate.

   e. Run tests without doing anything to the specimen.

18. The pancreas functions in the:

   a. endocrine and exocrine systems.

   b. renal and endocrine systems.

   c. pulmonary and exocrine systems.

   d. digestive and renal systems.

   e. pulmonary and vascular systems.

19. The salivary glands produce:

   a. creatinine.

   b. phosphates.

   c. glucose.

   d. lipase.

   e. amylase.

20. What is the body's normal pH range?

   a. 6.0 to 6.5

   b. 6.9 to 7.35

   c. 7.0 to 7.5

   d. 7.35 to 7.45

   e. 7.45 to 8.25

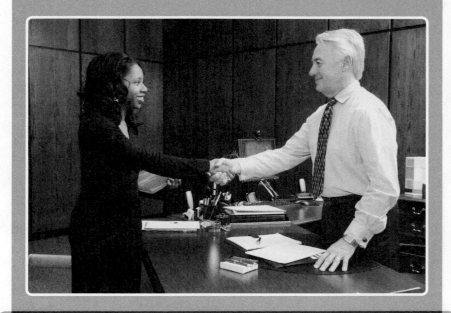

Career
Strategies

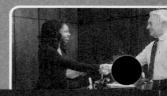

Making the Transition: Student to Employee

Chapter Checklist

- ☐ Read textbook chapter and take notes within the Chapter Notes outline. Answer the Learning Objectives as you reach them in the content, and then check them off.
- ☐ Work the Content Review questions—both Foundational Knowledge and Application.
- ☐ Perform the Active Learning exercise(s).

- ☐ Complete Professional Journal entries.
- ☐ Complete Skill Practice Activity(s) using Competency Evaluation Forms and Work Products, when appropriate.
- ☐ Take the Chapter Self-Assessment Quiz.
- ☐ Insert all appropriate pages into your Portfolio.

Learning Objectives

1. Spell and define the key terms.
2. Explain the purpose of the externship experience.
3. List your professional responsibilities during externship.
4. List personal and professional attributes necessary to ensure a successful externship.
5. Understand the importance of the evaluation process.
6. Determine your best career direction based on your skills and strengths.
7. Identify the steps necessary to apply for the right position and be able to accomplish those steps.

8. Draft an appropriate cover letter.
9. List the steps and guidelines in completing an employment application.
10. List guidelines for an effective interview that will lead to employment.
11. Identify the steps that you need to take to ensure proper career advancement.
12. Explain the process for recertification of a medical assisting credential.
13. Describe the importance of membership in a professional organization.

Chapter Notes

Note: Bold-faced headings are the major headings in the text chapter; headings in regular font are lower-level headings (i.e., the content is subordinate to, or falls "under," the major headings). Make sure you understand the key terms used in the chapter, as well as the concepts presented as Key Points.

TEXT SUBHEADINGS   **NOTES**

Introduction _____

_____

_____

☐ **LEARNING OBJECTIVE 1:** Spell and define the key terms.

_____

Externships _____

_____

Key Term: externship
Key Point:
• An **externship** is a training program that gives you the experience of working in a professional medical office under the supervision of a preceptor or supervisor who will help you to apply the theories and procedures you learned during classroom training.

☐ **LEARNING OBJECTIVE 2:** Explain the purpose of the externship experience.

_____

Types of Facilities _____

_____

Key Point:
• As a medical assisting student, you will experience an extensive scope of procedures during an externship in a general or family practice clinic or office.

Extern Sites _____

_____

Key Term: preceptor
Key Point:
• An ideal site should provide a variety of experiences, both in administrative (front office) and clinical (back office) procedures.

Externship Benefits _____

_____

_____

Benefits to the Student _____

_____

_____

Benefits to the Medical Assisting Program _____

_____

Key Point:
- Medical assisting programs also rely on the medical profession to aid in updating and revising the curriculum and course content to ensure that the methods and procedures presented to the students from year to year are current.

Benefits to the Externship Site _____

_____

_____

Externship Responsibilities _____

_____

_____

Responsibilities of the Student _____

_____

Key Points:
- You must be dependable.
- You must act in a professional manner.
- You must be well groomed and meet the program's dress code.

☐ **LEARNING OBJECTIVE 3:** List your professional responsibilities during externship.

Responsibilities of the Medical Assisting Program _____

_____

_____

Responsibilities of the Externship Site _____

_____

_____

Guidelines for a Successful Externship _____

_____

_____

_____

Procedural Performance _____

_____

_____

Key Point:
- You will be judged on your ability to measure up to the standard of care for an entry-level medical assistant.

Preparedness _____
_____
_____

Attendance _____
_____

Key Point:
- If at any time you will be late or will not be able to attend the site for any reason, you must notify both the externship coordinator and the site preceptor.

Appearance _____
_____

Key Point:
- You have only one opportunity to make a first impression.

Attitude _____
_____

Key Points:
- Much attitude is determined by how well you handle change and direction and how adaptable and flexible you are during difficult assignments.
- Your attitude determines your altitude.

☐ **LEARNING OBJECTIVE 4:** List personal and professional attributes necessary to ensure a successful externship.

Externship Documentation _____
_____

Key Point:
- Most programs use a time sheet or record of some sort to document your hours in the externship.

Externship Evaluations _____
_____
_____

Graduate Surveys _____
_____
_____

Employer Surveys _____
_____
_____

☐ **LEARNING OBJECTIVE 5:** Understand the importance of the evaluation process.

Establish the Job for You _____

_____

_____

Setting Employment Goals _____

_____

Key Points:
- The best way to set a goal and eventually get what you want is to study your strengths and weaknesses and from that self-knowledge design the best job for you.
- To win the position you want, you have to learn to sell yourself.

Self-Analysis _____

_____

_____

☐ **LEARNING OBJECTIVE 6:** Determine your best career direction based on your skills and strengths.

Finding the Right Job _____

_____

Key Term: networking
Key Point:
- Many studies show that most positions are never advertised in the media.

☐ **LEARNING OBJECTIVE 7:** Identify the steps necessary to apply for the right position and be able to accomplish those steps.

Applying for the Job _____

_____

_____

Answering Newspaper Advertisements _____

_____

_____

Preparing Your Résumé _____

_____

Key Term: résumé
Key Point:
- When you have chosen the people you want to use as references, be sure to ask their permission.

Preparing Your Cover Letter _____

_____

☐ **LEARNING OBJECTIVE 8:** Draft an appropriate cover letter.

Completing an Employment Application _____

_____

☐ **LEARNING OBJECTIVE 9:** List the steps and guidelines in completing an employment application.

The Interview _____

_____

Preparing for the Interview _____

Key Term: portfolio

Crucial Interview Questions _____

_____

Follow-Up _____

_____

☐ **LEARNING OBJECTIVE 10:** List guidelines for an effective interview that will lead to employment.

Leaving a Job _____

_____

Be a Lifelong Learner _____

_____

☐ **LEARNING OBJECTIVE 11:** Identify the steps that you need to take to ensure proper career advancement.

Recertification _____

_____

☐ **LEARNING OBJECTIVE 12:** Explain the process for recertification of a medical assisting credential.

Professionalism

☐ **LEARNING OBJECTIVE 13:** Describe the importance of membership in a professional organization.

Content Review

FOUNDATIONAL KNOWLEDGE

Externship Basics

1. What is the purpose of an externship?

2. Fill in the table to show the difference between primary care providers and general practice facilities.

Primary Care Provider	General Practice Facility

3. How will the site preceptor assist you in your externship?

4. List three responsibilities you will have during an externship.

a.

b.

c.

5. Your externship preceptor has said that you cannot receive permission to draw blood and perform other phlebotomy procedures. However, you know this is an area that you need to learn more about in a practical setting. How can you learn more about these procedures at your externship site if you cannot perform them yourself?

6. Preparation is Key

Personal preparation for your externship will save you many headaches once your experience is underway. What are the four main ways you can prepare yourself for your externship?

a. _____

b. _____

c. _____

d. _____

7. Appearance Matters

Review the descriptions below to see what three students wore on the first day of their medical assisting externships. Then decide if the student is dressed appropriately or inappropriately. If the student is dressed inappropriately, explain what changes you would recommend.

a. Marsha wore burgundy and navy scrubs along with a set of bangle bracelets, her favorite gemstone rings, and a pair of comfortable flip-flops.

_____

b. Lloyd also wore the required scrubs with a pair of clean white sneakers. His long dreadlocks were brushed away from his face and placed in a neat ponytail above his shoulders.

_____

c. Barry wore the required uniform and a pair of dark walking shoes. He even had his hairstylist color the tips of his spiked mohawk hair burgundy to match.

_____

Evaluating Externships

8. Your school will likely request that you fill out an evaluation form to determine if your externship site was effective for training. This helps the school decide if it's a good site for future externships. Review the list of questions below and place a check in the "Yes" or "No" column to show if it is a question that you should consider when filling out your site evaluation form on your externship.

	Yes	No
a. Was the overall experience positive or negative?		
b. Was my preceptor fun to be around?		
c. Did the office have a good cafeteria or break room?		
d. Were opportunities for learning abundant and freely offered or hard to obtain?		
e. Was my preceptor flexible about taking personal time during the day for phone calls and breaks?		
f. Were staff personnel open and caring or unwelcoming?		
g. Was the preceptor available and easily approachable or preoccupied and distant?		

9. During your externship, you realize that you really enjoy and are passionate about caring for sick children. You also know that you would like to explore medical careers that require further training beyond your medical assisting program. As you seek employment, what factors would you consider based on these two facts about yourself? What long-term goals would you set? What steps would you take once on the job? What other factors would you consider as you plan for your future?

_____

_____

Landing the Job

10. List five traditional sources of information for job openings.

a. _____

b. _____

c. _____

d. _____

e. _____

11. Circle the items that should be included on a résumé.

contact information	race	relevant volunteer work	birth date
experience	picture of yourself	list of professional goals	education

Ready, Set, Action!

12. Choose a more accurate action word from the box to replace the words in bold.

		Action Words			
generates	ensures	implement and maintain	interviews	records	articulates
draw and collect	prepares	selects	measures	assists	composes

a. **Helps** in examination and treatment of patients under the direction of a physician. _____

b. **Talks to** patients, **takes** vital signs (i.e., pulse rate, temperature, blood pressure, weight, and height), and **writes** information on patients' charts. _____

c. **Get** blood samples from patients and prepare specimens for laboratory analysis. _____

d. **Set up** treatment rooms for examination of patients. _____

Acing the Interview

13. Fill in the chart to explain what information you should include in the first, second, and third paragraphs of your cover letter.

a. First Paragraph	
b. Second Paragraph	
c. Third Paragraph	

14. Read each of the following tips for completing a job application. Place a check mark in the "Good Idea" column if the statement is a good idea, or rule, to follow when completing an application. Place a check mark in the "Bad Idea" column if the statement is not a good idea.

Best Practices for Completing an Application	Good Idea	Bad Idea
a. Read through application completely before beginning.		
b. Follow the instructions exactly.		
c. In the line for wage or salary desired, write highest pay possible.		
d. Answer every question. If the question does not apply to you, draw a line or write "N/A" so that the interviewer will know that you did not overlook the question.		
e. Use your best cursive writing.		
f. Highlight important information in red ink.		
g. Ask for two applications. Use the first one for practice.		

If you checked "Bad Idea" for any of the above, write the number and explain why.

_____

_____

15. Read the questions in the box. If you should ask them during an interview, place a check in the "Yes" column; if not, place a check in the "No" column.

Questions to Ask	Yes	No
a. What are the responsibilities of the position offered?		
b. What is the benefit package? Is there access to a 401(k) plan or other retirement plan? Health insurance? Life insurance?		
c. Is it acceptable to take three weeks off during the holiday season?		
d. How does the facility feel about continuing education? Is time off offered to employees to upgrade their skills? Does the facility subsidize the expense?		
e. Do I have to work with physicians who have bad attitudes?		
f. How many potlucks and happy hours does this office usually have?		
g. Is there a job performance or evaluation process?		

16. Explain what it means to be a lifelong learner.

_____

_____

17. How can you prepare for the process of recertification?

_____

_____

18. List two professional organizations to research and join while you are a student.

a. _____

b. _____

19. Match the following key terms to their definitions.

Key Terms	Definitions
a. externship _____	**1.** a teacher; one who gives direction, as in a technical matter
b. networking _____	**2.** an educational course that allows the student to obtain hands-on experience
c. portfolio _____	**3.** a system of personal and professional relationships through which to share information
d. preceptor _____	**4.** a document summarizing an individual's work experience or professional qualifications
e. résumé _____	**5.** a portable case containing documents

20. True or False? Determine whether the following statements are true or false. If false, explain why.

a. When you see dangerous practices, it is usually best to confront the employees first.

_____

_____

b. An Internet search is the best way to search for a job.

_____

_____

c. Include hobbies and personal interests on your résumé.

_____

_____

d. Write a long and detailed cover letter.

_____

_____

APPLICATION

Critical Thinking Practice

1. During an interview, you are asked to explain why your grades were low last semester. How would you answer this question honestly while still speaking about yourself fairly and objectively?

_____

_____

2. There are multiple gaps in your work history and your interviewer asks you to explain. One of the gaps is from relocation and other gaps are from taking time off to evaluate what you wanted to be doing. How would you explain this to your interviewer?

_____

_____

Patient Education

1. While working as an extern at a family care provider, you encounter an elderly patient who is uncomfortable with the fact that you as a student are participating in her care. What would you say to help her feel more comfortable?

_____

_____

Documentation

1. Your school would like to update its form to evaluate the externship experience for students. Make a list of 10 questions that should be included in this evaluation form to determine if it is a strong placement.

_____

_____

Active Learning

1. Write a list of your strengths and weaknesses as discussed in the chapter. Critically evaluate what you are able to contribute to the job and address your weaknesses. How can you work with these weaknesses to make them strengths? Now evaluate what kind of medical assisting job would best work with what you are already good at and how you would like to continue to grow in your professional development. Identify for yourself what type of job would be ideal for you.

2. Look for your ideal job in the newspaper, through an employment office, temping service, etc. Search carefully throughout your field noting what is available and what the current job market is like. Now write a résumé that is tailored to your ideal job. Write a cover letter and assemble your portfolio. Apply for this job when you are ready!

3. Practice interviewing with a fellow student. Make sure that you take turns asking questions so that you can both get to experience being on each side of the interview.

Professional Journal

REFLECT

(Prompts and Ideas: Are you nervous about job interviews? How can you calm yourself and gain the confidence that you need to answer the questions? What are you most looking forward to in your health care career?)

_____

_____

_____

_____

_____

_____

_____

PONDER AND SOLVE

1. You happen to know that dozens of other people have interviewed for the same position as you. You are nervous because this job is very important to you. Your interview has been going amazingly well despite your inner nervousness, and your interviewer asks you why she should hire you for this job. She asks why you would be the best person. You take a couple of seconds to consider these questions and then respond. What do you say?

_____

_____

_____

_____

_____

_____

2. You have been completing an externship at an obstetric clinic. You have really enjoyed all of the new experience and knowledge that you have acquired with this externship. However, you also feel that there were some inner workings at the office that required better management and more professionalism. When, where, and how would you communicate these observations?

_____

_____

_____

_____

_____

_____

EXPERIENCE

1. Writing a Résumé (Procedure 46-1).

   Record any common mistakes, lessons learned, and/or tips you discovered during your experience of practicing and demonstrating these skills:

_____

_____

_____

_____

_____

_____

Skill
Practice

PERFORMANCE OBJECTIVES:

1. Write a résumé to properly communicate skills and strengths (Procedure 46-1).

Name_____ Date _____ Time _____

Procedure 46-1:	WRITING A RÉSUMÉ

EQUIPMENT/SUPPLIES: Word processor, paper, personal information

STANDARDS: Given the needed equipment and a place to work, the student will perform this skill with _____% accuracy in a total of _____ minutes. *(Your instructor will tell you what the percentage and time limits will be before you begin practicing.)*

KEY: 4 = Satisfactory   0 = Unsatisfactory   NA = This step is not counted

PROCEDURE STEPS	SELF	PARTNER	INSTRUCTOR
1. At the top of the page, center your name, address, and phone numbers.	☐	☐	☐
2. List your education starting with the most current and working back. List graduation dates and areas of study. It is not necessary to go all the way back to elementary school.	☐	☐	☐
3. Using the chronological format, list your prior related work experience with dates, responsibilities, company, and supervisor's name.	☐	☐	☐
4. List any volunteer work with dates and places.	☐	☐	☐
5. List skills you possess including those acquired in your program and on your externship.	☐	☐	☐
6. List any certifications or awards received.	☐	☐	☐
7. List any information relevant to a certain position. Example: competence in spreadsheet applications for a job in a patient billing department.	☐	☐	☐
8. After obtaining permission and/or notifying the people, prepare a list of references with their addresses and phone contact information.	☐	☐	☐
9. Carefully proofread the resume for accuracy and typographical errors.	☐	☐	☐
10. Have someone else proofread the résumé for errors other than content.	☐	☐	☐
11. Print the résumé on high-quality paper.	☐	☐	☐

CALCULATION

Total Possible Points: _____
Total Points Earned: _____ Multiplied by 100 = _____ Divided by Total Possible Points = _____%

Pass   **Fail**
☐   ☐   Comments:

Student signature _____ Date _____
Partner signature _____ Date _____
Instructor signature _____ Date _____

Chapter Self-Assessment Quiz

1. Most externships range from:
   a. 160–240 hours a semester.
   b. 80–160 hours a semester.
   c. 200–240 hours a semester.
   d. 240–300 hours a semester.
   e. 260–300 hours a semester.

2. Preceptors are typically:
   a. physicians.
   b. nurses.
   c. graduate medical assistants.
   d. academic instructors.
   e. other students.

3. When responding to a newspaper advertisement, you should:
   a. mail your résumé and a portfolio.
   b. send your résumé by e-mail.
   c. phone right away to inquire about the job.
   d. follow the instructions in the advertisement.
   e. call to schedule an interview.

4. A CMA wishing to recertify must either retake the examination or complete:
   a. 60 hours of continuing education credits.
   b. 50 hours of continuing education credits.
   c. 100 hours of continuing education credits.
   d. 30 hours of continuing education credits.
   e. 75 hours of continuing education credits.

5. Two standard ways of listing experience on a résumé are:
   a. functional and chronological.
   b. functional and alphabetical.
   c. alphabetical and chronological.
   d. chronological and referential.
   e. referential and alphabetical.

6. During your externship, it is a good practice to arrive:
   a. a few minutes early.
   b. half an hour early.
   c. right on time.
   d. with enough time to beat traffic.
   e. as early as you can.

7. What is the appropriate length of a résumé?
   a. One page
   b. Two pages
   c. Three pages
   d. As long as it needs to be
   e. Check with the potential employer first

8. In addition to providing proof of general immunizations, what other vaccinations may be required before you begin your externship?
   a. Vaccination for strep throat
   b. Vaccination for cancer
   c. Vaccination for hepatitis B
   d. Vaccination for hepatitis C
   e. Vaccination for HIV

9. During your externship, you are expected to perform as:
   a. the student that you are; your preceptor will teach you the same skills as in the classroom.
   b. an experienced professional; your preceptor will expect you to perform every task perfectly.
   c. an entry-level employee; your preceptor will expect you to perform at the level of a new employee in the field.
   d. a patient; you have to see what it feels like to be on the receiving end of treatment.
   e. independently as possible; your preceptor will not have time to answer many questions.

10. Checking for telephone messages and arranging the day's appointments should be done:
    a. during your lunch break.
    b. at the close of the business day.
    c. after the office has opened.
    d. before the scheduled opening.
    e. between patients.

11. Fingernails should be kept short and clean to avoid:
    a. making your supervisor upset.
    b. accidentally scratching or harming a patient.
    c. transferring pathogens or ripping gloves.
    d. getting nail polish chips in lab samples.
    e. infecting sterile materials or surfaces.

12. Which document provides proof that tasks are performed and learning is taking place?

   a. Timesheet

   b. Journal

   c. Survey

   d. Evaluation

   e. Personal interview

13. Which document is used to improve performance and services offered to students?

   a. Timesheet

   b. Journal

   c. Survey

   d. Evaluation

   e. Personal interview

14. Membership in your professional allied health organization proves:

   a. that you are an allied health student.

   b. your level of professionalism and seriousness of purpose.

   c. that you will become a medical professional in two years.

   d. your willingness to network with other professionals.

   e. your interest in the medical field.

15. Which question should you avoid asking during an interview?

   a. Is there access to a 401(k) plan?

   b. Is tuition reimbursement available?

   c. How many weeks of vacation are available the first year?

   d. Are uniforms or lab coats worn?

   e. What are the responsibilities of this position?

16. If you decide to leave your job, it is a good idea to:

   a. tell your employer the day before you plan to leave.

   b. make sure your new job will pay more.

   c. get contact information for all of the new friends you made.

   d. finish all duties and tie up any loose ends.

   e. criticize employees during an exit interview.

17. If you are having a problem performing your assigned job duties, it is best to:

   a. volunteer for extra hours.

   b. inform your preceptor and instructor.

   c. ask for less challenging work.

   d. ask for a different externship site.

   e. switch your course of studies.

18. When anticipating calls from prospective employers, avoid:

   a. leaving silly or cute messages on your answering machine.

   b. telling family members or roommates that you are expecting important telephone calls.

   c. keeping a pen near the telephone at all times.

   d. checking messages on a regular basis.

   e. calling them every day after submitting your resume.

19. If bilingual applicants are encouraged to apply for a position you want, you should:

   a. learn simple greetings and act as if you can speak several languages.

   b. learn simple greetings and admit that you know a few words but are not fluent.

   c. do nothing; being bilingual is not important.

   d. avoid applying since you do not fluently speak another language.

   e. learn how to answer possible interview questions in two different languages.

20. Being a lifelong learner is a must for all medical professionals because:

   a. medical professionals have to recertify every five years.

   b. medical professionals are widely respected.

   c. changes in procedures, medical technologies, and legal issues occur frequently.

   d. changes in medical technologies are decreasing the need for medical professionals.

   e. medical professionals are required to change legal statutes once a year.